Alejandro F. Frangi · Julia A. Schnabel
Christos Davatzikos · Carlos Alberola-López
Gabor Fichtinger (Eds.)

Medical Image Computing and Computer Assisted Intervention – MICCAI 2018

21st International Conference
Granada, Spain, September 16–20, 2018
Proceedings, Part IV

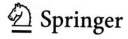 Springer

Editors
Alejandro F. Frangi (iD)
University of Leeds
Leeds
UK

Carlos Alberola-López (iD)
Universidad de Valladolid
Valladolid
Spain

Julia A. Schnabel
King's College London
London
UK

Gabor Fichtinger
Queen's University
Kingston, ON
Canada

Christos Davatzikos (iD)
University of Pennsylvania
Philadelphia, PA
USA

ISSN 0302-9743   ISSN 1611-3349   (electronic)
Lecture Notes in Computer Science
ISBN 978-3-030-00936-6   ISBN 978-3-030-00937-3   (eBook)
https://doi.org/10.1007/978-3-030-00937-3

Library of Congress Control Number: 2018909526

LNCS Sublibrary: SL6 – Image Processing, Computer Vision, Pattern Recognition, and Graphics

This Springer imprint is published by the registered company Springer Nature Switzerland AG
The registered company address is: Gewerbestrasse 11, 6330 Cham, Switzerland

More information about this series at http://www.springer.com/series/7412

Lecture Notes in Computer Science   11073

Commenced Publication in 1973
Founding and Former Series Editors:
Gerhard Goos, Juris Hartmanis, and Jan van Leeuwen

Editorial Board

Preface

We are very pleased to present the conference proceedings for the 21st International Conference on Medical Image Computing and Computer Assisted Intervention (MICCAI), which was successfully held at the Granada Conference Center, September 16–20, 2018 in Granada, Spain.

The conference also featured 40 workshops, 14 tutorials, and ten challenges held on September 16 or 20. For the first time, we had events co-located or endorsed by other societies. The two-day Visual Computing in Biology and Medicine (VCBM) Workshop partnered with EUROGRAPHICS[1], the one-day Biomedical Workshop Biomedical Information Processing and Analysis: A Latin American perspective partnered with SIPAIM[2], and the one-day MICCAI Workshop on Computational Diffusion on MRI was endorsed by ISMRM[3]. This year, at the time of writing this preface, the MICCAI 2018 conference had over 1,400 firm registrations for the main conference featuring the most recent work in the fields of:

- Reconstruction and Image Quality
- Machine Learning and Statistical Analysis
- Registration and Image Guidance
- Optical and Histology Applications
- Cardiac, Chest and Abdominal Applications
- fMRI and Diffusion Imaging
- Neuroimaging
- Computer-Assisted Intervention
- Segmentation

This was the largest MICCAI conference to date, with, for the first time, four volumes of *Lecture Notes in Computer Science* (LNCS) proceedings for the main conference, selected after a thorough double-blind peer-review process organized in several phases as further described below. Following the example set by the previous program chairs of MICCAI 2017, we employed the Conference Managing Toolkit (CMT)[4] for paper submissions and double-blind peer-reviews, the Toronto Paper Matching System (TPMS)[5] for automatic paper assignment to area chairs and reviewers, and Researcher.CC[6] to handle conflicts between authors, area chairs, and reviewers.

---

[1] https://www.eg.org.

[2] http://www.sipaim.org/.

[3] https://www.ismrm.org/.

[4] https://cmt.research.microsoft.com.

[5] http://torontopapermatching.org.

[6] http://researcher.cc.

In total, a record 1,068 full submissions (ca. 33% more than the previous year) were received and sent out to peer-review, from 1,335 original intentions to submit. Of those submissions, 80% were considered as pure Medical Image Computing (MIC), 14% as pure Computer-Assisted Intervention (CAI), and 6% as MICCAI papers that fitted into both MIC and CAI areas. The MICCAI 2018 Program Committee (PC) had a total of 58 area chairs, with 45% from Europe, 43% from the Americas, 9% from Australasia, and 3% from the Middle East. We maintained an excellent gender balance with 43% women scientists on the PC.

Using TPMS scoring and CMT, each area chair was assigned between 18 and 20 manuscripts using TPMS, for each of which they suggested 9–15 potential reviewers. Subsequently, 600 invited reviewers were asked to bid for the manuscripts they had been suggested for. Final reviewer allocations via CMT took PC suggestions, reviewer bidding, and TPMS scores into account, allocating 5–6 papers per reviewer. Based on the double-blind reviews, 173 papers (16%) were directly accepted and 314 papers (30%) were directly rejected – these decisions were confirmed by the handling area chair. The remaining 579 papers (54%) were invited for rebuttal. Two further area chairs were added using CMT and TPMS scores to each of these remaining manuscripts, who then independently scored these to accept or reject, based on the reviews, rebuttal, and manuscript, resulting in clear paper decisions using majority voting: 199 further manuscripts were accepted, and 380 rejected.

The overall manuscript acceptance rate was 34.9%. Two PC teleconferences were held on May 14, 2018, in two different time zones to confirm the final results and collect PC feedback on the peer-review process (with over 74% PC attendance rate). For the MICCAI 2018 proceedings, the 372 accepted papers[7] have been organized in four volumes as follows:

- Volume LNCS 11070 includes: Image Quality and Artefacts (15 manuscripts), Image Reconstruction Methods (31), Machine Learning in Medical Imaging (22), Statistical Analysis for Medical Imaging (10), and Image Registration Methods (21)
- Volume LNCS 11071 includes: Optical and Histology Applications (46); and Cardiac, Chest, and Abdominal Applications (59)
- Volume LNCS 11072 includes: fMRI and Diffusion Imaging (45); Neuroimaging and Brain Segmentation (37)
- Volume LNCS 11073 includes: Computer-Assisted Intervention (39) grouped into image-guided interventions and surgery; surgical planning, simulation and work flow analysis; and visualization and augmented reality; and Image Segmentation Methods (47) grouped into general segmentation methods; multi-organ segmentation; abdominal, cardiac, chest, and other segmentation applications.

We would like to thank everyone who contributed greatly to the success of MICCAI 2018 and the quality of its proceedings. These include the MICCAI Society, for support and insightful comments; and our sponsors for financial support and their presence on site. We are especially grateful to all members of the Program Committee for their diligent work in the reviewer assignments and final paper selection, as well as the 600

---

[7] One paper was withdrawn.

reviewers for their support during the entire process. Finally, and most importantly, we thank all authors, co-authors, students, and supervisors, for submitting and presenting their high-quality work which made MICCAI 2018 a greatly enjoyable, informative, and successful event. We are especially indebted to those reviewers and PC members who helped us resolve last-minute missing reviews at a very short notice.

We are looking forward to seeing you in Shenzhen, China, at MICCAI 2019!

August 2018

Julia A. Schnabel
Christos Davatzikos
Gabor Fichtinger
Alejandro F. Frangi
Carlos Alberola-López
Alberto Gomez Herrero
Spyridon Bakas
Antonio R. Porras

Organization

Organizing Committee

General Chair and Program Co-chair

Alejandro F. Frangi   University of Leeds, UK

General Co-chair

Carlos Alberola-López   Universidad de Valladolid, Spain

Associate to General Chairs

Antonio R. Porras   Children's National Medical Center,
           Washington D.C., USA

Program Chair

Julia A. Schnabel   King's College London, UK

Program Co-chairs

Christos Davatzikos   University of Pennsylvania, USA
Gabor Fichtinger   Queen's University, Canada

Associates to Program Chairs

Spyridon Bakas   University of Pennsylvania, USA
Alberto Gomez Herrero   King's College London, UK

Tutorial and Educational Chair

Anne Martel   University of Toronto, Canada

Tutorial and Educational Co-chairs

Miguel González-Ballester   Universitat Pompeu Fabra, Spain
Marius Linguraru   Children's National Medical Center,
           Washington D.C., USA
Kensaku Mori   Nagoya University, Japan
Carl-Fredrik Westin   Harvard Medical School, USA

Workshop and Challenge Chair

Danail Stoyanov   University College London, UK

Workshop and Challenge Co-chairs

Hervé Delingette	Inria, France
Lena Maier-Hein	German Cancer Research Center, Germany
Zeike A. Taylor	University of Leeds, UK

Keynote Lecture Chair

Josien Pluim   TU Eindhoven, The Netherlands

Keynote Lecture Co-chairs

Matthias Harders	ETH Zurich, Switzerland
Septimiu Salcudean	The University of British Columbia, Canada

Corporate Affairs Chair

Terry Peters   Western University, Canada

Corporate Affairs Co-chairs

Hayit Greenspan	Tel Aviv University, Israel
Despina Kontos	University of Pennsylvania, USA
Guy Shechter	Philips, USA

Student Activities Facilitator

Demian Wasserman   Inria, France

Student Activities Co-facilitator

Karim Lekadir   Universitat Pompeu-Fabra, Spain

Communications Officer

Pedro Lopes   University of Leeds, UK

Conference Management

DEKON Group

Program Committee

Ali Gooya	University of Sheffield, UK
Amber Simpson	Memorial Sloan Kettering Cancer Center, USA
Andrew King	King's College London, UK
Bennett Landman	Vanderbilt University, USA
Bernhard Kainz	Imperial College London, UK
Burak Acar	Bogazici University, Turkey

Carola Schoenlieb	Cambridge University, UK
Caroline Essert	University of Strasbourg/ICUBE, France
Christian Wachinger	Ludwig Maximilian University of Munich, Germany
Christos Bergeles	King's College London, UK
Daphne Yu	Siemens Healthineers, USA
Duygu Tosun	University of California at San Francisco, USA
Emanuele Trucco	University of Dundee, UK
Ender Konukoglu	ETH Zurich, Switzerland
Enzo Ferrante	CONICET/Universidad Nacional del Litoral, Argentina
Erik Meijering	Erasmus University Medical Center, The Netherlands
Gozde Unal	Istanbul Technical University, Turkey
Guido Gerig	New York University, USA
Gustavo Carneiro	University of Adelaide, Australia
Hassan Rivaz	Concordia University, Canada
Herve Lombaert	ETS Montreal, Canada
Hongliang Ren	National University of Singapore, Singapore
Ingerid Reinertsen	SINTEF, Norway
Ipek Oguz	University of Pennsylvania/Vanderbilt University, USA
Ivana Isgum	University Medical Center Utrecht, The Netherlands
Juan Eugenio Iglesias	University College London, UK
Kayhan Batmanghelich	University of Pittsburgh/Carnegie Mellon University, USA
Laura Igual	Universitat de Barcelona, Spain
Lauren O'Donnell	Harvard University, USA
Le Lu	Ping An Technology US Research Labs, USA
Li Cheng	A*STAR Singapore, Singapore
Lilla Zöllei	Massachusetts General Hospital, USA
Linwei Wang	Rochester Institute of Technology, USA
Marc Niethammer	University of North Carolina at Chapel Hill, USA
Marius Staring	Leiden University Medical Center, The Netherlands
Marleen de Bruijne	Erasmus MC Rotterdam/University of Copenhagen, The Netherlands/Denmark
Marta Kersten	Concordia University, Canada
Mattias Heinrich	University of Luebeck, Germany
Meritxell Bach Cuadra	University of Lausanne, Switzerland
Miaomiao Zhang	Washington University in St. Louis, USA
Moti Freiman	Philips Healthcare, Israel
Nasir Rajpoot	University of Warwick, UK
Nassir Navab	Technical University of Munich, Germany
Pallavi Tiwari	Case Western Reserve University, USA
Pingkun Yan	Rensselaer Polytechnic Institute, USA
Purang Abolmaesumi	University of British Columbia, Canada
Ragini Verma	University of Pennsylvania, USA
Raphael Sznitman	University of Bern, Switzerland
Sandrine Voros	University of Grenoble, France

Sotirios Tsaftaris	University of Edinburgh, UK
Stamatia Giannarou	Imperial College London, UK
Stefanie Speidel	National Center for Tumor Diseases (NCT) Dresden, Germany
Stefanie Demirci	Technical University of Munich, Germany
Tammy Riklin Raviv	Ben-Gurion University, Israel
Tanveer Syeda-Mahmood	IBM Research, USA
Ulas Bagci	University of Central Florida, USA
Vamsi Ithapu	University of Wisconsin-Madison, USA
Yanwu Xu	Baidu Inc., China

Scientific Review Committee

Amir Abdi	Martin Benning
Ehsan Adeli	Aïcha BenTaieb
Iman Aganj	Ruth Bergman
Ola Ahmad	Alessandro Bevilacqua
Amr Ahmed	Ryoma Bise
Shazia Akbar	Isabelle Bloch
Alireza Akhondi-asl	Sebastian Bodenstedt
Saad Ullah Akram	Hrvoje Bogunovic
Amir Alansary	Gerda Bortsova
Shadi Albarqouni	Sylvain Bouix
Luis Alvarez	Felix Bragman
Deepak Anand	Christopher Bridge
Elsa Angelini	Tom Brosch
Rahman Attar	Aurelien Bustin
Chloé Audigier	Irène Buvat
Angelica Aviles-Rivero	Cesar Caballero-Gaudes
Ruqayya Awan	Ryan Cabeen
Suyash Awate	Nathan Cahill
Dogu Baran Aydogan	Jinzheng Cai
Shekoofeh Azizi	Weidong Cai
Katja Bühler	Tian Cao
Junjie Bai	Valentina Carapella
Wenjia Bai	M. Jorge Cardoso
Daniel Balfour	Daniel Castro
Walid Barhoumi	Daniel Coelho de Castro
Sarah Barman	Philippe C. Cattin
Michael Barrow	Juan Cerrolaza
Deepti Bathula	Suheyla Cetin Karayumak
Christian F. Baumgartner	Matthieu Chabanas
Pierre-Louis Bazin	Jayasree Chakraborty
Delaram Behnami	Rudrasis Chakraborty
Erik Bekkers	Rajib Chakravorty
Rami Ben-Ari	Vimal Chandran

Catie Chang
Pierre Chatelain
Akshay Chaudhari
Antong Chen
Chao Chen
Geng Chen
Hao Chen
Jianxu Chen
Jingyun Chen
Min Chen
Xin Chen
Yang Chen
Yuncong Chen
Jiezhi Cheng
Jun Cheng
Veronika Cheplygina
Farida Cheriet
Minqi Chong
Daan Christiaens
Serkan Cimen
Francesco Ciompi
Cedric Clouchoux
James Clough
Dana Cobzas
Noel Codella
Toby Collins
Olivier Commowick
Sailesh Conjeti
Pierre-Henri Conze
Tessa Cook
Timothy Cootes
Pierrick Coupé
Alessandro Crimi
Adrian Dalca
Sune Darkner
Dhritiman Das
Johan Debayle
Farah Deeba
Silvana Dellepiane
Adrien Depeursinge
Maria Deprez
Christian Desrosiers
Blake Dewey
Jwala Dhamala
Qi Dou
Karen Drukker

Lei Du
Lixin Duan
Florian Dubost
Nicolas Duchateau
James Duncan
Luc Duong
Nicha Dvornek
Oleh Dzyubachyk
Zach Eaton-Rosen
Mehran Ebrahimi
Matthias J. Ehrhardt
Ahmet Ekin
Ayman El-Baz
Randy Ellis
Mohammed Elmogy
Marius Erdt
Guray Erus
Marco Esposito
Joset Etzel
Jingfan Fan
Yong Fan
Aly Farag
Mohsen Farzi
Anahita Fathi Kazerooni
Hamid Fehri
Xinyang Feng
Olena Filatova
James Fishbaugh
Tom Fletcher
Germain Forestier
Denis Fortun
Alfred Franz
Muhammad Moazam Fraz
Wolfgang Freysinger
Jurgen Fripp
Huazhu Fu
Yang Fu
Bernhard Fuerst
Gareth Funka-Lea
Isabel Funke
Jan Funke
Francesca Galassi
Linlin Gao
Mingchen Gao
Yue Gao
Zhifan Gao

Utpal Garain
Mona Garvin
Aimilia Gastounioti
Romane Gauriau
Bao Ge
Sandesh Ghimire
Ali Gholipour
Rémi Giraud
Ben Glocker
Ehsan Golkar
Polina Golland
Yuanhao Gong
German Gonzalez
Pietro Gori
Alejandro Granados
Sasa Grbic
Enrico Grisan
Andrey Gritsenko
Abhijit Guha Roy
Yanrong Guo
Yong Guo
Vikash Gupta
Benjamin Gutierrez Becker
Séverine Habert
Ilker Hacihaliloglu
Stathis Hadjidemetriou
Ghassan Hamarneh
Adam Harrison
Grant Haskins
Charles Hatt
Tiancheng He
Mehdi Hedjazi Moghari
Tobias Heimann
Christoph Hennersperger
Alfredo Hernandez
Monica Hernandez
Moises Hernandez Fernandez
Carlos Hernandez-Matas
Matthew Holden
Yi Hong
Nicolas Honnorat
Benjamin Hou
Yipeng Hu
Heng Huang
Junzhou Huang
Weilin Huang

Xiaolei Huang
Yawen Huang
Henkjan Huisman
Yuankai Huo
Sarfaraz Hussein
Jana Hutter
Seong Jae Hwang
Atsushi Imiya
Amir Jamaludin
Faraz Janan
Uditha Jarayathne
Xi Jiang
Jieqing Jiao
Dakai Jin
Yueming Jin
Bano Jordan
Anand Joshi
Shantanu Joshi
Leo Joskowicz
Christoph Jud
Siva Teja Kakileti
Jayashree Kalpathy-Cramer
Ali Kamen
Neerav Karani
Anees Kazi
Eric Kerfoot
Erwan Kerrien
Farzad Khalvati
Hassan Khan
Bishesh Khanal
Ron Kikinis
Hyo-Eun Kim
Hyunwoo Kim
Jinman Kim
Minjeong Kim
Benjamin Kimia
Kivanc Kose
Julia Krüger
Pavitra Krishnaswamy
Frithjof Kruggel
Elizabeth Krupinski
Sofia Ira Ktena
Arjan Kuijper
Ashnil Kumar
Neeraj Kumar
Punithakumar Kumaradevan

Manuela Kunz
Jin Tae Kwak
Alexander Ladikos
Rodney Lalonde
Pablo Lamata
Catherine Laporte
Carole Lartizien
Toni Lassila
Andras Lasso
Matthieu Le
Maria J. Ledesma-Carbayo
Hansang Lee
Jong-Hwan Lee
Soochahn Lee
Etienne Léger
Beatrice Lentes
Wee Kheng Leow
Nikolas Lessmann
Annan Li
Gang Li
Ruoyu Li
Wenqi Li
Xiang Li
Yuanwei Li
Chunfeng Lian
Jianming Liang
Hongen Liao
Ruizhi Liao
Roxane Licandro
Lanfen Lin
Claudia Lindner
Cristian Linte
Feng Liu
Hui Liu
Jianfei Liu
Jundong Liu
Kefei Liu
Mingxia Liu
Sidong Liu
Marco Lorenzi
Xiongbiao Luo
Jinglei Lv
Ilwoo Lyu
Omar M. Rijal
Pablo Márquez Neila
Henning Müller

Kai Ma
Khushhall Chandra Mahajan
Dwarikanath Mahapatra
Andreas Maier
Klaus H. Maier-Hein
Sokratis Makrogiannis
Grégoire Malandain
Anand Malpani
Jose Manjon
Tommaso Mansi
Awais Mansoor
Anne Martel
Diana Mateus
Arnaldo Mayer
Jamie McClelland
Stephen McKenna
Ronak Mehta
Raphael Meier
Qier Meng
Yu Meng
Bjoern Menze
Liang Mi
Shun Miao
Abhishek Midya
Zhe Min
Rashika Mishra
Marc Modat
Norliza Mohd Noor
Mehdi Moradi
Rodrigo Moreno
Kensaku Mori
Aliasghar Mortazi
Peter Mountney
Arrate Muñoz-Barrutia
Anirban Mukhopadhyay
Arya Nabavi
Layan Nahlawi
Ana Ineyda Namburete
Valery Naranjo
Peter Neher
Hannes Nickisch
Dong Nie
Lipeng Ning
Jack Noble
Vincent Noblet
Alexey Novikov

Ilkay Oksuz
Ozan Oktay
John Onofrey
Eliza Orasanu
Felipe Orihuela-Espina
Jose Orlando
Yusuf Osmanlioglu
David Owen
Cristina Oyarzun Laura
Jose-Antonio Pérez-Carrasco
Danielle Pace
J. Blas Pagador
Akshay Pai
Xenophon Papademetris
Bartlomiej Papiez
Toufiq Parag
Magdalini Paschali
Angshuman Paul
Christian Payer
Jialin Peng
Tingying Peng
Xavier Pennec
Sérgio Pereira
Mehran Pesteie
Loic Peter
Igor Peterlik
Simon Pezold
Micha Pfeifer
Dzung Pham
Renzo Phellan
Pramod Pisharady
Josien Pluim
Kilian Pohl
Jean-Baptiste Poline
Alison Pouch
Prateek Prasanna
Philip Pratt
Raphael Prevost
Esther Puyol Anton
Yuchuan Qiao
Gwénolé Quellec
Pradeep Reddy Raamana
Julia Rackerseder
Hedyeh Rafii-Tari
Mehdi Rahim
Kashif Rajpoot

Parnesh Raniga
Yogesh Rathi
Saima Rathore
Nishant Ravikumar
Shan E. Ahmed Raza
Islem Rekik
Beatriz Remeseiro
Markus Rempfler
Mauricio Reyes
Constantino Reyes-Aldasoro
Nicola Rieke
Laurent Risser
Leticia Rittner
Yong Man Ro
Emma Robinson
Rafael Rodrigues
Marc-Michel Rohé
Robert Rohling
Karl Rohr
Plantefeve Rosalie
Holger Roth
Su Ruan
Danny Ruijters
Juan Ruiz-Alzola
Mert Sabuncu
Frank Sachse
Farhang Sahba
Septimiu Salcudean
Gerard Sanroma
Emine Saritas
Imari Sato
Alexander Schlaefer
Jerome Schmid
Caitlin Schneider
Jessica Schrouff
Thomas Schultz
Suman Sedai
Biswa Sengupta
Ortal Senouf
Maxime Sermesant
Carmen Serrano
Amit Sethi
Muhammad Shaban
Reuben Shamir
Yeqin Shao
Li Shen

Bibo Shi
Kuangyu Shi
Hoo-Chang Shin
Russell Shinohara
Viviana Siless
Carlos A. Silva
Matthew Sinclair
Vivek Singh
Korsuk Sirinukunwattana
Ihor Smal
Michal Sofka
Jure Sokolic
Hessam Sokooti
Ahmed Soliman
Stefan Sommer
Diego Sona
Yang Song
Aristeidis Sotiras
Jamshid Sourati
Rachel Sparks
Ziga Spiclin
Lawrence Staib
Ralf Stauder
Darko Stern
Colin Studholme
Martin Styner
Heung-Il Suk
Jian Sun
Xu Sun
Kyunghyun Sung
Nima Tajbakhsh
Sylvain Takerkart
Chaowei Tan
Jeremy Tan
Mingkui Tan
Hui Tang
Min Tang
Youbao Tang
Yuxing Tang
Christine Tanner
Qian Tao
Giacomo Tarroni
Zeike Taylor
Kim Han Thung
Yanmei Tie
Daniel Toth

Nicolas Toussaint
Jocelyne Troccaz
Tomasz Trzcinski
Ahmet Tuysuzoglu
Andru Twinanda
Carole Twining
Eranga Ukwatta
Mathias Unberath
Tamas Ungi
Martin Urschler
Maria Vakalopoulou
Vanya Valindria
Koen Van Leemput
Hien Van Nguyen
Gijs van Tulder
S. Swaroop Vedula
Harini Veeraraghavan
Miguel Vega
Anant Vemuri
Gopalkrishna Veni
Archana Venkataraman
François-Xavier Vialard
Pierre-Frederic Villard
Satish Viswanath
Wolf-Dieter Vogl
Ingmar Voigt
Tomaz Vrtovec
Bo Wang
Guotai Wang
Jiazhuo Wang
Liansheng Wang
Manning Wang
Sheng Wang
Yalin Wang
Zhe Wang
Simon Warfield
Chong-Yaw Wee
Juergen Weese
Benzheng Wei
Wolfgang Wein
William Wells
Rene Werner
Daniel Wesierski
Matthias Wilms
Adam Wittek
Jelmer Wolterink

Ken C. L. Wong
Jonghye Woo
Pengxiang Wu
Tobias Wuerfl
Yong Xia
Yiming Xiao
Weidi Xie
Yuanpu Xie
Fangxu Xing
Fuyong Xing
Tao Xiong
Daguang Xu
Yan Xu
Zheng Xu
Zhoubing Xu
Ziyue Xu
Wufeng Xue
Jingwen Yan
Ke Yan
Yuguang Yan
Zhennan Yan
Dong Yang
Guang Yang
Xiao Yang
Xin Yang
Jianhua Yao
Jiawen Yao
Xiaohui Yao
Chuyang Ye
Menglong Ye
Jingru Yi
Jinhua Yu
Lequan Yu
Weimin Yu
Yixuan Yuan
Evangelia Zacharaki
Ernesto Zacur

Guillaume Zahnd
Marco Zenati
Ke Zeng
Oliver Zettinig
Daoqiang Zhang
Fan Zhang
Han Zhang
Heye Zhang
Jiong Zhang
Jun Zhang
Lichi Zhang
Lin Zhang
Ling Zhang
Mingli Zhang
Pin Zhang
Shu Zhang
Tong Zhang
Yong Zhang
Yunyan Zhang
Zizhao Zhang
Qingyu Zhao
Shijie Zhao
Yitian Zhao
Guoyan Zheng
Yalin Zheng
Yinqiang Zheng
Zichun Zhong
Luping Zhou
Zhiguo Zhou
Dajiang Zhu
Wentao Zhu
Xiaofeng Zhu
Xiahai Zhuang
Aneeq Zia
Veronika Zimmer
Majd Zreik
Reyer Zwiggelaar

Mentorship Program (Mentors)

Stephen Aylward   Kitware Inc., USA
Christian Barillot   IRISA/CNRS/University of Rennes, France
Kayhan Batmanghelich   University of Pittsburgh/Carnegie Mellon University,
                          USA
Christos Bergeles   King's College London, UK

Marleen de Bruijne	Erasmus Medical Center Rotterdam/University of Copenhagen, The Netherlands/Denmark
Cheng Li	University of Alberta, Canada
Stefanie Demirci	Technical University of Munich, Germany
Simon Duchesne	University of Laval, Canada
Enzo Ferrante	CONICET/Universidad Nacional del Litoral, Argentina
Alejandro F. Frangi	University of Leeds, UK
Miguel A. González-Ballester	Universitat Pompeu Fabra, Spain
Stamatia (Matina) Giannarou	Imperial College London, UK
Juan Eugenio Iglesias-Gonzalez	University College London, UK
Laura Igual	Universitat de Barcelona, Spain
Leo Joskowicz	The Hebrew University of Jerusalem, Israel
Bernhard Kainz	Imperial College London, UK
Shuo Li	University of Western Ontario, Canada
Marius G. Linguraru	Children's National Health System/George Washington University, USA
Le Lu	Ping An Technology US Research Labs, USA
Tommaso Mansi	Siemens Healthineers, USA
Anne Martel	Sunnybrook Research Institute, USA
Kensaku Mori	Nagoya University, Japan
Parvin Mousavi	Queen's University, Canada
Nassir Navab	Technical University of Munich/Johns Hopkins University, USA
Marc Niethammer	University of North Carolina at Chapel Hill, USA
Ipek Oguz	University of Pennsylvania/Vanderbilt University, USA
Josien Pluim	Eindhoven University of Technology, The Netherlands
Jerry L. Prince	Johns Hopkins University, USA
Nicola Rieke	NVIDIA Corp./Technical University of Munich, Germany
Daniel Rueckert	Imperial College London, UK
Julia A. Schnabel	King's College London, UK
Raphael Sznitman	University of Bern, Switzerland
Jocelyne Troccaz	CNRS/University of Grenoble, France
Gozde Unal	Istanbul Technical University, Turkey
Max A. Viergever	Utrecht University/University Medical Center Utrecht, The Netherlands
Linwei Wang	Rochester Institute of Technology, USA
Yanwu Xu	Baidu Inc., China
Miaomiao Zhang	Lehigh University, USA
Guoyan Zheng	University of Bern, Switzerland
Lilla Zöllei	Massachusetts General Hospital, USA

Sponsors and Funders

Platinum Sponsors

- NVIDIA Inc.
- Siemens Healthineers GmbH

Gold Sponsors

- Guangzhou Shiyuan Electronics Co. Ltd.
- Subtle Medical Inc.

Silver Sponsors

- Arterys Inc.
- Claron Technology Inc.
- ImSight Inc.
- ImFusion GmbH
- Medtronic Plc

Bronze Sponsors

- Depwise Inc.
- Carl Zeiss AG

Travel Bursary Support

- MICCAI Society
- National Institutes of Health, USA
- EPSRC-NIHR Medical Image Analysis Network (EP/N026993/1), UK

Contents – Part IV

**Computer Assisted Interventions: Surgical Planning, Simulation
and Work Flow Analysis**

**Computer Assisted Interventions: Visualization
and Augmented Reality**

**Image Segmentation Methods: General Image Segmentation Methods,
Measures and Applications**

Image Segmentation Methods: Abdominal Segmentation Methods

Image Segmentation Methods: Cardiac Segmentation Methods

Image Segmentation Methods: Chest, Lung and Spine Segmentation

Image Segmentation Methods: Other Segmentation Applications

Computer Assisted Interventions: Image Guided Interventions and Surgery

Uncertainty in Multitask Learning: Joint Representations for Probabilistic MR-only Radiotherapy Planning

Felix J. S. Bragman[1]([✉]), Ryutaro Tanno[1], Zach Eaton-Rosen[1], Wenqi Li[1], David J. Hawkes[1], Sebastien Ourselin[2], Daniel C. Alexander[1,3], Jamie R. McClelland[1], and M. Jorge Cardoso[1,2]

[1] Centre for Medical Image Computing, University College London, London, UK
f.bragman@ucl.ac.uk
[2] Biomedical Engineering and Imaging Sciences, King's College London, London, UK
[3] Clinical Imaging Research Centre, National University of Singapore, Singapore, Singapore

Abstract. Multi-task neural network architectures provide a mechanism that jointly integrates information from distinct sources. It is ideal in the context of MR-only radiotherapy planning as it can jointly regress a synthetic CT (synCT) scan and segment organs-at-risk (OAR) from MRI. We propose a probabilistic multi-task network that estimates: (1) *intrinsic* uncertainty through a heteroscedastic noise model for spatially-adaptive task loss weighting and (2) *parameter* uncertainty through approximate Bayesian inference. This allows sampling of multiple segmentations and synCTs that share their network representation. We test our model on prostate cancer scans and show that it produces more accurate and consistent synCTs with a better estimation in the variance of the errors, state of the art results in OAR segmentation and a methodology for quality assurance in radiotherapy treatment planning.

1 Introduction

Radiotherapy treatment planning (RTP) requires a magnetic resonance (MR) scan to segment the target and organs-at-risk (OARs) with a registered computed tomography (CT) scan to inform the photon attenuation. MR-only RTP has recently been proposed to remove dependence on CT scans as cross-modality registration is error prone whilst extensive data acquisition is labourious. MR-only RTP involves the generation of a synthetic CT (synCT) scan from MRI. This synthesis process, when combined with manual regions of interest and safety margins provides a deterministic plan that is dependent on the quality of the inputs. Probabilistic planning systems conversely allow the implicit estimation of dose delivery uncertainty through a Monte Carlo sampling scheme. A system that can sample synCT and OAR segmentations would enable the development of a fully end-to-end uncertainty-aware probabilistic planning system.

© Springer Nature Switzerland AG 2018
A. F. Frangi et al. (Eds.): MICCAI 2018, LNCS 11073, pp. 3–11, 2018.
https://doi.org/10.1007/978-3-030-00937-3_1

Past methods for synCT generation and OAR segmentation stem from multi-atlas propagation [1]. Applications of convolutional neural networks (CNNs) to CT synthesis from MRI have recently become a topic of interest [2,3]. Conditional generative adversarial networks have been used to capture fine texture details [2] whilst a CycleGAN has been exploited to leverage the abundance of unpaired training sets of CT and MR scans [3]. These methods however are fully deterministic. In a probabilistic setting, knowledge of the posterior over the network weights would enable sampling multiple realizations of the model for probabilistic planning whilst uncertainty in the predictions would be beneficial for quality control. Lastly, none of the above CNN methods segment OARs. If a model were trained in a multi-task setting, it would produce OAR segmentations and a synCT that are anatomically consistent, which is necessary for RTP.

Past approaches to multi-task learning have relied on uniform or hand-tuned weighting of task losses [4]. Recently, Kendall et al. [5] interpreted homoscedastic uncertainty as task-dependent weighting. However, homoscedastic uncertainty is constant in the task output and unrealistic for imaging data whilst yielding non-meaningful measures of uncertainty. Tanno et al. [6] and Kendall et al. [7] have raised the importance of modelling both *intrinsic* and *parameter* uncertainty to build more robust models for medical image analysis and computer vision. *Intrinsic* uncertainty captures uncertainty inherent in observations and can be interpreted as the irreducible variance that exists in the mapping of MR to CT intensities or in the segmentation process. *Parameter* uncertainty quantifies the degree of ambiguity in the model parameters given the observed data.

This paper makes use of [6] to enrich the multi-task method proposed in [5]. This enables modelling the spatial variation of *intrinsic* uncertainty via heteroscedastic noise across tasks and integrating *parameter* uncertainty via dropout [8]. We propose a probabilistic dual-task network, which operates on an MR image and simultaneously provides three valuable outputs necessary for probabilistic RTP: (1) synCT generation, (2) OAR segmentation and (3) quantification of predictive uncertainty in (1) and (2) (Fig. 2). The architecture integrates the methods of uncertainty modelling in CNNs [6,7] into a multi-task learning framework with hard-parameter sharing, in which the initial layers of the network are shared across tasks and branch out into task-specific layers (Fig. 1). Our probabilistic formulation not only provides an estimate of uncertainty over predictions from which one can stochastically sample the space of solutions, but also naturally confers a mechanism to spatially adapt the relative weighting of task losses on a voxel-wise basis.

2   Methods

We propose a probabilistic dual-task CNN algorithm which takes an MRI image, and simultaneously estimates the distribution over the corresponding CT image and the segmentation probability of the OARs. We use a heteroscedastic noise model and binary dropout to account for *intrinsic* and *parameter* uncertainty,

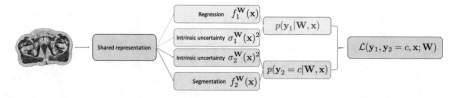

Fig. 1. Multi-task learning architecture. The predictive mean and variance $[f_i^{\mathbf{W}}(\mathbf{x}), \sigma_i^{\mathbf{W}}(\mathbf{x})^2]$ are estimated for the regression and segmentation. The task-specific likelihoods $p(\mathbf{y}_i|\mathbf{W}, \mathbf{x})$ are combined to yield the multi-task likelihood $p(\mathbf{y}_1, \mathbf{y}_2|\mathbf{W}, \mathbf{x})$.

respectively, and show that we obtain not only a measure of uncertainty over prediction, but also a mechanism for data-driven spatially adaptive weighting of task losses, which is integral in a multi-task setting. We employ a patch-based approach to perform both tasks, in which the input MR image is split into smaller overlapping patches that are processed independently. For each input patch $\mathbf{x}$, our dual-task model estimates the conditional distributions $p(\mathbf{y}_i|\mathbf{x})$ for tasks $i = 1, 2$ where $\mathbf{y}_1$ and $\mathbf{y}_2$ are the Hounsfield Unit and OAR class probabilities. At inference, the probability maps over the synCT and OARs are obtained by stitching together outputs from appropriately shifted versions of the input patches.

Dual-Task Architecture. We perform multi-task learning with hard-parameter sharing [9]. The model shares the initial layers across the two tasks to learn an invariant feature space of the anatomy and branches out into four task-specific networks with separate parameters (Fig. 1). There are two networks for each task (regression and segmentation). Where one aims to performs CT synthesis (regression) or OAR segmentation, and the remaining models *intrinsic* uncertainty associated to the data and the task.

The rationale behind shared layers is to learn a joint representation between two tasks to regularise the learning of features for one task by using cues from the other. We used a high-resolution network architecture (HighResNet) [10] as the shared trunk of the model for its compactness and accuracy shown in brain parcellation. HighResNet is a fully convolutional architecture that utilises dilated convolutions with increasing dilation factors and residual connections to produce an end-to-end mapping from an input patch ($\mathbf{x}$) to voxel-wise predictions ($\mathbf{y}$). The final layer of the shared representation is split into two task-specific compartments (Fig. 1). Each compartment consists of two fully convolutional networks which operate on the output of representation network and together learn task-specific representation and define likelihood function $p(\mathbf{y}_i|\mathbf{W}, \mathbf{x})$ for each task $i = 1, 2$ where $\mathbf{W}$ denotes the set of all parameters of the model.

Task Weighting with Heteroscedastic Uncertainty. Previous probabilistic multitask methods in deep learning [5] assumed constant intrinsic uncertainty per task. In our context, this means that the inherent ambiguity present across synthesis or segmentation does not depend on the spatial locations within an image. This is a highly unrealistic assumption as these tasks can be more challenging on some anatomical structures (e.g. tissue boundaries) than others. To capture potential spatial variation in intrinsic uncertainty, we adapt the *heteroscedastic* (data-dependent) noise model to our multitask learning problem.

For the CT synthesis task, we define our likelihood as a normal distribution $p(\mathbf{y}_1|\mathbf{W}, \mathbf{x}) = \mathcal{N}(f_1^{\mathbf{W}}(\mathbf{x}), \sigma_1^{\mathbf{W}}(\mathbf{x})^2)$ where mean $f_1^{\mathbf{W}}(\mathbf{x})$ and variance $\sigma_1^{\mathbf{W}}(\mathbf{x})^2$ are modelled by the regression output and uncertainty branch as functions of the input patch $\mathbf{x}$ (Fig. 1). We define the task loss for CT synthesis to be the negative log-likelihood (NLL) $\mathcal{L}_1(\mathbf{y}_1, \mathbf{x}; \mathbf{W}) = \frac{1}{2\sigma_1^{\mathbf{W}}(\mathbf{x})^2}||\mathbf{y}_1 - f_1^{\mathbf{W}}(\mathbf{x})||^2 + \log \sigma_1^{\mathbf{W}}(\mathbf{x})^2$. This loss encourages assigning high-uncertainty to regions of high errors, enhancing the robustness of the network against noisy labels and outliers, which are prevalent at organ boundaries especially close to the bone.

For the segmentation, we define the classification likelihood as softmax function of scaled logits i.e. $p(\mathbf{y}_2|\mathbf{W}, \mathbf{x}) = \text{Softmax}(f_2^{\mathbf{W}}(\mathbf{x})/2\sigma_2^{\mathbf{W}}(\mathbf{x})^2)$ where the segmentation output $f_2^{\mathbf{W}}(\mathbf{x})$ is scaled by the uncertainty term $\sigma_2^{\mathbf{W}}(\mathbf{x})^2$ before softmax (Fig. 1). As the uncertainty $\sigma_2^{\mathbf{W}}(\mathbf{x})^2$ increases, the Softmax output approaches a uniform distribution, which corresponds to the maximum entropy discrete distribution. We simplify the scaled Softmax likelihood by considering an approximation in [5], $\frac{1}{\sigma^2}\sum_{c'}\exp(\frac{1}{2\sigma_2^{\mathbf{W}}(\mathbf{x})^2}f_{2,c'}^{\mathbf{W}}(\mathbf{x})) \approx$ $\left(\sum_{c'}\exp(f_{2,c'}^{\mathbf{W}}(\mathbf{x}))\right)^{1/2\sigma_2^{\mathbf{W}}(\mathbf{x})^2}$ where c' denotes a segmentation class. This yields the NLL task-loss of the form $\mathcal{L}_2(\mathbf{y}_2 = c, \mathbf{x}; \mathbf{W}) \approx \frac{1}{2\sigma_2^{\mathbf{W}}(\mathbf{x})^2}\text{CE}(f_2^{\mathbf{W}}(\mathbf{x}), \mathbf{y}_2 = c) + \log \sigma_2^{\mathbf{W}}(\mathbf{x})^2$, where CE denotes cross-entropy.

The joint likelihood factorises over tasks such that $p(\mathbf{y}_1, \mathbf{y}_2|\mathbf{W}, \mathbf{x}) = \prod_i^2 p(\mathbf{y}_i|\mathbf{W}, \mathbf{x})$. We can therefore derive the NLL loss for the dual-task model as

$$\mathcal{L}(\mathbf{y}_1, \mathbf{y}_2 = c, \mathbf{x}; \mathbf{W}) = \frac{||\mathbf{y}_1 - f_1^{\mathbf{W}}(\mathbf{x})||^2}{2\sigma_1^{\mathbf{W}}(\mathbf{x})^2} + \frac{\text{CE}(f_2^{\mathbf{W}}(\mathbf{x}), \mathbf{y}_2 = c)}{2\sigma_2^{\mathbf{W}}(\mathbf{x})^2} + \log\left(\sigma_1^{\mathbf{W}}(\mathbf{x})^2\sigma_2^{\mathbf{W}}(\mathbf{x})^2\right)$$

where both task losses are weighted by the inverse of heteroscedastic intrinsic uncertainty terms $\sigma_i^{\mathbf{W}}(\mathbf{x})^2$, that enables automatic weighting of task losses on a per-sample basis. The log-term controls the spread.

Parameter Uncertainty with Approximate Bayesian Inference. In data-scarce situations, the choice of best parameters is ambiguous, and resorting to a single estimate without regularisation often leads to overfitting. Gal et al. [8] have shown that dropout improves the generalisation of a NN by accounting for *parameter* uncertainty through an approximation of the posterior distribution over its weights $q(\mathbf{W}) \approx p(\mathbf{W}|\mathbf{X}, \mathbf{Y}_1, \mathbf{Y}_2)$ where $\mathbf{X} = \{\mathbf{x}^{(1)}, \dots, \mathbf{x}^{(N)}\}$, $\mathbf{Y}_1 = \{\mathbf{y}_1^{(1)}, \dots, \mathbf{y}_1^{(N)}\}$, $\mathbf{Y}_2 = \{\mathbf{y}_2^{(1)}, \dots, \mathbf{y}_2^{(N)}\}$ denote the training data. We also use binary dropout in our model to assess the benefit of modelling parameter uncertainty in the context of our multitask learning problem.

During training, for each input (or minibatch), network weights are drawn from the approximate posterior $w' \sim q(\mathbf{W})$ to obtain the multi-task output $\mathbf{f}^{w'}(\mathbf{x}) := [f_1^{w'}(\mathbf{x}), f_2^{w'}(\mathbf{x}), \sigma_1^{w'}(\mathbf{x})^2, \sigma_2^{w'}(\mathbf{x})^2]$. At test time, for each input patch $\mathbf{x}$ in an MR scan, we collect output samples $\{\mathbf{f}^{w^{(t)}}(\mathbf{x})\}_{t=1}^{T}$ by performing T

stochastic forward-passes with $\{w^{(t)}\}_{t=1}^{T} \sim q(\mathbf{W})$. For the regression, we calculate the expectation over the T samples in addition to the variance, which is the *parameter* uncertainty. For the segmentation, we compute the expectation of class probabilities to obtain the final labels whilst *parameter* uncertainty in the segmentation is obtained by considering variance of the stochastic class probabilities on a class basis. The final predictive uncertainty is the sum of the *intrinsic* and *parameter* uncertainties.

Implementation Details. We implemented our model within the NiftyNet framework [11] in TensorFlow. We trained our model on randomly selected 152×152 patches from 2D axial slices and reconstructed the 3D volume at test time. The representation network was composed of a convolutional layer followed by 3 sets of twice repeated dilated convolutions with dilation factors $[1, 2, 4]$ and a final convolutional layer. Each layer (l) used a 3×3 kernel with features $f_R = [64, 64, 128, 256, 2048]$. Each task-specific branch was a set of 5 convolutional layers of size $[256_{l=1,2,3,4}, n_{i,l=5}]$ where $n_{i,l=5}$ is equal to 1 for regression and σ and equal to the number of segmentation classes. The first two layers were 3×3 kernels whilst the final convolutional layers were fully connected. A Bernouilli drop-out mask with probability $p = 0.5$ was applied on the final layer of the representation network. We minimised the loss using ADAM with a learning rate 10^{-3} and trained up to 19000 iterations with convergence of the loss starting at 17500. For the stochastic sampling, we performed model inference 10 times at iterations 18000 and 19000 leading to a set of $T = 20$ samples.

3   Experiments and Results

Data. We validated on 15 prostate cancer patients, who each had a T2-weighted MR (3T, $1.46 \times 1.46 \times 5\text{mm}^3$) and CT scan (140kVp, $0.98 \times 0.98 \times 1.5\text{mm}^3$) acquired on the same day. Organ delineation was performed by a clinician with labels for the left and right femur head, bone, prostate, rectum and bladder. Images were resampled to isotropic resolution. The CT scans were spatially aligned with the T2 scans prior to training [1]. In the segmentation, we predicted labels for the background, left/right femur head, prostate, rectum and bladder.

Experiments. We performed 3-fold cross-validation and report statistics over all hold-out sets. We considered the following models: (1) baseline networks for regression/segmentation (M1), (2) baseline network with drop-out (M2a), (3) the baseline with drop-out and heteroscedastic noise (M2b), (4) multi-task network using homoscedastic task weighting (M3) [5] and (5) multi-task network using task-specific heteroscedastic noise and drop-out (M4). The baseline networks used only the representation network with $1/2f_R$ and a fully-connected layer for the final output to allow a fair comparison between single and multi-task networks. We also compared our results against the current state of the art in atlas propagation (AP) [1], which was validated on the same dataset.

Model Performance. An example of the model output is shown in Fig. 2. We calculated the Mean Absolute Error (MAE) between the predicted and reference scans across the body and at each organ (Table 1). The fuzzy DICE score

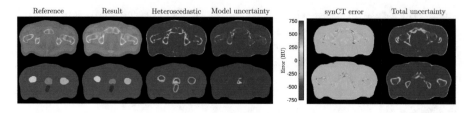

Fig. 2. Model output. *Intrinsic* and *parameter* uncertainty both correlate with regions of high contrast (bone in the regression, organ boundary for segmentation). Note the correlation between model error and the predicted uncertainty.

between the probabilistic segmentation and the reference was calculated for the segmentation (Table 1). Best performance was in our presented method (M4) for the regression across all masks except at the bladder. Application of the multi-task heteroscedastic network with drop-out (M4) produced the most consistent synCT across all models with the lowest average MAE and the lowest variation across patients (43.3 ± 2.9 versus 45.7 ± 4.6 [1] and 44.3 ± 3.1 [5]). This was significant lower when compared to M1 ($p < 0.001$) and M2 ($p < 0.001$). This was also observed at the bone, prostate and bladder ($p < 0.001$). Whilst differences at $p < 0.05$ were not observed versus M2b and M3, the consistent lower MAE and standard deviation across patients in M4 demonstrates the added benefit of modelling heteroscedastic noise and the inductive transfer from the segmentation task. We performed better than the current state of the art in atlas propagation, which used both T1 and T2-weighted scans [1]. Despite equivalence with the state of the art (Table 1), we did not observe any significant differences

Table 1. Model comparison. Bold values indicate when a model was significantly worse than M4 $p < 0.05$. No data was available for significance testing with AP. M2b was statistically better $p < 0.05$ than M4 in the prostate segmentation.

Models	All	Bone	L femur	R femur	Prostate	Rectum	Bladder
Regression - synCT - Mean Absolute Error (HU)							
M1	**48.1(4.2)**	**131(14.0)**	78.6(19.2)	**80.1(19.6)**	**37.1(10.4)**	63.3(47.3)	**24.3(5.2)**
M2a	**47.4(3.0)**	**130(12.1)**	78.0(14.8)	77.0(13.0)	**36.5(7.8)**	67(44.6)	**24.1(7.5)**
M2b [7]	44.5(3.6)	128(17.1)	75.8(20.1)	74.2(17.4)	31.2(7.0)	56.5(45.5)	17.8(4.7)
M3 [5]	44.3(3.1)	126(14.4)	74.0(19.5)	73.7(17.1)	29.4(4.7)	58.4(48.0)	18.2(3.5)
AP [1]	45.7(4.6)	125(10.3)	-	-	-	-	-
M4 (ours)	43.3(2.9)	121(12.6)	69.7(13.7)	67.8(13.2)	28.9(2.9)	55.1(48.1)	18.3(6.1)
Segmentation - OAR - Fuzzy DICE score							
M1	-	-	0.91(0.02)	0.90(0.04)	0.67(0.12)	0.70(0.15)	0.92(0.05)
M2a	-	-	0.85(0.03)	0.90(0.04)	0.66(0.12)	0.69(0.13)	0.90(0.07)
M2b [7]	-	-	0.92(0.02)	0.92(0.01)	0.77(0.07)	0.74(0.13)	0.92(0.03)
M3 [5]	-	-	0.92(0.02)	0.92(0.02)	0.73(0.07)	0.76(0.10)	0.93(0.02)
AP [1]	-	-	0.89(0.02)	0.90(0.01)	0.73(0.06)	0.77(0.06)	0.90(0.03)
M4 (ours)	-	-	0.91(0.02)	0.91(0.02)	0.70(0.06)	0.74(0.12)	0.93(0.04)

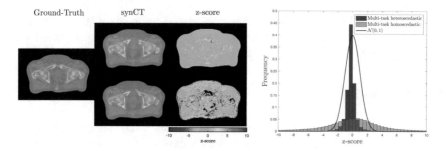

Fig. 3. Analysis of uncertainty estimation. (a) synCTs and z-scores for the a subject between M4 (top) and M3 (bottom) models. (b) z-score distribution of all patients (15) between both models.

between our model and the baselines despite an improvement in mean DICE at the prostate and rectum (0.70 ± 0.06 and 0.74 ± 0.12) versus the baseline M1 (0.67 ± 0.12, 0.70 ± 0.15). The *intrinsic uncertainty* (Fig. 2) models the uncertainty specific to the data and thus penalises regions of high error leading to an under-segmentation yet with higher confidence in the result.

Uncertainty Estimation for Radiotherapy. We tested the ability of the proposed network to better predict associated uncertainties in the synCT error. To verify that we produce clinically viable samples for treatment planning, we quantified the distribution of regression z-scores for the multi-task heteroscedastic and homoscedastic models. In the former, the total predictive uncertainty is the sum of the *intrinsic* and *parameter* uncertainties. This leads to a better approximation of the variance in the model. In contrast, the total uncertainty in the latter reduces to the variance of the stochastic test-time samples. This is likely to lead to a miscalibrated variance. A χ^2 goodness of fit test was performed, showing that the homoscedastic z-score distribution is not normally distributed (0.82 ± 0.54, $p < 0.01$) in contrast to the heteroscedastic model (0.04 ± 0.84, $p > 0.05$). This is apparent in Fig. 3 where there is greater confidence in the synCT produced by our model in contrast the homoscedastic case.

The predictive uncertainty can be exploited for quality assurance (Fig. 4). There may be issues whereupon time differences have caused variations in bladder and rectum filling across MR and CT scans causing patient variability in the

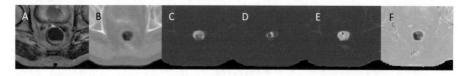

Fig. 4. Uncertainty in problematic areas. (a) T2 with reference segmentation, (b) synCT with localised error, (c) *intrinsic* uncertainty, (d) *parameter* uncertainty, (e) total predictive uncertainty and (f) error in HU (range [−750HU, 750HU]).

training data. This is exemplified by large errors in the synCT at the rectum (Fig. 4) and quantified by large localise z-scores (Fig. 4f), which correlate strongly with the *intrinsic* and *parameter* uncertainty across tasks (Figs. 2 and 4).

4   Conclusions

We have proposed a probabilistic dual-network that combines uncertainty modelling with multi-task learning. Our network extends prior work in multi-task learning by integrating heteroscedastic uncertainty modelling to naturally weight task losses and maximize inductive transfer between tasks. We have demonstrated the applicability of our network in the context of MR-only radiotherapy treatment planning. The model simultaneously provides the generation of synCTs, the segmentation of OARs and quantification of predictive uncertainty in both tasks. We have shown that a multi-task framework with heteroscedastic noise modelling leads to more accurate and consistent synCTs with a constraint on anatomical consistency with the segmentations. Importantly, we have demonstrated that the output of our network leads to consistent anatomically correct stochastic synCT samples that can potentially be effective in treatment planning.

Acknowledgements. FB, JM, DH and MJC were supported by CRUK Accelerator Grant A21993. RT was supported by Microsoft Scholarship. ZER was supported by EPSRC Doctoral Prize. DA was supported by EU Horizon 2020 Research and Innovation Programme Grant 666992 and EPSRC Grant M020533, M006093 and J020990. We thank NVIDIA Corporation for hardware donation.

References

1. Burgos, N., et al.: Iterative framework for the joint segmentation and CT synthesis of MR images: application to MRI-only radiotherapy treatment planning. Phys. Med. Biol. **62**, 4237 (2017)
2. Nie, D., et al.: Medical image synthesis with context-aware generative adversarial networks. arXiv:1612.05362
3. Wolterink, J.M., Dinkla, A.M., Savenije, M.H.F., Seevinck, P.R., van den Berg, C.A.T., Išgum, I.: Deep MR to CT synthesis using unpaired data. In: Tsaftaris, S.A., Gooya, A., Frangi, A.F., Prince, J.L. (eds.) SASHIMI 2017. LNCS, vol. 10557, pp. 14–23. Springer, Cham (2017). https://doi.org/10.1007/978-3-319-68127-6_2
4. Moeskops, P., et al.: Deep learning for multi-task medical image segmentation in multiple modalities. In: Ourselin, S., Joskowicz, L., Sabuncu, M.R., Unal, G., Wells, W. (eds.) MICCAI 2016. LNCS, vol. 9901, pp. 478–486. Springer, Cham (2016). https://doi.org/10.1007/978-3-319-46723-8_55
5. Kendall, A., et al.: Multi-task learning using uncertainty to weigh losses for scene geometry and semantics. In: CVPR (2018)
6. Tanno, R., et al.: Bayesian image quality transfer with CNNs: exploring uncertainty in dMRI super-resolution. In: Descoteaux, M., Maier-Hein, L., Franz, A., Jannin, P., Collins, D.L., Duchesne, S. (eds.) MICCAI 2017. LNCS, vol. 10433, pp. 611–619. Springer, Cham (2017). https://doi.org/10.1007/978-3-319-66182-7_70

7. Kendall, A., Gal, Y.: What uncertainties do we need in Bayesian deep learning for computer vision? In: NIPS, pp. 5580–5590 (2017)
8. Gal, Y., Ghahramani, Z.: Dropout as a Bayesian approximation: representing model uncertainty in deep learning. In: ICML, pp. 1050–1059 (2016)
9. Caruana, R.: Multitask learning: a knowledge-based source of inductive bias. In: ICML (1993)
10. Li, W., Wang, G., Fidon, L., Ourselin, S., Cardoso, M.J., Vercauteren, T.: On the compactness, efficiency, and representation of 3D convolutional networks: brain parcellation as a pretext task. In: Niethammer, M., Styner, M., Aylward, S., Zhu, H., Oguz, I., Yap, P.-T., Shen, D. (eds.) IPMI 2017. LNCS, vol. 10265, pp. 348–360. Springer, Cham (2017). https://doi.org/10.1007/978-3-319-59050-9_28
11. Gibson, E., et al.: NiftyNet: a deep-learning platform for medical imaging. Comput. Methods Programs Biomed. **158**, 113-122 (2018)

A Combined Simulation and Machine Learning Approach for Image-Based Force Classification During Robotized Intravitreal Injections

Andrea Mendizabal[1,2(✉)], Tatiana Fountoukidou[3], Jan Hermann[3],
Raphael Sznitman[3], and Stephane Cotin[1]

[1] Inria, Strasbourg, France
andrea.mendizabal@inria.fr
[2] University of Strasbourg, ICube, Strasbourg, France
[3] ARTORG Center, University of Bern, Bern, Switzerland

Abstract. Intravitreal injection is one of the most common treatment strategies for chronic ophthalmic diseases. The last decade has seen the number of intravitreal injections dramatically increase, and with it, adverse effects and limitations. To overcome these issues, medical assistive devices for robotized injections have been proposed and are projected to improve delivery mechanisms for new generation of pharmacological solutions. In our work, we propose a method aimed at improving the safety features of such envisioned robotic systems. Our vision-based method uses a combination of 2D OCT data, numerical simulation and machine learning to estimate the range of the force applied by an injection needle on the sclera. We build a Neural Network (NN) to predict force ranges from Optical Coherence Tomography (OCT) images of the sclera directly. To avoid the need of large training data sets, the NN is trained on images of simulated deformed sclera. We validate our approach on real OCT images collected on five *ex vivo* porcine eyes using a robotically-controlled needle. Results show that the applied force range can be predicted with 94% accuracy. Being real-time, this solution can be integrated in the control loop of the system, allowing for in-time withdrawal of the needle.

1 Introduction

Intravitreal injections are one of the most frequent surgical interventions in opthalmology with more than 4 million injections in 2014 alone [1]. This procedure is used, for instance, in the treatment of age-related macular degeneration for injecting vascular endothelial growth factor inhibitors. Similarly, intravitreal therapy is also used in the treatment of diabetic maculopathy and retinopathy. With the increasing prevalence of diabetic patients and aging demographics, the demand for such intravitreal therapy is growing significantly.

© Springer Nature Switzerland AG 2018
A. F. Frangi et al. (Eds.): MICCAI 2018, LNCS 11073, pp. 12–20, 2018.
https://doi.org/10.1007/978-3-030-00937-3_2

At the same time, robotic assistance in ophthalmology offers the ability to improve manipulation dexterity, along with shorter and safer surgeries [2]. Ullrich *et al.* [1] has also proposed a robotized intravitreal injection device capable of assisting injections into the vitreous cavity, whereby faster injections in safer conditions are projected. Designing such robotic systems involves significant hurdles and challenges however. Among others, accurate force sensing represents an important topic, whereby the force required to puncture the sclera with a needle is very small and measuring this force is essential for the safety of the patient.

For many devices, force sensing plays a central role in the control loop and safety system of surgical robots [3]. The use of force sensors and force-based control algorithms allows for higher quality human-machine interaction, more realistic sensory feedback and telepresence. Beyond this, it can facilitate the deployment of important safety features [4]. Considerable amount of work relying on force sensors has previously been done, focusing on the development of miniaturized sensors to ease their integration with actual systems. In addition, they must be water resistant, sterilizable and insensitive to changes in temperature [5]. The major limitation of standard force sensors is thus the associated cost, since most surgical tools are disposable [4]. Alternatively, qualitative estimation of forces based on images has been proposed in the past [5,6]. Mura *et al.* presented a vision-based haptic feedback system to assist the movement of an endoscopic device using 3D maps. Haouchine *et al.* estimates force feedback in robot assisted surgery using a biomechanical model of the organ in addition to the 3D maps. In contrast, including detailed material characteristics allows precise quantitative assessment of forces but calculating the properties of the materials still remains highly complex [7]. Recent research have proposed the use of neural networks for force estimation, such as in [8] where interaction forces using recurrent neural networks are estimated from camera acquisitions, kinematic variables and the deformation mappings. In a follow up, [7] used a neuro-vision based approach for estimating applied forces. In this approach tissue surface deformation is reconstructed by minimizing an energy functional.

In contrast, our method consists in estimating the force, based only on an OCT image of the deformation of the eye sclera. The method relies on a deep learning classifier for estimating quantiles of forces during robotized intravitreal injections. Our contribution hence consists of two critical stages. We first build a biomechanical model of the sclera in order to generate virtually infinite force-OCT image pairs for training any supervised machine learning method. In particular, we will show that this allows us to avoid the need for large data sets of real OCT images. Second, we train end-to-end, a two-layer image classifier algorithm with the synthetic images and the corresponding forces. This allows a very simple estimation process to take place, without the need of a specific image feature extraction method beforehand [7,8]. The consequence of this two-stage process to produce synthetic data for training a NN is the ability to classify force ranges with 94% accuracy. We validate this claim on real OCT images collected on five *ex vivo* porcine eyes using a robotically-controlled needle.

2   Method

Deep learning has already been proposed to improve existent features of robotic assisted surgeries such as instrument detection and segmentation [9]. A key requirement for deep learning methods to work is the high amount of data to train on. Since for the moment, intravitreal injections are manually performed, there is no available information on the force applied by the needle. In this paper, we build a numerical model of the relevant part of the eye to generate images of the deformed sclera under needle-induced forces. The simulations are parametrized to match experimental results and compensate for the lack of real data.

2.1   Numerical Simulation for Fast Data Generation

Biomechanical model: The deformation of the sclera under needle-induced forces can be approximated by modeling the eye as an elastic material, shaped like a half-sphere subject to specific boundary conditions. Since applied forces and resulting deformations remain small, we choose a linear relationship between strain ϵ and stress σ, known as Hooke's law (1):

$$\sigma = 2\mu\epsilon + \lambda tr(\epsilon)I \tag{1}$$

where λ and μ are the Lamé coefficients that can be determined from the Young's modulus $\mathbf{E}$ and Poisson's ratio $\boldsymbol{\nu}$ of the material. The linearity of Hooke's law leads us to a simple relation $\sigma = \mathbf{C}\epsilon$ where $\mathbf{C}$ is the linear elasticity constitutive matrix of homogeneous and isotropic materials. Boundary conditions are then added. Dirichlet boundary conditions are used to prevent rigid body motion of the sclera, while a constant pressure is applied on the inner domain boundary to simulate the intraocular pressure (IOP). The IOP plays an important role in the apparent stiffness of the eye and its variability is well studied, as high eye pressure can be an indication for glaucoma. The external force due to IOP is simply given by $F = S \times P$ where S is the surface area of the eye given in m^2 and P the IOP in Pa. The external forces of the system are formed by the IOP, the force induced by the needle and gravity. Scleral thickness also plays an important role in the deformation of the sclera so it has to be taken into account.

Finite Element simulation: We solve the equation for the constitutive model using a finite element method. To discretize the eyeball, which we consider as nearly spherical, we generated a quadrilateral surface mesh of a half sphere of radius $12\,\mathrm{mm}$, discretized using the Catmull-Clark subdivision method. This quadrilateral surface is then extruded according to the scleral thickness to generate almost regular hexahedra. The deformation is specified by the nodal displacements $\mathbf{u}$ and the nodal forces $\mathbf{f}$, according to the following equation:

$$\mathbf{Ku} = \mathbf{f_p} + \mathbf{f_g} + \mathbf{f_n} \tag{2}$$

Force class 0   Force class 1   Force class 2

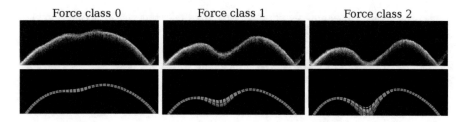

Fig. 1. Real OCT images of the sclera and their corresponding simulated images for the three different force ranges.

The matrix $\mathbf{K}$ is the stiffness matrix, and can be computed thanks to the elastic parameters of the material $\mathbf{E}$ and $\boldsymbol{\nu}$. $\mathbf{E}$ is Young's modulus and is a measure of the stiffness of the material while $\boldsymbol{\nu}$ is Poisson's ratio and estimates the compressibility of the material. According to the values in the literature [10] we set $\mathbf{E} = 0.25$ MPa and $\boldsymbol{\nu} = 0.45$. To model the needle pushing on the sclera, we apply a local force $\mathbf{f_n}$ on a subset of nodes within a small region of interest near the virtual needle tip. $\mathbf{f_g}$ is the force due to gravity, and $\mathbf{f_p}$ the force normal to the surface due to the IOP. To compute accurately the deformation of the sclera, the finite element mesh needs to be sufficiently fine ($14,643$ hexahedral elements in our case), resulting in about $5\,$s of computation to obtain the solution of the deformation. Since we need to repeat thousands of times this type of computation in order to generate the training data set, we take advantage of the linearity of the model and pre-compute the inverse of $\mathbf{K}$. This significantly speeds up the generation of the training data. In Fig. 1 are shown different examples of the output of the simulation (bottom) matching the OCT images (top). The simulated images correspond to a 2D cross-section of the entire 3D mesh.

2.2   Neural Network Image Classification

Our goal is to create an artificial NN model to predict the force based solely on a single OCT image of the deformation. Using cross sectional OCT images allows one to visualize millimeters beneath the surface of the sclera and therefore provides information about the induced deformation. Using 2D OCT B-scans over 3D scans is preferred here as can be acquired at high-frame rates using low cost hardware [11]. Instead of estimating the force as a scalar value, we opt to estimate an interval of forces in order to be less sensitive to exact force values. As such, we set up our inference problem as a classification task where a probability for a class label (i.e. a force interval) is desired.

Given our above simulation model, we can now train our prediction model with virtually an *infinite* amount of data. In our case, the forces applied in the experiments varied between 0.0 N to 0.08325 N. To ensure quality of the simulations (i.e. small displacements) forces going from 0.0 N to 0.06 N were applied on the Finite Element mesh of the sclera. The objective being the in-time withdrawal of the needle to limit scleral damage, we decided to label the forces only using three classes. The classes are such that the first one translates no danger at damaging the sclera, the second means that a considerable force is being applied and the last class triggers the alarm to withdraw the needle. If we set the alarm threshold to 0.03 N, we have the following class ranges (see Fig. 1 for the deformation corresponding to each class):

- Class 0: force values smaller than 0.005 N
- Class 1: force values from 0.005 N to 0.03 N
- Class 2: force values bigger than 0.03 N

Our NN then consists of three layers (an input layer, a fully connected hidden layer and an output layer). The input layer has 5600 neurons and the hidden and output layers have 600 neurons. The output layer is softmax activated. ReLu activation was used as well as a 0.8 dropout factor between layers. For training, we used Gradient descent optimization and the cross-entropy loss function. The network was implemented using Tensorflow and the Keras Python library and was trained from scratch. Validation was performed on unseen simulated images.

3   Results

In this section we first report the real data acquisition on *ex vivo* porcine eyes. Then, the virtually generated data set and the following training are presented. And last, we validate the NN on unseen real data.

3.1   Experimental Set-Up

To validate the ability of the NN on real data, we collected pairs of force-OCT images from *ex vivo* porcine eyes. Five porcine eyes were obtained from the local abattoir and transported in ice. Experiments began within 3 h of death and were completed between 4 and 10 h postmortem. During the experiments the eyes were moisturized with water. For the experiments, the eyes were fixed with super glue on a 3D-printed holder to ensure fixed boundary conditions on the lower half of the eyeball. The IOP was measured with a tonometer. For all the eyes the IOP was close to 2 mmHg (i.e. 266 Pa). The IOP is low since it decreases dramatically after death [12] and no fluid injection was made during the experiments. A medical robot [3] was used to guide a needle while measuring the applied force. A 22G Fine-Ject needle (0.7 × 30 mm) was mounted at the tip of the end effector of the robot. The needle was placed as close as possible to the B-scan but without intersecting it to avoid shadows on OCT images. The margin between the needle and the B-scan was taken into account in the simulation. The robot moved towards the center of the eye (i.e. normally to the sclera) and forces in the direction of movement were continuously recorded with a sensor. To collect OCT images an imaging system was used to record B-scans over time. The OCT device used 840 nm ± 40 nm wavelength light source, with an A-scan rate of 50 kHz and 12 bits per pixel. The resulting 2D image had a resolution of 512 ×512 pixels, corresponding to roughly 15 × 4 mm. As the images were acquired at a lower rate than the forces, the corresponding forces were averaged over the imaging time for each frame (i.e. two seconds after the starting moment of the line move). Overall, 54 trials were performed. For each eye, one position near the corneal-scleral limbus was chosen and several line moves were performed in the same direction.

3.2   Data Generation for Neural Network Training

Measurements on ten porcine eyes are made to estimate the thickness of the sclera at the locations where the forces are applied. The values range from 460 μm to 650 μm with a mean value of 593 μm. From the literature [13], the thickness near corneal-scleral limbus is estimated to be between 630 μm and 1030 μm. Hence, we simulated scleras of five different thicknesses: 400 μm, 500 μm, 600 μm, 700 μm and 800 μm. The IOP is the same for all the eyes in the experiments so it is fixed at 266 Pa for all simulations. For the smallest thickness, we generated 3200 images of deformed scleras undergoing the stated IOP and forces going from 0.0 N to 0.045 N. For each of the other four thicknesses, we generated 4000 images of deformed scleras where the forces vary from 0.0 N to 0.06 N at different random locations. For each thickness, the simulation took approximatively half an hour. Overall, a data set of 19200 synthetic images was generated within 2 h and a half (see Fig. 2(b)). The generated images look like images in Fig. 1 below. This images are post-processed with a contour detection algorithm using OpenCV functions and binarized to obtain the images used to train the NN (see Fig. 2(b)).

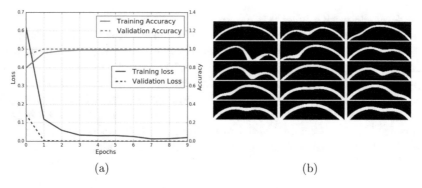

(a)   (b)

Fig. 2. (a) Loss and Accuracy curves for training and validation sets. (b) Fragment of the training data set generated by our numerical simulation.

To train the NN, the data set is split such that 90% of the images are for training and the remaining 10% for validating. Hence, the NN is trained on 17280 images and validated on the other 1920 images. In Fig. 2(a) the accuracy and loss of the model are shown on both training and validation data sets over each epoch. The validation accuracy curve shows 100% accuracy when classifying unseen synthetic images. This curve is above the training accuracy curve probably because of the high dropout applied during the training.

3.3   Tests on Unseen Data

The aim of our work is to classify force ranges from real OCT images of the deformed scleras. All the OCT images obtained during the experiments (see Fig. 3(a)) are blurred and thresholded to obtain similar images to the synthetic ones (see Figs. 3(b) and 2(b)).

Now that the OCT images look like the simulated ones they can be given as input to the NN for predictions. For each OCT acquisition, the force measured by the robot is converted into a class label (going from 0 to 2) and is considered as the ground truth (target class). The performance of the classification is given in the confusion matrix in Table 1. Each raw of the table gives the instances in a target class and each column the instances in a predicted class. For each class, the correct decisions are highlighted in red. Overall the accuracy of the classifier is 94%.

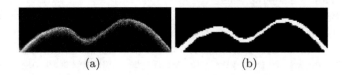

(a)   (b)

Fig. 3. (a) Unprocessed OCT image. (b) Blurred and thresholded OCT image.

A force class with label 0 is understood as a very small force meaning that there is no risk of damaging the sclera. On the contrary, a force class with label 1 means the sclera is being considerably deformed (forces in this range go from 0.005 N to 0.03 N) and a force class with label 2 means that the sclera is potentially being damaged and a withdrawal of the needle is advised. With the eyes used during the experiments, the lowest precision of the NN was found for target class 0 (71%). For target class 2, the precision is of 100%. It is not dramatic if forces of range 0 and 1 are misclassified since the risk of damaging the sclera with forces so close to the alarm threshold is almost null (assuming

Table 1. Confusion matrix

Prediction / Target	Class 0	Class 1	Class 2	Precision
Class 0	5	2	0	0.71
Class 1	0	14	1	0.93
Class 2	0	0	32	1.00
Recall	1.00	0.88	0.97	

the threshold is correctly set). On the other hand it is essential that the forces of range 2 are predicted correctly.

4   Conclusion and Discussion

In this paper, we have proposed a method aimed at improving the safety features of upcoming robotized intravitreal injections. Our vision-based method combining numerical simulation and Neural Networks, predicts the range of the force applied by a needle using only 2D images of the scleral deformation with high accuracy. It indicates in real-time the need to withdraw the needle as soon as a certain alarm threshold is reached. To avoid the need of large training data sets, the NN is trained on synthetic images from a simulated deformed sclera.

It is worth mentioning that more complex scenarios could be simulated such as different eye sizes, variable needle insertion angles and different intraocular pressures. We also propose to improve the simulated images to better match real surgical scenarios. In particular it seems important to add the shadows induced by the needle in the OCT image. From an imaging point of view, we know that the predictions of the NN are very sensitive to the image framing and scaling. To address this issue, we plan to randomly crop each simulated image, and enlarge the data set with it. We might also train a Convolutional Neural Network to reduce sensitivity to image properties and allow for more accurate predictions.

References

1. Ullrich, F., Michels, S., Lehmann, D., Pieters, R.S., Becker, M., Nelson, B.J.: Assistive device for efficient intravitreal injections. Ophthalmic Surg. Lasers Imaging Retina, Healio **47**(8), 752–762 (2016)
2. Meenink, H., et al.: Robot-assisted vitreoretinal surgery. pp. 185–209, October 2012
3. Weber, S., et al.: Instrument flight to the inner ear, March 2017
4. Haidegger, T., Beny, B., Kovcs, L., Beny, Z.: Force sensing and force control for surgical robots. Proceedings of the 7th IFAC Symposium on Modelling and Control in Biomedical Systems, pp. 401–406, August 2009
5. Haouchine, N., Kuang, W., Cotin, S., Yip, M.: Vision-based force feedback estimation for robot-assisted surgery using instrument-constrained biomechanical 3D maps. IEEE Robot. Autom. Lett. **3**, 2160–2165 (2018)
6. Mura, M., et al.: Vision-based haptic feedback for capsule endoscopy navigation: a proof of concept. J. Micro-Bio Robot. **11**, 35–45 (2016). https://doi.org/10.1007/s12213-016-0090-2
7. Aviles, A.I., Alsaleh, S., Sobrevilla, P., Casals, A.: Sensorless force estimation using a neuro-vision-based approach for robotic-assisted surgery, pp. 86–89, April 2015
8. Aviles, A.I., Marban, A., Sobrevilla, P., Fernandez, J., Casals, A.: A recurrent neural network approach for 3D vision-based force estimation, pp. 1–6, October 2014
9. Pakhomov, D., Premachandran, V., Allan, M., Azizian, M., Navab, N.: Deep residual learning for instrument segmentation in robotic surgery, March 2017
10. Asejczyk-Widlicka, M., Pierscionek, B.: The elasticity and rigidity of the outer coats of the eye. Bristish J. Ophthalmol. **92**, 1415–1418 (2008)

11. Apostolopoulos, S., Sznitman, R.: Efficient OCT volume reconstruction from slit-lamp microscopes. IEEE Trans. Biomed. Eng. **64**(10), 2403–2410 (2017)
12. Gnay, Y., Basmak, H., Kenan Kocaturk, B., Sahin, A., Ozdamar, K.: The importance of measuring intraocular pressure using a tonometer in order to estimate the postmortem interval. Am. J. Forensic Med. Pathol. **31**, 151–155 (2010)
13. Olsen, T., Sanderson, S., Feng, X., Hubbard, W.C.: Porcine sclera: thickness and surface area. Invest. Ophthalmol. Vis. Sci. **43**, 2529–2532 (2002)

Learning from Noisy Label Statistics: Detecting High Grade Prostate Cancer in Ultrasound Guided Biopsy

Shekoofeh Azizi[1(✉)], Pingkun Yan[2], Amir Tahmasebi[3], Peter Pinto[4], Bradford Wood[4], Jin Tae Kwak[5], Sheng Xu[4], Baris Turkbey[4], Peter Choyke[4], Parvin Mousavi[6], and Purang Abolmaesumi[1]

[1] University of British Columbia, Vancouver, Canada
shazizi@ece.ubc.ca
[2] Rensselaer Polytechnic Institute, Troy, USA
[3] Philips Research North America, Cambridge, USA
[4] National Institutes of Health, Bethesda, USA
[5] Sejong University, Seoul, Korea
[6] Queen's University, Kingston, Canada

Abstract. The ubiquity of noise is an important issue for building computer-aided diagnosis models for prostate cancer biopsy guidance where the histopathology data is sparse and not finely annotated. We propose a solution to alleviate this challenge as a part of Temporal Enhanced Ultrasound (TeUS)-based prostate cancer biopsy guidance method. Specifically, we embed the prior knowledge from the histopathology as the soft labels in a two-stage model, to leverage the problem of diverse label noise in the ground-truth. We then use this information to accurately detect the grade of cancer and also to estimate the length of cancer in the target. Additionally, we create a Bayesian probabilistic version of our network, which allows evaluation of model uncertainty that can lead to any possible misguidance during the biopsy procedure. In an *in vivo* study with 155 patients, we analyze data from 250 suspicious cancer foci obtained during fusion biopsy. We achieve the average area under the curve of 0.84 for cancer grading and mean squared error of 0.12 in the estimation of tumor in biopsy core length.

Keywords: Temporal enhanced ultrasound · Prostate cancer
Recurrent neural networks

1 Introduction

The ultimate diagnosis for prostate cancer is through histopathology analysis of prostate biopsy, guided by either Transrectal Ultrasound (TRUS), or fusion of TRUS with multi-parametric Magnetic Resonance Imaging (mp-MRI) [14,15]. Computer-aided diagnosis models for detection of prostate cancer and guidance of biopsy involve both ultrasound (US)- and mp-MRI-based tissue

© Springer Nature Switzerland AG 2018
A. F. Frangi et al. (Eds.): MICCAI 2018, LNCS 11073, pp. 21–29, 2018.
https://doi.org/10.1007/978-3-030-00937-3_3

characterization. mp-MRI has high sensitivity in detection of prostate lesions but low specificity [1,10], hence, limiting its utility in detecting disease progression over time [15]. US-based tissue characterization methods focus on the analysis of texture [11] and spectral features [7] within a single ultrasound frame, Doppler imaging and elastography [13]. Temporal Enhanced Ultrasound (TeUS), involving a time-series of ultrasound RF frames captured from insonification of tissue over time [6], has enabled the depiction of patient-specific cancer likelihood maps [2,3,5,12]. Despite promising results in detecting prostate cancer, accurate characterization of aggressive lesions from indolent ones is an open problem and requires refinement.

The goodness of models built based on all the above analyses depends on detailed, noise-free annotations of ground-truth labels from pathology. However, there are two key challenges with the ground-truth. First, histopathology data used for training of the models is sparsely annotated with the inevitable ubiquity of noise. Second, the heterogeneity in morphology and pathology of the prostate itself contributes as a source of inaccuracy in labeling.

In this paper, we propose a method to address the challenge of sparse and noisy histopathology ground-truth labels to improve TeUS-based prostate biopsy guidance. The contributions of the paper are: (1) Employing prior histopathology knowledge to estimate ground-truth probability vectors as soft labels. We then use these soft labels as a replacement for the sparse and noisy labels for training a two-stage Recurrent Neural Networks (RRN)-based model; (2) Using the new ground-truth probability vectors to accurately estimate the tumor in biopsy core length; and (3) A strategy for the depiction of new patient-specific colormaps for biopsy guidance using the estimated model uncertainty.

2   Materials

Data Acquisition and Preprocessing. We use TeUS data from 250 biopsy targets of 155 subjects. All subjects were identified as suspicious for cancer in a preoperative mp-MRI examination. The subjects underwent MRI-guided ultrasound biopsy using UroNav (Invivo Corp., FL) MR-US fusion system [14]. Prior to biopsy sampling from each target, the ultrasound transducer is held steady for 5 seconds to obtain $T = 100$ frames of TeUS RF data. This procedure is followed by firing the biopsy gun to acquire a tissue specimen. Histopathology information of each biopsy core is used as the gold-standard for generating a label for that core. For each biopsy target, we analyze an area of $2\,mm \times 10\,mm$ around the target, along with the projected needle path. We divide this region into 80 equally-sized Regions of Interest (ROIs) of $0.5\,mm \times 0.5\,mm$. For each ROI, we generate a sequence of TeUS data, $\mathbf{x}^{(i)} = (x_1^{(i)}, ..., x_T^{(i)}), T = 100$ by averaging over all the time series values within a given ROI of an ultrasound frame (Fig. 2). An individual TeUS sequence is constituted of echo-intensity values $x_t^{(i)}$ for each time step, t. We also augment the training data ($\mathcal{D}_{train}$) by generating ROIs using a sliding window of size $0.5\,mm \times 0.5\,mm$ over the target region with the step size of $0.1\ mm$, which results in 1,536 ROIs per target.

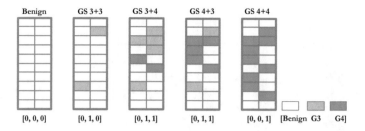

Fig. 1. Illustration of noisy and not finely annotated ground-truth label. The exact location of the cancerous ROI in the core, the ratio of the different Gleason grade, and the exact location of the Gleason grades are unknown and noisy. The bottom vectors show one of the possible multi-label binarization approaches.

Ground-Truth Labeling. Histopathology reports include the length of cancer in the biopsy core and a Gleason Score (GS) [13]. The GS is reported as a summation of the Gleason grades of the two most common cancer patterns in the tissue specimen. Gleason grades range from 1 (normal) to 5 (aggressive cancerous). The histopathology reports a measure of the statistical distribution of cancer in the cancer foci. The ground-truth is noisy and not finely annotated to show the exact location of the cancerous tissue in the core (Fig. 1). Therefore, the exact grade of each ROI in a core is not available while the overarching goal is to determine the ROI-level grade of the specimen. In our dataset, 78 biopsy cores are cancerous with GS $3+3$ or higher, where 26 of those are labeled as clinically significant cancer with GS $\geq 4+3$. The remaining 172 cores are benign.

3 Method

3.1 Discriminative Model

Let $\mathcal{D} = \{(\mathbf{x}^{(i)}, \mathbf{y}^{(i)})\}_{i=1}^{|\mathcal{D}|}$ represent the collection of all ROIs, where $\mathbf{x}^{(i)}$ is the ith TeUS sequence with length T and is labeled as $\mathbf{y}^{(i)})$ corresponding to a cancer grade. The objective is to develop a probabilistic model to discriminate between cancer grades using noisy and not well-annotated data in $\mathcal{D}$. For this purpose, we propose a two-stage approach to consider the diverse nature of noise in the ground-truth labeling: benign vs. all grades of cancer and the mixture of cancer grades. The goal of the first stage is to mine the data points with non-cancerous tissue in the presence of possible noise where several theoretical studies have shown the robustness of the binary classification accuracy to the simple and symmetric label noise [8]. The goal of the second stage is to learn from the noisy label statistic in cancerous cores by suppressing the influence of noise using a soft label. In the core of the approach, we use deeply connected RNN layers to explicitly model the temporal information in TeUS followed by a fully connected layer to map the sequence to a posterior over classes. Each RNN layer includes $T = 100$ homogeneous hidden units (*i.e.*, traditional/vanilla RNN, LSTM or GRU cells) to capture temporal changes in data. Given the

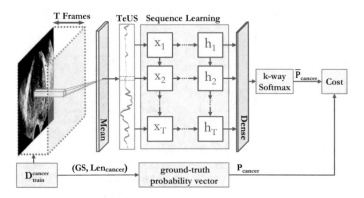

Fig. 2. Overview of the second stage of the method: the goal of is to assign a patho-logical score to a sample. To mitigate the problem of noisy labels, we embed the length of the cancer in the ground-truth probability vector as a soft label.

input sequence $\mathbf{x} = (x_1, , ..., x_T)$, RNN computes the hidden vector sequence $\mathbf{h} = (h_1, , ..., h_T)$ in the sequence learning step. This hidden vector, $\mathbf{h}$ is a function of the input sequence $\mathbf{x}$, model parameters, Θ, and time.

Stage 1: Detection of Benign Samples: Let $y_b^{(i)} \in \{0, 1\}$ indicate the corresponding binary label for $\mathbf{x}^{(i)}$, where zero and one indicate benign and cancer outcome, respectively. We aim to learn a mapping from $\mathbf{x}^{(i)}$ to $y_b^{(i)}$ in a supervised manner. After the sequence learning step, the final node generates the posterior probability for the given sequence:

$$\overline{y}_b^{(i)} = \arg\max_j \mathcal{S}(\mathbf{z}_j^{(i)}), \; j \in \{0, 1\}, \; \mathbf{z}^{(i)} = \mathbf{W}_s^T \mathbf{h} + \mathbf{b}_s, \tag{1}$$

where $\mathbf{W}_s$ and $\mathbf{b}_s$ are the weight and bias of the fully-connected layer and $\mathcal{S}$ is the softmax function, which in our binary classification case is equivalent to the logistic function, and $\overline{y}_b^{(i)}$ indicates the predicted label. The optimization criterion for the network is to minimize the binary cross-entropy between $y_b^{(i)}$ and $\overline{y}_b^{(i)}$ over all training samples.

Stage 2: Grading of Cancerous Samples: The goal of this stage is to assign a pathological score to $\mathcal{D}_{train}^{cancer} = \{(\mathbf{x}^{(i)}, y_b^{(i)} \in \mathcal{D}_{train} \mid y_b^{(i)} = 1\}_{i=1}^N$. Here, unlike the first stage, we are facing a multi-label classification task with sparse labeling (Fig. 1). The histopathology reports include two informative parts: (1) Gleason score which implies any of the possible labels $\Omega \in \{Benign, G3, G4\}$ for all ROIs within a core, where all or at least two of these patterns can happen at the same time; (2) The measured length of cancerous tissues ($\mathcal{L}en$) in a typical core length ($\mathcal{L}en^{typical}$) of 18.0 mm. We propose a new approach for ground-truth probability vector generation, enabling the soft labeling instead of the traditional label encoding methods. For this purpose, using $\mathcal{D}_{train}^{cancer}$ the output of sequence learning step $\mathbf{h}$ is fed into a k-way softmax function, which produces a probability distribution over the k possible class labels ($k = 3$). Suppose $\mathcal{L}en^{(i)}$ represents the length of cancer for the core that $\mathbf{x}^{(i)}$ belongs to. The ground-truth probability vector of the ith ROI is defined as $\mathbf{p}^{(i)} = [p_1^{(i)}, ..., p_k^{(i)}]$. To estimate these probabilities we define the normalized cancer percentage as $\mathbf{C}^{(i)} = \mathcal{L}en^{(i)}/\mathcal{L}en^{typical}$ ($\mathbf{C}^{(i)} \in [0, 1]$). For $k = 3$:

$$\mathbf{p}^{(i)} = \left[p_1^{(i)} = (1 - \mathbf{C}^{(i)}), p_2^{(i)} = \omega \times \mathbf{C}^{(i)}, p_3^{(i)} = (1 - \omega) \times \mathbf{C}^{(i)} \right] \qquad (2)$$

where ω is the cancer regularization factor to control the inherent ratio between pattern G3 and G4 in a way that for the cores with GS $3 + 4$ label, ω be greater than 0.5 to imply a higher probability of having pattern G3 than the G4 and vice-versa. For ROIs which originate from the cores with GS $3 + 3$ or $4 + 4$ readings, ω is set to 1 and 0, respectively. The cost function to be minimized is defined as:

$$J = \frac{1}{|\mathcal{D}_{train}^{cancer}|} \sum_{i=1}^{N} \sum_{k=1}^{K} (\mathbf{p}_k^{(i)} - \overline{\mathbf{p}}_k^{(i)})^2 \qquad (3)$$

where $\overline{\mathbf{p}}^{(i)} = [\overline{p}_1^{(i)}, ..., \overline{p}_k^{(i)}]$ is the predictive probability vector.

3.2 Cancer Grading and Tumor in Core Length Estimation

Suppose $\mathcal{C} = \{(\mathbf{x}^{(i)}, y_b^{(i)})\}_{i=1}^{|\mathcal{C}|}$ represent the collection of all labeled ROIs surrounding a target core, where $\mathcal{C} \in \mathcal{D}_{test}$, $|\mathcal{C}| = 80$, $\mathbf{x}^{(i)}$ represents the ith TeUS sequence of the core, and $y_b^{(i)}$ indicates the corresponding binary label. Using the probability output of the first stage model for each ROI, we assign a binary label to each target core. The label is calculated using a majority voting based on the predicted labels of all ROIs surrounding the target. We define the predicted label for each ROI, $\overline{y}_b^{(i)}$, as 1, when $P(y_b^{(i)}|\mathbf{x}^{(i)}) \geq 0.5$, and as 0 otherwise. The probability of a given core being cancerous based on the cancerous ROIs within that core is $\mathcal{P}_b = \sum_{i=1}^{|\mathcal{C}|} I(\overline{\mathbf{y}}^{(i)} = 1)/|\mathcal{C}|$. A binary label of 1 is assigned to a core, when $\mathcal{P}_b \geq 0.5$. For the cores with prediction of the cancer, we use the output the second stage model to both predict the cancer length and determine a GS for the test core. Suppose $\mathbf{p}_m^{(i)} = \left[p_1^{(i)}, p_2^{(i)}, p_3^{(i)} \right]$ represents the predictive probability output of ith TeUS sequence in the second stage. We define the average predictive probability as $\mathcal{P}^m = \sum_{i=1}^{|\mathcal{C}|} \mathbf{p}_m^{(i)}/|\mathcal{C}|$. Following the histopathology guidelines, to determine a GS for a cancerous test core, $\mathcal{Y}$, we define the core as "GS 4+3 or higher" when $\mathbf{P}_m^{(3)} \geq \mathbf{P}_m^{(2)}$ and otherwise as "GS 3+4 or lower". Furthermore, based on Eq. (2), we can estimate the predicted length of cancer for this core as $\mathcal{L}en^{\mathcal{C}} = (1 - \mathbf{P}_{(1)}^m) \times \mathcal{L}en^{typical}$.

3.3 Model Uncertainty Estimation

We also aim to estimate the model uncertainty in detection of cancer for the areas outside the cancer foci, where the annotation is not available. The key to estimating model uncertainty is the posterior distribution $P(\Theta|\mathcal{D})$, also referred to a Bayesian inference [9]. Here, we follow the idea in [9] to approximate model uncertainty using Monte Carlo dropout (MC dropout). Given a new input $\mathbf{x}^{(i)}$, we compute the model output with stochastic dropouts at each layer. That is, randomly dropout each hidden unit with certain probability p. This procedure is repeated B times, and we obtain $\{\overline{y}_b^{*(1)}, ..., \overline{y}_b^{*(B)}\}$. Then, the model uncertainty can be approximated by the sample variance, $1/B\sum_{j=1}^{B}(\overline{y}_b^{*(j)} - \hat{y}_b^{*(j)})^2$, where $\hat{y}_b^{*(j)}$ is the average of $\overline{y}_b^{*(j)}$ values.

4   Experiments and Results

Data Division and Model Selection: Data is divided into mutually exclusive patient sets for training, $\mathcal{D}_{train}$, and test, $\mathcal{D}_{test}$. Training data is made up of 80 randomly selected cores from patients with homogeneous tissue regions where the number of cancerous and non-cancerous cores are equal. The test data consists of 170 cores, where 130 cores are labeled as benign, 29 cores with $GS \leq 3+4$, and 12 cores with $GS \geq 4+3$. Given the data augmentation strategy in Sect. 2, we obtain a total number of $80 \times 1,536 = 122,880$ training samples ($N = |\mathcal{D}_{train}| = 122,880$). We use 20% of $\mathcal{D}_{train}$ data as the held-out validation sets ($\mathcal{D}_{val}$) to perform the grid search over the number of RNN hidden layers, $n_h \in \{1, 2\}$, batch size, $b_s \in \{64, 128\}$, and initial learning rate, $lr \in \{0.01 - 0.0001\}$, and cancer regularization factor, ω, with three different optimization algorithms, SGD, RMSprop and *Adam*. Results from hyperparameter search demonstrate that network structures with two RNN hidden layers outperform other architectures. Furthermore, for the vanilla RNN, $b_s = 128$, $lr = 0.0001$; for LSTM, $b_s = 64$, $lr = 0.0001$; and for GRU, $b_s = 128$, $lr = 0.01$ generate the optimum models. For all models, $d_r = 0.2$, $l_reg = 0.0001$ generate the lowest loss and the highest accuracy in $\mathcal{D}_{val}$. Also, $\omega = 0.7$ for GS $3+4$ and $\omega = 0.3$ for GS $4+3$ result in the highest performance. After model selection, we use the whole $\mathcal{D}_{train}$ for training a model for the first stage and $\mathcal{D}_{train}^{cancer}$ for the second stage model.

Comparative Method and Baselines: We use standard evaluation metrics as prior approaches [2,4] to quantify our results. We assess the inter-class area under the receiver operating characteristic curve (AUC) for detection of Benign vs. $GS \geq 3+4$ (AUC_1), Benign vs. $GS \geq 4+3$ (AUC_2), and $GS \geq 3+4$ vs. $GS \geq 4+3$ (AUC_3). Table 1 shows the performance comparison between the proposed approach and the following baselines. To substantiate the proposed soft ground-truth label in the second stage of our approach, we replace $\mathbf{p}^{(i)}$ with the labels from multi-label binarization as shown in Fig. 1 (**BL-1**). Also, to justify the necessity of a two-stage approach to tackle the noise, we use the labels from multi-label binarization (**BL-2**) and the weighted version (**BL-3**) in a single stage approach; after the sequence learning step we feed the output to a fully-connected layer with a 3-way softmax function. To generate the weighted version of multi-label binarization labels, for GS $3+4$, the encoded vector is defined as $[0, 0.7, 0.3]$,

Table 1. Model performance for classification of cores in the test data (N = 170)

Method	AUC_1	AUC_2	AUC_3	Average AUC
LSTM	0.96	0.96	**0.86**	**0.93**
GRU	0.92	0.92	**0.84**	**0.89**
Vanilla RNN	0.76	0.76	0.70	0.74
BL-1	0.96	0.96	0.68	0.86
BL-2	0.75	0.68	0.58	0.67
BL-3	0.82	0.84	0.65	0.77
LSTM + GMM-Clustering	0.60	0.74	0.69	0.68
DBN + GMM-Clustering	0.68	0.62	0.60	0.63

and for GS $4+3$ the encoded vector is $[0, 0.3, 0.7]$. We have also implemented the GMM-clustering method proposed by [4]. We have used the learned feature vector from Deep Belied Network (DBN) method [4] and our best RNN structure (LSTM) to feed the proposed GMM-clustering method. The results suggest that the proposed strategy using both LSTM and GRU cells can lead to a statistically significant improvement in the performance ($p < 0.05$), which is mainly due to a superior performance of our proposed approach in the separation of GS $\geq 3+4$ from GS $\geq 4+3$. It is worthwhile mentioning that core-based approaches like multi-instance learning and traditional multi-class classification are not feasible due to the small number of samples. Also, in the lack of a more clean and reliable dataset, direct modeling of the noise level is not pragmatic [8].

Tumor in Core Length Estimation: Fig. 3 shows the scatter plot of the reported tumor in core length in histopathology vs. the predicted tumor in core length using LSTM cells. The graph shows the correlation between the prediction and histopathology report (correlation coefficient $= 0.95$). We also calculate the mean squared error (MSE) as the measure of our performance in cancer length estimation where we achieve MSE of 0.12 in the estimation of tumor length.]

Cancer Likelihood Colormaps: Fig. 4(a) shows an example of a cancer likelihood map for biopsy guidance derived from the output of the proposed two-stages approach. Figure 4(b) shows the corresponding estimated uncertainty map generated from the proposed uncertainty estimation method ($p = 0.5$, $B = 100$). Uncertainty is measured as the sample variance for each ROI and normalized to the whole prostate region uncertainty. The level of uncertainty is color-coded using a blue-red spectrum where the blue shows a low level of uncertainty and the dark red indicates the highest level of uncertainty. The uncertainty colormap along with the cancer likelihood map can be used as an effective strategy to harness the possible misguidance during the biopsy.

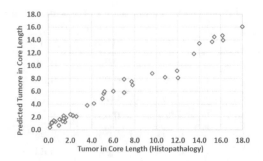

Fig. 3. Scatter plot of the reported tumor in core length in histopathology vs. the predicted tumor in core length

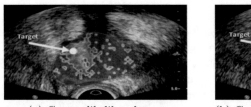

(a) Cancer likelihood map   (b) Corresponding uncertainty map

Fig. 4. (a) Cancer likelihood maps overlaid on B-mode image, along with the projected needle path in TeUS data (GS $\geq 4 + 3$) and centered on the target. ROIs of size 0.5×0.5 mm^2 for which we detect the Gleason grade of 4 and 3 are colored in red and yellow, respectively. The non-cancerous ROIs are colored as blue. (b) The red boundary shows the segmented prostate in MRI projected in TRUS coordinates.[blue=low uncertainty, red=high uncertainty

5   Conclusion

In this paper, we addressed the problem of sparse and noisy histopathology-based ground-truth labels by employing the ground-truth probability vectors as soft labels. These soft labels were estimated by embedding the prior histopathology knowledge about the length of cancer in our two-stage model. The results suggest that soft labels can help the learning process by suppressing the influence of noisy labels and can be used to accurately estimate the length of the suspicious cancer foci. Furthermore, possible misguidance in biopsy is highlighted by the proposed uncertainty measure. Future work will be focused on the analysis of the source of the uncertainty and integrate the proper solution in the framework.

References

1. Ahmed, H.U., et al.: Diagnostic accuracy of multi-parametric MRI and TRUS biopsy in prostate cancer (PROMIS). Lancet **389**(10071), 815–822 (2017)
2. Azizi, S., Bayat, S., Abolmaesumi, P., Mousavi, P., et al.: Detection and grading of prostate cancer using temporal enhanced ultrasound: combining deep neural networks and tissue mimicking simulations. IJCARS **12**(8), 1293–1305 (2017)

3. Azizi, S., et al.: Classifying cancer grades using temporal ultrasound for transrectal prostate biopsy. In: Ourselin, S., Joskowicz, L., Sabuncu, M.R., Unal, G., Wells, W. (eds.) MICCAI 2016. LNCS, vol. 9900, pp. 653–661. Springer, Cham (2016). https://doi.org/10.1007/978-3-319-46720-7_76

4. Azizi, S., Mousavi, P., et al.: Detection of prostate cancer using temporal sequences of ultrasound data: a large clinical feasibility study. Int. J. CARS **11**, 947 (2016). https://doi.org/10.1007/s11548-016-1395-2

5. Azizi, S., et al.: Ultrasound-based detection of prostate cancer using automatic feature selection with deep belief networks. In: Navab, N., Hornegger, J., Wells, W.M., Frangi, A.F. (eds.) MICCAI 2015. LNCS, vol. 9350, pp. 70–77. Springer, Cham (2015). https://doi.org/10.1007/978-3-319-24571-3_9

6. Bayat, S., Azizi, S., Daoud, M., et al.: Investigation of physical phenomena underlying temporal enhanced ultrasound as a new diagnostic imaging technique: theory and simulations. IEEE Trans. UFFC **65**(3), 400–410 (2017)

7. Feleppa, E., Porter, C., Ketterling, J., Dasgupta, S., Ramachandran, S., Sparks, D.: Recent advances in ultrasonic tissue-type imaging of the prostate. In: André, M.P. (ed.) Acoustical imaging, vol. 28, pp. 331–339. Springer, Dordrecht (2007). https://doi.org/10.1007/1-4020-5721-0_35

8. Frénay, B., Verleysen, M.: Classification in the presence of label noise. IEEE Trans. Neural Netw. Learn. Syst. **25**(5), 845–869 (2014)

9. Gal, Y., Ghahramani, Z.: Dropout as a Bayesian approximation: representing model uncertainty in deep learning. In: Machine Learning, pp. 1050–1059 (2016)

10. Kasivisvanathan, V.: Prostate evaluation for clinically important disease: Sampling using image-guidance or not? (PRECISION). Eur. Urol. Suppl. **17**(2), e1716–e1717 (2018)

11. Llobet, R., Pérez-Cortés, J.C., Toselli, A.H.: Computer-aided detection of prostate cancer. Int. J. Med. Inf. **76**(7), 547–556 (2007)

12. Moradi, M., Abolmaesumi, P., Siemens, D.R., Sauerbrei, E.E., Boag, A.H., Mousavi, P.: Augmenting detection of prostate cancer in transrectal ultrasound images using SVM and RF time series. IEEE TBME **56**(9), 2214–2224 (2009)

13. Nelson, E.D., Slotoroff, C.B., Gomella, L.G., Halpern, E.J.: Targeted biopsy of the prostate: the impact of color doppler imaging and elastography on prostate cancer detection and Gleason score. Urology **70**(6), 1136–1140 (2007)

14. Siddiqui, M.M., et al.: Comparison of MR/US fusion-guided biopsy with US-guided biopsy for the diagnosis of prostate cancer. JAMA **313**(4), 390–397 (2015)

15. Singer, E.A., Kaushal, A., et al.: Active surveillance for prostate cancer: past, present and future. Curr. Opin. Oncol. **24**(3), 243–250 (2012)

A Feature-Driven Active Framework for Ultrasound-Based Brain Shift Compensation

Jie Luo[1,2(✉)], Matthew Toews[3], Ines Machado[1], Sarah Frisken[1],
Miaomiao Zhang[4], Frank Preiswerk[1], Alireza Sedghi[1], Hongyi Ding[5],
Steve Pieper[1], Polina Golland[6], Alexandra Golby[1], Masashi Sugiyama[2,5],
and William M. Wells III[1,6]

[1] Brigham and Women's Hospital, Harvard Medical School, Boston, USA
[2] Graduate School of Frontier Sciences, The University of Tokyo, Kashiwa, Japan
[3] Ecole de Technologie Superieure, University of Quebec, Montreal, Canada
[4] Computer Science and Engineering Department,
Lehigh University, Bethlehem, USA
[5] Center for Advanced Intelligence Project, RIKEN, Tokyo, Japan
[6] Computer Science and Artificial Intelligence Laboratory, MIT, Cambridge, USA
jluo5@bwh.harvard.edu

Abstract. A reliable Ultrasound (US)-to-US registration method to compensate for brain shift would substantially improve Image-Guided Neurological Surgery. Developing such a registration method is very challenging, due to factors such as the tumor resection, the complexity of brain pathology and the demand for fast computation. We propose a novel feature-driven active registration framework. Here, landmarks and their displacement are first estimated from a pair of US images using corresponding local image features. Subsequently, a Gaussian Process (GP) model is used to interpolate a dense deformation field from the sparse landmarks. Kernels of the GP are estimated by using variograms and a discrete grid search method. If necessary, the user can actively add new landmarks based on the image context and visualization of the uncertainty measure provided by the GP to further improve the result. We retrospectively demonstrate our registration framework as a robust and accurate brain shift compensation solution on clinical data.

Keywords: Brain shift · Active image registration
Gaussian process · Uncertainty

1 Introduction

During neurosurgery, Image-Guided Neurosurgical Systems (IGNSs) provide a patient-to-image mapping that relates the preoperative image data to an intraoperative patient coordinate system, allowing surgeons to infer the locations of their surgical instruments relative to preoperative image data and helping them

© Springer Nature Switzerland AG 2018
A. F. Frangi et al. (Eds.): MICCAI 2018, LNCS 11073, pp. 30–38, 2018.
https://doi.org/10.1007/978-3-030-00937-3_4

to achieve a radical tumor resection while avoiding damage to surrounding functioning brain tissue.

Commercial IGNSs assume a rigid registration between preoperative imaging and patient coordinates. However, intraoperative deformation of the brain, also known as brain shift, invalidates this assumption. Since brain shift progresses during surgery, the rigid patient-to-image mapping of IGNS becomes less and less accurate. Consequently, most surgeons only use IGNS to make a surgical plan but justifiably do not trust it throughout the entire operation [1,2].

Related Work. As one of the most important error sources in IGNS, intraoperative brain shift must be compensated in order to increase the accuracy of neurosurgeries. Registration between the intraoperative MRI (iMRI) image and preoperative MRI (preMRI) image (preop-to-intraop registration) has been a successful strategy for brain shift compensation [3–6]. However, iMRI acquisition is disruptive, expensive and time consuming, making this technology unavailable for most clinical centers worldwide. More recently, 3D intraoperative Ultrasound (iUS) appears to be a promising replacement for iMRI. Although some progress has been made by previous work on preMRI-to-iUS registration [7–13], yet there are still no clinically accepted solutions and no commercial neuro-navigation systems that provide brain shift compensation. This is due to three reasons: (1) Most non-rigid registration methods can not handle artifacts and missing structures in iUS; (2) The multi-modality of preMRI-to-iUS registration makes the already difficult problem even more challenging; (3) A few methods [14] can achieve a reasonable alignment, yet they take around 50 min for an US pair and are too slow to be clinically applicable. Another shortcoming of existing brain shift compensation approaches is the lack of an uncertainty measure. Brain shift is a complex spatio-temporal phenomenon and, given the state of registration technology and the importance of the result, it seems reasonable to expect an indication (e.g. error bars) of the confidence level in the estimated deformation.

In this paper, we propose a novel feature-driven active framework for brain shift compensation. Here, landmarks and their displacement are first estimated from a pair of US images using corresponding local image features. Subsequently, a Gaussian Process (GP) model [15] is used to interpolate a dense deformation field from the sparse landmarks. Kernels of the GP are estimated by using variograms and a discrete grid search method. If necessary, for areas that are difficult to align, the user can actively add new landmarks based on the image context and visualization of the uncertainty measure provided by the GP to further improve the registration accuracy. We retrospectively demonstrate the efficacy of our method on clinical data.

Contributions and novelties of our work can be summarized as follows:

1. The proposed feature-based registration is robust for aligning iUS image pairs with missing correspondence and is fast.
2. We explore applying the GP model and variograms for image registration.
3. Registration uncertainty in transformation parameters can be naturally obtained from the GP model.

4. To the best of our knowledge, the proposed active registration strategy is the first method to actively combine user expertise in brain shift compensation.

2 Method

2.1 The Role of US-to-US Registration

In order to alleviate the difficulty of preop-to-intraop registration, instead of directly aligning iMRI and iUS images, we choose an iterative compensation approach which is similar to the work in [16].

As shown in Fig. 1 the acquisition processes for pre-duraUS (preUS) and post-resectionUS (postUS) take place before opening the dura and after (partial) tumor resection, respectively. Since most brain-shift occurs after taking the preUS, a standard multi-modal registration may be suffice to achieve a good alignment T_{multi} between preMRI and preUS [12]. Next, we register the preUS to postUS using the proposed feature-driven active framework to acquire a deformable mapping T_{mono}. After propagating T_{multi} and T_{mono} to the preMRI, surgeons may use it as an updated view of anatomy to compensate for brain shift during the surgery.

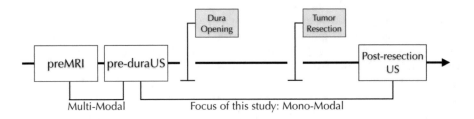

Fig. 1. Pipeline of the US-based brain shift compensation.

2.2 Feature-Based Registration Strategy

Because of tumor resection, compensating for brain shift requires non-rigid registration algorithms capable of aligning structures in one image that have no correspondences in the other image. In this situation, many image registration methods that take into account the intensity pattern of the entire image will become trapped in incorrect local minima.

We therefore pursue a Feature-Based Registration (FBR) strategy due to its robustness in registering images with missing correspondence [17]. FBR mainly consists of 3 steps: feature-extraction, feature-matching and dense deformation field estimation. An optional "active registration" step can be added depending on the quality of FBR.

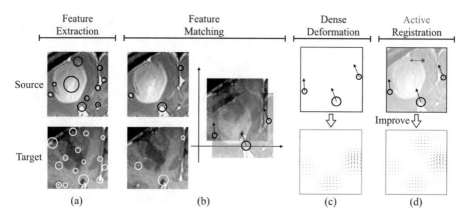

Fig. 2. Pipeline of the feature-based active preUS-to-postUS registration.

Feature Extraction and Matching. As illustrated in Fig. 2(a) and (b), distinctive local image features are automatically extracted and identified as key-points on preUS and postUS images. An automatic matching algorithm searches for a corresponding postUS key-point for each key-point on the preUS image [17].

For a matched key-point pair, let $\mathbf{x}_i$ be the coordinates of the preUS key-point and $\mathbf{x}_i^{\text{post}}$ be the coordinate of its postUS counterpart. We first use all matched PreUS key-points as landmarks, and perform a land-mark based preUS-to-postUS affine registration to obtain a rough alignment. $\mathbf{x}_i^{\text{post}}$ becomes $\mathbf{x}_i^{\text{affine}}$ after the affine registration. The displacement vector, which indicates the movement of landmark $\mathbf{x}_i$ due to the brain shift process, can be calculated as $\mathbf{d}(\mathbf{x}_i) = \mathbf{x}_i^{\text{affine}} - \mathbf{x}_i$. where $\mathbf{d} = [d_x, d_y, d_z]$.

Dense Deformation Field. The goal of this step is to obtain a dense deformation field from a set of N sparse landmark and their displacements $\mathcal{D} = \{(\mathbf{x}_i, \mathbf{d}_i), i = 1 : N\}$, where $\mathbf{d}_i = \mathbf{d}(\mathbf{x}_i)$ is modeled as a observation of displacements.

In the GP model, let $\mathbf{d}(\mathbf{x})$ be the displacement vector for the voxel at location $\mathbf{x}$ and define a prior distribution as $d(\mathbf{x}) \sim \text{GP}(\text{m}(\mathbf{x}), \text{k}(\mathbf{x}, \mathbf{x}'))$, where m($\mathbf{x}$) is the mean function, which usually is set to 0, and the GP kernel $\mathbf{k}(\mathbf{x}, \mathbf{x}')$ represents the spatial correlation of displacement vectors.

By the modeling assumption, all displacement vectors follow a joint Gaussian distribution $p(\mathbf{d} \mid \mathbf{X}) = \mathcal{N}(\mathbf{d} \mid \mu, \mathbf{K})$, where $K_{ij} = \mathbf{k}(\mathbf{x}, \mathbf{x}')$ and $\mu = (\text{m}(\mathbf{x}_1), ..., \text{m}(\mathbf{x}_N))$. As a result, the displacement vectors $\mathbf{d}$ for known landmarks and N_* unknown displacement vectors $\mathbf{d}_*$ at location $\mathbf{X}_*$, which we want to predict, have the following relationship:

$$\begin{pmatrix} \mathbf{d} \\ \mathbf{d}_* \end{pmatrix} \sim \text{GP}\left(\begin{pmatrix} \mu \\ \mu_* \end{pmatrix}, \begin{pmatrix} \mathbf{K} & \mathbf{K}_* \\ \mathbf{K}_*^T & \mathbf{K}_{**} \end{pmatrix} \right) \tag{1}$$

In Eq. 1, $\mathbf{K} = \text{k}(\mathbf{X}, \mathbf{X})$ is the $N \times N$ matrix, $\mathbf{K}_* = \text{k}(\mathbf{X}, \mathbf{X}_*)$ is a similar $N \times N_*$ matrix, and $\mathbf{K}_{**} = \text{k}(\mathbf{X}_*, \mathbf{X}_*)$ is a $N_* \times N_*$ matrix. The mean $\mu_* = [\mu_{*x}, \mu_{*y}, \mu_{*z}]$

represents values of voxel-wise displacement vectors and can be estimated from the posterior Gaussian distribution $p(\mathbf{d}_* \mid \mathbf{X}_*, \mathbf{X}, \mathbf{d}) = \mathcal{N}(\mathbf{d}_* \mid \mu_*, \Sigma_*)$ as

$$\mu_* = \mu(\mathbf{X}_*) + \mathbf{K}_*^T \mathbf{K}^{-1}(\mathbf{d} - \mu(\mathbf{X})). \tag{2}$$

Given $\mu(\mathbf{X}) = \mu(\mathbf{X}_*) = 0$, we can obtain the dense deformation field for the preUS image by assigning $\mu_{*x}, \mu_{*y}, \mu_{*z}$ to d_x, d_y and d_z, respectively.

Active Registration. Automatic approaches may have difficulty in the preop-to-intraop image registration, especially for areas near the tumor resection site. Another advantage of the GP framework is the possibility of incorporating user expertise to further improve the registration result.

From Eq. 1, we can also compute the covariance matrix of the posterior Gaussian $p(\mathbf{d}_* \mid \mathbf{X}_*, \mathbf{X}, \mathbf{d})$ as

$$\Sigma_* = \mathbf{K}_{**} - \mathbf{K}_*^T \mathbf{K}^{-1} \mathbf{K}_*. \tag{3}$$

Entries on the diagonal of Σ_* are the marginal variances of predicted values. They can be used as an uncertainty measure to indicates the confidence in the estimated transformation parameters.

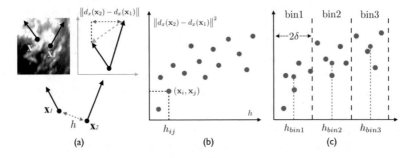

Fig. 3. (a) $\|d_x(\mathbf{x}_2) - d_x(\mathbf{x}_1)\|$ and h; (b) Empirical variogram cloud; (c) Variogram cloud divided into bins with their means marked as blue.

If users are not satisfied by the FBR alignment result, they could manually, guided by the image context and visualization of registration uncertainty, add new corresponding pairs of key-points to drive the GP towards better results.

2.3   GP Kernel Estimation

The performance of GP registration depends exclusively on the suitability of the chosen kernels and its parameters. In this study, we explore two schemes for the kernel estimation: Variograms and discrete grid search.

Variograms. The variogram is a powerful geostatistical tool for characterizing the spatial dependence of a stochastic process [18]. While being briefly mentioned in [19], it has not yet received much attention in the medical imaging field.

In the GP registration context, where $\mathbf{d}(\mathbf{x})$ is modelled as a random quantity, variograms can measure the extent of pairwise spatial correlation between displacement vectors with respect to their distance, and give insight into choosing a suitable GP kernel.

In practice, we estimate the empirical variogram of landmarks' displacement vector field using

$$\hat{\gamma}(h \pm \delta) := \frac{1}{2|N(h \pm \delta)|} \sum_{(i,j) \in N(h \pm \delta)} \|\mathbf{d}(\mathbf{x}_i) - \mathbf{d}(\mathbf{x}_j)\|^2. \tag{4}$$

For the norm term $\|\mathbf{d}(\mathbf{x}_i) - \mathbf{d}(\mathbf{x}_j)\|$, we separate its 3 components d_x d_y d_z and construct 3 variograms respectively. As shown in Fig. 3(a), for displacement vectors $\mathbf{d}(x_1)$ and $\mathbf{d}(x_2)$, $\|d_x(\mathbf{x}_2) - d_x(\mathbf{x}_1)\|$ is the vector difference with respect to the $\mathbf{x}$ axis, etc. h represents the distance between two key-points.

To construct an empirical variogram, the first step is to make a variogram cloud by plotting $\|d(\mathbf{x}_2) - d(\mathbf{x}_1)\|^2$ and h_{ij} for all displacement pairs. Next, we divide the variogram cloud into bins with a bin width setting to 2δ. Lastly, the mean of each bin is calculated and further plotted with the mean distance of that bin to form an empirical variogram. Figure 4(a) shows an empirical variogram of a real US image pair that has 71 corresponding landmarks.

In order to obtain the data-driven GP kernel function, we further fit a smooth curve, generated by pre-defined kernel functions, to the empirical variogram. As shown in Fig. 4(b), a fitted curve is commonly described by the following characteristics:

Nugget The non-zero value at $h = 0$.
   Sill The value at which the curve reaches its maximum.
Range The value of distance h where the sill is reached.

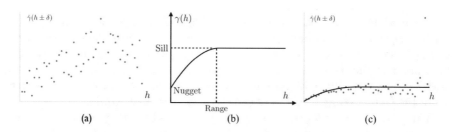

(a)   (b)   (c)

Fig. 4. (a) X-axis empirical variogram of a US images pair; (b) Sill, range and nugget; (c) Fitting a continuous model to an empirical variogram.

Fitting a curve to an empirical variogram is implemented in most geostatistics software. A popular choice is choosing several models that appear to have the right shape and use the one with smallest weighted squared error [18]. In this study, we only test Gaussian curves

$$\gamma(h) = c_0 + c\{1 - exp(-\frac{h^2}{a})\}. \tag{5}$$

Here, c_0 is the nugget, $c = \text{Sill} - c_0$ and a is the model parameter. Once the fitted curve is found, we can obtain a from the equation (5) and use it as the Gaussian kernel scale in the GP interpolation.

Discrete Grid Search. The variogram scheme often requires many landmarks to work well [18]. For US pairs that have fewer landmarks, we choose predefined Gaussian kernels, and use cross validation to determine the scale parameter in a discrete grid search fashion [15].

3   Experiments

The experimental dataset consists of 6 sets 3D preUS and postUS image pairs. The US signals were acquired on a BK Ultrasound 3000 system that is directly connected to the Brainlab VectorVision Sky neuronavigaton system during surgery. Signals were further reconstructed as 3D volume using the PLUS [20] library in 3D Slicer [21] (Table 1).

Table 1. Registration evaluation results (in mm)

	Landmarks	Before Reg.	Affine	Thin-plate	Variograms	GaussianK
Patient 1	123	5.56 ± 1.05	2.99 ± 1.21	1.79 ± 0.70	2.11 ± 0.74	1.75 ± 0.68
Patient 2	71	3.35 ± 1.22	2.08 ± 1.13	2.06 ± 1.18	2.06 ± 1.12	1.97 ± 1.05
Patient 3	49	2.48 ± 1.56	1.93 ± 1.75	1.25 ± 1.95	n/a	1.23 ± 1.77
Patient 4	12	4.40 ± 1.79	3.06 ± 2.35	1.45 ± 1.99	n/a	1.42 ± 2.04
Patient 5	64	2.91 ± 1.33	1.86 ± 1.24	1.29 ± 1.17	n/a	1.33 ± 1.40
Patient 6	98	3.29 ± 1.09	2.12 ± 1.16	2.02 ± 1.21	2.05 ± 1.40	1.96 ± 1.38

We used the mean euclidean distance between the predicted and ground truth of key-points' coordinates, measured in mm, for the registration evaluation. During the evaluation, we compared: affine, thin-plate kernel FBR, variograms FBR and gaussian kernel FBR. For US pairs with fewer than 50 landmarks, we used leave-one-out cross validation, otherwise we used 5-fold cross validation. All of the compared methods were computed in less than 10 min.

The pre-defined Gaussian kernel with discrete grid search generally yield better result than the variogram scheme. This is reasonable as the machine learning approach stresses the prediction performance, while the geostatistical variogram favours the interpretability of the model. Notice that the cross validation strategy is not an ideal evaluation, this could be improved by using manual landmarks in public datasets, such as RESECT [22] and BITE [23].

In addition, we have performed preliminary tests on active registration as shown in Fig. 5, which illustrate the use of a colour map of registration uncertainty to guide the manual placement of 3 additional landmarks to improve the registration. By visual inspection, we can see the alignment of tumor boundary substantially improved.

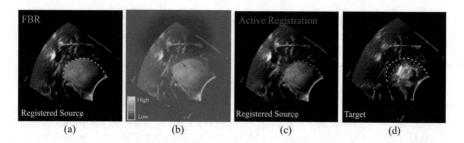

Fig. 5. (a) FBR result of the preUS with a tumor boundary outlined in green; (b) Overlaying the visualization of uncertainty on the preUS image. A characteristic of GP is that voxels near landmarks tend to have smaller uncertainty. In this example, all landmarks happen to be located near the large sulcus, hence the incertitude looks high everywhere else except around the sulcus. (c) Active registration result of the preUS with a tumor boundary outlined in blue; (d) Overlaying the green and blue tumor boundary on the target image.

4 Discussion

One key point of our framework is the "active registration" idea that aims to overcome the limitation of automatic image registration. Human and machines have complementary abilities; we believe that the element of simple user interaction should be added to the pipeline for some challenging medical imaging applications. Although the proposed method is designed for brain shift compensation, it is also applicable to other navigation systems that require tracking of tissue deformation. The performance of FBR is highly correlated with the quality of feature matching. In future works, we plan to test different matching algorithms [24], and also perform more validation with public datasets.

Acknowledgement. MS was supported by the International Research Center for Neurointelligence (WPI-IRCN) at The University of Tokyo Institutes for Advanced Study. This work was also supported by NIH grants P41EB015898 and P41EB015902.

References

1. Gerard, I.J., et al.: Brain shift in neuronavigation of brain tumors: a review. Med. Image Anal. **35**, 403–420 (2017)
2. Bayer, S., et al.: Intraoperative imaging modalities and compensation for brain shift in tumor resection surgery. Int. J. Biomed. Imaging **2017** (2017). Article ID. 6028645
3. Hata, N., Nabavi, A., Warfield, S., Wells, W., Kikinis, R., Jolesz, F.A.: A volumetric optical flow method for measurement of brain deformation from intraoperative magnetic resonance images. In: Taylor, C., Colchester, A. (eds.) MICCAI 1999. LNCS, vol. 1679, pp. 928–935. Springer, Heidelberg (1999). https://doi.org/10.1007/10704282_101
4. Clatz, O., et al.: Robust nonrigid registration to capture brain shift from intraoperative MRI. IEEE TMI **24**(11), 1417–1427 (2005)

5. Vigneron, L.M., et al.: Serial FEM/XFEM-based update of preoperative brain images using intraoperative MRI. Int. J. Biomed. Imaging **2012** (2012). Article ID. 872783

6. Drakopoulos, F., et al.: Toward a real time multi-tissue adaptive physics-based non- rigid registration framework for brain tumor resection. Front. Neuroinf. **8**, 11 (2014)

7. Gobbi, D.G., Comeau, R.M., Peters, T.M.: Ultrasound/MRI overlay with image warping for neurosurgery. In: Delp, S.L., DiGoia, A.M., Jaramaz, B. (eds.) MICCAI 2000. LNCS, vol. 1935, pp. 106–114. Springer, Heidelberg (2000). https://doi.org/10.1007/978-3-540-40899-4_11

8. Arbel, T., et al.: Automatic non-linear MRI-ultrasound registration for the correction of intra-operative brain deformations. Comput. Aided Surg. **9**, 123–136 (2004)

9. Pennec, X., et al.: Tracking brain deformations in time sequences of 3D US images. Pattern Recogn. Lett. **24**, 801–813 (2003)

10. Letteboer, M.M.J., Willems, P.W.A., Viergever, M.A., Niessen, W.J.: Non-rigid Registration of 3D ultrasound images of brain tumours acquired during neurosurgery. In: Ellis, R.E., Peters, T.M. (eds.) MICCAI 2003. LNCS, vol. 2879, pp. 408–415. Springer, Heidelberg (2003). https://doi.org/10.1007/978-3-540-39903-2_50

11. Reinertsen, I., Descoteaux, M., Drouin, S., Siddiqi, K., Collins, D.L.: Vessel driven correction of brain shift. In: Barillot, C., Haynor, D.R., Hellier, P. (eds.) MICCAI 2004. LNCS, vol. 3217, pp. 208–216. Springer, Heidelberg (2004). https://doi.org/10.1007/978-3-540-30136-3_27

12. Fuerst, B., et al.: Automatic ultrasound-MRI registration for neurosurgery using 2D and 3D LC^2 metric. Med. Image Anal. **18**(8), 1312–1319 (2014)

13. Rivaz, H., Collins, D.L.: Deformable registration of preoperative MR, pre-resection ultrasound, and post-resection ultrasound images of neurosurgery. IJCARS **10**, 1017–1028 (2015)

14. Ou, Y., et al.: DRAMMS: deformable registration via attribute matching and mutual-saliency weighting. Med. Image Anal. **15**, 622–639 (2011)

15. Rasmussen, C.E., Williams, C.: Gaussian Processes for Machine Learning. MIT Press, Cambridge (2006)

16. Riva, M., et al.: 3D intra-op US and MR image guidance: pursuing an ultrasound-based management of brainshift to enhance neuronavigation. IJCARS **12**(10), 1711–1725 (2017)

17. Toews, M., Wells, W.M.: Efficient and robust model-to-image alignment using 3D scale-invariant features. Med. Image Anal. **17**, 271–282 (2013)

18. Cressie, N.A.C.: Statistics for Spatial Data, p. 900. Wiley, Hoboken (1991)

19. Ruiz-Alzola, J., Suarez, E., Alberola-Lopez, C., Warfield, S.K., Westin, C.-F.: Geostatistical medical image registration. In: Ellis, R.E., Peters, T.M. (eds.) MICCAI 2003. LNCS, vol. 2879, pp. 894–901. Springer, Heidelberg (2003). https://doi.org/10.1007/978-3-540-39903-2_109

20. Lasso, A., et al.: PLUS: open-source toolkit. IEEE TBE **61**(10), 2527–2537 (2014)

21. Kikinis, R., et al.: 3D Slicer. Intraoper. Imaging IGT **3**(19), 277–289 (2014)

22. Xiao, Y., et al.: RESECT: a clinical database. Med. Phys. **44**(7), 3875–3882 (2017)

23. Mercier, L., et al.: BITE: on-line database. Med. Phys. **39**(6), 3253–3261 (2012)

24. Jian, B., Vemuri, B.C.: Robust point set registration using Gaussian mixture models. IEEE TPAMI **33**(8), 1633–1645 (2011)

Soft-Body Registration of Pre-operative 3D Models to Intra-operative RGBD Partial Body Scans

Richard Modrzejewski[1,2]([envelope]), Toby Collins[2], Adrien Bartoli[1],
Alexandre Hostettler[2], and Jacques Marescaux[2]

[1] EnCoV, Institut Pascal, UMR 6602, CNRS/UBP/SIGMA,
63000 Clermont-Ferrand, France
Richard.modrzejewski@gmail.com

[2] IRCAD and IHU-Strasbourg, 1 Place de l'Hopital, 67000 Strasbourg, France

Abstract. We present a novel solution to soft-body registration between a pre-operative 3D patient model and an intra-operative surface mesh of the patient lying on the operating table, acquired using an inexpensive and portable depth (RGBD) camera. The solution has several clinical applications, including skin dose mapping in interventional radiology and intra-operative image guidance. We propose to solve this with a robust non-rigid registration algorithm that handles partial surface data, significant posture modification and patient-table collisions. We investigate several unstudied and important aspects of this registration problem. These are the benefits of heterogeneous versus homogeneous biomechanical models and the benefits of modeling patient/table interaction as collision constraints. We also study how abdominal registration accuracy varies as a function of scan length in the caudal-cranial axis.

1 Introduction, Background and Contributions

An ongoing and major objective in computer-assisted abdominal interventional radiology and surgery is to robustly register pre-operative 3D images such as MR or CT, or 3D models built from these images, to intra-operative data. There are two broad clinical objectives for this. The first is to facilitate automatic radiation dose mapping and monitoring in fluoroscopy-guided procedures [1,2], using a pre-operative model as a reference. The most important aspect is registering the skin exposed to primary radiation. Good registration would enable dose exposure monitoring across the patient's skin, and across multiple treatments. The second clinical objective is to achieve interventional image guidance using pre-operative 3D image data if interventional 3D imaging is unavailable. Recently methods have been proposed to register a pre-operative 3D model using external color [3] or depth+color (RGBD) images [4–7], capturing the external intra-operative body shape and posture of the patient, operating table and surrounding structures. The advantages of registering with color or RGBD cameras is they are very low-cost, very safe, compact, and large regions of the patient's

© Springer Nature Switzerland AG 2018
A. F. Frangi et al. (Eds.): MICCAI 2018, LNCS 11073, pp. 39–46, 2018.
https://doi.org/10.1007/978-3-030-00937-3_5

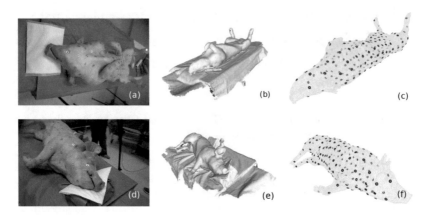

Fig. 1. Porcine dataset. (a) Example of supine position, (b) RGBD scan corresponding to (a), (c) CT model corresponding to (a) with segmented surface markers. (d–f) equivalent images with a right-lateral position.

body can be imaged in real-time. They also facilitate 'body see-through' AR visualization using hand-held devices such as tablets or head-mounted displays Their disadvantage is that the internal anatomy cannot be imaged. Therefore we can only establish correspondence (data association) on the patient's visible surface, which can be difficult particularly in the abdominal region, where the skin has few distinguishing geometrical features. The second main difficulty are large occluded regions. For example, for patients in the supine position the posterior is never visible to the camera. Because of these difficulties, previous registration methods that use external cameras have been limited to rigid registration [3–7]. These methods cannot handle soft-body deformation, which is unavoidable and often difficult to precisely control. Such deformation can be significant, which is particularly true when the patient's lying position is different. For example, CT and MR are mainly acquired in the supine position, but the procedure may require the patient in lateral or prone positions. We show our solution can improve registration accuracy with strong posture changes.

The main contributions of this paper are both technical and scientific. Technically, this is the first solution to soft-body patient registration using a preoperative CT model and 3D surface meshes built from multiple external RGBD images. We build on much existing work on fast, soft-body registration using surface-based constraints. The approaches most robust to missing data, occlusions and outliers, are currently iterative methods based on robust Iterative Closest Point (ICP) [8–11]. These work by interleaving data association with deformable model fitting, while simultaneously detecting and rejecting false point matches. These methods have been applied to solve other medical registration problems including laparoscopic organ registration [9], and registering standing humans with RGBD surface meshes e.g. [11]. We extend these works in the following ways: (1) to model table-patient interaction via table reconstruction and collision reasoning, (2) outlier filtering to avoid false correspondences.

Scientifically, it is well known that measuring soft-body registration accuracy with real data is notoriously difficult, but essential. In related papers quantitative evaluation is performed using virtual simulations, with simplified and not always accurate modeling of the physics and data. We have designed a systematic series of experiments to quantitatively asses registration accuracy using real porcine models in different body postures. The ethically-approved dataset consists of a pig in 20 different postures, with 197 thin metal disc markers (10 mm diameter, 2 mm width) fixed over the pig's body. For each posture there is a CT image, an RGBD body scan and the marker centroids. The centroids were excluded from the biomechanical models, preventing them being exploited for registration. We could then answer important and unstudied questions:

– Does modeling patient/table collision improve registration results? Is this posture dependent? Are the improvements mainly at the contact regions?
– Does using a heterogeneous biomechanical model improve registration compared to a heterogeneous model? This tells us whether accurate biomechanical modeling of different tissue classes/bones are required.
– How much of the abdominal region is required in the CT image for good registration? We study this by varying image size in the caudal-cranial axis.

We also demonstrate qualitatively our registration algorithm on a human patient in real operating room conditions for CT-guided percutaneous tumor ablation. This result is the first of its kind.

2 Methods

2.1 Biomechanical Model Description

We take as input a generic biomechanical mesh model representing the patient's body (either partial or full-body). We denote the model's surface vertices corresponding to the patient's skin as $\mathcal{V}_s$, and the interior vertices as $\mathcal{V}_I$. We use $f(\mathbf{p}; \mathbf{x}) : \mathbb{R}^3 \rightarrow \mathbb{R}^3$ to denote the transform of a 3D point $\mathbf{p}$ in 3D patient coordinates to patient scan coordinates, provided by the biomechanical model. This is parameterized by an unknown vector $\mathbf{x}$, and our task is to recover it. In our experiments we model $E_M(\mathbf{x})$ using a mass-spring model generated from segmentations provided by [12]. We used Tetgen to generate tetrahedral meshes from surface triangles, which formed the interior vertex set $\mathcal{V}_I$. We emphasize that the algorithm is compatible with any first order differentiable biomechanical model.

2.2 Intra-operative Patient Scanning and Segmentation

We scan the patient using a hand-held RGBD camera (Orbic Astra Pro), that is swept over the patient by an assistant. Another option for scanning would be to use ceiling-mounted RGBD cameras, however this has some limitations. The cost is higher, there may be line-of-sight problems, and closer-range scanning is not

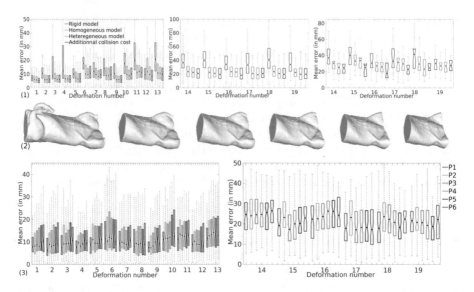

Fig. 2. NLD of markers for different configurations: row (1) small posture changes (left), large changes (center) and markers localized only on the table (right), row (3) different section sizes (corresponding to row (2)), from P1 (biggest section) to P6 (smallest section), with supine postures (left) and lateral postures (right).

generally possible (<1 m), which limits depthmap accuracy. We reconstruct 3D surface meshes from the RGBD video using an existing reconstruction method [13] but any other method could be used. The scanning process can be performed in approximately 10 s, allowing it to be done during a single breath hold to circumvent breathing artifacts. To reduce occlusions, we perform scanning before surgical coverings are placed. We denote the fused output by the vertex set $\mathcal{Q}$. When using [13] this is typically of size $O(10^5)$. We model the table as a planar surface with a flat thin padded top layer, which is valid in most real conditions. We use the distance $t \in \mathbb{R}^+$ mm to denote the maximal compression the padded layer can undergo for any patient, which can be measured once *a priori*. We fit a plane in the form $ax + by + cz + d = 0$ to the points in $\mathcal{Q}$ corresponding to the table top. This is done using RANSAC, where the largest planar region is found within a maximal depth of 1 m to the camera. This heuristic is used to eliminate the ground plane.

2.3 Registration Problem Formulation

We formulate the problem as iterative energy minimization based on [8,9]. The energy has the form $E(\mathbf{x}) = E_M(\mathbf{x}) + \lambda_{ICP} E_{ICP}(\mathbf{x}; \mathcal{V}_s, \mathcal{Q}) + E_{collision}(\mathbf{x}; \mathcal{V}_s, \mathcal{V}_I)$, where $\lambda_{ICP} \in \mathbb{R}^+$ is the ICP weight. The term E_{ICP} is the *ICP energy*, which attracts the model's transformed surface vertices $\mathcal{V}_s$ to fit to their closest vertices in $\mathcal{Q}$, while simultaneously handling mismatches, which are in practice inevitable. We compute the closest vertices using fast matching on the GPU, using the computer vision library OpenCV. We then filter out matches that are strongly likely to be outliers (e.g. matches to surrounding objects on the table, or the table itself). This filter is derived from [13], by measuring the angle between surface normals of the matched points, and rejecting each match which disagrees by a tolerance threshold τ_N. We set this to 45 degrees. We denote the remaining matches by the set $\{(\mathbf{p}_i, \mathbf{q}_i)\}$, $\mathbf{p}_i \in \mathcal{V}_s$, $\mathbf{q}_i \in \mathcal{Q}$. We define E_{ICP} as:

$$E_{ICP}(\mathbf{x}; \mathcal{V}_s, Q) = \sum_i \rho_h \left(\mathbf{n}_i^\top (f(\mathbf{p}_i) - \mathbf{q}_i) \right) \qquad (1)$$

where $\mathbf{n}_i$ denotes the normal of point $\mathbf{q}_i$ and ρ_h denotes the Huber norm. This defines a *point-to-plane distance* function, which improves convergence in ICP by allowing surfaces to slice across each other during optimization [14]. The Huber norm is used to reduce the influence of any remaining outlier matches on the energy function. This is essential to achieve good robustness.

The term $E_{collision}$ is the table collision energy, which prevents model vertices penetrating the table. We assume that the patient's body is always above the table, which is valid is practically all cases. Collision is handled by forcing all model vertices to exist above the table at a state of maximum pad compression. We do this using a *signed distance-to-table* function $d(\mathbf{p})$. For a planar table this is $d(\mathbf{p}) = [a, b, c]\mathbf{p} + d - t$. The extension to non-planar tables can be handled by modifying $d(\mathbf{p})$ according to the table's shape. We define the penalty as:

$$E_{collision}(\mathbf{x}; \mathcal{V}_s, \mathcal{V}_I) = \sigma_k \sum_{\mathbf{p} \in \mathcal{V}_s \cup \mathcal{V}_I} \max(d(\mathbf{p}), 0) \qquad (2)$$

where σ_k is the penalty coefficient. At each iteration σ_k is increased by a factor of 10. At convergence the collision constraint is exactly enforced. To avoid incorrect data association with the table, we eliminate all ICP matches that associate points on the scan that correspond to the table. This is done with a distance-to-table threshold τ with a default of 10 mm.

2.4   Optimization and Initialization

We adopt the method in [15] to reduce the deformable model's deformation space, exploiting the fact that feasible deformations tend to be mostly smooth. This works by performing a modal analysis using the model's volumetric Laplacian $\mathbf{L}$. The eigenvectors of $\mathbf{L}^\top \mathbf{L}$ with lowest eigenvalues correspond to the smoothest modes of variation. The reduced model is parameterized by $\mathbf{x}$ with a default length of 200. We optimize $E(\mathbf{x})$ iteratively using a stiff-to-flexible strategy [8,9], which is important to avoid local minima. Initially the model is kept rigid, by setting λ_{ICP} to small value (1.1 in our experiments). We then optimize $E(\mathbf{x})$ using a single Gauss-Newton iteration, and increase λ_{ICP} by a factor (we use a default of 1.2). We then repeat the process, truncating λ_{ICP} to a maximal value, which we set to 10 times the initial value. We continue until convergence is detected or a maximum number of iterations is reached (we use a limit of 50 iterations). We initialize using a roughly-estimated rigid transform. This is currently done by 6 manual landmark correspondences between the model's surface and the scanned surface, then running Horn's algorithm in OpenCV. In future works, automated landmarks extraction can also be used (computed using 2D features learnt [16] for instance). Landmark assocations can be added to Eq. (2) with an extra energy term, with a similar form as the ICP term but with point-to-point distances and fixed associations. In the experimental results we did not include this to validate the performance of ICP-only association.

3   Experimental Results

3.1   Quantitative Analysis with Porcine Datasets

We performed this using a euthanized 50 kg pig with 197 metal markers (1 cm diameter) quasi-uniformly arranged over its skin (Fig. 1). A reference CT was made in the supine position, discretized using Tetgen into 19069 3D vertices corresponding to 87524 tetrahedron. We then moved the pig to 19 different positions, representing different intra-operative poses, on a CT table (13 supine (Fig. 1a), 4 left-lateral (Fig. 1d) and 2 right-lateral). For each position we took a CT image and a corresponding RGBD scan. We compared soft-body registration with rigid ICP registration. This allowed us to measure the impact of modeling soft-body deformation. Several conditions were tested: the first was where the full reference CT was used to build the biomechanical model, and we compared accuracy using either a homogeneous biomechanical model and a heterogeneous model. We implemented the latter with two classes (bone and other), where the stiffness of bone springs were 100 times stronger than the other class, to mimic rigid body motion). We further tested with and without table collision. The error metric we used is the Nearest Landmark distance (NLD). It is infeasible to determine real matches between all markers, so nearest neighbours were used as proxies. These were computed after registration by matching each marker in the reference CT to its nearest neighbour in the CT associated with a given RGBD scan. As the average spacing was large (approximately 50 mm) compared to the observed errors, the NLD approximates well the true endpoint error.

In the first row of Fig. 2 left, we show the marker endpoint error for the 13 supine positions averaged over all 197 markers. Here the pig's deformation is smaller than in the lateral positions. We observe a considerable improvement using the soft-body models in most cases. There is no substantial improvement in the first case, the reason being that the body posture was more similar to the reference CT posture. We observe a general small improvement using the heterogeneous model and with the addition of table collision constraints. In the first row of Fig. 2 middle, we show similar results for the lateral positions. We generally observe a larger improvement with the heterogeneous versus homogeneous model, justifying its use for large deformations caused by posture change. However there is little to no improvement using the collision constraints. In the first row of Fig. 2 right, we show NLD for the lateral postures, measured only at the markers in contact with the table. Here we can see a general small improvement

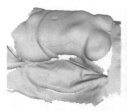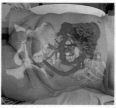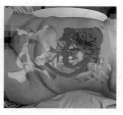

Fig. 3. Results with a human patient in a live operating room. The RGBD scan (left), rigid registration (middle) and deformable registration (right).

using the collision constraints, indicating they can improve localized registration accuracy at the table/skin interface. The errors are larger than Fig. 2 middle because they represent completely hidden regions. We then studied the influence of the size of the abdominal region in the reference CT on registration accuracy. Five reference models were tested by cropping the CT in the caudal-cranial axis with six lengths (80 cm to 35 cm) centered on the abdomen, labeled P1 to P6. These are shown from left to right in Fig. 2, row 3. We measured registration accuracy using only the markers in the 35 cm section (79 markers). This was to measure the influence of having more geometric information surrounding the abdominal region (hips, arms, shoulders ...). For this the heterogeneous model was used with collision constraints. The results for the supine positions are given in Fig. 2, bottom left. The results for the lateral positions are given in Fig. 2, bottom right. We see a general reduction in registration accuracy with increased cropping of the reference CT. The problem is caused by the reduced geometrical information needed to 'anchor' the deformation at geometrically distinct regions. This is clearly present when we move from P1 to P2, where arms and shoulders regions are cropped out.

3.2   Qualitative Analysis with a Human Patient

We tested our method in our local hospital for registering a human patient under general anesthetic, before undergoing a percutaneous radio frequency tumor ablation (Fig. 3). The idea was to check the reliability of our registration in computer-assisted percutaneous surgery by visually checking the position of the organs, and by assessing the surface fit. The patient was 58 years old. From her CT scans, a model containing 4383 vertices and 19362 tetrahedron was extracted and 13 organs were segmented and seen in the AR view. Results are presented using AR visualization, using a standard external calibrated RGB camera on a tripod. Both registration and AR visualization were performed live during the operation. We see an improved result through deformable registration, clearly demonstrated by inspecting the patient's silhouette contours. This is the first time soft-body registration has been performed using an intra-operative abdominal RGBD scan of a human patient in an operating theater.

4   Conclusion

We have presented a low-cost method to perform soft-body registration between partial or full-body pre-operative 3D models and intra-operative, partial RGBD scans. We have quantitatively evaluated using a challenging real porcine dataset, which is the first of its kind and will be made public. The achieved accuracy is sufficient for interventional radiation skin dose modeling [1]. It may also be sufficient for rough AR visualization of internal structures, as we have demonstrated with a real patient. In future work we will investigate the impact of more detailed biomechanical models and evaluate internal registration accuracy using segmented anatomical structures.

References

1. Johnson, P.B., Borrego, D., Balter, S., Johnson, K., Siragusa, D., Bolch, W.E.: Skin dose mapping for fluoroscopically guided interventions. Med. Phys. **38**, 5490–5499 (2011)
2. Rodas, N.L., Bert, J., Visvikis, D., De Mathelin, M., Padoy, N.: Pose optimization of a C-arm imaging device to reduce intraoperative radiation exposure of staff and patient during interventional procedures. In: ICRA (2017)
3. Mahmoud, N.: On-patient see-through augmented reality based on visual SLAM. Int. J. Comput. Assist. Radiol. Surg. **12**, 1–11 (2017)
4. Macedo, M.C.F., Apolinário Jr., A.L., Souza, A.C.S., Giraldi, G.A.: High-quality on-patient medical data visualization in a markerless augmented reality environment. J. Interact. Syst. **5**, 41–52 (2014)
5. Lee, J.D., Huang, C.H., Huang, T.C., Hsieh, H.Y., Lee, S.T.: Medical augmented reality using a markerless registration framework. ESA **39**, 5286–5294 (2012)
6. Chen, X.: Development of a surgical navigation system based on augmented reality using an optical see-through head-mounted display. Biomed. Inf. **55**, 124–131 (2015)
7. Tully, S.T.: BodySLAM: localization and mapping for surgical guidance (2012)
8. Amberg, B., Romdhani, S., Vetter, T.: Optimal step nonrigid ICP algorithms for surface registration. In: CVPR (2007)
9. Collins, T., et al.: A system for augmented reality guided laparoscopic tumour resection with quantitative ex-vivo user evaluation. In: Peters, T., et al. (eds.) CARE 2016. LNCS, vol. 10170, pp. 114–126. Springer, Cham (2017). https://doi.org/10.1007/978-3-319-54057-3_11
10. Petit, A., Lippiello, V., Siciliano, B.: Real-time tracking of 3D elastic objects with an RGB-D sensor. In: IROS (2015)
11. Huang, Q.X., Adams, B., Wicke, M., Guibas, L.J.: Non-rigid registration under isometric deformations. In: Eurographics Symposium on Geometry Processing (2008)
12. IRCAD: Visiblepatient. https://www.visiblepatient.com/
13. Izadi, S., et al.: KinectFusion. In: ISMAR (2011)
14. Segal, A., Haehnel, D., Thrun, S.: Generalized-ICP. In: RSA (2009)
15. Collins, T., Bartoli, A., Bourdel, N., Canis, M.: Robust, real-time, dense and deformable 3D organ tracking in laparoscopic videos. In: Ourselin, S., Joskowicz, L., Sabuncu, M.R., Unal, G., Wells, W. (eds.) MICCAI 2016. LNCS, vol. 9900, pp. 404–412. Springer, Cham (2016). https://doi.org/10.1007/978-3-319-46720-7_47
16. Cao, Z., Simon, T., Wei, S.E., Sheikh, Y.: Realtime multi-person 2D pose estimation using part affinity fields. In: CVPR (2017)

Automatic Classification of Cochlear Implant Electrode Cavity Positioning

Jack H. Noble[1,2(✉)], Robert F. Labadie[2], and Benoit M. Dawant[1]

[1] Department of Electrical Engineering and Computer Science, Vanderbilt University, Nashville, TN 37235, USA
jack.noble@vanderbilt.edu
[2] Department of Otolaryngology – Head and Neck Surgery, Vanderbilt University Medical Center, Nashville, TN 37232, USA

Abstract. Cochlear Implants (CIs) restore hearing using an electrode array that is surgically implanted into the intra-cochlear cavities. Research has indicated that each electrode can lie in one of several cavities and that location is significantly associated with hearing outcomes. However, comprehensive analysis of this phenomenon has not been possible because the cavities are not directly visible in clinical CT images and because existing methods to estimate cavity location are not accurate enough, labor intensive, or their accuracy has not been validated. In this work, a novel graph-based search is presented to automatically identify the cavity in which each electrode is located. We test our approach on CT scans from a set of 34 implanted temporal bone specimens. High resolution μCT scans of the specimens, where cavities are visible, show our method to have 98% cavity classification accuracy. These results indicate that our methods could be used on a large scale to study the link between electrode placement and outcome, which could lead to advances that improve hearing outcomes for CI users.

Keywords: Cochlear implant · Graph search · Scalar location

1 Introduction

Cochlear implants (CIs) are considered the standard of care treatment for profound hearing loss [1]. CIs use an array of electrodes surgically implanted into the cochlea (see Fig. 1) to directly stimulate the auditory nerve, inducing the sensation of hearing. Although CIs have been remarkably successful, speech recognition ability remains highly variable across CI recipients. Research has indicated that each electrode can lie in one of several intra-cochlear cavities and that array cavity location is significantly associated with hearing outcomes [2–6]. However, comprehensive analysis of this phenomenon has not been possible because the cavity position for each individual electrode has been unknown. Electrode position is generally unknown in surgery because the array is blindly threaded into a small opening of the cochlea. To analyze the relationship between electrode position and outcome, several groups have proposed post-operative imaging techniques. But these processes have been relatively imprecise because visual assessment in CT images can only indicate coarse array positioning,

© Springer Nature Switzerland AG 2018
A. F. Frangi et al. (Eds.): MICCAI 2018, LNCS 11073, pp. 47–54, 2018.
https://doi.org/10.1007/978-3-030-00937-3_6

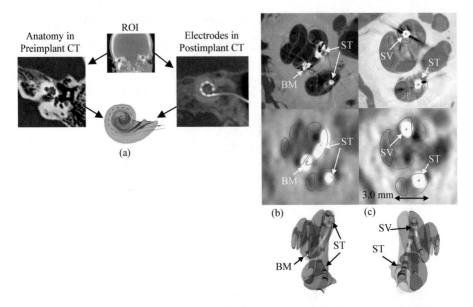

Fig. 1. (a) Pre-processing flow chart. The position of the electrodes relative to intracochlear anatomy (ST = red, modiolus = green) is found by registering preimplant CT anatomy segmentations to postimplant CT electrode localizations. In (b) and (c) different electrode position classifications for two cases are shown in μCT (top row) and CT (middle row) overlaid with automatic, CT-based anatomy localizations (ST = red, SV = blue). The bottom row shows automatic anatomy and electrode localizations in 3D.

e.g., whether or not the array is entirely within one internal cavity of the cochlea, rather than specifying cavity location for each individual electrode. Thus, studies have concluded that electrode position and outcomes are correlated but conclusions are vague and conflict across studies regarding precise relationships, such as the relationship between outcomes and the number of electrodes that lie in each cavity. Dataset size has also been limited in many studies, in part due to the amount of manual effort that must be undertaken to analyze the images when automatic techniques are not available. In the current work, we propose a fully automatic approach for localizing the cavity position of individual CI electrodes. Such an approach could permit analysis on large numbers of datasets to better study the relationship between electrode position and outcome, which may lead to advances in implant design or surgical techniques.

To determine the cavity in which each electrode is located, we start with an accurate but imperfect localization of the centroid of each electrode and segmentations of the principal intra-cochlear cavities, the scala tympani (ST) and scala vestibuli (SV) (see Fig. 1). The electrodes are automatically localized in postimplantation CT [7, 8], where the electrode array can be well visualized; the intra-cochlear cavities are automatically localized in preimplantation CT [9], where there are no implant related artifacts present and the cochlea can be visualized; and the two results are registered as shown in Fig. 1a. While the external walls of the cochlea are visible in CT, the borders between the intra-cochlear cavities are not directly visible due to the micron scale of the structures separating the cavities as shown in Fig. 1b. Thus, we use a technique where the external walls of the cochlea are used as landmarks to estimate the invisible borders of the intracochlear cavities. To do this, a statistical shape model was constructed using high resolution μCT imaging of cochleae specimens where intracochlear borders are visible. μCT can be acquired for specimens but not *in vivo* due to radiation and size considerations. The external wall portion of the model is fitted to the walls of the cochlea visible in the patient CT image, and the model statistically estimates the shape and position of the intracochlear cavities based on the wall shape.

It is possible to directly estimate the cavity location of each electrode using these data. However, while these techniques to localize the cavities and the electrodes have been shown to be accurate, they are prone to small errors, and small localization errors can result in cavity classification errors. In this work, we present the first validation study on the use of these image processing techniques for electrode cavity classification. As our results will show, classification of the cavity position of each electrode using these data can be done more accurately by using a method that is robust to errors in the localization results. We present a novel graph search-based algorithm that is robust to localization errors to classify the cavity position of each contact. We validate our approach with a set of 34 cochlea specimens. For each specimen, we run our automatic algorithm on pre- and postimplantation CTs. We compute the accuracy of our results by comparing them to the ground truth cavity location, which is defined using high resolution μCT imaging.

2 Methods

To more robustly estimate the cavity position of each electrode compared to direct estimation based on the image processing results, we assume that the classification of neighboring electrodes on the array should be relatively consistent. In other words, if both flanking electrodes in a group of three lie within and distant to the border of the scala tympani, it is highly likely that the central electrode also lies in the scala tympani. To implement a search that exploits this heuristic, we develop a graph search-based classification solution that permits defining penalties for class transitions between electrodes and finding a solution that globally optimizes our classification criteria. The graph $G = \{V, E\}$ we have designed is shown in Fig. 2. This is a directed-acyclic graph where the N middle columns of nodes correspond to the N electrodes in the array, and the three rows of the N middle columns correspond to the three possible cavity classifications for each electrode (ST = scala tympani, SV = scala vestibuli, and BM = basilar membrane). The ST and SV classifications correspond to electrodes that fall within the scala tympani or scala vestibuli. The BM classification corresponds to electrodes that have violated the basilar membrane that separates the ST and SV and sit between the ST and SV in the region where the BM was located preimplantation. Electrodes belonging to these three classifications are shown in CT and μCT and in 3D in Fig. 1b.

The graph is designed such that a path from the seed to the endnode will include one and only one of the three nodes that belong to each of the N electrodes. Thus, with this graph, a path that connects the seed to the endnode also implies a cavity

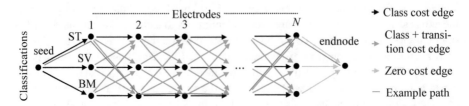

Fig. 2. Graph (black, green, and gray) that is used to classify the cavity location of each of the N electrodes. One possible path through the graph is shown in red.

classification for each electrode. An example path is shown in red in Fig. 2. This example path implies a ST cavity classification for electrodes 1 and N and a BM classification for electrodes 2 and 3 because it passes through the top (ST) row in the columns corresponding to electrodes 1 and N, and through the bottom (BM) row for electrodes, 2 and 3. To use this graph to find an accurate cavity classification, we need to define appropriate cost values for the set of edges E. Then we can use standard graph searching methods, such as Dijkstra's algorithm [10], to find the path with the globally minimum cost.

We define two types of cost for our edge cost function, "class cost" and "transition cost," which are the electrode classification cost, and the class transition cost. Let $C(V_j)$ and $P(V_j)$ represent the cavity classification and the electrode associated with node V_j, respectively. Then, the class cost for an edge $E_{i,j}$ connecting node V_i to V_j represents the cost for assigning the electrode represented by V_j, $P(V_j)$, to the cavity classification associated with V_j, $C(V_j)$, and is defined by

$$\text{class}(V_j) = \begin{cases} D_{ST}(P(V_j)) - d_{\min} + \alpha & C(V_j) = ST \\ D_{SV}(P(V_j)) - d_{\min} + \alpha & C(V_j) = SV \\ |D_{ST}(P(V_j)) - D_{SV}(P(V_j))| & C(V_j) = BM \end{cases}, \tag{1}$$

where

$$d_{\min} = \min(D_{ST}(P(V_j)), D_{SV}(P(V_j))), \tag{2}$$

D_{ST} and D_{SV} are signed-distance map representations of the scala tympani and scala vestibuli computed using fast marching techniques [11] with negative distances in the structure foreground and positive distances in the background, $D(P)$ is the value of the signed distance map at electrode P, and α is a parameter tuned as described in the following section that controls the width of the region between the scala tympani and vestibuli that is considered to be the basilar membrane region. If the electrode $P(V_j)$ falls 0.5α mm within the border of the scala vestibuli, then $D_{SV}(P(V_j)) = -0.5\alpha$, $D_{ST}(P(V_j)) \geq 0.5\alpha$, $d_{\min} = -0.5\alpha$, and $|D_{ST}(P(V_j)) - D_{SV}(P(V_j))| \geq \alpha$. In this case, the classification cost for assigning $P(V_j)$ to SV, BM, or ST, would be α, $\geq \alpha$, and $\geq 2\alpha$. Thus, the highest cost is assigned to ST classification. If the electrode sits farther than 0.5α mm from the scala tympani, the second highest cost would be to BM classification.

Otherwise SV and BM are assigned equal cost because the electrode falls on the border between the SV and the α mm wide BM region we have defined between the ST and SV.

The transition cost for edge $E_{i,j}$ represents the cost for transitioning classifications from $C(V_i)$ to $C(V_j)$ and is defined by

$$\text{transition}(V_i, V_j) = \left\{ \begin{array}{ll} \beta & C(V_i) \neq C(V_j) \\ 0 & C(V_i) = C(V_j) \end{array} \right\}, \tag{3}$$

where β is a constant to punish class inconsistency among neighboring electrodes and is tuned as described in the following section. The overall cost function is defined as

$$cost(E_{i,j}) = \left\{ \begin{array}{ll} \text{class}(V_j) + \text{transition}(V_i, V_j) & C(V_i) \neq C(V_j) \\ \text{class}(V_j) & C(V_i) = C(V_j) \text{ or } C(V_i) = \text{seed} \\ 0 & C(V_j) = \text{endnode} \end{array} \right\},$$

where these three types of edges are shown as green, black, and gray edges in the graph in Fig. 2.

Finally, it is also common for some electrodes to be outside the cochlea when the surgeon stops inserting the array prior to those electrodes entering the cochlea. To detect which electrodes are outside of the cochlea, we find the first electrode in the array that falls within the foreground of the ST or SV segmentations and classify all previous electrodes as falling outside of the cochlea.

Parameter Selection and Validation. We trained parameters and evaluated our approach simultaneously using a leave-one-out validation study. In this process, our two parameters α and β were tuned using 33 of the 34 datasets and then tested on the left-out dataset. This process was repeated so that the method was tested on each of the 34 datasets while leaving that testing set out of the training process. To train our parameters, first, heuristic tuning was done on one case. We started with values 0.3 and 0.15 for α and β and found 0.2 and 0.3 to lead to better results. Then, these values were used as initial values when performing the parameter optimization in all cases. For each testing case, these parameters were iteratively optimized on the training dataset until converging to a local classification error minimum. Classification errors were defined as the sum of incorrect cavity classifications relative to the ground truth classification across all training sets. The ground truth cavity classification for each electrode was defined by visual inspection of the raw high resolution μCT images, where cavity borders are visible, in an interactive viewer with three 2D orthogonal planar views without the benefit of the automated image processing data. Within each iteration of the parameter search, each parameter was independently varied from its initial value in the range $[-0.125, 0.125]$ in steps of 0.025. A new value for the parameter was selected as the value that resulted in minimum overall error. Because the cost function is discrete, it often can result in multiple equal minima. When separate multiple minima were present, preference was given to the minimum closest to the initial value. When three or more adjacent values resulted in identical minimal error, preference was given to values that were not adjacent to non-minimal values in order to choose values that corresponded to locations within, rather than on the edge of, the minimum region.

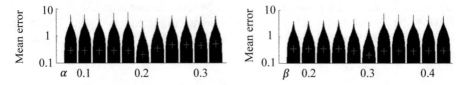

Fig. 3. Violin plots of classification errors made in the entire dataset when sweeping parameters α (left) and β (right) around their final values.

Table 1. Confusion matrices and classification results of the leave-one-out experiment, when using the final selected parameters on the entire dataset, and when not using the proposed graph search method.

		Results with leave-one-out				Results with final parameters				Results without graph search			
		OC	ST	SV	BM	OC	ST	SV	BM	OC	ST	SV	BM
Ground Truth	OC	32	2	0	0	32	2	0	0	32	0	0	2
	ST	1	506	2	0	1	506	2	0	1	458	2	48
	SV	0	0	30	0	0	0	30	0	0	0	27	3
	BM	0	5	0	0	0	2	0	3	0	2	0	3
Sensitivity (%)		94.1	99.4	100.0	0.0	94.1	99.4	100.0	60.0	94.1	90.0	90.0	60.0
Specificity (%)		99.8	89.9	99.6	100.0	99.8	94.2	99.6	100.0	99.8	97.1	99.6	90.8

3   Results

A local optimum of both parameters was successfully obtained for every leave-one-out parameter search. In 1 of 34 test cases (case #12), the parameter search selected α and β as 0.175 and 0.3. In the remaining 33 of 34 test cases, the parameter search converged to values of 0.2 and 0.3. Thus, these values appear to correspond to a stable optimum and we select them as the final parameter values. Violin plots of the number of classification errors for each dataset when sweeping these parameters around their final parameter values is shown in Fig. 3. The mean of the number of errors for each case is shown as a red cross for each parameter value. As can be seen in the figure, values of 0.2 and 0.3 for α and β correspond to a clear local minimum of classification error.

Overall classification results are shown in Table 1. When using the trained parameters found in the leave-one-out tests, we achieve overall classification accuracy of 98%, and excellent specificity and sensitivity for the ST, SV, and Out of Cochlea (OC) classifications. However, our method achieves 0% sensitivity for the BM class. This is because the BM class is highly underrepresented in our dataset, with all of the only 5 BM electrodes belonging to case #12. Thus, when leave-one-out testing on case #12, there were zero BM electrodes in the training set, and it is unsurprising that the resulting leave-one-out trained α was selected low enough to lead to 0% BM sensitivity. When using the final selected parameters on the whole dataset, overall accuracy is 99% and BM sensitivity is 60%, which is still low but unsurprising considering the BM class is only represented by 5 of 578 electrodes in our dataset.

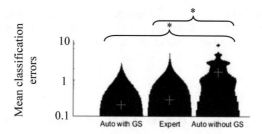

Fig. 4. Final results shown as violin plots of the proposed automatic method with graph search (GS), expert determination of the cavity positioning, and automatic cavity localization without the graph search method we propose.

We also compared the leave-one-out classification results to expert classification and automatic classification using the image processing data directly without the benefit of the robustness-boosting graph search method we propose. These results are shown as violin plots in Fig. 4 and confusion matrix in Table 1. Expert classification of cavity position for each electrode was done by inspection of the CT images and image processing data (electrode localization and anatomy segmentation) in an interactive viewer with 3D views and three 2D orthogonal planar views without the benefit of the high resolution μCT. The expert classification results are found to have a slightly higher mean error than our proposed method, although this difference was not found to be statistically significant using a paired t-test. Both the proposed method and expert classification perform statistically significantly better ($p < 1e-4$) than automatic classification without the graph search method proposed in this work.

4   Conclusions

In this work, we have proposed a novel and fully automatic method for identification of the cavity position of intracochlear electrodes. Our experiments show that our method has high classification accuracy. Compared to expert cavity identification, our method produces comparable results. Compared to non-robust cavity identification techniques, our method produces significantly more accurate results. Our approach is also fast, requiring less than a second of processing time after a 5 min procedure is used to automatically localize the anatomical structures and electrode array.

While overall classification accuracy is high, our method results in poor sensitivity for BM classification because this class is inadequately represented in our dataset. In future work, we will expand our ground truth dataset to attempt to obtain more examples of electrodes located in the BM region to explore whether our method can achieve acceptable BM classification sensitivity when using a more balanced training dataset. We also plan to apply our method to large numbers of clinical datasets to facilitate studying how the location of individual electrodes correlates with outcomes with the goal of developing technologies that can improve hearing outcomes with CIs.

Acknowledgements. This work was supported in part by grants R01DC014037 and R01DC014462 from the NIDCD. The content is solely the responsibility of the authors and does not necessarily represent the official views of this institute.

References

1. "Cochlear Implants," National Institute on Deafness and Other Communication Disorders, No. 11–4798 (2011)
2. Verbist, B.M., Frijns, J.H.M., Geleijns, J., van Buchem, M.A.: Multisection CT as a valuable tool in the postoperative assessment of cochlear implant patients. Am J Neuroradiol **26**, 424–429 (2005)
3. Aschendorff, A., et al.: Quality control after cochlear implant surgery by means of rotational tomography. Otol. Neurotol. **26**, 34–37 (2005)
4. Skinner, M.W., et al.: In vivo estimates of the position of advanced bionics electrode arrays in the human cochlea. Ann. Otol. Rhinol. Laryngol. Suppl. **197**, 2–24 (2007)
5. Wanna, G.B., et al.: Assessment of electrode placement and audiologic outcomes in bilateral cochlear implantation. Otol. Neurotol. **32**, 428–432 (2011)
6. Wanna, G.B., et al.: Impact of electrode design and surgical approach on scalar location and cochlear implant outcomes. Laryngoscope **124**(S6), S1–S7 (2014)
7. Noble, J.H., Dawant, B.M.: Automatic graph-based localization of cochlear implant electrodes in CT. In: Navab, N., Hornegger, J., Wells, W.M., Frangi, A.F. (eds.) MICCAI 2015. LNCS, vol. 9350, pp. 152–159. Springer, Cham (2015). https://doi.org/10.1007/978-3-319-24571-3_19
8. Zhao, Y., Dawant, B.M., Labadie, R.F., Noble, J.H.: Automatic localization of cochlear implant electrodes in CT. In: Golland, P., Hata, N., Barillot, C., Hornegger, J., Howe, R. (eds.) MICCAI 2014. LNCS, vol. 8673, pp. 331–338. Springer, Cham (2014). https://doi.org/10.1007/978-3-319-10404-1_42
9. Noble, J.H., Labadie, R.F., Majdani, O., Dawant, B.M.: Automatic segmentation of intra-cochlear anatomy in conventional CT. IEEE Trans. on Biomedical. Eng. **58**(9), 2625–2632 (2011)
10. Dijkstra, E.W.: A note on two problems in connexion with graphs. Numer. Math. **1**, 269–271 (1959)
11. Sethian, J.A.: Level Set Methods and Fast Marching Methods, 2nd edn. Cambridge University Press, Cambridge (1999)

X-ray-transform Invariant Anatomical Landmark Detection for Pelvic Trauma Surgery

Bastian Bier[1,2(✉)], Mathias Unberath[2], Jan-Nico Zaech[1,2], Javad Fotouhi[2], Mehran Armand[3], Greg Osgood[4], Nassir Navab[2], and Andreas Maier[1]

[1] Pattern Recognition Lab, Friedrich-Alexander-Universität Erlangen-Nürnberg, Erlangen, Germany
bastian.bier@fau.de
[2] Computer Aided Medical Procedures, Johns Hopkins University, Baltimore, USA
[3] Applied Physics Laboratory, Johns Hopkins University, Baltimore, USA
[4] Department of Orthopaedic Surgery, Johns Hopkins Hospital, Baltimore, USA

Abstract. X-ray image guidance enables percutaneous alternatives to complex procedures. Unfortunately, the indirect view onto the anatomy in addition to projective simplification substantially increase the task-load for the surgeon. Additional 3D information such as knowledge of anatomical landmarks can benefit surgical decision making in complicated scenarios. Automatic detection of these landmarks in transmission imaging is challenging since image-domain features characteristic to a certain landmark change substantially depending on the viewing direction. Consequently and to the best of our knowledge, the above problem has not yet been addressed. In this work, we present a method to automatically detect anatomical landmarks in X-ray images independent of the viewing direction. To this end, a sequential prediction framework based on convolutional layers is trained on synthetically generated data of the pelvic anatomy to predict 23 landmarks in single X-ray images. View independence is contingent on training conditions and, here, is achieved on a spherical segment covering $120°\times90°$ in LAO/RAO and CRAN/CAUD, respectively, centered around AP. On synthetic data, the proposed approach achieves a mean prediction error of 5.6 ± 4.5 mm. We demonstrate that the proposed network is immediately applicable to clinically acquired data of the pelvis. In particular, we show that our intra-operative landmark detection together with pre-operative CT enables X-ray pose estimation which, ultimately, benefits initialization of image-based 2D/3D registration.

1 Introduction

X-ray image guidance during surgery has enabled percutaneous alternatives to complicated procedures reducing the risk and discomfort for the patient. This

---

B. Bier, M. Unberath, N. Navab and A. Maier—These authors have contributed equally and are listed in alphabetical order.

© Springer Nature Switzerland AG 2018
A. F. Frangi et al. (Eds.): MICCAI 2018, LNCS 11073, pp. 55–63, 2018.
https://doi.org/10.1007/978-3-030-00937-3_7

benefit for the patient comes at the cost of an increased task-load for the surgeon, who has no direct view on the anatomy but relies on indirect feedback through X-ray images. These suffer from the effects of projective simplification; particularly the absence of depth cues, and vanishing anatomical landmarks depending on the viewing direction. Therefore, many X-rays from different views are required to ensure correct tool trajectories [1]. Providing additional, "implicit 3D" information during these interventions can drastically ease the mental mapping from 2D images to 3D anatomy [2,3]. In this case, implicit 3D information refers to data that is not 3D as such but provides meaningful contextual information related to prior knowledge of the surgeon.

A promising candidate for implicit 3D information are the positions of anatomical landmarks in X-ray images. Landmark or key point detection is well understood in computer vision, where robust feature descriptors disambiguate correspondences between images, finally enabling purely image-based pose retrieval. Unfortunately, the above concept defined for reflection imaging does not translate directly to transmission imaging, since the appearance of the same anatomical landmark can vary substantially depending on the viewing direction. Consequently and to the best of our knowledge, X-ray-transform invariant anatomical landmark detection has not yet been investigated. However, successful translation of the above concept to X-ray imaging bears great potential to aid fluoroscopic guidance.

In this work, we propose an automatic, purely image-based method to detect anatomical landmarks in X-ray images independent of the viewing direction. Landmarks are detected using a sequential prediction framework [4] trained on synthetically generated images. Based on landmark knowledge, we can (a) identify corresponding regions between arbitrary views of the same anatomy and (b) estimate pose relative to a pre-procedurally acquired volume without the need for calibration. We evaluate our approach on synthetic validation data and demonstrate that it generalizes to unseen clinical X-rays of the pelvis without the need of re-training. Further, we argue that the accuracy of our detections in clinical X-rays may benefit the initialization of 2D/3D registration.

While automatic approaches to detect anatomical landmarks are not unknown in literature, all previous work either focuses on 3D image volumes [5] or 2D X-ray images acquired from *a single predefined* pose [6,7]. In contrast to the proposed approach that restricts itself to implicit 3D information, several approaches exist that introduce explicit 3D information. These solutions rely on external markers to track the tools or the patient in 3D [8], consistency conditions to estimate relative pose between X-ray images [9], or 2D/3D registration of pre-operative CT to intra-operative X-ray to render multiple views simultaneously [8,10]. While these approaches have proven helpful, they are not widely accepted in clinical practice. The primary reasons are disruptions to the surgical workflow [3], susceptibility to both truncation and initialization due to the low capture range of the optimization target [11].

2   Method

Background: Recently, sequential prediction frameworks proved effective in estimating human pose from RGB images [4]. The architecture of such network is shown in Fig. 1. Given a single image, the network predicts belief maps b_t^p for each anatomical landmark $p \in \{1,\dots,P\}$. The core idea of the network is that belief maps are predicted in stages $t \in \{1,\dots,T\}$ using both local image information and long-range contextual dependencies of landmark distributions given the belief of the previous stage. In the first stage of the network, the initial belief b_1^p is predicted only based on local image evidence x using a block of convolutional and pooling layers. In subsequent stages $t \geqslant 2$, belief maps are obtained using local image features x' and the belief maps of the preceding stage. Over all stages, the weights of x' are shared. The cost function is defined as the sum of L2-distances between the ground truth $b_*^p(z)$ and the predicted belief maps accumulated over all stages. The ground truth belief maps are normal distributions centered around the ground truth location of that landmark. The network design results in the following properties: (1) In each stage, the predicted belief maps of the previous stage can resolve ambiguities that appear due to locality of image features. The network can learn that certain landmarks appear in characteristic configurations only. (2) To further leverage this effect, each output pixel exhibits a large receptive field on the input image of 160×160. This enables learning of implicit spatial dependencies between landmarks over long distances. (3) Accumulating the loss over the predicted belief in multiple stages diminishes the effect of vanishing gradients that complicates learning in large networks.

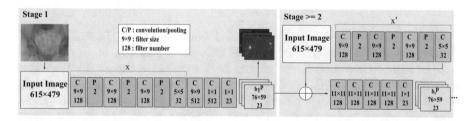

Fig. 1. Network architecture: In subsequent stages, landmarks are predicted from belief maps of the previous stage and image features of the input image. Adapted from [4].

X-ray Transform Invariant Landmark Detection: We exploit the aforementioned advantages of sequential prediction frameworks for the detection of anatomical landmarks in X-ray images independent of their viewing direction. Our assumption is that anatomical landmarks exhibit strong constraints and thus characteristic patterns even in presence of arbitrary viewing angles. In fact, this assumption may be even stronger compared to human pose estimation if limited anatomy, such as the pelvis, is considered due to rigidity. Within this paper and as a first proof-of-concept, we study anatomical landmarks on the pelvis. We devise a network adapted from [4] with six stages to simultaneously predict 23 belief maps per X-ray image that are used for landmark location extraction (Fig. 1). Implementation was done in tensorflow, with a learning rate of 0.00001, and a batchsize of one. Optimization was performed using Adam over 30 epochs (convergence reached).

Predicted belief maps b_t^p are averaged over all stages prior to estimating the position of the landmarks yielding the averaged belief map b^p. We define the landmark position l_p as the position with the highest response in b^p. Landmarks with responses $b^p < 0.4$ are discarded since they may be outside the field of view or not reliably recognized.

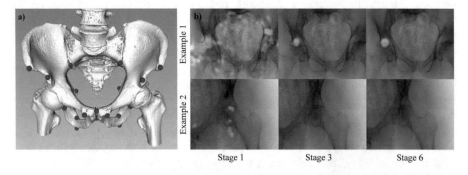

Fig. 2. Uncertainty in the local feature detection after stage 1 is resolved in subsequent stages. This is shown for a symmetric response (Example 1, anterior inferior iliac spine) and for a landmark not in the FOV (Example 2, tip of femoral head).

Training data is synthetically generated from full body CTs from the NIH Cancer Imaging Archive [12]. In total, 20 CTs (male and female patients) were cropped to an ROI around the pelvis and 23 anatomical landmark positions were annotated manually in 3D. Landmarks were selected to be clinically meaningful and clearly identifiable in 3D; see Fig. 2(a). From these volumes and 3D points, projection images and projected 2D positions were created, respectively. X-rays had 615×479 pixels with an isotropic pixel size of 0.616 mm. The belief maps were downsampled eight times. During projection generation augmentation was applied: We used random translations in all three axes, variation of the source-to-isocenter distance, and horizontal flipping of the projections. Further and most importantly, we sampled images on a spherical segment with a range of 120° in LAO/RAO and 90° in CRAN/CAUD centered around AP, which approximates the range of variation in X-ray images during surgical procedures on the pelvis [13]. The forward projector computes material-dependent line integral images, which are then converted to synthetic X-rays [14]. A total of 20.000 X-rays with corresponding ground truth belief maps were generated. Data was split $18 \times 1 \times 1$-fold in training, testing, and validation. We ensured that images of one patient are not shared among sets.

3   Experiments and Results

3.1   Synthetic X-Rays

Experiment: For evaluation, we uniformly sampled projections from our testing volume on a spherical segment covering the same angular range used in training. The angular increment between samples was $5°$, soure-to-isocenter distance was 750 mm, and source-to-detector distance was 1200 mm.

Confidence Development: In Fig. 2 the refinement of the belief maps is shown for two examples. After the first stage, several areas in the X-ray image have a high response due to the locality of feature detection. With increasing stages, the belief in the correct landmark location is increased.

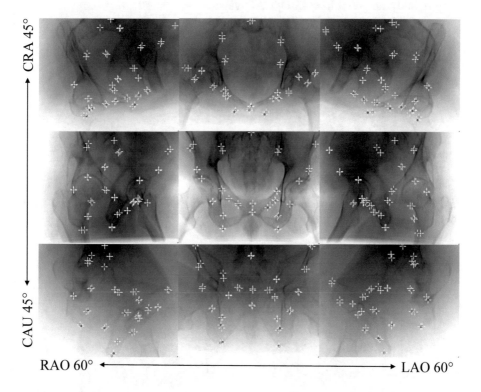

Fig. 3. Detection results over the sampled sphere. White and red marker positions indicate ground truth and predicted landmark location, respectively.

Qualitative Results: In Fig. 3, example X-rays covering the whole angular range are shown. Visually, one notices very good overall agreement between the predicted and true landmark locations[1].

---

[1] https://camp.lcsr.jhu.edu/miccai-2018-demonstration-videos/.

Belief Map Response and Prediction Error: The maximum belief is an indicator for the quality of a detected landmark. Figure 4 shows the correlation between belief map response and prediction error. As motivated previously, we define a landmark as *detected* if the maximum belief is ≥ 0.4. Then, the mean prediction error with respect to ground truth is 9.1 ± 7.4 pixels (5.6 ± 4.5 mm).

View Invariance: The view invariance of landmark detection is illustrated in the spherical plot in Fig. 4. We define accuracy as the ratio of landmarks with an error < 15 pixels to all detected landmarks in that view. The plot indicates that detection is slightly superior in AP compared to lateral views. To provide intuition on this observation, we visualize the maximum belief of two representative landmarks as a function of viewing direction in Fig. 5. While the first landmark is robust to changes in viewing direction, the second landmark is more reliably detected in CAUD/RAO views.

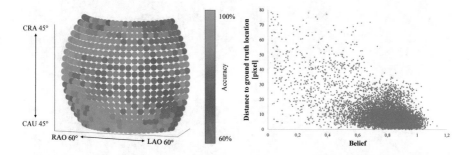

Fig. 4. Left: detection accuracy in dependence of the viewing direction. Right: correlation between belief and prediction error.

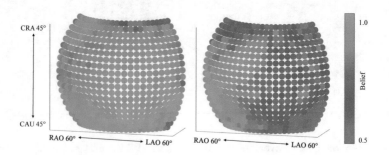

Fig. 5. Belief distribution of two single landmarks. Each landmark has it own detection belief distribution over the sphere.

3.2 Real X-Rays

Landmark Detection: Real X-ray images of a cadaver study were used to test generality of our model *without* re-training. Sample images of our landmark detection are shown in Fig. 6, top row. Visually, the achieved predictions are in very good agreement with the expected outcome. Even in presence of truncation, landmarks on the visible anatomy are still predicted accurately, see Fig. 6(c). A failure case of the network is shown in Fig. 6(d), where a surgical tool in the field of view impedes landmark prediction.

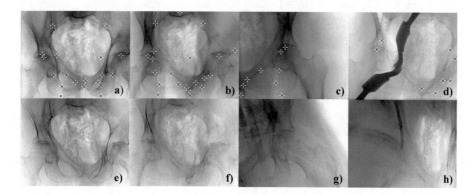

Fig. 6. Top: landmark predictions on clinical X-rays. Bottom: generated projection images after X-ray pose was retrieved using the detections.

Applications in 2D/3D Registration: As candidate clinical application, we study initialization of 2D/3D registration between pre-operative CT and intra-operative X-ray of cadaver data based on landmarks. Anatomical landmarks are manually labeled in 3D CT and automatically extracted from 2D X-ray images using the proposed method. Since correspondences between 2D detections and 3D references are known, the X-ray pose yielding the current view can be estimated in closed form [15]. To increase robustness of the estimation and because belief of a landmark may depend on viewing direction, only landmarks with a belief above 0.7 (but at least 6) are used. The estimated projection matrix is verified via forward projection of the volume in that geometry (Fig. 6, bottom row). While initialization performs well in standard cases where most landmarks are visible and detected, performance deteriorates slightly in presence of truncation due to the lower amount of reliable landmarks, and exhibits poor performance if landmark detection is challenged by previously unseen scenarios, such as tools in the image.

4   Discussion and Conclusions

We presented an approach to automatically detect anatomical landmarks in X-rays invariant of their viewing direction to benefit orthopedic surgeries by providing implicit 3D information. Our results are very promising but some limitations remain. (1) As shown in Fig. 6(d), the performance of our method is susceptible to scenarios not included in training, such as surgical tools in the image.

(2) Lateral views of the pelvis exhibit slightly worse prediction performance compared to AP-like views. We attribute this behavior to more drastic overlap of the anatomy and lower amount of training samples seen by the network. We are confident that this effect can be compensated by increasing the angular range during training while limiting validation to the current range. Since some landmarks are equally well predicted over the complete angular range, the concept of maximum belief is powerful in selecting reliable landmarks for further processing. (3) Downsampling of ground truth belief map limits the accuracy of the detection despite efforts to increase accuracy, e. g. sub-pixel maximum detection. Detecting anatomical landmarks proved essential in automatic image parsing in diagnostic imaging, but may receive considerable attention in image-guided interventions as new approaches, such as this one, strive for clinically acceptable performance. In addition to 2D/3D registration, we anticipate applications for the proposed approach in clinical tasks that inherently involve X-ray images from multiple orientations, in particular K-wire placement.

Acknowledgments. The authors gratefully acknowledge funding support from NIH 5R01AR065248-03.

References

1. Stöckle, U., Schaser, K., König, B.: Image guidance in pelvic and acetabular surgery-expectations, success and limitations. Injury **38**(4), 450–462 (2007)
2. Starr, R., Jones, A., Reinert, C., Borer, D.: Preliminary results and complications following limited open reduction and percutaneous screw fixation of displaced fractures of the acetabulum. Injury **32**, SA45–50 (2001)
3. Härtl, R., Lam, K.S., Wang, J., Korge, A., Audigé, F.K.L.: Worldwide survey on the use of navigation in spine surgery. World Neurosurg. **379**(1), 162–172 (2013)
4. Wei, S.E., Ramakrishna, V., Kanade, T., Sheikh, Y.: Convolutional pose machines. In: CVPR, pp. 4724–4732 (2016)
5. Ghesu, F.C., Georgescu, B., Mansi, T., Neumann, D., Hornegger, J., Comaniciu, D.: An artificial agent for anatomical landmark detection in medical images. In: Ourselin, S., Joskowicz, L., Sabuncu, M.R., Unal, G., Wells, W. (eds.) MICCAI 2016. LNCS, vol. 9902, pp. 229–237. Springer, Cham (2016). https://doi.org/10. 1007/978-3-319-46726-9_27
6. Wang, C.W., Huang, C.T., Hsieh, M.C.: Evaluation and comparison of anatomical landmark detection methods for cephalometric x-ray images: a grand challenge. Trans. Med. Imaging **34**(9), 1890–1900 (2015)
7. Chen, C., Xie, W., Franke, J., Grutzner, P., Nolte, L.P., Zheng, G.: Automatic x-ray landmark detection and shape segmentation via data-driven joint estimation of image displacements. Med. Image Anal. **18**(3), 487–499 (2014)
8. Markelj, P., Tomaževič, D., Likar, B., Pernuš, F.: A review of 3D/2D registration methods for image-guided interventions. Med. Image Anal. **16**(3), 642–661 (2012)
9. Aichert, A., Berger, M., Wang, J., Maass, N., Doerfler, A., Hornegger, J., Maier, A.K.: Epipolar consistency in transmission imaging. IEEE Trans. Med. Imag. **34**(11), 2205–2219 (2015)
10. Tucker, E., et al.: Towards clinical translation of augmented orthopedic surgery: from pre-op CT to intra-op x-ray via RGBD sensing. In: SPIE Medical Imaging (2018)

11. Hou, B., et al.: Predicting slice-to-volume transformation in presence of arbitrary subject motion. In: Descoteaux, M., Maier-Hein, L., Franz, A., Jannin, P., Collins, D.L., Duchesne, S. (eds.) MICCAI 2017. LNCS, vol. 10434, pp. 296–304. Springer, Cham (2017). https://doi.org/10.1007/978-3-319-66185-8_34

12. Roth, H., et al.: A new 2.5D representation for lymph node detection in CT. The Cancer Imaging Archive (2015)

13. Khurana, B., Sheehan, S.E., Sodickson, A.D., Weaver, M.J.: Pelvic ring fractures: what the orthopedic surgeon wants to know. Radiographics **34**(5), 1317–1333 (2014)

14. Unberath, M., et al.: DeepDRR-a catalyst for machine learning in fluoroscopy-guided procedures. In: Frangi, A.F., et al. (eds.) MICCAI 2018. LNCS, vol. 11073, pp. 98–106. Springer, Heidelberg (2018)

15. Hartley, R.I., Zisserman, A.: Multiple View Geometry in Computer Vision. Cambridge University Press, Cambridge (2004). ISBN 0521540518

Endoscopic Navigation in the Absence of CT Imaging

Ayushi Sinha[1]([✉]), Xingtong Liu[1], Austin Reiter[1], Masaru Ishii[2],
Gregory D. Hager[1], and Russell H. Taylor[1]

[1] The Johns Hopkins University, Baltimore, USA
sinha@jhu.edu
[2] Johns Hopkins Medical Institutions, Baltimore, USA

Abstract. Clinical examinations that involve endoscopic exploration of the nasal cavity and sinuses often do not have a reference image to provide structural context to the clinician. In this paper, we present a system for navigation during clinical endoscopic exploration in the absence of computed tomography (CT) scans by making use of shape statistics from past CT scans. Using a deformable registration algorithm along with dense reconstructions from video, we show that we are able to achieve submillimeter registrations in in-vivo clinical data and are able to assign confidence to these registrations using confidence criteria established using simulated data.

1 Introduction

Endoscopic explorations of the nasal cavity and sinuses are generally not accompanied by a reference computed tomography (CT) image since CT image acquisition exposes patients to high doses of ionizing radiation and is, therefore, avoided unless necessary. Clinicians performing the exploration must rely entirely on the endoscopic camera for visualization and, therefore, must cope with restricted field of view. In order to reduce reliance on experience or memory and to provide additional context information, we have developed a system that enables navigation without the need for accompanying patient CT or other similar imaging and associates a confidence measure to the navigation being provided. Further, our system does not introduce any additional devices than those already used in clinical endoscopic exploration. Therefore, the clinician is not responsible for anything in addition to the endoscope.

Most navigation systems that have been developed are intended for surgical use [1,2]. For surgical navigation, there is almost always access to preoperative CT scans, which have high contrast between air, bone, and soft tissue. This allows surgeons to better understand their location, the proximity to surrounding bones and soft tissue, and the thickness of surrounding bones, enabling them to make more informed decisions during surgery and prevent harm to critical structures nearby, like the brain, eyes, optic nerves, carotid arteries, etc.

The main difference between these previous methods and the method presented here is the absence of patient specific CT scans. In order to make up

© Springer Nature Switzerland AG 2018
A. F. Frangi et al. (Eds.): MICCAI 2018, LNCS 11073, pp. 64–71, 2018.
https://doi.org/10.1007/978-3-030-00937-3_8

for this absence, we utilize past CT scans to build statistical shape models of relevant structures. Statistically derived shapes are then deformably registered to dense reconstructions of anatomy visible in endoscopic video, and statistical confidence measures are automatically assigned to the registrations. The registration accomplishes two tasks simultaneously. First, it aligns the endoscopic video to the statistically derived shape, giving the clinician more information about where surrounding structures may be. Second, it deforms the statistically derived shape to fit the structure obtained from video and, in effect, *estimates the patient CT*. The confidence measure further informs the clinician on when and how much the navigation system can be trusted, and also allows the navigation system to attempt to improve itself if its current registration estimate has low confidence. We perform two experiments to evaluate our framework. First, we establish that our framework can compute submillimeter registrations and reliably assign confidence to the registrations using simulated data. Second, we evaluate our framework on in-vivo clinical data, and use the confidence criteria to assign confidence to the registrations.

2 Method

To build statistical shape models (SSMs), we automatically segment 53 publicly available head CTs [3–6] by transferring 3D meshes extracted from manually created labels in a template CT image to the 53 CTs using deformation fields produced by an intensity-based CT-CT registration algorithm [7]. With some improvement to these initial segmentations using the method described in [8], we obtain reliably segmented structures in all CTs along with reliable correspondences. These correspondences allow us to build SSMs of the segmented structures using established methods like principal component analysis (PCA) [9]:

$$\boldsymbol{\Sigma}_{\text{SSM}} = \frac{1}{\mathbf{n}_s} \sum_{j=1}^{\mathbf{n}_s} (\mathbf{V}_j - \bar{\mathbf{V}})^{\mathbf{T}} (\mathbf{V}_j - \bar{\mathbf{V}}) = [\mathbf{m}_1 \dots \mathbf{m}_{\mathbf{n}_s}] \begin{bmatrix} \lambda_1 & & \\ & \ddots & \\ & & \lambda_{\mathbf{n}_s} \end{bmatrix} [\mathbf{m}_1 \dots \mathbf{m}_{\mathbf{n}_s}]^{\mathbf{T}},$$

(1)

where $\mathbf{V}_j$ is the stacked vector of vertices, $\mathbf{V} = [\mathbf{v}_1 \ \mathbf{v}_2 \dots \mathbf{v}_{\mathbf{n}_v}]^{\mathbf{T}}$, for the jth mesh, $\bar{\mathbf{V}}$ is the mean shape computed by averaging the $\mathbf{n}_v$ corresponding vertices over $\mathbf{n}_s$ shapes, $\bar{\mathbf{V}} = \frac{1}{n_s} \sum_{j=1}^{n_s} \mathbf{V}_j$, and $\boldsymbol{\Sigma}_{\text{SSM}}$ is the shape covariance matrix. An eigen decomposition of $\boldsymbol{\Sigma}_{\text{SSM}}$ produces the principal modes of variation, $\mathbf{m}$, and the mode weights, λ, which represent the amount of variation along the corresponding $\mathbf{m}$ (Eq. 1). PCA enables any new shape, $\mathbf{V}^*$, that is in correspondence with the shapes used to build the SSM, to be estimated using $\bar{\mathbf{V}}$, $\mathbf{m}$ and λ: $\tilde{\mathbf{V}}^* = \bar{\mathbf{V}} + \sum_{j=1}^{\mathbf{n}_m} s_j \mathbf{w}_j$, where $\tilde{\mathbf{V}}^*$ is the estimated $\mathbf{V}^*$, $1 \leq \mathbf{n}_m < \mathbf{n}_s$ is some specified number of modes, $\mathbf{w}_j = \sqrt{\lambda_j} \mathbf{m}_j$ are the weighted modes of variation, and s_j are the shape parameters in units of standard deviation (SD) which can be obtained by projecting the mean subtracted $\mathbf{V}^*$ onto the weighted modes.

These shape parameters, $\mathbf{s} = \{s_j\}$, can be incorporated into probabilistic models of registration to enable optimization over $\mathbf{s}$ in addition to other registration parameters [10]. In particular, we evaluate the deformable extension of the

generalized iterative most likely oriented point (G-IMLOP) algorithm, an iterative rigid registration algorithm [11]. The generalized *deformable* iterative most
likely oriented point (GD-IMLOP) algorithm extends G-IMLOP, which incorporates an anisotropic Gaussian noise model and an anisotropic Kent noise model
to account for measurement errors in position and orientation, respectively [11].
Assuming both position and orientation errors are zero-mean, independent and
identically distributed, the match likelihood function for each oriented point, $\mathbf{x}$,
transformed by a current similarity transform, $[a, \mathbf{R}, \mathbf{t}]$, is defined as [11]:

$$
f_{\text{match}}(\mathbf{x}; \mathbf{y}, \boldsymbol{\Sigma}_{\mathbf{x}}, \boldsymbol{\Sigma}_{\mathbf{y}}, \kappa, \beta, \hat{\gamma}_1, \hat{\gamma}_2, a, \mathbf{R}, \mathbf{t}) = \frac{1}{\sqrt{(2\pi)^3 |\boldsymbol{\Sigma}|} \cdot c(\kappa, \beta)}
$$

$$
\cdot e^{-\frac{1}{2}(\mathbf{y_p}-a\mathbf{R}\mathbf{x_p}-\mathbf{t})^{\mathbf{T}}\boldsymbol{\Sigma}^{-1}(\mathbf{y_p}-a\mathbf{R}\mathbf{x_p}-\mathbf{t})-\kappa\hat{\mathbf{y}}_{\mathbf{n}}^{\mathbf{T}}\mathbf{R}\hat{\mathbf{x}}_{\mathbf{n}}+\beta\left(\left(\hat{\gamma}_1^{\mathbf{T}}\mathbf{R}\hat{\mathbf{x}}_{\mathbf{n}}\right)^2-\left(\hat{\gamma}_2^{\mathbf{T}}\mathbf{R}\hat{\mathbf{x}}_{\mathbf{n}}\right)^2\right)} . \tag{2}
$$

This function finds the $\mathbf{y} = (\mathbf{y_p}, \hat{\mathbf{y}}_{\mathbf{n}})$ that maximizes the likelihood of a match
with $\mathbf{x} = (\mathbf{x_p}, \hat{\mathbf{x}}_{\mathbf{n}})$. $\boldsymbol{\Sigma} = \mathbf{R}\boldsymbol{\Sigma}_{\mathbf{x}}\mathbf{R}^{\mathbf{T}} + \boldsymbol{\Sigma}_{\mathbf{y}}$, where $\boldsymbol{\Sigma}_{\mathbf{x}}$ and $\boldsymbol{\Sigma}_{\mathbf{y}}$ are the covariance
matrices representing the measurement noise associated with $\mathbf{x}$ and $\mathbf{y}$, $\kappa = \frac{1}{\sigma^2}$
is the concentration parameter of the orientation noise model, where σ is the
SD of orientation noise, and $\beta = e\frac{\kappa}{2}$ controls the anisotropy of the orientation
noise model along with $\hat{\gamma}_1$ and $\hat{\gamma}_2$, which are the major and minor axes that
define the directions of the elliptical level sets of the Kent distribution on the
unit sphere [11,12]. $\hat{\mathbf{y}}_{\mathbf{n}}$, $\hat{\gamma}_1$, $\hat{\gamma}_2$ are orthogonal and $e \in [0, 1]$ is the eccentricity of
the noise model.

Correspondences are computed by minimizing the negative log likelihood
of f_{match} [10]. The main difference in the correspondence phases of G-IMLOP
and GD-IMLOP is that GD-IMLOP computes matched points on the current
deformed shape. Outlier rejection is performed after each correspondence phase.
Under the assumption of generalized Gaussian noise, the square Mahalanobis
distance is approximately distributed as a chi-square distribution with 3 degrees
of freedom (DOF) [11]. Therefore, a match is labeled an outlier if this distance
exceeds the value of a chi-square inverse cumulative density function (CDF)
with 3 DOF at some probability p. That is, if for any corresponding $\mathbf{x}$ and $\mathbf{y}$,
$(\mathbf{y_p} - a\mathbf{R}\mathbf{x_p} - \mathbf{t})^{\mathbf{T}}\boldsymbol{\Sigma}^{-1}(\mathbf{y_p} - a\mathbf{R}\mathbf{x_p} - \mathbf{t}) > \text{chi2inv}(p, 3)$, then that match is an
outlier. Here, we set $p = 0.95$. Matches that are not rejected as outliers using
this test, are evaluated for orientation consistency. Here, a match is an outlier
if $\hat{\mathbf{y}}_{\mathbf{n}}^{\mathbf{T}}\mathbf{R}\hat{\mathbf{x}}_{\mathbf{n}} < \cos(\theta_{\text{thresh}})$, where $\theta_{\text{thresh}} = 3\sigma_{\text{circ}}$ and σ_{circ} is the circular SD
computed using the mean angular error between all correspondences.

Matches that pass these two tests are inliers and a registration between these
points is computed by minimizing the following cost function with respect to the
transformation and shape parameters [10]:

$$
\mathbf{T} = \underset{[a, \mathbf{R}, \mathbf{t}], \mathbf{s}}{\operatorname{argmin}} \left(\frac{1}{2} \sum_{i=1}^{n_{\text{data}}} \left((\mathbf{T}_{\text{ssm}}(\mathbf{y}_{\mathbf{p}_i}) - a\mathbf{R}\mathbf{x}_{\mathbf{p}_i} - \mathbf{t})^{\mathbf{T}}\boldsymbol{\Sigma}^{-1}(\mathbf{T}_{\text{ssm}}(\mathbf{y}_{\mathbf{p}_i}) - a\mathbf{R}\mathbf{x}_{\mathbf{p}_i} - \mathbf{t}) \right) + \right.
$$

$$
\left. \sum_{i=1}^{n_{\text{data}}} \kappa_i(1 - \hat{\mathbf{y}}_{\mathbf{n}_i}^{\mathbf{T}}\mathbf{R}\hat{\mathbf{x}}_{\mathbf{n}_i}) - \sum_{i=1}^{n_{\text{data}}} \beta_i \left(\left(\hat{\gamma}_{1i}^{\mathbf{T}}\mathbf{R}^{\mathbf{T}}\hat{\mathbf{y}}_{\mathbf{n}i}\right)^2 - \left(\hat{\gamma}_{2i}^{\mathbf{T}}\mathbf{R}^{\mathbf{T}}\hat{\mathbf{y}}_{\mathbf{n}i}\right)^2 \right) + \frac{1}{2} \sum_{j=1}^{n_{\text{m}}} \|s_j\|_2^2 \right), \tag{3}
$$

where n_{data} is the number of inlying data points, $\mathbf{x}_i$. This first term in Eq. 3 minimizes the Mahalanobis distance between the positional components of the correspondences, $\mathbf{x_{p_i}}$ and $\mathbf{y_{p_i}}$. $T_{\text{ssm}}(\cdot)$, a term introduced in the registration phase, is a transformation, $T_{\text{ssm}}(\mathbf{y_{p_i}}) = \sum_{j=1}^{3} \mu_i^{(j)} T_{\text{ssm}}(\mathbf{v}_i^{(j)})$, that deforms the matched points, $\mathbf{y}_i$, based on the current $\mathbf{s}$ deforming the model shape [10]. Here, $T_{\text{ssm}}(\mathbf{v}_i) = \bar{\mathbf{v}}_i + \sum_{j=1}^{\mathbf{n}_m} s_j \mathbf{w}_j^{(i)}$, and $\mu_i^{(j)}$ are the 3 barycentric coordinates that describe the position of $\mathbf{y}_i$ on a triangle on the model shape [10]. The second and third terms minimize the angular error between the orientation components of corresponding points, $\hat{\mathbf{x}}_{\mathbf{n}_i}$ and $\hat{\mathbf{y}}_{\mathbf{n}_i}$, while respecting the anisotropy in the orientation noise. The final term minimizes the shape parameters to find the smallest deformation required to modify the model shape to fit the data points, $\mathbf{x}_i$ [10]. $\mathbf{s}$ is initialized to 0, meaning the registration begins with the statistically mean shape. The objective function (Eq. 3) is optimized using a nonlinear constrained quasi-Newton based optimizer, where the constraint is used to ensure that $\mathbf{s}$ are found within ± 3 SDs, since this interval explains 99.7% of the variation.

Once the algorithm has converged, a final set of tests is performed to assign confidence to the computed registration. For position components, this is similar to the outlier rejection test, except now the sum of the square Mahalanobis distance is compared against the value of a chi-square inverse CDF with $3n_{\text{data}}$ DOF [11]; i.e., confidence in a registration begins to degrade if

$$E_p = \sum_{i=1}^{n_{\text{data}}} (\mathbf{y_{p_i}} - a\mathbf{R}\mathbf{x_{p_i}} - \mathbf{t})^{\mathbf{T}} \Sigma^{-1} (\mathbf{y_{p_i}} - a\mathbf{R}\mathbf{x_{p_i}} - \mathbf{t}) > \text{chi2inv}(p, 3n_{\text{data}}). \quad (4)$$

If a registration is successful according to Eq. 4, it is further tested for orientation consistency using a similar chi-square test by approximating the Kent distribution as a 2D wrapped Gaussian [12]. Registration confidence degrades if

$$E_o = \sum_{i=1}^{n_{\text{data}}} \begin{bmatrix} \cos^{-1}(\hat{\mathbf{y}}_{\mathbf{n}_i}{}^{\mathbf{T}}\mathbf{R}\hat{\mathbf{x}}_{\mathbf{n}_i}) \\ \sin^{-1}(\hat{\gamma}_{1_i}{}^{\mathbf{T}}\mathbf{R}^{\mathbf{T}}\hat{\mathbf{y}}_{\mathbf{n}_i}) \\ \sin^{-1}(\hat{\gamma}_{2_i}{}^{\mathbf{T}}\mathbf{R}^{\mathbf{T}}\hat{\mathbf{y}}_{\mathbf{n}_i}) \end{bmatrix}^{\mathbf{T}} \begin{bmatrix} \kappa_i & 0 & 0 \\ 0 & \kappa_i - 2\beta_i & 0 \\ 0 & 0 & \kappa_i + 2\beta_i \end{bmatrix} \begin{bmatrix} \cos^{-1}(\hat{\mathbf{y}}_{\mathbf{n}_i}{}^{\mathbf{T}}\mathbf{R}\hat{\mathbf{x}}_{\mathbf{n}_i}) \\ \sin^{-1}(\hat{\gamma}_{1_i}{}^{\mathbf{T}}\mathbf{R}^{\mathbf{T}}\hat{\mathbf{y}}_{\mathbf{n}_i}) \\ \sin^{-1}(\hat{\gamma}_{2_i}{}^{\mathbf{T}}\mathbf{R}^{\mathbf{T}}\hat{\mathbf{y}}_{\mathbf{n}_i}) \end{bmatrix}$$
$$> \text{chi2inv}(p, 2n_{\text{data}}), \quad (5)$$

since $\hat{\mathbf{y}}_{\mathbf{n}_i}$ must align with $\hat{\mathbf{x}}_{\mathbf{n}_i}$, but remain orthogonal to $\hat{\gamma}_{1_i}$ and $\hat{\gamma}_{2_i}$. p is set to 0.95 for **very confident** success classification. As p increases, the confidence in success classification decreases while that in failure classification increases.

3   Experimental Results and Discussion

Two experiments are conducted to evaluate this system: one using simulated data where ground truth is known, and one using in-vivo clinical data where ground truth is not known. Registrations are computed using $\mathbf{n}_m \in \{0, 10, 20, 30, 40, 50\}$ modes. At 0 modes, this algorithm is essentially G-IMLOP with an additional scale component in the optimization.

3.1   Experiment 1: Simulation

In this experiment, we performed a leave-one-out evaluation using shape models of the right nasal cavity extracted from 53 CTs. 3000 points were sampled from the section of the left out mesh that would be visible to an endoscope inserted into the cavity. Anisotropic noise with SD $0.5 \times 0.5 \times 0.75 \, \text{mm}^3$ and $10°$ with $e = 0.5$ was added to the position and orientation components of the points, respectively, since this produced realistic point clouds compared to in-vivo data with higher uncertainty in the z-direction. A rotation, translation and scale are applied to these points in the intervals $[0, 10]$ mm, $[0, 10]°$ and $[0.95, 1.05]$, respectively. 2 offsets are sampled for each left out shape. GD-IMLOP makes slightly more generous noise assumptions with SDs $1 \times 1 \times 2 \, \text{mm}^3$ and $30°$ ($e = 0.5$) for position and orientation noise, respectively, and restricts scale optimization to within $[0.9, 1.1]$. A registration is considered successful if the total registration error (tRE), computed using the Hausdorff distance (HD) between the left-out shape and the estimated shape transformed to the frame of the registered points, is below 1 mm. The success or failure of the registrations is compared to the outcome predicted by the algorithm. Further, the HD between the left-out and estimated shapes in the same frame is used to evaluate errors in reconstruction.

Results over all modes, using $p = 0.95$, show that E_p is less strict than E_o (Fig. 1), meaning that although E_p identifies all successful registrations correctly, it also allows many unsuccessful registrations to be labeled successful. E_o, on the other hand, correctly classifies fewer successful registrations, but does not label any failed registrations as successful. Therefore, registrations with $E_p < \text{chi2inv}(0.95, 3n_{\text{data}})$ and $E_o < \text{chi2inv}(0.95, 2n_{\text{data}})$ can be **very confidently** classified as successful. The average tRE produced by registrations in this category over all modes was 0.34 (± 0.03) mm. At $p = 0.9975$, more successful registrations were correctly identified (Fig. 1, right). These registrations can be **confidently** classified as successful with mean tRE increasing to 0.62 (± 0.03) mm. Errors in correct classification creep in with $p = 0.9999$, where 3 out of 124 registrations are incorrectly labeled successful. These registrations can be **somewhat confidently** classified as successful with mean tRE increasing

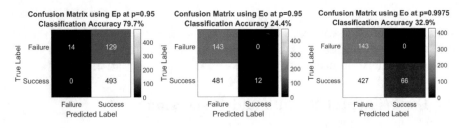

Fig. 1. Left: using only E_p, all successful registration pass the chi-square inverse test at $p = 0.95$. However, many failed registrations also pass this test. Using $p = 0.9975$ produces the same result. Middle: on the other hand, using only E_o, no failed registrations pass the chi-square inverse test at $p = 0.95$, but very few successful registrations pass the test. Right: using $p = 0.9975$, more successful registrations pass the test.

slightly to 0.78 (±0.04) mm. Increasing p to 0.999999 further decreases classification accuracy. 10 out of 121 registrations in this category are incorrectly classified as successful with mean tRE increasing to 0.8 (±0.05) mm. These registrations can, therefore, be classified as successful with **low confidence**. The mean tRE for the remaining registrations increases to over 1 mm at 1.31 (±0.85) mm, with no registration passing the E_p threshold except for registrations using 0 modes. Of these, however, 0 are correctly classified as successful. Therefore, although about half of all registrations in this category are successful, there can be **no confidence** in their correct classification. Figure 2 (left and middle) shows the distribution of tREs in these categories for registrations using 30 and 50 modes.

GD-IMLOP can, therefore, compute successful registrations between a statistically mean right nasal cavity mesh and points sampled only from part of the left-out meshes, and reliably assign confidence to these registrations. Further, GD-IMLOP can accurately estimate the region of the nasal cavity where points are sampled from, while errors gradually deteriorate away from this region, e.g., towards the front of the septum since points are not sampled from this region (Fig. 2, right). Overall, the mean shape estimation error was 0.77 mm.

3.2 Experiment 2: In-Vivo

For the in-vivo experiment, we collected anonymized endoscopic videos of the nasal cavity from consenting patients under an IRB approved study. Dense point clouds were produced from single frames of these videos using a modified version of the learning-based photometric reconstruction technique [13] that uses registered structure from motion (SfM) points to train a neural network to predict dense depth maps. Point clouds from different nearby frames in a sequence were aligned using the relative camera motion from SfM. Small misalignments due to errors in depth estimation were corrected using G-IMLOP with scale to produce a dense reconstruction spanning a large area of the nasal passage. GD-IMLOP is executed with 3000 points sampled from this dense reconstruction assuming noise with SDs $1 \times 1 \times 2\,\text{mm}^3$ and $30°$ ($e = 0.5$) for position and orientation

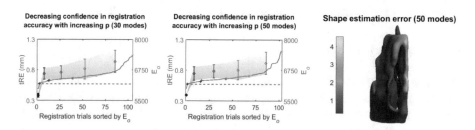

Fig. 2. Left and middle: mean tRE and standard deviation increase as E_o increases. The dotted red line corresponds to chi2inv$(0.95, 2n_{\text{data}})$, below which registrations are classified **very confidently** as successful. Beyond this threshold, confidence gradually degrades. The pink bar indicates that none of these registrations passed the E_p test. Right: average error at each vertex computed over all left-out trials using 50 modes.

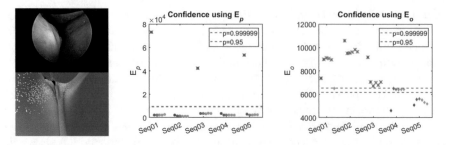

Fig. 3. Left: visualization of the final registration and reconstruction for Seq01 using 50 modes. Middle and right: E_p and E_o for all registrations, respectively, plotted for each sequence. Per sequence, from left to right, the plot points indicate scores achieved using 0-50 modes at increments of 10. Crossed out plot points indicate rejected registrations.

data, respectively, and with scale and shape parameter optimization restricted to within $[0.7, 1.3]$ and ± 1 SD, respectively. We assign confidence to the registrations based on the tests explained in Sect. 2 and validated in Sect. 3.1.

All registrations run with 0 modes terminated at the maximum iteration threshold of 100, while those run using modes converged at an average 10.36 iterations in 26.03 s. Figure 3 shows registrations using increasing modes from left to right for each sequence plotted against E_p (middle) and E_o (right). All deformable registration results pass the E_p test as they fall below the $p = 0.95$ threshold (Fig. 3, middle) using the chi-square inverse test. However, several of these fail the E_o test (Fig. 3, right). Deformable registrations on sequence 01 using 50 modes and on sequence 04 for all except 30 modes pass this test with **low confidence**. Using 30 modes, the registration on sequence 04 passes **somewhat confidently**. The rigid registration on sequence 04 (the only rigid registration to pass both E_p and E_o) and all deformable registrations on sequence 05 pass this test **very confidently**. Although, the rigid registration on sequence 05 passes this test very confidently, E_p already labels it a failed registration. Successful registrations produced a mean residual error of 0.78 (± 0.07) mm. Visualizations of successful registrations also show accurate alignment (Fig. 3, left).

4   Conclusion

We show that GD-IMLOP is able to produce submillimeter registrations in both simulation and in-vivo experiments, and assign confidence to these registrations. Further, it can accurately predict the anatomy where video data is available. In the future, we hope to learn statistics from thousands of CTs to better cover the range of anatomical variations. Additional features like contours can also be used to further improve registration and to add an additional test to evaluate the success of the registration based on contour alignment. Using improved statistics and reconstructions from video along with confidence assignment, this approach can be extended for use in place of CTs during endoscopic procedures.

Acknowledgment. This work was funded by NIH R01-EB015530, NSF Graduate Research Fellowship Program, an Intuitive Surgical, Inc. fellowship, and JHU internal funds.

References

1. Mirota, D.J., Ishii, M., Hager, G.D.: Vision-based navigation in image-guided interventions. Ann. Rev. Biomed. Eng. **13**(1), 297–319 (2011)
2. Azagury, D.E., et al.: Real-time computed tomography-based augmented reality for natural orifice transluminal endoscopic surgery navigation. Brit. J. Surg. **99**(9), 1246–1253 (2012)
3. Beichel, R.R., et al.: Data from QIN-HEADNECK. The Cancer Imaging Archive (2015)
4. Bosch, W.R., Straube, W.L., Matthews, J.W., Purdy, J.A.: Data from head-neck_cetuximab. The Cancer Imaging Archive (2015)
5. Clark, K., et al.: The cancer imaging archive (TCIA): maintaining and operating a public information repository. J. Digit. Imaging **26**(6), 1045–1057 (2013)
6. Fedorov, A., et al.: DICOM for quantitative imaging biomarker development: a standards based approach to sharing clinical data and structured PET/CT analysis results in head and neck cancer research. PeerJ **4**, e2057 (2016)
7. Avants, B.B., Tustison, N.J., Song, G., Cook, P.A., Klein, A., Gee, J.C.: A reproducible evaluation of ANTs similarity metric performance in brain image registration. NeuroImage **54**(3), 2033–2044 (2011)
8. Sinha, A., Reiter, A., Leonard, S., Ishii, M., Hager, G.D., Taylor, R.H.: Simultaneous segmentation and correspondence improvement using statistical modes. In: Proceedings of SPIE, vol. 10133, pp. 101 331B–101 331B–8 (2017)
9. Cootes, T.F., Taylor, C.J., Cooper, D.H., Graham, J.: Active shape models their training and application. Comp. Vis. Image Underst. **61**, 38–59 (1995)
10. Sinha, A., et al.: The deformable most-likely-point paradigm. Med. Image Anal. (Submitted)
11. Billings, S.D., Taylor, R.H.: Generalized iterative most likely oriented-point (G-IMLOP) registration. Int. J. Comput. Assist. Radiol. Surg. **10**(8), 1213–1226 (2015)
12. Mardia, K.V., Jupp, P.E.: Directional statistics. Wiley Series in Probability and Statistics, pp. 1–432. Wiley, Hoboken (2008)
13. Reiter, A., Leonard, S., Sinha, A., Ishii, M., Taylor, R.H., Hager, G.D.: Endoscopic-CT: learning-based photometric reconstruction for endoscopic sinus surgery. In: Proceedings of SPIE, vol. 9784, pp. 978 418–978 418–6 (2016)

A Novel Mixed Reality Navigation System for Laparoscopy Surgery

Jagadeesan Jayender[1,2(✉)], Brian Xavier[3], Franklin King[1],
Ahmed Hosny[3], David Black[4], Steve Pieper[5], and Ali Tavakkoli[1,2]

[1] Brigham and Women's Hospital, Boston, MA 02115, USA
jayender@bwh.harvard.edu
[2] Harvard Medical School, Boston, MA 02115, USA
[3] Boston Medical School, Boston, MA 02115, USA
[4] Fraunhofer MEVIS, Bremen, Germany
[5] Isomics, Inc., Boston, MA 02115, USA

Abstract. OBJECTIVE: To design and validate a novel mixed reality head-mounted display for intraoperative surgical navigation. DESIGN: A mixed reality navigation for laparoscopic surgery (MRNLS) system using a head mounted display (HMD) was developed to integrate the displays from a laparoscope, navigation system, and diagnostic imaging to provide context-specific information to the surgeon. Further, an immersive auditory feedback was also provided to the user. Sixteen surgeons were recruited to quantify the differential improvement in performance based on the mode of guidance provided to the user (laparoscopic navigation with CT guidance (LN-CT) versus mixed reality navigation for laparoscopic surgery (MRNLS)). The users performed three tasks: (1) standard peg transfer, (2) radiolabeled peg identification and transfer, and (3) radiolabeled peg identification and transfer through sensitive wire structures. RESULTS: For the more complex task of peg identification and transfer, significant improvements were observed in time to completion, kinematics such as mean velocity, and task load index subscales of mental demand and effort when using the MRNLS ($p < 0.05$) compared to the current standard of LN-CT. For the final task of peg identification and transfer through sensitive structures, time taken to complete the task and frustration were significantly lower for MRNLS compared to the LN-CT approach. CONCLUSIONS: A novel mixed reality navigation for laparoscopic surgery (MRNLS) has been designed and validated. The ergonomics of laparoscopic procedures could be improved while minimizing the necessity of additional monitors in the operating room.

Keywords: Mixed-reality · Surgical navigation · Laparoscopy surgery
Audio navigation · Visual navigation · Ergonomics

This project was supported by the National Institute of Biomedical Imaging and Bioengineering of the National Institutes of Health through Grant Numbers P41EB015898 and P41RR019703, and a Research Grant from Siemens-Healthineers USA.

© Springer Nature Switzerland AG 2018
A. F. Frangi et al. (Eds.): MICCAI 2018, LNCS 11073, pp. 72–80, 2018.
https://doi.org/10.1007/978-3-030-00937-3_9

1   Introduction

For several years now, surgeons have been aware of the greater physical stress and mental strain during minimally invasive surgery (MIS) compared to their experience with open surgery [1, 2]. Limitations of MIS include lack of adequate access to the anatomy, perceptual challenges and poor ergonomics [3]. The laparoscopic view only provides surface visualization of the anatomy. The internal structures are not revealed on white light laparoscopic imaging, preventing visualization of underlying sensitive structures. This limitation could lead to increased minor or major complications. To overcome this problem, the surrounding structures can be extracted from volumetric diagnostic or intraprocedural CT/MRI/C-arm CT imaging and augmented with the laparoscopic view [4–6]. However, interpreting and fusing the models extracted from volumetric imaging with the laparoscopic images by the surgeon intraoperatively is time-consuming and could add stress to an already challenging procedure. Presenting the information to the surgeon in an intuitive way is key to avoiding information overload for better outcomes [7]. Ergonomics also plays an important role in laparoscopic surgery. It not only improves the performance of the surgeon but also minimizes the physical stress and mental demand [8]. A recent survey of 317 laparoscopic surgeons reported that an astonishing 86.9% of MIS surgeons suffered from physical symptoms of pain or discomfort [9]. Typically, during laparoscopic surgery, the display monitor is placed outside the sterile field at a particular height and distance, which forces the surgeon to work in a direction not in line with the viewing direction. This causes eye-strain and physical discomfort of the neck, shoulders, and upper extremities. Continuous viewing of the images on a monitor can lead to prolonged contraction of the extraocular and ciliary muscles, which can lead to eye-strain [9]. This paper aims to address the problem of improving the image visualization and ergonomics of MIS procedures by taking advantage of advances in the area of virtual, mixed and augmented reality.

2   Mixed Reality Navigation for Laparoscopy Surgery

A novel MRNLS application was developed using the combination of an Oculus Rift Development Kit 2 virtual reality headset, modified to include two front-facing pass-through cameras, navigation system, auditory feedback and a virtual environment created and rendered using the Unity environment.

2.1   Mixed-Reality Head Mounted Display (HMD)

The Oculus Rift Development Kit 2 (DK2) is a stereoscopic head-mounted virtual reality display that uses a 1920 × 1080 pixel display (960 × 1080 pixels per eye) in combination with lenses to produce a stereoscopic image for the user with an approximately 90° horizontal field of view. The headset also features 6 degrees of freedom rotational and positional head tracking achieved via gyroscope, accelerometer, magnetometer, and infrared LEDs with an external infrared camera. A custom fitted mount for the DK2 was designed and created to hold two wide-angle fisheye lens cameras, as shown in Fig. 1. The cameras add the ability to provide a stereoscopic real-world view to the user. The field of view for each camera was set to 90° for this mixed reality application. The double-camera mount prototype was 3D printed allowing for adjusting the interpupillary distance as well as the angle of inclination for convergence between the 2 cameras. These adjustments were designed to be independent of one another. Camera resolution was at 640 × 480 pixels each. It was found that the interpupillary distance had the greatest contribution to double vision - and was hence adjusted differently from one user to another. The prototype was designed to be as lightweight and stable as possible to avoid excessive added weight to the headset and undesired play during head motion respectively. An existing leap motion attachment was used to attach the camera mount to the headset.

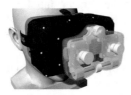 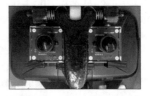

Fig. 1. (left) CAD model showing the camera attachment. (right) 3D printed attachment on the Oculus Rift.

2.2 Mixed Reality Navigation Software

A virtual environment was created using Unity 3D and rendered to the Oculus Rift headset worn by the user (Fig. 2). As seen in Fig. 3, a real-world view provided by the mounted cameras is virtually projected in front of the user. Unlike the real-world view, virtual objects are not tethered to the user's head movements. The combination of a real-world view and virtual objects creates a mixed reality environment for the user. Multiple virtual monitors are arranged in front of the user displaying a laparoscope camera view, a navigation view, and diagnostic/intraprocedural images.

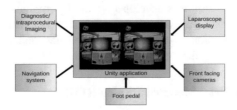

Fig. 2. Software layout of the mixed reality navigation for laparoscopic surgery.

Diagnostic/Intraprocedural Images. A custom web server module was created for 3D Slicer allowing for external applications to query and render DICOM image data to the headset. Similar to the VR diagnostic application [ref-withheld], we have developed a web server module in 3D Slicer to forward volume slice image data to the MR application, created using the Unity game engine. The Unity application created a scene viewable within the HMD and query the 3D Slicer Web Server module for a snapshot of image slice windows, which is then displayed and arrayed within the Unity scene. The Unity application renders the scene stereoscopically with distortion and chromatic aberration compensating for the DK2's lenses. At startup, image datasets were arrayed hemispherically at a distance allowing for a quick preview of the image content, but not at the detail required for in-depth examination. Using a foot pedal while placing the visual reticule on the images brings the image window closer to allow for in-depth examination.

Surgical Navigation Module (iNavAMIGO). The iNavAMIGO module was built using the Wizard workflow using Qt and C++. The advantage of this workflow is that it allows the user to step through the different steps of setting up the navigation system in a systematic method. The Wizard workflow consists of the following steps – (a) Pre-operative planning, (b) Setting up the OpenIGTLink Server and the Instruments, (c) Calibration of the tool, (d) Patient to Image Registration, (e) Setting up Displays, (f) Postoperative Assessment, and (g) Logging Data.

Setting up the OpenIGTLink Server and the Instruments. In this step, an OpenIGTLink server is initiated to allow for the communication with the EndoTrack module. The EndoTrack module is a command line module that interfaces to the electromagnetic tracking system (Ascension Technologies, Vermont, USA) to track the surgical instruments in real-time. Further an additional server is setup to communicate with a client responsible for the audio feedback. Visualization Toolkit (VTK) models of the grasper and laparoscope are created and set to observe the sensor transforms. Motion of the sensor directly controls the display of the instrument models in 3D Slicer.

Calibration and Registration. Since the EM sensors are placed at an offset from the instrument tip, calibration algorithms are developed to account for this offset. The calibration of the instruments is performed using a second sensor that computes the offset of the instrument tip from the sensor location. Although the iNavAMIGO module supports a number of algorithms to register the EM to imaging space, in this work we have used fiducial-based landmark registration algorithm to register the motion of the instruments with respect to the imaging space.

Displays. The display consists of three panes – the top view shows the three-dimensional view of the instruments and the peg board. This view also displays the distance of the grasper from the target and the orthogonal distance of the grasper from the target. The bottom left view shows the virtual laparoscopic view while the bottom right view shows the three-dimensional view from the tip of the grasper instrument. The instrument-display models and the two bottom views are updated in real-time and displayed to the user. The display of the navigation software is captured using a video capture card (Epiphan DVI2PCI2, Canada) and imported into the Unity game development platform. Using the VideoCapture API in Unity, the video from the navigation software is textured and layered into the Unity Scene. The navigation display pane is placed in front of the user at an elevation angle of $-30°$ within the HMD (Fig. 3 (right)).

Laparoscopic and Camera View. Video input from both front-facing cameras mounted on the HMD was received by the Unity application via USB. The video input was then projected onto a curved plane corresponding to the field of view of the webcams in order to undistort the image. A separate camera view was visible to each eye creating a real-time stereoscopic pass-through view of the real environment from within the virtual environment. Laparoscopic video input was also received by the Unity application via a capture card (Epiphan DVI2PCI2, Canada). The laparoscopic video appears as a texture on an object acting as a virtual monitor. Since the laparoscopy video is the primary imaging modality, this video is displayed on the virtual monitor placed 15° below the eye level at 100 cm from the user. The virtual monitor for the laparoscopy video is also be placed directly in line with the hands of the surgeon to minimize the stress on the back, neck and shoulder muscles, see Fig. 3 (right).

2.3   Audio Navigation System

The auditory feedback changes corresponding to the grasper motion in 3DOFs. In basic terms, up-and-down (elevation) changes are mapped to the pitch of a tone that alternates with a steady tone so that the two pitches can be compared. Changes in left-and-right motion (azimuth) are mapped to the stereo position of the sound output, such that feedback is in both ears when the grasper is centered. Finally, the distance of the tracked grasper to the target is mapped to the inter-onset interval of the tones, such that approaching the target results in a decrease in inter-onset interval; the tones are played faster. The synthesized tone consists of three triangle oscillators, for which the amplitude and frequency ratios are 1, 0.5, 0.3 and 1, 2, and 4, respectively. The frequency of the moving base tone is mapped to changes in elevation. The pitches range from note numbers 48 to 72 on the Musical Instrument Digital Interface (MIDI). These correspond to a frequency range of 130.81 Hz to 523.25 Hz, respectively. Pitches are quantized to a C-major scale. For the y axis (elevation), the frequency f of the moving base tone changes as per the elevation angle. The pitch of the reference tone is MIDI note 60 (261.62 Hz). Thus, the moving tone and reference tone are played in a repeating alternating fashion, so that the user can compare the pitches and manipulate the pitch of the moving tone such that the two pitches are the same and elevation $y = 0$. Movement along the azimuth (x-axis) is mapped to the stereo position of the output synthesizer signal. Using this mapping method, the tip of the grasper is imagined as the 'listener,' and the target position is the sound source, so that the grasper should be navigated towards the sound source.

3   Experimental Methods

A pilot study was conducted to validate the use of the head mounted device based mixed reality surgical navigation environment in the operating room simulated by a FLS skills training box. IRB approval was waived for this study.

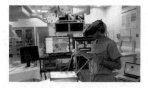 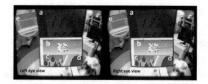

Fig. 3. (left) User with the MRNLS performing the trial (right) view provided to the user through the HMD. Virtual monitors show the laparoscopy view (panel a - red hue) and the navigation system display (panel b, c, d). The surrounding environment (label e) can also be seen through the HMD.

Participants were asked to complete a series of peg transfer tasks on a previously validated FLS skills trainer, the Ethicon TASKit - Train Anywhere Skill Kit (Ethicon Endo-Surgery Cincinnati, OH, USA). Modifications were made to the Ethicon TASKit to incrementally advance the difficulty of the tasks as well as to streamline data acquisition (see Fig. 4 (left)). Two pegboards were placed in the box instead of one to increase the yield of each trial. The pegboards were placed inside a plastic container that was filled with water, red dye, and cornstarch to simulate decreased visibility for the operator and increased reliance on the navigation system. Depending on the task, visualization and navigation would be performed using laparoscopic navigation with CT imaging (LN-CT, standard of care) or mixed reality navigation (MRNLS).

Tasks 1 and 2 - Peg Transfer. Using standardized instructions, participants were briefed on the task goals of transferring all pegs from the bottom six posts to the top six posts and then back to their starting position. This task was done on two pegboards using the LN-CT (task 1) and then repeated using the head mounted device (task 2). No additional information or navigation system was given to the participants while wearing the head mounted device other than the laparoscopic camera feed. To determine time and accuracy of each trial, grasper kinematics were recorded from the grasper sensor readings, including path length, velocity, acceleration, and jerk.

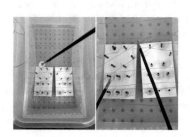 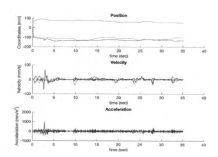

Fig. 4. (left) Example trajectory of the grasper as recorded by the EM sensor.

Tasks 3 and 4 - "Tumor" Peg Identification and Transfer. Tasks 3 and 4 were designed as a modified peg transfer with a focus on using the navigation system and all information to identify and select a target "tumor" peg from surrounding normal pegs, which were visually similar to the "tumor" peg but distinct on CT images. Participants were instructed to use the given navigation modalities to identify and lift the "tumor" peg on each pegboard and transfer it to the last row at the top of the pegboard. Task 3 had participants use the standard approach of laparoscopy and CT guidance (LN-CT), whereas task 4 was done with the laparoscopic feed, audio navigation, and 3D renderings integrated on the mixed reality HMD environment, i.e., the MRNLS. Metrics recorded included time to completion, peg drops, incorrect peg selections, and probe kinematics such as path length, velocity, acceleration, and jerk.

Tasks 5 and 6 - "Tumor" Peg Identification and Transfer Through Sensitive Structures. For the final two tasks, modifications were made to the laparoscopic skills trainer box to stress the navigation system and recreate possible intraoperative obstacles such as vasculature, nerves, and ducts. Using a plastic frame and conductive wire, an intricate structure was made that could easily be attached for tasks 5 and 6. The structure held the conductive wire above the pegboards in three random, linear tiers (Fig. 4 (left)). A data acquisition card (Sensoray S826, OR, USA) was used to asynchronously detect contact with the wires by polling the digital input ports at a sampling rate of 22 Hz. Contact between the grasper and the wires could then be registered and tracked over time. Operators were asked to identify the radiolabeled "tumor" peg and transfer this peg to the last row on the pegboards. However, in this task they were also instructed to do so while minimizing contact with the sensitive structures. In task 5, participants used the current standard approach of LN-CT, while in task 6, they used the proposed MRNLS system with fully integrated audio feedback, 3D render-based, and image guided navigation environment viewed on the HMD.

Participants. A total of 16 surgeons with different experience levels in laparoscopic surgery volunteered to participate in the study and were assigned to novice or experienced subject groups. Novice surgical subjects included participants who performed more than 10 laparoscopic surgeries as the secondary operator but less than 100 laparoscopic surgeries as the primary operator. Experienced subjects were those who performed more than 100 laparoscopic surgeries as primary operator.

Questionnaire and Training Period. Following each task, participants were asked to complete a NASA Task Load Index questionnaire to assess the workload of that approach on six scales: mental demand, physical demand, temporal demand, performance, effort, and frustration.

Statistical Analysis. The Wilcoxon signed-rank test for non-parametric analysis of paired sample data was used to compare the distributions of metrics for all participants by task. The Mann-Whitney U test was used to compare distributions in all metrics between novice and expert cohorts. $P < 0.05$ was considered statistically significant.

4   Results and Discussion

Figure 4 (right) shows an example trajectory of one of the trials, from which the kinematic parameters have been derived.

Tasks 1 and 2

On the initial baseline peg transfer task with no additional navigational modalities, participants took longer to complete the task when viewing the laparoscopic video feed on the mixed reality HMD, as part of the MRNLS (standard: 166.9 s; mixed reality: 210.1 s; P = 0.001). On cohort analysis, expert participants showed higher significance in time to completion than novices (P = 0.004, P = 0.011). Additionally, there was no difference in number of peg drops or kinematic parameters such as the mean velocity, mean acceleration, and mean jerks per subject amongst all participants or by expertise. During these baseline tasks, mental demand, physical demand, and frustration were significantly increased (P < 0.05) when using the mixed reality HMD environment with mildly significant decrease in perceived performance (P = 0.01). However, effort and temporal demand showed no significant differences amongst all subjects nor novices and experts.

Tasks 3 and 4

Compared to the standard LN-CT in task 3, all participants showed significant decrease in time to completion with the aid of the MRNLS (decrease in time = −20.03 s, P = 0.017). When comparing the addition of the MRNLS in task 4 to the standard approach in novice and expert participants, novice participants showed significant improvements in mean velocity, mean acceleration, and mean jerks between tasks 3 and 4, compared to only mean velocity in experts. Mental demand was significantly decreased when combining the results of both novice and expert participants (P = 0.022) and there was near significance for performance (P = 0.063) and effort (P = 0.089) for the MRNLS.

Tasks 5 and 6

Tasks 5 and 6 were designed to compare the standard LN-CT and proposed MRNLS on a complex, modified task. These final tasks again demonstrated significantly faster time to completion when using the MRNLS in task 8 (100.74 s) versus the LN-CT in task 7 (131.92 s; P = 0.044.) All other kinematic metrics such as average velocity, acceleration, jerks, as well as time in contact with sensitive wire structures, peg drops, or incorrect selections showed no significant difference between navigation modalities for all participants, novices, or experts. Amongst novice participants, there was a decrease in the means of time to completion (−45.5 s), time in contact (−14.5 s), and path length (−432.5 mm) while amongst experts there was a smaller decrease in these metrics (−20.1 s, 2.12 s, −163.1 mm) for the MRNLS. Novices were twice as likely to make an incorrect selection using LN-CT versus MRNLS, however, and experts were 3 times as likely. According to the NASA Task Load Index values, the effort that participants reported to complete the task was significantly lower using the MRNLS compared to the LN-CT (Difference of 1.375, P = 0.011). Upon analysis by expert group, this significance is present among the novice participants but not among expert participants (Novices: −2.57, P = 0.031; Experts: −0.44; P = 0.34). There was a similar result for frustration that was near significance (All participants: −1.38, P = 0.051; Novices: −2.43, P = 0.063; Experts: −0.22, P = 1).

5 Conclusion

We have validated the use of a novel mixed reality head mounted display navigation environment for the intraoperative surgical navigation use. Although further studies are warranted, we find the use of this novel surgical navigation environment proves ready for in-vivo trials with the objective of additionally showing added benefits with respect to surgical success, complication rates, and patient-reported outcomes.

References

1. Patkin, M., Isabel, L.: Ergonomics, engineering and surgery of endosurgical dissection. J. R. Coll. Surg. Edinb. **40**(2), 120–132 (1995)
2. Kant, I.J., et al.: A survey of static and dynamic work postures of operating room staff. Int. Arch. Occup. Environ. Health **63**(6), 423–428 (1992)
3. Keehner, M.M., et al.: Spatial ability, experience, and skill in laparoscopic surgery. Am. J. Surg. **188**(1), 71–75 (2004)
4. Fuchs, H., et al.: Augmented reality visualization for laparoscopic surgery. In: Wells, W.M., Colchester, A., Delp, S. (eds.) MICCAI 1998. LNCS, vol. 1496, pp. 934–943. Springer, Heidelberg (1998). https://doi.org/10.1007/BFb0056282
5. Mountney, P., Fallert, J., Nicolau, S., Soler, L., Mewes, Philip W.: An augmented reality framework for soft tissue surgery. In: Golland, P., Hata, N., Barillot, C., Hornegger, J., Howe, R. (eds.) MICCAI 2014. LNCS, vol. 8673, pp. 423–431. Springer, Cham (2014). https://doi.org/10.1007/978-3-319-10404-1_53
6. Shuhaiber, J.H.: Augmented reality in surgery. Arch. Surg. **139**(2), 170–174 (2004)
7. Dixon, B.J., et al.: Surgeons blinded by enhanced navigation: the effect of augmented reality on attention. Surg. Endosc. **27**(2), 454–461 (2013)
8. Erfanian, K., et al.: In-line image projection accelerates task performance in laparoscopic appendectomy. J. Pediatr. Surg. **38**(7), 1059–1062 (2003)
9. Park, A., Lee, G., et al.: Patients benefit while surgeons suffer: an impending epidemic. J. Am. Coll. Surg. **210**(3), 306–313 (2010)

Respiratory Motion Modelling
Using cGANs

Alina Giger[1], Robin Sandkühler[1], Christoph Jud[1(✉)], Grzegorz Bauman[1,2],
Oliver Bieri[1,2], Rares Salomir[3], and Philippe C. Cattin[1]

[1] Department of Biomedical Engineering, University of Basel, Allschwil, Switzerland
{alina.giger,christoph.jud}@unibas.ch
[2] Department of Radiology, Division of Radiological Physics,
University Hospital Basel, Basel, Switzerland
[3] Image Guided Interventions Laboratory, University of Geneva,
Geneva, Switzerland

Abstract. Respiratory motion models in radiotherapy are considered as one possible approach for tracking mobile tumours in the thorax and abdomen with the goal to ensure target coverage and dose conformation. We present a patient-specific motion modelling approach which combines navigator-based 4D MRI with recent developments in deformable image registration and deep neural networks. The proposed regression model based on conditional generative adversarial nets (cGANs) is trained to learn the relation between temporally related US and MR navigator images. Prior to treatment, simultaneous ultrasound (US) and 4D MRI data is acquired. During dose delivery, online US imaging is used as surrogate to predict complete 3D MR volumes of different respiration states ahead of time. Experimental validations on three volunteer lung datasets demonstrate the potential of the proposed model both in terms of qualitative and quantitative results, and computational time required.

Keywords: Respiratory motion model · 4D MRI · cGAN

1 Introduction

Respiratory organ motion causes serious difficulties in image acquisition and image-guided interventions in abdominal or thoracic organs, such as liver or lungs. In the field of radiotherapy, respiration induced tumour motion has to be taken into account in order to precisely deliver the radiation dose to the target volume while sparing the surrounding healthy tissue and organs at risk. With the introduction of increasingly precise radiation delivery systems, such as pencil beam scanned (PBS) proton therapy, suitable motion mitigation techniques are required to fully exploit the advantages which come with conformal dose delivery [2]. Tumour tracking based on respiratory motion modelling provides a potential solution to these problems, and as a result a large variety of motion models and surrogate data have been proposed in recent years [7].

© Springer Nature Switzerland AG 2018
A. F. Frangi et al. (Eds.): MICCAI 2018, LNCS 11073, pp. 81–88, 2018.
https://doi.org/10.1007/978-3-030-00937-3_10

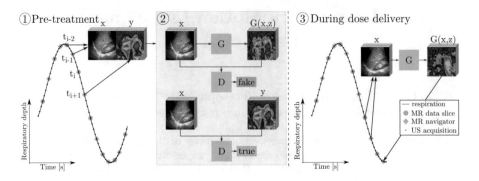

Fig. 1. Schematics of the motion modelling pipeline. See Sect. 2 for details.

In this work we present an image-driven and patient-specific motion modelling approach relying on 2D ultrasound (US) images as surrogate data. The proposed approach is targeted primarily but not exclusively at PBS proton therapy of lung tumours. We combine hybrid US and magnetic resonance imaging (MRI), navigator-based 4D MRI methods [12] and recent developments in deep neural networks [4,6] into a motion modelling pipeline as illustrated in Fig. 1. In a pre-treatment phase, a regression model between abdominal US images and 2D deformation fields of MR navigator scans is learned using the conditional adversarial network presented in [6]. During dose delivery, US images are used as inputs to the trained model in order to generate the corresponding navigator deformation field, and hence to predict a 3D MR volume of the patient.

Artificial neural networks (ANN) have previously been investigated for time-series prediction in image-guided radiotherapy in order to cope with system latencies [3,5]. While these approaches rely on relatively simple network architectures, such as multilayer perceptrons with one hidden layer only, a more recent work combines fuzzy logic and an ANN with four hidden layers to predict intra- and inter-fractional variations of lung tumours [8]. Common to the aforementioned methods is that the respiratory motion was retrieved from external markers attached to the patients' chest, either measured with fluoroscopy [5] or LED sensors and cameras [8]. However, external surrogate data might suffer from a lack of correlation between the measured respiratory motion and the actual internal organ motion [12]. To overcome these limitations, the use of US surrogates for motion modelling offers a potential solution. In [9], anatomical landmarks extracted from US images in combination with a population-based statistical shape model are used for spatial and temporal prediction of the liver. Our work has several distinct advantages over [9]: we are able to build patient-specific and dense volume motion models without the need for manual landmark annotation. Moreover, hybrid US/MR imaging has been investigated for out-of-bore synthesis of MR images [10]. A single-element US transducer was used for generating two orthogonal MR slices.

The proposed image-driven motion modelling approach has only become feasible with recent advances in deep learning, in particular with the introduction of generative adversarial nets (GANs) [4]. In this framework, two models are trained simultaneously while competing with each other: a generative model G aims to fool an adversarially trained discriminator D, while the latter learns to distinguish between real and generated images. Conditional GANs (cGANs) have shown to be suitable for a multitude of image-to-image translation tasks due to their generic formulation of the loss function [6]. We exploit the properties of cGANs in order to synthesize deformation fields of MR images given 2D US images as inputs.

While all components used within the proposed motion modelling framework have been presented previously, to the best of our knowledge, this is the first approach which suggests to integrate deep neural networks into the field of respiratory motion modelling and 4D MR imaging. We believe the strength of this work lies in the novelty of the motion modelling pipeline and underline two contributions: First, we investigate the practicability of cGANs for medical images where only relatively small training sets are available. Second, we present a patient-specific motion model which is capable of predicting complete MR volumes within reasonable time for image-guided radiotherapy. Moreover, thanks to the properties of the applied 4D MRI method and the availability of ground truth MR scans, we are able to quantitatively validate the prediction accuracy of the proposed approach within a proof-of-concept study.

2   Method

Although MR navigators have been proved to be suitable surrogate data for 4D MR imaging and motion modelling [7,12], this imaging modality is often not available during dose delivery in radiotherapy. Inspired by image-to-image translation, one could think of a two step process to overcome this limitation: first, a cGAN is trained to learn the relation between surrogate images available during treatment and 2D MR images. Second, following the 4D MRI approach of [12], an MR volume is stacked after registering the generated MR navigator to a master image. The main idea of the approach proposed here is to join these two steps into one by learning the relation between abdominal US images and the corresponding deformation fields of 2D MR navigator slices. Directly predicting navigator deformation fields has the major benefit that image registration during treatment is rendered obsolete as it is inherently learned by the neural network. Since this method is sensitive to the US imaging plane, we assume that the patient remains in supine position and does not stand up between the pre-treatment data acquisition and the dose delivery. The motion modelling pipeline consists of three main steps as illustrated in Fig. 1 and explained below.

2.1   Data Acquisition and Image Registration

Simultaneous US/MR imaging and the interleaved MR acquisition scheme for 4D MR imaging [12] constitute the first key component as shown in step ① of Fig. 1. For 4D MRI, free respiration acquisition of the target volume is performed using dynamic 2D MR images in sequential order. Interleaved to these so-called data slices, a 2D navigator scan at fixed slice position is acquired. All MR navigator slices are registered to an arbitrary master navigator image in order to obtain 2D deformation fields. Following the slice stacking approach, the data slices representing the organ of interest in the most similar respiration state are grouped to form a 3D MR volume. The respiratory state of the data slices is determined by comparing the deformation fields of the embracing navigator slices. For further details on 4D MRI, we refer to [12]. Unlike [12], deformable image registration of the navigator slices is performed using the approach proposed in [11], which was specifically developed for mask-free lung image registration.

We combine the 4D MRI approach with simultaneous acquisition of US images in order to establish temporal correspondence between the MR navigators and the US surrogate data. For the US image to capture the respiratory motion, an MR-compatible US probe is placed on the subject's abdominal wall such that the diaphragm's motion is clearly visible. The US probe is fastened tightly by means of a strap passed around the subject's chest.

2.2   Training of the Neural Network

We apply image-to-image translation as proposed in [6] in order to learn the regression model between navigator deformation fields and US images. The cGAN is illustrated in step ② of Fig. 1: the generator G learns the mapping from the recorded US images x and a random noise vector z to the deformation field y, i.e. $G : \{x, z\} \mapsto y$. The discriminator D learns to classify between real and synthesised image pairs. For the network to be able to distinguish between mid-cycle states during inhalation and exhalation, respectively, we introduce gradient information by feeding two consecutive US images as input to the cGAN. Since the deformation field has two components, one in x and one y direction, the network is trained for two input and two output channels. Moreover, instead of learning the relation between temporally corresponding data of the two imaging modalities, we introduce a time shift: given the US images at times t_{i-2} and t_{i-1}, we aim to predict the deformation field at time t_{i+1}. Together with the previously generated deformation field at time t_{i-1}, we are then able to reconstruct an MR volume at t_i as the estimates of the embracing navigators are known. In real-time applications, this time shift allows for system latency compensation.

2.3   Real-Time Prediction of Deformation Fields and Stacking

During dose delivery, US images are continuously acquired and fed to the trained cGAN (see step ③ in Fig. 1). The generated deformation fields at times t_{i-1} and t_{i+1} are used to generate a complete MR volume at time t_i by stacking the MR data slices acquired in step ①, analogous to [12].

3   Experiments and Results

Data Acquisition. The data used in this work was tailored to develop a motion model of the lungs with abdominal US images of the liver and the diaphragm as surrogates. Three hybrid US/MR datasets of two healthy volunteers were acquired on a 1.5 Tesla MR-scanner (MAGNETOM Aera, Siemens Healthineers, Erlangen, Germany) using an ultra-fast balanced steady-state free precession (uf-bSSFP) pulse sequence [1] with the following parameters: flip angle $\alpha = 35°$, TE = 0.86 ms, TR = 1.91 ms, pixel spacing 2.08 mm, slice thickness 8 mm, spacing between slices 5.36 mm, image dimensions $192 \times 190 \times 32$ (rows $\times$ columns $\times$ slice positions). Coronal multi-slice MR scans were acquired in sequential order at a temporal resolution of $f_{MR} = 2.5$ Hz which drops to $f_{MR}/2 = 1.25$ Hz for data slices and navigators considered separately. Simultaneous US imaging was performed at $f_{US} = 20$ Hz using a specifically developed MR-compatible US probe and an Acuson clinical scanner (Antares, Siemens Healthineers, Mountain View, CA). Although the time sampling points of the MR and the US scans did not exactly coincide, we assumed that corresponding image pairs represent the lungs at sufficiently similar respiration states since f_{US} was considerably higher than f_{MR}. The time horizon for motion prediction was $t_h = 1/f_{MR} = 400$ ms.

For each dataset, MR images were acquired for a duration of 9.5 min resulting in 22 dynamics or complete scans of the target volume. Two datasets of the same volunteer were acquired after the volunteer had been sitting for a couple of minutes and the US probe was removed and repositioned. We treat these datasets separately since the US imaging plane and the position of the volunteer within the MR bore changed. The number of data slices and navigators per dataset was $N = 704$ each. Volunteer 2 was advised to breath irregularly for the last couple of breathing cycles. However, we excluded these data for the quantitative analysis below. The datasets were split into $N_{train} = 480$ training images and $N_{test} = \{224, 100, 110\}$ test images for datasets $\{1, 2, 3\}$, respectively. We assumed that the training data represents the pretreatment data as described in Sect. 2.1. It comprised the first 6.4 min or 15 dynamics of the dataset.

Training Details. We adapted the PyTorch implementation for paired image-to-image translation [6] in order for the network to cope with medical images and data with two input and two output channels. The US and MR images were cropped and resized to 256×256 pixels. We used the U-Net based generator architecture, the convolutional PatchGAN classifier as discriminator and default training parameters as proposed in [6]. For each dataset, the network was trained from scratch using the training sets described above and training was stopped after 20 epochs or roughly 7 min.

Validation. For each consecutive navigator pair of the test set a complete MR volume was stacked using the data slices of the training set as possible candidates. In the following, we compare our approach with a reference method and introduce the following notation: RDF is referred to as the reference stacking method using the deformation fields computed on the actually recorded MR navigator slices, and GDF denotes the proposed approach based on the generated deformation fields obtained as a result of the cGAN.

The 2D histogram in Fig. 2 shows the correlation of the slices selected either by RDF or GDF. The bins represent the dynamics of the acquisition and a strong

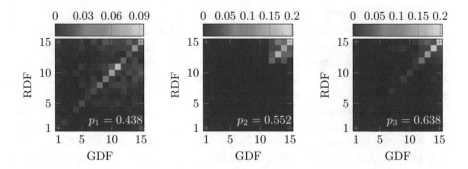

Fig. 2. Slice selection illustrated as joint histogram for reference and generated deformation fields, respectively. From left to right: datasets 1 to 3.

diagonal line is to be expected if the two methods select the same data slices for stacking. The sum over the diagonals, that is the percentage of equally selected slices, is indicated as p_k for dataset $k \in \{1, 2, 3\}$. For all datasets the diagonal is clearly visible and the matching rates are in the range of 43.8% to 63.8%. While these numbers give a first indication of whether the generated deformation fields are able to stack reasonable volumes, they are not a quantitative measure of quality: two different but very similar data slices could be picked by the two methods which would lead to off-diagonal entries but without affecting the image quality of the generated MR volumes.

The histograms for datasets 2 and 3 suggest a further conclusion: the data slices used for stacking are predominantly chosen from the last four dynamics of the training sets (96.5% and 81.7%). Visual inspection of the US images in dataset 2 revealed that one dominant vessel structure appeared more clearly starting from dynamic 11 onwards. This might have been caused by a change in the characteristics of the organ motion, such as organ drift, or a shift of the US probe and emphasises the need for internal surrogate data.

Qualitative comparison of a sample deformation field is shown in Fig. 3a where the reference and the predicted deformations are overlaid. Satisfactory alignment can be observed with the exception of minor deviations in the region of the intestine and the heart. Visual inspection of the stacked volumes by either of the two methods RDF and GDF revealed only minor discontinuities in organ boundaries and vessel structures.

Quantitative results were computed on the basis of image comparison: Each navigator pair of the test set embraces a data slice acquired at a specific slice position. We computed the difference between the training data slice selected for stacking and the actually acquired MR image representing the ground truth. The error was quantified as mean deformation field after 2D registration was performed using the same registration method as in Sect. 2.1 [11]. The median error lies below 1 mm and the maximum error below 3 mm for all datasets and both methods. The average prediction accuracy can compete with previously reported

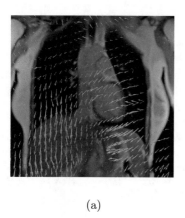

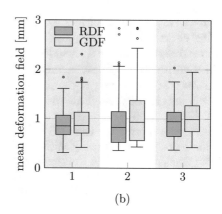

(a)   (b)

Fig. 3. Qualitative and quantitative results. (a) Sample motion field of dataset 2 with reference (green) and predicted (yellow) deformations, and (b) error distribution quantified as mean deformation field.

values [9]. Comparing RDF and GDF, slightly better results were achieved for the reference method which is, however, not available during treatment.

The proposed method required a mean computation time of 20 ms for predicting the deformation field on a NVIDIA Tesla V100 GPU, and 100 ms for slice selection and stacking on a standard CPU. With a prediction horizon of $t_h = 400$ ms, the motion model is real-time applicable and allows for online tracking of the target volume.

4   Discussion and Conclusion

We presented a novel motion modelling framework which is persuasive in several perspectives: the motion model relies on internal surrogate data, it is patient-specific and capable of predicting dense volume information within reasonable computation time for real-time applications, while training of the regression model can be performed within 7 min only.

We are aware, though, that the proposed approach demands further investigation: It shares the limitation with most motion models that respiration states which have not been observed during pretreatment imaging cannot be reconstructed during dose delivery. This includes in particular, extreme respiration depth or baseline shifts due to organ drift. Also, the motion model is sensitive to the US imaging plane, and a small shift of the US probe may have adverse effects on the outcome. Therefore, the proposed framework requires the patients to remain in supine position with the probe attached to their chests. Future work will aim to alleviate this constraint by, for example, investigating the use of skin tattoos for a precise repositioning of the US probe. Furthermore, the motion model relies on a relatively small amount of training data which bears the danger of overfitting. The current implementation of the cGAN includes dropout but one could consider to additionally apply data augmentation on the input images. Further effort will be devoted towards the development of effective data augmentation strategies and must include a thorough investigation of the robustness of cGANs within the context of motion modelling. Moreover, the formulation of a control criterion which is capable of detecting defective deformation fields or MR volumes is considered an additional necessity in future works.

Acknowledgement. We thank Tony Lomax, Miriam Krieger, and Ye Zhang from the Centre for Proton Therapy at the Paul Scherrer Institute (PSI), Switzerland, and Pauline Guillemin from the University of Geneva, Switzerland, for fruitful discussions and their assistance with the data acquisition. This work was supported by the Swiss National Science Foundation, SNSF (320030_163330/1).

References

1. Bieri, O.: Ultra-fast steady state free precession and its application to in vivo 1H morphological and functional lung imaging at 1.5 tesla. Magn. Reson. Med. **70**(3), 657–663 (2013)
2. De Ruysscher, D., Sterpin, E., Haustermans, K., Depuydt, T.: Tumour movement in proton therapy: solutions and remaining questions: a review. Cancers **7**(3), 1143–1153 (2015)
3. Goodband, J., Haas, O., Mills, J.: A comparison of neural network approaches for on-line prediction in IGRT. Med. Phys. **35**(3), 1113–1122 (2008)
4. Goodfellow, I., et al.: Generative adversarial nets. In: Advances in neural information processing systems, pp. 2672–2680 (2014)
5. Isaksson, M., Jalden, J., Murphy, M.J.: On using an adaptive neural network to predict lung tumor motion during respiration for radiotherapy applications. Med. Phys. **32**(12), 3801–3809 (2005)
6. Isola, P., Zhu, J.Y., Zhou, T., Efros, A.A.: Image-to-Image Translation with Conditional Adversarial Networks. In: CVPR (2017)
7. McClelland, J.R., Hawkes, D.J., Schaeffter, T., King, A.P.: Respiratory motion models: a review. Med. Image Anal. **17**(1), 19–42 (2013)
8. Park, S., Lee, S.J., Weiss, E., Motai, Y.: Intra-and inter-fractional variation prediction of lung tumors using fuzzy deep learning. IEEE J. Transl. Eng. Health Med. **4**, 1–12 (2016)
9. Preiswerk, F., et al.: Model-guided respiratory organ motion prediction of the liver from 2D ultrasound. Med. Image Anal. **18**(5), 740–751 (2014)
10. Preiswerk, F.: Hybrid MRI-ultrasound acquisitions, and scannerless real-time imaging. Magn. Reson. Med. **78**(3), 897–908 (2017)
11. Sandkühler, R., Jud, C., Pezold, S., Cattin, P.C.: Adaptive graph diffusion regularisation for discontinuity preserving image registration. In: Klein, S., Staring, M., Durrleman, S., Sommer, S. (eds.) WBIR 2018. LNCS, vol. 10883, pp. 24–34. Springer, Cham (2018). https://doi.org/10.1007/978-3-319-92258-4_3
12. von Siebenthal, M., Szekely, G., Gamper, U., Boesiger, P., Lomax, A., Cattin, P.: 4D MR imaging of respiratory organ motion and its variability. Phys. Med. Biol. **52**(6), 1547 (2007)

Physics-Based Simulation to Enable Ultrasound Monitoring of HIFU Ablation: An MRI Validation

Chloé Audigier[1,2(✉)], Younsu Kim[2], Nicholas Ellens[1], and Emad M. Boctor[1,2]

[1] Department of Radiology, Johns Hopkins University, Baltimore, MD, USA
caudigi1@jhmi.edu
[2] Department of Computer Science, Johns Hopkins University, Baltimore, MD, USA

Abstract. High intensity focused ultrasound (HIFU) is used to ablate pathological tissue non-invasively, but reliable and real-time thermal monitoring is crucial to ensure a safe and effective procedure. It can be provided by MRI, which is an expensive and cumbersome modality.

We propose a monitoring method that enables real-time assessment of temperature distribution by combining intra-operative ultrasound (US) with physics-based simulation. During the ablation, changes in acoustic properties due to rising temperature are monitored using an external US sensor. A physics-based HIFU simulation model is then used to generate 3D temperature maps at high temporal and spatial resolutions. Our method leverages current HIFU systems with external low-cost and MR-compatible US sensors, thus allowing its validation against MR thermometry, the gold-standard clinical temperature monitoring method.

We demonstrated *in silico* the method feasibility, performed sensitivity analysis and showed experimentally its applicability on phantom data using a clinical HIFU system. Promising results were obtained: a mean temperature error smaller than $1.5\,°C$ was found in four experiments.

1 Introduction

In the past two decades, high intensity focused ultrasound (HIFU) has been used with generally good success for the non-invasive ablation of tumors in the prostate, uterus, bone, and breasts [1], along with the ablation of small volumes of neurological tissue for the treatment of essential tremor and Parkinson disease [2]. Even though its use has considerably expanded, a major limitation is still the lack of detailed and accurate real-time thermal information, needed to detect the boundary between ablated and non-ablated zones. The clinical end-point being to ensure a complete ablation while preserving as much healthy tissue as possible. This kind of information can be provided with $\pm1\,°C$ accuracy by MRI [3], routinely used to guide HIFU in clinical settings [4].

However high temporal and spatial resolutions are needed to accommodate with the small and non-uniform ablation shape and to detect unexpected off-target heating. This is challenging to achieve over a large field of view with MRI

© Springer Nature Switzerland AG 2018
A. F. Frangi et al. (Eds.): MICCAI 2018, LNCS 11073, pp. 89–97, 2018.
https://doi.org/10.1007/978-3-030-00937-3_11

as the scan time limits the volume coverage and spatial resolution. Typically, one to four adjacent slices perpendicular and one slice parallel to the acoustic beam path, with a voxel size of $2 \times 2 \times 5$ mm, at 0.1–1 Hz are acquired. Moreover, this modality is expensive, cumbersome, and subject to patient contraindications due to claustrophobia, non-MRI safe implants or MR contrast material.

Compared to MRI, ultrasound (US) offers higher temporal and spatial resolutions, low cost, safety, mobility and ease of use. Several heat-induced echo-strain approaches relying on successive correlation of RF images, have been proposed for US thermometry [5]. Despite good results in benchtop experiments, they suffer from low SNR, uncertainties in the US speckles, weak temperature sensitivity and have failed to translate to clinical applications, mainly due to their high sensitivity to motion artifacts, against which the proposed method is robust since it relies on direct measurements in the microsecond range.

We present an inexpensive yet comprehensive method for ablation monitoring, that enables real-time assessment of temperature and therefore thermal dose distributions, via an integrative approach. Intra-operative time-of-flight (TOF) US measurements and patient-specific biophysical simulation are combined for mutual benefits. Each source of information alone has disadvantages. Accurate simulation of an ablation procedure requires the knowledge of patient-specific parameters, which might not be easy to acquire [6]. US thermometry alone is not robust enough to fully meet the clinical requirements for assessing the progression of *in-vivo* tissue ablation. We propose to leverage conventional HIFU system with external low-cost and MR-compatible US sensors to provide in addition to ablation, real-time US temperature monitoring. Indeed, as HIFU deposits acoustic thermal dosage, invaluable intra-operative information is usually omitted. With rising temperature and ablation progression, acoustic properties such as the speed of sound (SOS) and attenuation coefficient vary. This affects the TOF carried by the US pressure waves going through the ablation zone and propagating to the opposite end, which we intend to record by simply integrating US sensors. Moreover, the proposed approach allows to use MRI for validation.

US thermometry through tomographic SOS reconstruction from direct TOF measurements has previously been proposed [7]. But for HIFU monitoring, the tomographic problem is ill-posed. First, it is rank deficient as the acquired TOF data is sparse: equal to the number of HIFU elements: 256 with common clinical HIFU system, times the number of sensors employed. However, we aim to reconstruct the temperature at the voxel level. Moreover, the relationship between SOS and temperature is tissue-specific and linear only until a certain point (around 55–60 °C). To tackle these, we propose to incorporate prior knowledge of biological and physical phenomena in thermal ablation through patient-specific computational modeling. 3D thermal maps at a high temporal and spatial resolution as well as TOF variations during ablation progression are simulated.

In this paper, we introduced the proposed method, presented simulation experiments and sensitivity analysis to evaluate its feasibility. *In vitro* validation against MRI in 4 phantom experiments were also performed.

2   Methods

HIFU ablation consists in the transmission of high intensity US pressure waves by all the HIFU elements. Each wave passes through the tissue with little effect and propagates to the opposite end. At the focal point where the beams converge, the energy reaches a useful thermal effect. By integrating external MR-compatible US sensors placed on the distal surface of the body (Fig. 1A), our method records invaluable direct time-of-flight (TOF) information, related to local temperature changes. Therefore, a large US thermometric cone defined by the HIFU aperture and the US external sensor is covered (Fig. 1B).

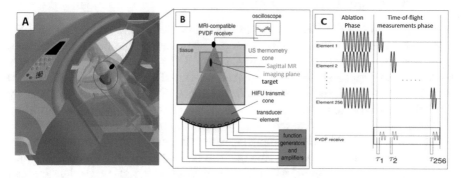

Fig. 1. The system setup (A) a 3D rendering showing the HIFU system embedded in the patient bed, external MR-compatible ultrasound (US) sensors, and MRI gantry. (B) a zoomed-in schematic diagram highlights individually controlled HIFU elements, US sensor, both HIFU transmit cone and US thermometry cone, and the sagittal MR imaging plane. (C) timing diagram shows both HIFU ablation and monitoring phases.

2.1   Biophysical Modeling of HIFU Thermal Ablation

HIFU is modeled in two steps, ultrasound propagation followed by heat transfer.

Ultrasound Propagation: The nonlinear US wave propagation in heterogeneous medium is simulated based on a pseudo-spectral computation of the wave equation in k-space [8]. The US pressure field $p(\mathbf{x},t)$ [Pa] is computed during the ablation and monitoring phases.

Heat Source Term: $Q(\mathbf{x},t)$ [W/m^3] is computed from the US pressure as [9]:

$$Q(\mathbf{x},t) = \frac{\alpha f}{\rho_t c}|p(\mathbf{x},t)|^2 \tag{1}$$

where α [Np/(m MHz)] is the acoustic absorption coefficient, f [MHz] the HIFU frequency, ρ_t [kg/m^3], the tissue density and c [m/s] the speed of sound.

Heat Transfer Model: From a 3D anatomical image acquired before ablation, the temperature $T(\mathbf{x}, t)$ evolution is computed in each voxel by solving the bioheat equation, as proposed in the Pennes model [10]:

$$\rho_t c_t \frac{\partial T(\mathbf{x}, t)}{\partial t} = Q(\mathbf{x}, t) + \nabla \cdot (d_t T(\mathbf{x}, t)) + R(T_{b0} - T(\mathbf{x}, t)) \tag{2}$$

where c_t [J/(kg K)], d_t [W/(m K)] are the tissue heat capacity and conductivity. T_{b0} is the blood temperature. R is the reaction coefficient, modeling the blood perfusion, which is set to zero in this study, as we deal with a phantom.

2.2   Ultrasound Thermal Monitoring

From the Forward Model: The biophysical model generates longitudinal 3D temperature maps, which can be used to plan and/or monitor the ablation. They are also converted into heterogeneous SOS maps given a temperature-to-SOS curve (Fig. 2 shows such a curve measured in a phantom). Thus, US wavefronts are simulated as emitted from each HIFU element and received by the US sensor with temperature-induced changes in their TOF. For monitoring, the recorded TOFs are compared to those predicted by the forward model: if they are similar, then the ablation is going as expected and the simulated temperature maps can be used. If the values diverge, the ablation should be stopped. Thus, insufficient ablation in the target region and unexpected off-target heating can now be detected during the procedure.

From tomographic SOS Reconstruction: During each monitoring phase t_m, 3D SOS volumes are reconstructed by optimizing Eq. 3 using the acquired TOF, provided that the number of equations is at least equal to the number of unknowns, i.e. the SOS in each voxel of the 3D volume. As the acquired TOF data is limited, additional constraints are needed. To reduce the number of unknowns, we created layer maps M_{t_m}. Each M_{t_m} includes N_{t_m} different layers grouping voxels expected to have the same temperature according to the forward model.

$$\min_x \|Sx - TOF_{aquired}\|^2 \quad \text{subject to} \quad A_{eq} \cdot x = b_{eq},$$
$$A_{ineq} \cdot x \leq b_{ineq}, \tag{3}$$
$$SOS_{min} \leq 1/x \leq SOS_{max}$$

where the vector x represents the inverse of the SOS, the matrix S contains the intersection lengths through each voxel for the paths between the HIFU elements and the US sensor, $\mathcal{P}_{\mathcal{HIFU} \rightarrow \mathcal{US}}$. Constraints between voxels in the same layer (A_{eq}, b_{eq}) and different layers (A_{ineq}, b_{ineq}) are computed based on M_{t_m}. The solution is also bounded by a feasible SOS range. From the estimated SOS, the temperature can be recovered using a temperature-to-SOS curve (Fig. 2).

3   Experiments and Results

We used a clinical MR-HIFU system (Sonalleve V2, Profound Medical, Toronto, Canada) providing in real-time 2 MR temperature images in the coronal and sagittal planes for comparison. We reprogrammed the HIFU system [11] to perform three consecutive cycles consisting of a heating phase at 50 W and 1.2 MHz (all elements continuous wave) for 10 s and a monitoring phase with an element-by-element acoustic interrogation at 2 W (40 cycle pulses, 128 elements sequentially) for 24 s to determine TOF (Fig. 1C). We fabricated a receiving US sensor, made of a 2.5-mm diameter tube of Lead Zirconate Titate material (PZT-5H). A 3-m long wire is connected to an oscilloscope located outside of the MR room. The US sensor was placed on top of the phantom, about 15 cm from the transducer and was localized using TOF measured prior to ablation. The sensor produced negligible artifacts on the MR images (Fig. 2, left).

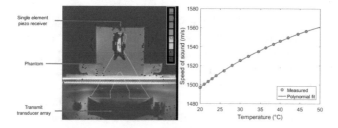

Fig. 2. (Left) experimental setup: HIFU is performed on a phantom under MR thermometry. The MR-compatible US sensor is placed on top of the phantom to acquire time-of-flight (TOF) data during the monitoring phase of the modified protocol. (Right) the phantom-specific temperature-to-SOS curve.

3.1   Sensitivity Analysis

The protocol described above was simulated using the forward model with both the ablation and monitoring phases. The US propagation and heat transfer are computed on the same Cartesian grid including a perfect match layer (PML = 8), with a spatial resolution of $\delta x = 1.3$ mm, different time steps: $\delta t = 12.5\,\mu$s and $\delta t = 0.1$ s respectively, and using the optimized CPU version of k-Wave 1.2.1[1]. Temperature images of $1.3 \times 1.3 \times 1.3$ mm were generated every 1 s by the forward model. Layer maps M_{t_m} were generated with a temperature step of $0.6\,°$C. For example, at the end of the third ablation phase t_3, when the maximal temperature is reached, a map of $N_{t_3} = 26$ layers was generated.

Effect of US Element Location: As the US sensor defines the US thermometry cone, its location with respect to the HIFU system and to the heated region highly affects the monitoring temperature accuracy. To study this effect, we

---

[1] http://www.k-wave.org.

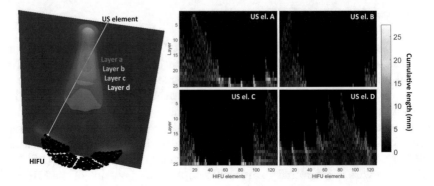

Fig. 3. (Left) one path from one HIFU element to the US receiver going through the layer map is displayed over a simulated temperature image. 4 layers with $a < b < c < d$ are shown. (Right) matrices I made of the cumulative length of the intersection of $\mathcal{P}_{\mathcal{HIFU} \rightarrow \mathcal{US}}$ with each of the layers in M_{t_3} are shown for 4 US sensor positions.

simulated 4 different US sensor locations at the phantom top surface, 1 cm away from each other in each direction (the same setting was replicated in the phantom experiment, as detailed below). For each sensor location, we computed a matrix I, made of the cumulative length of the intersection of $\mathcal{P}_{\mathcal{HIFU} \rightarrow \mathcal{US}}$ with each of the layers of M_{t_3}. From the example illustrated in Fig. 3, it can be observed that at location A and D, most of the layers are covered by several paths. However, at location B, most of the paths from the central HIFU elements are not going through any layers, making it more difficult to reconstruct accurately SOS maps. This is also true for location C although to a lesser extent.

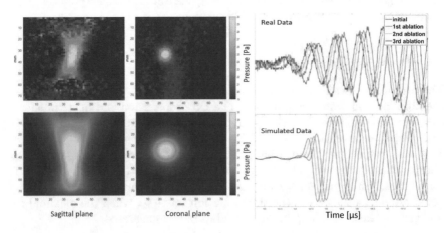

Fig. 4. (Left) MR (top) and simulated (bottom) thermal images compare qualitatively well in a ROI of 75×75 mm, centered around the targeted region. (Right) measured (top) and simulated (bottom) TOF from HIFU element 241 to the US sensor in position A. Delays of 0.1, 0.2, 0.3 μs occur after the first, second and third heating phases.

Effect of the Number of US Elements: Multiple US sensors receiving simultaneously TOF at different locations can be used to improve the method accuracy, as the matrix I is less sparse. As it can be observed in Fig. 3, a better sampling of the layers (less zeros in I) can be achieved with certain combination of the 4 sensors. For example, by combining US sensors at location A and B, information about the outer layers 23 to 25, is obtained with high cumulative lengths by the HIFU elements 36 to 112 from the US sensor at location A, whereas information about the inner layer 1 comes from location B.

3.2   Phantom Feasibility Study

Four experiments with different US sensor locations were performed on an isotropic and homogeneous phantom made of 2%-agar and 2%-silicon-dioxide. Its specific temperature-to-SOS curve was measured pre-operatively (Fig. 2). First, the acquired MR thermal images and the ones generated by the forward model were compared. As shown in Fig. 4 at t_3, temperature differences in a ROI of 75×75mm were $0.7 \pm 1.2\,^{\circ}\text{C}$ and $1.6 \pm 1.9\,^{\circ}\text{C}$ on average, with a maximum of $6.7\,^{\circ}\text{C}$ and $11.7\,^{\circ}\text{C}$ in the coronal and sagittal planes, respectively. TOF simulated at baseline and after the first, second and third heating phases were in agreement with the measures (Fig. 4). The delays caused by the temperature changes were computed by cross-correlation between signals received before and during ablation.

To evaluate *in vitro* the effect of multiple sensors acquiring TOF simultaneously, individual measurements obtained sequentially at the 4 different locations were grouped to mimic the monitoring by 2, 3 or 4 sensors. It was possible since

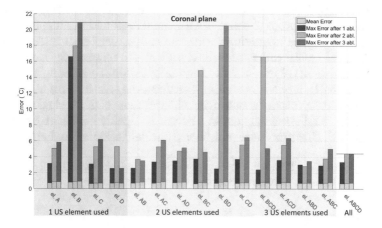

Fig. 5. Error between the temperature estimated by the SOS reconstruction algorithm and the coronal MR image. The TOF from 1, 2, 3 or 4 sensors are used. The mean error in yellow is lower than $1\,^{\circ}\text{C}$ in each case. The max error at t_1, t_2 and t_3 appears in blue, cyan and pink. The overall max error decreases when we increase the number of elements, as shown by the black horizontal lines.

we waited for the phantom to return to room temperature between each experiment. We analyzed all the combinations using 1, 2, 3 and 4 sensors. In each of the 15 scenarios, temperature images are generated using the tomographic SOS reconstruction and compared to MRI. As illustrated in Fig. 5 for the coronal plane, the algorithm accuracy highly depends on the position and number of the US sensors, as predicted in the above sensitivity analysis study. The overall max error decreases with the number of US elements employed. Similar results were obtained in the sagittal plane, with a mean error lower than $1.5\,°C$ in each case.

4   Discussion and Conclusion

In this work, we used nominal parameters from the literature, but the biophysical model handles the presence of blood, different tissue types, and can be personalized to simulate patient-specific ablation responses to improve its accuracy *in vivo* [6]. As the simulation runs fast, model parameters could be personalized from intra-operative measurements during a first ablation phase and then used in the following phases. Different temperature-to-SOS curves could also be used.

As the heating is paused during monitoring, this period is desired to be as short as possible. To be more effective, one could minimize the switching time while cycling through the HIFU elements without inducing cross-talk. One could also sonicate pulses from multiple elements at once and deconvolve the received signals geometrically. Finally, we could investigate whether a smaller subset of the HIFU elements could be sufficient for temperature monitoring.

In conclusion, we have shown that biophysical model simulating the effect of treatment on patient-specific data, can be combined with US information directly recorded from HIFU signals to reconstruct intra-operative 3D thermal maps. This method demonstrated low temperature error when compared to MRI. While this work is a proof of concept with simulation and preliminary but solid phantom results, *in vivo* experiments are warranted to determine the viability of this US thermal monitoring approach. It promises to increase the safety, efficacy and cost-effectiveness of non-invasive thermal ablation. By offering an affordable alternative to MRI, it will for example transform the treatment of uterine fibroid into an outpatient procedure, improving the workflow of gynecologists who typically diagnose the disease but cannot perform MR-guided HIFU. By shifting the guidance to US, this procedure will be more widely adopted and employed.

Acknowledgments. This work was supported by the National Institute of Health (R01EB021396) and the National Science Foundation (1653322).

References

1. Escoffre, J.-M., Bouakaz, A.: Therapeutic Ultrasound, vol. 880. Springer, Cham (2016). https://doi.org/10.1007/978-3-319-22536-4
2. Magara, A., Bühler, R., Moser, D., Kowalski, M., Pourtehrani, P., Jeanmonod, D.: First experience with MR-guided focused ultrasound in the treatment of Parkinson's disease. J. Ther. Ultrasound **2**(1), 11 (2014)

3. Quesson, B., de Zwart, J.A., Moonen, C.T.: Magnetic resonance temperature imaging for guidance of thermotherapy. JMRI **12**(4), 525–533 (2000)
4. Fennessy, F.M., et al.: Uterine leiomyomas: MR imaging-guided focused ultrasound surgery-results of different treatment protocols. Radiology **243**(3), 885–893 (2007)
5. Seo, C.H., Shi, Y., Huang, S.W., Kim, K., O'Donnell, M.: Thermal strain imaging: a review. Interface Focus. **1**(4), 649–664 (2011)
6. Audigier, C., et al.: Parameter estimation for personalization of liver tumor radiofrequency ablation. In: Yoshida, H., Näppi, J., Saini, S. (eds.) International MICCAI Workshop on Computational and Clinical Challenges in Abdominal Imaging, pp. 3–12. Springer, Heidelberg (2014). https://doi.org/10.1007/978-3-319-13692-9_1
7. Basarab-Horwath, I., Dorozhevets, M.: Measurement of the temperature distribution in fluids using ultrasonic tomography. Ultrason. Symp. **3**, 1891–1894 (1994)
8. Treeby, B.E., Cox, B.T.: k-wave: MATLAB toolbox for the simulation and reconstruction of photoacoustic wave fields. J. Biomed. Opt. **15**(2), 021314–021314 (2010)
9. Nyborg, W.L.: Heat generation by ultrasound in a relaxing medium. J. Acoust. Soc. Am. **70**(2), 310–312 (1981)
10. Pennes, H.H.: Analysis of tissue and arterial blood temperatures in the resting human forearm. J. Appl. Physiol. **85**(1), 5–34 (1998)
11. Zaporzan, B., Waspe, A.C., Looi, T., Mougenot, C., Partanen, A., Pichardo, S.: MatMRI and MatHIFU: software toolboxes for real-time monitoring and control of MR-guided HIFU. J. Ther. Ultrasound **1**(1), 7 (2013)

DeepDRR – A Catalyst for Machine Learning in Fluoroscopy-Guided Procedures

Mathias Unberath[1]([✉]), Jan-Nico Zaech[1,2], Sing Chun Lee[1], Bastian Bier[1,2],
Javad Fotouhi[1], Mehran Armand[3], and Nassir Navab[1]

[1] Computer Aided Medical Procedures, Johns Hopkins University, Baltimore, USA
unberath@jhu.edu
[2] Pattern Recognition Lab, Friedrich-Alexander-Universität Erlangen-Nürnberg,
Erlangen, Germany
[3] Applied Physics Laboratory, Johns Hopkins University, Baltimore, USA

Abstract. Machine learning-based approaches outperform competing methods in most disciplines relevant to diagnostic radiology. Interventional radiology, however, has not yet benefited substantially from the advent of deep learning, in particular because of two reasons: (1) Most images acquired during the procedure are never archived and are thus not available for learning, and (2) even if they were available, annotations would be a severe challenge due to the vast amounts of data. When considering fluoroscopy-guided procedures, an interesting alternative to true interventional fluoroscopy is *in silico* simulation of the procedure from 3D diagnostic CT. In this case, labeling is comparably easy and potentially readily available, yet, the appropriateness of resulting synthetic data is dependent on the forward model. In this work, we propose Deep-DRR, a framework for fast and realistic simulation of fluoroscopy and digital radiography from CT scans, tightly integrated with the software platforms native to deep learning. We use machine learning for material decomposition and scatter estimation in 3D and 2D, respectively, combined with analytic forward projection and noise injection to achieve the required performance. On the example of anatomical landmark detection in X-ray images of the pelvis, we demonstrate that machine learning models trained on DeepDRRs generalize to unseen clinically acquired data without the need for re-training or domain adaptation. Our results are promising and promote the establishment of machine learning in fluoroscopy-guided procedures.

Keywords: Monte Carlo simulation · Volumetric segmentation
Beam hardening · Image-guided procedures

M. Unberath and J.-N. Zaech—Both authors contributed equally and are listed in alphabetical order.

A. F. Frangi et al. (Eds.): MICCAI 2018, LNCS 11073, pp. 98–106, 2018.
https://doi.org/10.1007/978-3-030-00937-3_12

1   Introduction

The advent of convolutional neural networks (ConvNets) for classification, regression, and prediction tasks, currently most commonly referred to as deep learning, has brought substantial improvements to many well studied problems in computer vision, and more recently, medical image computing. This field is dominated by diagnostic imaging tasks where (1) all image data are archived, (2) learning targets, in particular annotations of any kind, exist traditionally [1] or can be approximated [2], and (3) comparably simple augmentation strategies, such as rigid and non-rigid displacements [3], ease the limited data problem.

Unfortunately, the situation is more complicated in interventional imaging, particularly in 2D fluoroscopy-guided procedures. First, while many X-ray images are acquired for procedural guidance, only very few radiographs that document the procedural outcome are archived suggesting a severe lack of meaningful data. Second, learning targets are not well established or defined; and third, there is great variability in the data, e. g. due to different surgical tools present in the images, which challenges meaningful augmentation. Consequently, substantial amounts of clinical data must be collected and annotated to enable machine learning for fluoroscopy-guided procedures. Despite clear opportunities, in particular for prediction tasks, very little work has considered learning in this context [4–7].

A promising approach to tackling the above challenges is *in silico* fluoroscopy generation from diagnostic 3D CT, most commonly referred to as digitally reconstructed radiographs (DRRs) [4,5]. Rendering DRRs from CT provides fluoroscopy in known geometry, but more importantly: Annotation and augmentation can be performed on the 3D CT substantially reducing the workload and promoting valid image characteristics, respectively. However, machine learning models trained on DRRs do not generalize to clinical data since traditional DRR generation, e. g. as in [4,8], does not accurately model X-ray image formation. To overcome this limitation we propose DeepDRR, an easy-to-use framework for realistic DRR generation from CT volumes targeted at the machine learning community. On the example of view independent anatomical landmark detection in pelvic trauma surgery [9], we demonstrate that training on DeepDRRs enables direct application of the learned model to clinical data without the need for re-training or domain adaptation.

2   Methods

2.1   Background and Requirements

DRR generation considers the problem of finding detector responses given a particular imaging geometry according to Beer-Lambert law [10]. Methods for *in silico* generation of DRRs can be grouped in analytic and statistical approaches, i. e. ray-tracing and Monte Carlo (MC) simulation, respectively. Ray-tracing algorithms are computationally efficient since the attenuated photon fluence of a detector pixel is determined by computing total attenuation along a 3D line that then applies to all photons emitted in that direction [8]. Commonly, ray-tracing only considers a single material in the mono-energetic case and thus fails to model beam hardening. In addition and since ray-tracing is analytic, statistical processes during image formation, such as scattering, cannot be modeled. Conversely, MC methods simulate single photon transport by evaluating the probability of photon-matter interaction, the sequence of which determines attenuation [11]. Since the probability of interaction is inherently material and energy dependent, MC simulations require material decomposition in CT that is usually achieved by thresholding of CT values (Houndfield units, HU) [12] and spectra of the emitter [11]. As a consequence, MC is very realistic. Unfortunately, for training-set-size DRR generation on conventional hardware, MC is prohibitively expensive. As an example, accelerated MC simulation [11] on an NVIDIA Titan Xp takes $\approx$ 4h for a single X-ray image with 10^{10} photons. To leverage the advantages of MC simulations in clinical practice, the medical physics community provides further acceleration strategies if prior knowledge on the problem exists. A well studied example is variance reduction for scatter correction in cone-beam CT, since scatter is of low frequency [13].

Unfortunately, several challenges remain that hinder the implementation of realistic *in silico* X-ray generation for machine learning applications. We have identified the following fundamental challenges at the interface of machine learning and medical physics that must be overcome to establish realistic simulation in the machine learning community: (1) Tools designed for machine learning must seamlessly integrate with the common frameworks. (2) Training requires many images so data generation must be fast and automatic. (3) Simulation must be realistic: Both analytic and statistic processes such as beam-hardening and scatter, respectively, must be modeled.

2.2   DeepDRR

Overview: We propose DeepDRR, a Python, PyCUDA, and PyTorch-based framework for fast and automatic simulation of X-ray images from CT data. It consists of 4 major modules: (1) Material decomposition in CT volumes using a deep segmentation ConvNet; (2) A material- and spectrum-aware ray-tracing forward projector; (3) A neural network-based Rayleigh scatter estimation; and (4) Quantum and electronic readout noise injection. The individual steps of DeepDRR are visualized schematically in Fig. 1 and explained in greater detail in the remainder of this section. The fully automated pipeline is open source available for download[1].

Material Decomposition: Material decomposition in 3D CT for MC simulation is traditionally accomplished by thresholding, since a given material has a characteristic HU range [12]. This works well for large HU discrepancies, e.g. air ($[-1000]$ HU) and bone ($[200, 3000]$ HU), but may fail otherwise, particularly

---

[1] Github link: https://github.com/mathiasunberath/DeepDRR.

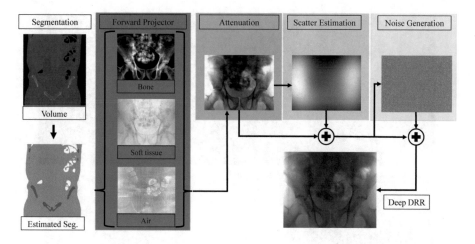

Fig. 1. Schematic overview of DeepDRR.

between soft tissue ($[-150, 300]$ HU) and bone in presence of low mineral density. This is problematic since, despite similar HU, the attenuation characteristic of bone is substantially different of soft tissue [10]. Within this work, we use a deep volumetric ConvNet adapted from [3] to automatically decompose air, soft tissue, and bone in CT volumes. The ConvNet is of encoder-decoder structure with skip-ahead connections to retain information of high spatial resolution while enabling large receptive fields. The ConvNet is trained on patches with $128 \times 128 \times 128$ voxels with voxel sizes of $0.86 \times 0.86 \times 1.0$ mm yielding a material map $M(\boldsymbol{x})$ that assigns a candidate material to each 3D point $\boldsymbol{x}$. We used the multi-class Dice loss as the optimization target. 12 whole-body CT data were manually annotated, and then split: 10 for training, and 2 for validation and testing. Training was performed over 600 epochs until convergence where, in each epoch, one patch from every volume was randomly extracted. During application, patches of $128 \times 128 \times 128$ voxels are fed-forward with stride of 64 since only labels for the central $64 \times 64 \times 64$ voxels are accepted.

Analytic Primary Computation: Once segmentations of the considered materials $M = \{\text{air, soft tissue, bone}\}$ are available, the contribution of each material to the total attenuation density at detector position $\boldsymbol{u}$ are computed using a given geometry (defined by projection matrix $\boldsymbol{P} \in \mathbb{R}^{3 \times 4}$) and X-ray spectral density $p_0(E)$ via ray-tracing:

$$p(\boldsymbol{u}) = \int p(E, \boldsymbol{u}) \mathrm{d}E$$

$$= \int p_0(E) \exp \left(\sum_{m \in M} \delta\left(m, M(\boldsymbol{x})\right) (\mu/\rho)_m(E) \int \rho(\boldsymbol{x}) \, \mathrm{d}\boldsymbol{l_u} \right) \mathrm{d}E, \quad (1)$$

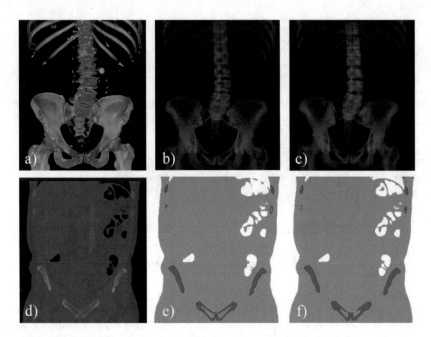

Fig. 2. Representative results of the segmentation ConvNets. From left to right, the columns show input volume, manual segmentation, and ConvNet result. The top rows shows volume renderings of the bony anatomy and respective label, while the bottom row shows a coronal slice through the volumes.

where $\delta\left(\cdot,\cdot\right)$ is the Kronecker delta, $\boldsymbol{l_u}$ is the 3D ray connecting the source position and 3D location of detector pixel $\boldsymbol{u}$ determined by $\boldsymbol{P}$, $(\mu/\rho)_m(E)$ is the material and energy dependent linear attenuation coefficient [10], and $\rho(\boldsymbol{x})$ is the material density at position $\boldsymbol{x}$ derived from HU values. The projection domain image $p(\boldsymbol{u})$ is then used as input to our scatter prediction ConvNet.

Learning-Based Scatter Estimation: Traditional scatter estimation relies on variance-reduced MC simulations [13], which requires a complete MC setup. Recent approaches to scatter estimation via ConvNets outperform kernel based methods [14] while retaining the low computational demand. In addition, they inherently integrate with deep learning software environments. We define a ten layer ConvNet, where the first six layers generate Rayleigh scatter estimates and the last four layers, with 31×31 kernels and a single channel, ensure smoothness. The network was trained on 330 images generated via MC simulation [11], augmented by random rotations and reflections. The last three layers were trained using pre-training of the preceding layers. The input to the network is downsampled to 128×128 pixels.

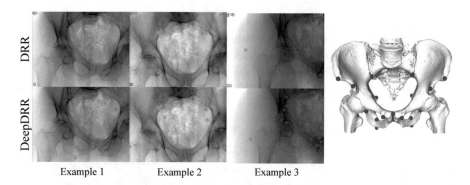

Fig. 3. Anatomical landmark detection on real data using the method detailed in [9]. Top row: Detections of a model trained on conventional DRRs. Bottom row: Detections of a model trained on the proposed DeepDRRs. No domain adaption or re-training was performed. Right-most image: Schematic illustration of desired landmark locations.

Noise Injection: After adding scatter, $p(\boldsymbol{u})$ expresses the energy deposited by a photon in detector pixel $\boldsymbol{u}$. The number of photons is estimated as:

$$N(\boldsymbol{u}) = \sum_E \frac{p(E, \boldsymbol{u})}{E} N_0 \,, \tag{2}$$

to obtain the number of registered photons $N(\boldsymbol{u})$ and perform realistic noise injection. In Eq. 2, N_0 (potentially location dependent $N_0(\boldsymbol{u})$, e.g. due to bow-tie filters) is the emitted number of photons per pixel. Noise in X-ray images is a composite of uncorrelated quantum noise due to photon statistics that becomes correlated due to pixel crosstalk, and correlated readout noise [15]. Due to beam hardening, the spectrum arriving at any detector pixel differs. To account for this fact in the Poisson noise model, we compute a mean photon energy for each pixel by $\bar{E}(\boldsymbol{u})$ and estimate quantum noise as $\bar{E}/N_0(p_{Poisson}(N) - N)$, where $p_{Poisson}$ is the Poisson generating function. Since real flat panel detectors suffer from pixel crosstalk, we correlate the quantum noise of neighboring pixels by convolving the noise signal with a blurring kernel [15]. The second major noise component is electronic readout noise. Electronic noise is signal independent and can be modeled as additive Gaussian noise with correlation along rows due to sequential readout [15]. Finally, we obtain a realistically simulated DRR.

3 Experiments and Results

3.1 Framework Validation

Since forward projection and noise injection are analytic processes, we only assess the prediction accuracy of the proposed ConvNets for volumetric segmentation and projection domain scatter estimation. For volumetric segmentation of air, soft tissue, and bone in CT volumes, we found a misclassification rate of

$(2.03 \pm 3.63)\,\%$ which is in line with results reported in previous studies using this architecture [3]. Representative results on the test set are shown in Fig. 2. For scatter estimation, the evaluation on a test set consisting of 30 image yielded a normalized mean squared error of 9.96 %. For 1000 images with $620 \times 480\,\mathrm{px}$, the simulation per image took $0.56\,\mathrm{s}$ irrespective of number of emitted photons.

3.2 Task-Based Evaluation

Fundamentally, the goal of DeepDRR is to enable the learning of models on synthetically generated data that generalizes to unseen clinical fluoroscopy without re-training or other domain adaptation strategies. To this end, we consider anatomical landmark detection in X-ray images of the pelvis from arbitrary views [9]. The authors annotated 23 anatomical landmarks in CT volumes of the pelvis (Fig. 3, last column) and generated DRRs with annotations on a spherical segment covering 120° and 90° in RAO/LAO and CRAN/CAUD, respectively. Then, a sequential prediction framework is learned and, upon convergence, used to predict the 23 anatomical landmarks in unseen, real X-ray images of cadaver studies. The network is learned twice: First, on conventionally generated DRRs assuming a single material and mono-energetic spectrum, and second, on Deep-DRRs as described in Sect. 2.2. Images had 615×479 pixels with 0.616^2 mm pixel size. We used the spectrum of a tungsten anode operated at $120\,\mathrm{kV}$ with $4.3\,\mathrm{mm}$ aluminum and assumed a high-dose acquisition with $5 \cdot 10^5$ photons per pixel. In Fig. 3 we show representative detections of the sequential prediction framework on unseen, clinical data acquired using a flat panel C-arm system (Siemens Cios Fusion, Siemens Healthcare GmbH, Germany) during cadaver studies. As expected, the model trained on conventional DRRs (upper row) fails to predict anatomical landmark locations on clinical data, while the model trained on DeepDRRs produces accurate predictions even on partial anatomy. In addition, we would like to refer to the comprehensive results reported in [9] that were achieved using training on the proposed DeepDRRs.

4 Discussion and Conclusion

We proposed DeepDRR, a framework for fast and realistic generation of synthetic X-ray images from diagnostic 3D CT, in an effort to ease the establishment of machine learning-based approaches in fluoroscopy-guided procedures. The framework combines novel learning-based algorithms for 3D material decomposition from CT and 2D scatter estimation with fast, analytic models for energy and material dependent forward projection and noise injection. On a surrogate task, i. e. the prediction of anatomical landmarks in X-ray images of the pelvis, we demonstrate that models trained on DeepDRRs generalize to clinical data without the need of re-training or domain adaptation, while the same model trained on conventional DRRs is unable to perform. Our future work will focus on improving volumetric segmentation by introducing more materials, in particular metal, and scatter estimation that could benefit from a larger training set size. In conclusion, we understand realistic *in silico* generation of X-ray images, e. g. using the proposed framework, as a catalyst designed to benefit the implementation of machine learning in fluoroscopy-guided procedures. Our framework seamlessly integrates with the software environment currently used for machine learning and will be made open-source at the time of publication[2].

References

1. Kooi, T., et al.: Large scale deep learning for computer aided detection of mammographic lesions. Med. Image Anal. **35**, 303–312 (2017)
2. Roy, A.G., Conjeti, S., Sheet, D., Katouzian, A., Navab, N., Wachinger, C.: Error corrective boosting for learning fully convolutional networks with limited data. In: Descoteaux, M., Maier-Hein, L., Franz, A., Jannin, P., Collins, D.L., Duchesne, S. (eds.) MICCAI 2017. LNCS, vol. 10435, pp. 231–239. Springer, Cham (2017). https://doi.org/10.1007/978-3-319-66179-7_27
3. Milletari, F., Navab, N., Ahmadi, S.A.: V-Net: fully convolutional neural networks for volumetric medical image segmentation. In: 2016 Fourth International Conference on 3D Vision (3DV), pp. 565–571. IEEE (2016)
4. Li, Y., Liang, W., Zhang, Y., An, H., Tan, J.: Automatic lumbar vertebrae detection based on feature fusion deep learning for partial occluded C-arm X-ray images. In: 2016 IEEE 38th Annual International Conference of the Engineering in Medicine and Biology Society (EMBC), pp. 647–650. IEEE (2016)
5. Terunuma, T., Tokui, A., Sakae, T.: Novel real-time tumor-contouring method using deep learning to prevent mistracking in X-ray fluoroscopy. Radiol. Phys. Technol. **11**, 43–53 (2017)
6. Ambrosini, P., Ruijters, D., Niessen, W.J., Moelker, A., van Walsum, T.: Fully automatic and real-time catheter segmentation in X-ray fluoroscopy. In: Descoteaux, M., Maier-Hein, L., Franz, A., Jannin, P., Collins, D.L., Duchesne, S. (eds.) MICCAI 2017. LNCS, vol. 10434, pp. 577–585. Springer, Cham (2017). https://doi.org/10.1007/978-3-319-66185-8_65
7. Ma, H., Ambrosini, P., van Walsum, T.: Fast prospective detection of contrast inflow in X-ray angiograms with convolutional neural network and recurrent neural network. In: Descoteaux, M., Maier-Hein, L., Franz, A., Jannin, P., Collins, D.L., Duchesne, S. (eds.) MICCAI 2017. LNCS, vol. 10435, pp. 453–461. Springer, Cham (2017). https://doi.org/10.1007/978-3-319-66179-7_52
8. Russakoff, D.B., et al.: Fast generation of digitally reconstructed radiographs using attenuation fields with application to 2D–3D image registration. IEEE Trans. Med. Imaging **24**(11), 1441–1454 (2005)
9. Bier, B., et al.: X-ray-transform invariant anatomical landmark detection for pelvic trauma surgery. In: Frangi, A.F., et al. (eds.) MICCAI 2018. LNCS, vol. 11073, pp. 55–63. Springer, Heidelberg (2018)
10. Hubbell, J.H., Seltzer, S.M.: Tables of X-ray mass attenuation coefficients and mass energy-absorption coefficients 1 keV to 20 MeV for elements Z = 1 to 92 and 48 additional substances of dosimetric interest. Technical report, National Institute of Standards and Technology (1995)

---

[2] The source code available at this link: https://github.com/mathiasunberath/DeepDRR.

11. Badal, A., Badano, A.: Accelerating Monte Carlo simulations of photon transport in a voxelized geometry using a massively parallel graphics processing unit. Med. Phys. **36**(11), 4878–4880 (2009)
12. Schneider, W., Bortfeld, T., Schlegel, W.: Correlation between CT numbers and tissue parameters needed for Monte Carlo simulations of clinical dose distributions. Phys. Med. Biol. **45**(2), 459 (2000)
13. Sisniega, A., et al.: Monte carlo study of the effects of system geometry and anti-scatter grids on cone-beam CT scatter distributions. Med. Phys. **40**(5) (2013)
14. Maier, J., Sawall, S., Kachelrieß, M.: Deep scatter estimation (DSE): feasibility of using a deep convolutional neural network for real-time X-ray scatter prediction in cone-beam CT. In: SPIE Medical Imaging, SPIE (2018)
15. Zhang, H., Ouyang, L., Ma, J., Huang, J., Chen, W., Wang, J.: Noise correlation in CBCT projection data and its application for noise reduction in low-dose CBCT. Med. Phys. **41**(3) (2014)

Exploiting Partial Structural Symmetry for Patient-Specific Image Augmentation in Trauma Interventions

Javad Fotouhi[1,2(✉)], Mathias Unberath[1,2], Giacomo Taylor[1],
Arash Ghaani Farashahi[2], Bastian Bier[1], Russell H. Taylor[2],
Greg M. Osgood[3], Mehran Armand[2,3,4], and Nassir Navab[1,2,5]

[1] Computer Aided Medical Procedures, Johns Hopkins University, Baltimore, USA
javad.fotouhi@jhu.edu
[2] Laboratory for Computational Sensing and Robotics, Johns Hopkins University,
Baltimore, USA
[3] Department of Orthopaedic Surgery, Johns Hopkins Hospital, Baltimore, USA
[4] Applied Physics Laboratory, Johns Hopkins University, Baltimore, USA
[5] Computer Aided Medical Procedures, Technische Universität München,
Munich, Germany

Abstract. In unilateral pelvic fracture reductions, surgeons attempt to reconstruct the bone fragments such that bilateral symmetry in the bony anatomy is restored. We propose to exploit this "structurally symmetric" nature of the pelvic bone, and provide intra-operative image augmentation to assist the surgeon in repairing dislocated fragments. The main challenge is to automatically estimate the desired plane of symmetry within the patient's pre-operative CT. We propose to estimate this plane using a non-linear optimization strategy, by minimizing Tukey's biweight robust estimator, relying on the partial symmetry of the anatomy. Moreover, a regularization term is designed to enforce the similarity of bone density histograms on both sides of this plane, relying on the biological fact that, even if injured, the dislocated bone segments remain within the body. The experimental results demonstrate the performance of the proposed method in estimating this "plane of partial symmetry" using CT images of both healthy and injured anatomy. Examples of unilateral pelvic fractures are used to show how intra-operative X-ray images could be augmented with the forward-projections of the mirrored anatomy, acting as objective road-map for fracture reduction procedures.

Keywords: Symmetry · Robust estimation · Orthopedics · X-ray · CT

1 Introduction

The main objective in orthopedic reduction surgery is to restore the correct alignment of the dislocated or fractured bone. In both unilateral and bilateral

---

J. Fotouhi, M. Unberath and G. Taylor—These authors are regarded as joint first authors.

© Springer Nature Switzerland AG 2018
A. F. Frangi et al. (Eds.): MICCAI 2018, LNCS 11073, pp. 107–115, 2018.
https://doi.org/10.1007/978-3-030-00937-3_13

fractures, surgeons attempt to re-align the fractures to their natural biological alignment. In the majority of cases, there are no available anatomical imaging data prior to injury, and CT scans are only acquired after the patient is injured to identify the fracture type and plan the intervention. Therefore, no reference exists to identify the correct and natural alignment of the bone fragments. Instead, surgeons use the opposite healthy side of the patient as reference, and aim at producing symmetry across the sagittal plane [1]. It is important to mention that, although the healthy pelvic bone is not entirely symmetric, surgeons aim at aligning the bone fragments to achieve structural and functional symmetry. For orthopedic traumatologists, the correct length, alignment, and rotation of extremities are also verified by comparing to the contralateral side. Examples of other fields of surgery that use symmetry for guidance include crainiofacial [2] and breast reconstruction surgeries [3].

Self-symmetry assessment is only achievable if the fractures are not bilateral, so that the contralateral side of the pelvis is intact. According to pelvis fracture classification, a large number of fracture reduction cases are only unilateral [4]. Consequently, direct comparison of bony structures across the sagittal plane is possible in a large number of orthopedic trauma interventions.

CT-based statistical models from a population of data are particularly important when patient-specific pre-operative CT images are not present. In this situation, statistical modeling and deformable registration enable 3D understanding of the underlying anatomy using only 2D intra-operative imaging. Statistical shape models are used to extrapolate and predict the unknown anatomy in partial and incomplete medical images [5]. In the aforementioned methods, instead of patient self-correlation, relations to a population of data are exploited for identifying missing anatomical details.

In this work, we hypothesize that there is a high structural correlation across the sagittal plane of the pelvis. Quantitative 3D measurements on healthy pelvis data indicate that 78.9% of the distinguishable anatomical landmarks on the pelvis are symmetric [6], and the asymmetry in the remaining landmarks are still tolerated for fracture reduction surgery [7]. To exploit the partial symmetry, we automatically detect the desired plane of symmetry using Tukey's biweight distance measure. In addition, a novel regularization term is designed that ensures a similar distribution of bone density on both sides of the plane. Regularization is important when the amount of bone dislocation is large, and Tukey's cost cannot solely drive the symmetry plane to the optimal pose. After identifying the partial symmetry, the CT volume is mirrored across the symmetry plane which then allows simulating the ideal bone fragment configurations. This information is provided intra-operatively to the surgeon, by overlaying the C-arm X-ray image with a forward-projection of the mirrored volume.

The proposed approach relies on pre-operative CT scans of the patient. It is important to note that acquiring pre-operative CT scans is standard practice in severe trauma and fracture reduction cases. Therefore, it is valid to assume that pre-operative imaging is available for the types of fractures discussed in this manuscript, namely illiac wing, superior and inferior pubic ramus, lateral compression, and vertical shear fractures. In this paper, we introduce an approach that enables the surgeon to use patient CT scans intra-operatively, without explicitly visualizing the 3D data, but instead using 2D image augmentation on commonly used X-ray images.

2   Materials and Methods

2.1   Problem Formulation

The plane of symmetry of an object $O \subseteq \mathbb{R}^3$ is represented using an involutive isometric transformation $\mathbf{M}(g) \in E_o(3)$, such that $E_o(3) = \{h \in E(3) \mid h(O) = O\}$, where $E(3)$ is the 3D Euclidean group, consisting of all isometries of $\mathbb{R}^3$ which map $\mathbb{R}^3$ onto $\mathbb{R}^3$. The transformation $\mathbf{M}(g)$ mirrors the object O across the plane as; $\mathbf{o_{-x}} = \mathbf{M}(g)\,\mathbf{o_x}$, where $\mathbf{o_x} \subseteq \mathbb{P}^3$ and $\mathbf{o_{-x}} \subseteq \mathbb{P}^3$ are sub-volumes of object O on opposite sides of the symmetry plane, and are defined in the 3D projective space $\mathbb{P}^3$. Assuming the plane of symmetry is the Y-Z plane, $\mathbf{M}(g)$ is given by $\mathbf{M}(g) := g\,\mathbf{F}_x\,g^{-1}$, where $\mathbf{F}_x$ is reflection about the X-axis, and $g \in SE(3)$, where $SE(3)$ is the 3D special Euclidean group. We propose to estimate $\mathbf{M}(g)$ by minimizing a distance function $D(\mathbf{M}(g))$ as:

$$\arg \min_{g} D(\mathbf{M}(g)) := d_I(\mathbf{o_x}, \mathbf{M}(g)\mathbf{o_x}) + \lambda\, d_D(\mathbf{o_x}, \mathbf{M}(g)\mathbf{o_x}), \qquad (1)$$

combining an intensity-based distance measure $d_I(.)$, and a regularization term $d_D(.)$ based on the bone density distribution. The term λ in Eq. 1 is a relaxation factor, and $\lambda, d_I(.), d_D(.) \in \mathbb{R}$. Derivations of $d_I(.)$ and $d_D(.)$ are explained in Sects. 2.2 and 2.3, respectively. In Sect. 2.4, we suggest an approach to incorporate the knowledge from the plane of symmetry, and provide patient-specific image augmentation in fracture reduction interventions.

2.2   Robust Loss for Estimation of Partial Symmetry

The CT data of a pelvis only exhibits partial symmetry, as several regions within the CT volume may not have a symmetric counterpart on the contralateral side. These outlier regions occur either due to dislocation of the bone fragments, or asymmetry in the natural anatomy. To estimate the plane of "partial symmetry", we suggest to minimize a disparity function that is robust with respect to outliers, and only considers the partial symmetry present in the volumetric data. The robustness to outlier is achieved by down-weighting the error measurements associated to potential outlier regions. To this end, we estimate the plane of partial symmetry by minimizing Tukey's beweight loss function defined as [8]:

$$d_I(\mathbf{o_x}, \mathbf{M}(g)\mathbf{o_x}) = \sum_{i=1}^{|\Omega_s|} \frac{\rho(e_i(\mathbf{M}(g)))}{|\Omega_s|},$$

$$\rho(e_i(\mathbf{M}(g))) = \begin{cases} e_i(\mathbf{M}(g)) \left[1 - \left(\frac{e_i(\mathbf{M}(g))}{c}\right)^2\right]^2 & ;\, |e_i(\mathbf{M}(g))| \leqslant c, \\ 0 & ;\, \text{otherwise,} \end{cases} \qquad (2)$$

with Ω_s being the spatial domain of CT elements. The threshold of assigning data elements as outlier is defined by a constant factor c that is inversely proportional to the down-weight assigned to outliers. As suggested in the literature, $c = 4.685$ provides high asymptotic efficiency [8]. The residual error for the i-th voxel element is $e_i(\mathbf{M}(g))$ and is defined as following:

$$e_i(\mathbf{M}(g)) = \frac{|\mathrm{CT}(o_{x_i}) - \mathrm{CT}(\mathbf{M}(g)o_{x_i})|}{S}. \tag{3}$$

In Eq. 3, o_{x_i} is the i-th voxel element, $\mathrm{CT}(o_{x_i})$ is the intensity of o_{x_i}, and S is the scaling factor corresponding to the median absolute deviation of residuals.

2.3 Bone Density Histogram Regularization

In fractured bones, the distribution of bone material inside the body will remain nearly unaffected. Based on this fact, we hypothesize that the distribution of bone intensities, i.e. histograms of bone Hounsfield Unit (HU), on the opposite sides of the plane of symmetry remains similar in presence of fracture (example shown in Fig. 1). Therefore, we design a regularization term based on normalized mutual information as follows [9]:

$$d_D(\mathbf{o_x}, \mathbf{M}(g)\mathbf{o_x}) = -\frac{H(\mathrm{CT}(\mathbf{o_x})) + H(\mathrm{CT}(\mathbf{M}(g)\mathbf{o_x}))}{H(\mathrm{CT}(\mathbf{o_x}), \mathrm{CT}(\mathbf{M}(g)\mathbf{o_x})))}, \tag{4}$$

where $H(.)$ is the entropy of voxels' HU distribution. Minimizing the distance function in Eq. 4 is equivalent to increasing the similarity between the distributions of bone on the opposing sides of the plane of partial symmetry.

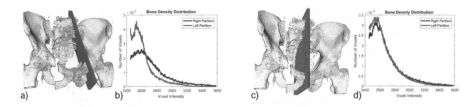

Fig. 1. Bone intensity histograms are shown in **(a–b)** and **(c–d)** before and after estimating the plane of partial symmetry.

2.4 Patient-Specific Image Augmentation

After estimating the plane of partial symmetry, the CT volume is mirrored across this plane to construct a patient-specific CT volume representing the bony structures "as if they were repaired". It is important to note that, although the human pelvic skeleton is not entirely symmetric, it is common in trauma interventions to consider it as symmetric, and use the contralateral side as reference.

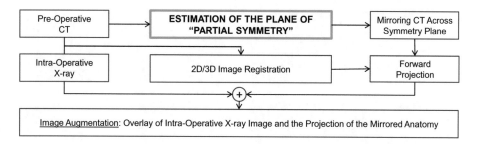

Fig. 2. Workflow for patient-specific image augmentation based on partial symmetry

To assist the orthopedic surgeon in re-aligning bone fragments, we propose to augment intra-operative X-ray images with the bone contours from the mirrored CT volume. This step requires generation of digitally reconstructed radiographs (DRRs) from views identical to the one acquired intra-operatively using a C-arm. Hence, 2D/3D image registration is employed to estimate the projection geometry between the X-ray image and CT data. This projective transformation is then used to forward-project and generate DRR images from the same viewing angle that the X-ray image was acquired. Finally, we augment the X-ray image with the edge-map acquired from the DRR that will then serve as a road-map for re-aligning the fragmented bones. The proposed workflow is shown in Fig. 2.

3   Experimental Validation and Results

We conducted experiments on synthetic and real CT images of healthy and fractured data. For all experiments, the optimization was performed using bound constrained by quadratic approximation algorithm, where the maximum number of iterations was set to 100. The regularization term λ in Eq. 1 was set to 0.5 which allowed $d_I(.)$ to be the dominant term driving the similarity cost, and $d_D(.)$ to serve as a data fidelity term.

Performance Evaluation on Synthetic Data: A synthetic 3D data of size 100^3 voxels and known plane of symmetry was generated. The synthetic volume was perfectly symmetric along the Y-Z plane, where the intensities of each voxel was proportional to its Y and Z coordinate in the volume. We evaluated the performance of the Tukey-based cost $d_I(.)$ with respect to noise and outliers, and compared the outcome to NCC-based cost. The results are shown in Fig. 3.

Estimating the Plane of Partial Symmetry on non-Fractured Data: The plane of partial symmetry was estimated for twelve CT datasets with no signs of fractures or damaged bone. Four of the volumes were lower torso cadaver CT data, and eight were from subjects with Sarcoma. After estimating the plane of partial symmetry, the CT volumes were mirrored across the estimated plane. We then identified the following 4 anatomical landmarks and measured the distance between each landmark on the original volume to the corresponding landmark on

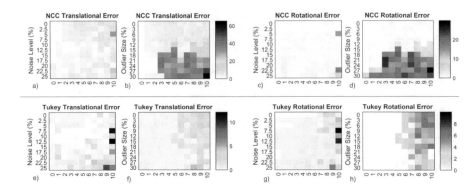

Fig. 3. The performance of Tukey-based distance measure is evaluated against noise level and amount of outlier. The horizontal axis indicates the relative pose of the symmetry plane at the initial step with respect to the ground-truth, where the initialization parameters were increased with the increments of 2 voxels translation and 2° rotation along each 3D axis. The amount of outlier was varied between 0% to 30% of the size of the entire volume, and the Gaussian noise between 0% to 25% of the highest intensity in the volume. **(a–d)** and **(e–h)** show the performance of NCC and Tukey robust estimator, respectively. It is important to note that different heat-map color scales are used for NCC and Tukey to demonstrate the changes within each sub-plot.

the mirrored CT volume: $\mathbf{L}_1$: anterior superior iliac spine, $\mathbf{L}_2$: posterior superior iliac spine, $\mathbf{L}_3$: ischial spine, and $\mathbf{L}_4$: ischial ramus. Results of this experiment using NCC, Tukey robust estimator $d_I(.)$, and regularized Tukey $d_I(.) + \lambda d_D(.)$ distance functions are shown in Table 1.

Table 1. Errors in estimation of partial symmetry were measured using four anatomical landmarks. The values in the table are in mm units, and are shown as mean ± SD. The final row are the results of our proposed method.

	$\mathbf{L}_1$	$\mathbf{L}_2$	$\mathbf{L}_3$	$\mathbf{L}_4$
NCC	12.8 ± 7.15	11.5 ± 10.7	7.81 ± 5.08	7.12 ± 5.20
Tukey	6.79 ± 3.95	6.95 ± 5.34	4.63 ± 2.60	4.75 ± 1.85
Regularized Tukey	$\mathbf{3.85 \pm 1.79}$	$\mathbf{4.06 \pm 3.32}$	$\mathbf{3.16 \pm 1.41}$	$\mathbf{2.77 \pm 2.13}$

Estimating the Plane of Partial Symmetry on Fractured Data: We simulated three different fractures - *i.e.* iliac wing, pelvic ring, and vertical shear fractures (shown in Fig. 4(a–c)) - and evaluated the performance of the proposed solution in presence of bone dislocation. These three fractures were applied to three different volumes, and in total nine fractured CT volumes were generated. The error measurements are presented in Table 2.

Intra-operative Image Augmentation: After estimating the plane of partial symmetry, we mirrored the healthy side of the pelvis across the plane of partial

Table 2. Error measurements on fractured data in mm units.

	L_1	L_2	L_3	L_4
Iliac wing fracture				
NCC	26.4 ± 14.3	20.1 ± 14.2	14.9 ± 9.17	10.2 ± 1.04
Tukey	6.36 ± 3.40	6.80 ± 4.10	6.90 ± 5.86	4.89 ± 1.29
Regularized Tukey	$\mathbf{3.60 \pm 2.93}$	$\mathbf{3.30 \pm 3.13}$	$\mathbf{4.01 \pm 1.24}$	$\mathbf{2.06 \pm 0.92}$
Pelvic ring fracture				
NCC	39.2 ± 39.9	27.0 ± 23.9	26.6 ± 32.5	25.4 ± 31.0
Tukey	4.54 ± 2.39	6.14 ± 5.88	6.28 ± 3.81	3.68 ± 0.81
Regularized Tukey	$\mathbf{2.17 \pm 1.37}$	$\mathbf{3.75 \pm 3.17}$	$\mathbf{2.03 \pm 0.73}$	$\mathbf{1.98 \pm 0.99}$
Vertical shear fracture				
NCC	28.1 ± 15.1	16.6 ± 11.9	21.7 ± 6.91	19.7 ± 6.02
Tukey	15.8 ± 7.66	10.9 ± 8.48	11.1 ± 3.54	11.4 ± 5.52
Regularized Tukey	$\mathbf{5.46 \pm 2.04}$	$\mathbf{3.52 \pm 2.63}$	$\mathbf{4.85 \pm 1.86}$	$\mathbf{5.28 \pm 2.89}$

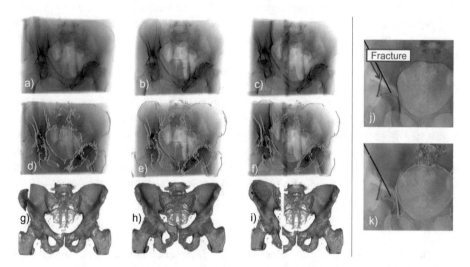

Fig. 4. (**a–c**) are simulated iliac wing, pelvic ring, and vertical shear fractures, respectively. Image augmentations are shown in (**d–f**). The red arrows indicate the fracture location in the pelvis. The green contours represent the desired bone contours to achieve bilateral symmetry. (**g–h**) show the 3D visualization of the fractures, where red color indicates regions that were rejected as outliers using Tukey's robust estimator. The intra-operative X-ray image in (**j**) is augmented with the edge-map of the DRR generated from the mirrored volume using the projection geometry estimated from 2D/3D X-ray to CT image registration(**k**).

symmetry. In Fig. 4(d–f) we present the superimposition of the fractured data shown in Fig. 4(a–c) with the edge-map extracted from gradient-weighted DRRs. Moreover, we preformed 2D/3D intensity-based registration between the pre-operative CT and the intra-operative X-ray (Fig. 4j), and used the estimated projection geometry to generate DRRs and augment the X-ray image of the fractured bone. The augmentation is shown in Fig. 4k.

4   Discussion and Conclusion

This work presents a novel method to estimate partial structural symmetry in CT images of fractured pelvises. We used Tukey's biweight robust estimator which prevents outlier voxel elements from having large effects on the similarity measure. Moreover, Tukey's distance function is regularized by enforcing high similarity in bilateral bone HU distribution. The experimental results on synthetic data indicate that Tukey-based similarity cost outperformed NCC-based similarity cost substantially in the presence of noise and outliers. The results in Table 1 show an average landmark error of 5.78 mm and 3.46 mm using Tukey- and regularized Tukey-based cost, respectively. Similarly for fractured data presented in Table 2, the mean error reduced from 7.91 mm to 3.50 mm after including the regularization term.

In conclusion, we proposed to incorporate the knowledge from partial symmetry and provide intra-operative image augmentation to assist orthopedic surgeons in re-aligning the bone fragments with respect to bilateral symmetry. Our work relies on pre-operative CT images and is only applicable to surgical interventions where pre-operative 3D imaging exist. This solution enables patient-specific image augmentation which is not possible using statistical atlases. Using atlases for this application requires a large population of patient pelvis data for different age, sex, race, disease, etc. which are not available.

References

1. Bellabarba, C., Ricci, W.M., Bolhofner, B.R.: Distraction external fixation in lateral compression pelvic fractures. J. Orthop. Trauma 14(7), 475–482 (2000)
2. Vannier, M.W., Marsh, J.L., Warren, J.O.: Three dimensional CT reconstruction images for craniofacial surgical planning and evaluation. Radiology 150(1), 179–184 (1984)
3. Edsander-Nord, A., Brandberg, Y., Wickman, M.: Quality of life, patients' satisfaction, and aesthetic outcome after pedicled or free tram flap breast surgery. Plastic Reconstr. Surg. 107(5), 1142–53 (2001)
4. Tile, M.: Acute pelvic fractures: I. causation and classification. JAAOS-J. Am. Acad. Orthop. Surg. 4(3), 143–151 (1996)
5. Chintalapani, G., et al.: Statistical atlas based extrapolation of CT data. In: Medical Imaging 2010: Visualization, Image-Guided Procedures, and Modeling. Vol. 7625, p. 762539. International Society for Optics and Photonics (2010)
6. Boulay, C., et al.: Three-dimensional study of pelvic asymmetry on anatomical specimens and its clinical perspectives. J. Anat. 208(1), 21–33 (2006)

7. Shen, F., Chen, B., Guo, Q., Qi, Y., Shen, Y.: Augmented reality patient-specific reconstruction plate design for pelvic and acetabular fracture surgery. Int. J. Comput. Assist. Radiol. Surg. **8**(2), 169–179 (2013)
8. Huber, P.J.: Robust statistics. In: Lovric, M. (ed.) International Encyclopedia of Statistical Science, pp. 1248–1251. Springer, Heidelberg (2011). https://doi.org/10.1007/978-3-642-04898-2_594
9. Studholme, C., Hill, D.L., Hawkes, D.J.: An overlap invariant entropy measure of 3D medical image alignment. Pattern Recogn. **32**(1), 71–86 (1999)

Intraoperative Brain Shift Compensation Using a Hybrid Mixture Model

Siming Bayer[1](✉), Nishant Ravikumar[1], Maddalena Strumia[2],
Xiaoguang Tong[3], Ying Gao[4], Martin Ostermeier[2], Rebecca Fahrig[2],
and Andreas Maier[1]

[1] Pattern Recognition Lab, Friedrich-Alexander University, Martenstaße 3,
91058 Erlangen, Germany
siming.bayer@fau.de
[2] Siemens Healthcare GmbH, Siemensstr. 1, 91301 Forchheim, Germany
[3] Tianjin Huanhu Hospital, Jizhao Road 6, Tianjin 300350, China
[4] Siemens Healthcare Ltd, Wanjing Zhonghuan Nanlu, Beijing 100102, China

Abstract. Brain deformation (or *brain shift*) during neurosurgical procedures such as tumor resection has a significant impact on the accuracy of neuronavigation systems. Compensating for this deformation during surgery is essential for effective guidance. In this paper, we propose a method for *brain shift* compensation based on registration of vessel centerlines derived from preoperative C-Arm cone beam CT (CBCT) images, to intraoperative ones. A hybrid mixture model (HdMM)-based non-rigid registration approach was formulated wherein, Student's t and Watson distributions were combined to model positions and centerline orientations of cerebral vasculature, respectively. Following registration of the preoperative vessel centerlines to its intraoperative counterparts, B-spline interpolation was used to generate a dense deformation field and warp the preoperative image to each intraoperative image acquired. Registration accuracy was evaluated using both synthetic and clinical data. The former comprised CBCT images, acquired using a deformable anthropomorphic brain phantom. The latter meanwhile, consisted of four 3D digital subtraction angiography (DSA) images of one patient, acquired before, during and after surgical tumor resection. HdMM consistently outperformed a state-of-the-art point matching method, coherent point drift (CPD), resulting in significantly lower registration errors. For clinical data, the registration error was reduced from 3.73 mm using CPD to 1.55 mm using the proposed method.

1 Introduction

Brain shift compensation is imperative during neurosurgical procedures such as tumor resection as the resulting deformation of brain parenchyma significantly affects the efficacy of preoperative plans, central to surgical guidance. Conventional image-guided navigation systems (IGNS) model the skull and its contents

© Springer Nature Switzerland AG 2018
A. F. Frangi et al. (Eds.): MICCAI 2018, LNCS 11073, pp. 116–124, 2018.
https://doi.org/10.1007/978-3-030-00937-3_14

as rigid objects and do not compensate for soft tissue deformation induced during surgery. Consequently, non-rigid registration is essential to compensate to update surgical plans, and ensure precision during image-guided neurosurgery.

C-arm computed tomography (CT) is a state-of-the-art imaging system, capable of acquiring high resolution and high contrast 3D images of cerebral vasculature in real time. However, in contrast to other intraoperative imaging systems such as magnetic resonance (MR), ultrasound (US), laser range scanners and stereo vision cameras, few studies have investigated the use of C-arm CT in an interventional setting for *brain shift* compensation [1]. The advantages of C-arm interventional imaging systems are, they do not require special surgical tools as with MR and provide high resolution images (unlike MR and US). Additionally, they enable recovery of soft tissue deformation within the brain, rather than just the external surface (as with laser range imaging and stereo vision cameras). The downsides are a slight increase in X-ray and contrast agent dose.

Recently, Smit-Ockeleon et al. [5] employed B-spline based elastic image registration to compensate for *brain shift*, using pre- and intraoperative CBCT images (although, not during surgical tumor resection). Coherent point drift (CPD) [8], a state-of-the-art non-rigid point set registration approach was used in [3] and [7], for *brain shift* compensation. Both studies used thin plate splines (TPS)-based interpolation to warp the preoperative image to its intraoperative counterparts, based on the initial sparse displacement field estimated using CPD. Although [3] demonstrated the superiority of CPD compared to conventional point matching approaches such as iterative closest point (ICP), a fundamental drawback of the former in an interventional setting is that it lacks automatic robustness to outliers. To overcome this limitation, Ravikumar et al. [10] proposed a probabilistic point set registration approach based on Student's t-distributions and Von-Mises-Fisher distributions for group-wise shape registration.

In this paper we propose a vessel centerlines-based registration framework for intraoperative *brain shift* compensation at different stages of neurosurgery, namely, at dura-opening, during tumor resection, and following tumor removal. The main contributions of our work are: (1) a feature based registration framework that enables the use of 3D digital subtraction angiography (DSA) images and 3D CBCT acquired using C-arm CT, for *brain shift* compensation; (2) the formulation of a probabilistic non-rigid registration approach, using a hybrid mixture model (HdMM) that combines Student's t-distributions ($\mathcal{S}$, for automatic robustness to outliers) to model spatial positions, and Watson distributions ($\mathcal{W}$) to model the orientation of vessel centerlines; and (3) to the best of our knowledge, this is the first paper exploring the use of pre-, intra-, and post-surgery 3D DSA for *brain shift* compensation in a real patient.

2   Materials and Methods

This study investigates the use of C-Arm CT, which captures 3D cerebral vasculature, as pre- and intraoperative image modalities for *brain shift* compensation during surgical tumor resection. Vessel centerlines were extracted from pre- and intraoperative images automatically using Frangi's vesselness filter [4] and a homotopic thinning algorithm proposed in [6]. The registration pipeline we followed is: (1) rigid and non-rigid registration, (2) an optional resection detection and registration refinement step, and (3) B-Spline image warping.

Hybrid Mixture Model-Based Registration: The extracted centerlines are represented as 6D hybrid point sets, comprising spatial positions and their associated undirected unit vectors representing the local orientation of vessels. Preoperative centerlines are registered to their intraoperative counterparts using a pair-wise, hybrid mixture model-based rigid and non-rigid registration approach. Rigid registration is used to initialize the subsequent non-rigid step, in all experiments conducted. Recently, [10] proposed a similar approach for group-wise shape registration. Here, hybrid shape representations which combined spatial positions and their associated (consistently oriented) surface normal vectors are employed to improve registration accuracy for complex geometries. However, their approach is designed to model directional data using Von-Mises-Fisher (vmF) distributions and correspondingly required the surface normal vectors to be consistently oriented. vmF distributions lack antipodal symmetry and consequently are not suitable to model axial data such as vessel centerlines. We propose a variant of this registration approach that incorporates Watson distributions (whose probability density is the same in either direction along its mean axis) in place of vmFs, to address this limitation.

Registration of the preoperative (Source) and intraoperative (Target) vessel centerlines is formulated as a probability density estimation problem. Hybrid points defining the Source are regarded as the centroids of a HdMM, which is fit to those defining the Target, regarded as its data points. This is achieved by maximizing the log-likelihood (llh) function, using expectation-maximization (EM). The desired rigid and non-rigid transformations are estimated during the maximization (M)-step of the algorithm. By assuming the spatial position ($\mathbf{x}_i$) and centerline orientation ($\mathbf{n}_i$) components of each hybrid point in the Target set to be conditionally independent, their joint probability density function (PDF) can be approximated as a product of the individual conditional densities. The PDF of an undirected 3D unit vector $\mathbf{n}_i$ sampled from the jth component's Watson distribution in a HdMM, with a mean $\mathbf{m}_j$, is expressed as: $p(\pm\mathbf{n}_i|\mathbf{m}_j,\kappa_j) = M(\frac{1}{2},\frac{D}{2},\kappa_j)^{-1}\exp^{\kappa_j(\mathbf{m}_j{}^T\mathbf{n}_i)^2}$. Here, κ_j and $M(\cdot)$ represent the dispersion parameters and confluent hypergeometric function, respectively.

$$\log(\mathbf{T} \mid \mathcal{T},\Theta_p,\Theta_d) = \sum_{i=1}^{N}\log\sum_{j=1}^{M}\pi_j\mathcal{S}(\mathbf{x}_i \mid \mathcal{T}\boldsymbol{\mu}_j,\nu_j,\sigma^2)\mathcal{W}(\mathbf{n}_i \mid \mathcal{T}\mathbf{m}_j,\kappa_j) \quad (1a)$$

$$Q(\Theta_p^{t+1} \mid \Theta_p^t) = \sum_{i,j=1}^{N,M} -P_{i,j}^\star\frac{||\mathbf{x}_i - (\boldsymbol{\mu}_j + v(\boldsymbol{\mu}_j))||^2}{2\sigma^2} + \frac{\lambda}{2}\mathrm{Tr}\{\mathbf{W}^T\mathbf{G}\mathbf{W}\} \quad (1b)$$

Assuming all $i = 1...N$ hybrid points in the Target ($\mathbf{T}$) to be independent and identically distributed, and as data points generated by an $j = 1...M$-component mixture model (defining the Source), the *llh* is expressed as shown in Eq. 1a. Here, $\boldsymbol{\mu}_j$ and π_j represent the spatial position and mixture coefficient of the jth component in the HdMM. In the first stage, rigid transformation ($\mathcal{T}$) and model parameters associated with the Student's t-distributions in the mixture ($\Theta_p = \{\nu_j, \sigma^2\}$), namely, translation, rotation, scaling, and degrees of freedom (ν_j), variance (σ^2), respectively, are updated in the M-step similarly to [9]. In the second stage, the desired non-rigid transformation ($\mathcal{T}$) is expressed as a linear combination of radial basis functions, and the associated parameters are estimated as described in [8]. Tikhonov regularization is employed to ensure that the estimated deformation field is smooth. The resulting cost function that is maximized to estimate the desired non-rigid transformation is expressed as shown in Eq. 1b. Here, Q represents the expected *llh*, t represents the current EM-iteration, $P^\star$ represents the corrected posterior probabilities estimated in the expectation (E)-step (as described in [9]), v is the displacement function mapping the Source to the Target, λ controls the smoothness enforced on the deformation field and $\mathbf{W}$ and $\mathbf{G}$ represent the weights associated with the radial basis functions and the Gaussian kernel, respectively. During both rigid and non-rigid registration, parameters associated with the Watson distributions ($\Theta_d = \{\kappa_j\}$) are estimated as described in [2].

Resection Detection and Registration Refinement: While the Student's t-distributions in the proposed framework provide automatic robustness to outliers, it is difficult to cope with large amounts of missing data in the Target relative to the Source, as is the case during and following tumor resection. Consequently, we formulated a mechanism for refining the correspondences, in order to accommodate for the missing data during registration. This was achieved by detecting and excluding points in the Source that lie within the resected region in the Target, following both rigid and non-rigid registration. The refined correspondences in the Source were subsequently non-rigidly registered (henceforth referred to as HdMM+) to the Target, to accommodate for the missing data and improve the overall registration accuracy. Points within the resected region were identified by first building a 2D feature space for each point in the Source. The selected features comprised: the minimum euclidean distance between each Source point and the points in the Target; and the number of points in the Target which had been assigned posterior probabilities greater than $1e^{-5}$, for each point in the Source. Subsequently, PCA was used to reduce the dimensionality of this feature space and extract the first principal component. Finally, automatic histogram clipping using Otsu-thresholding was performed on the first principal component, to identify and exclude points within the resected region.

3   Experiments and Results

Data Acquisition: A deformable anthropomorphic brain phantom Fig. 1, (manufactured by True Phantom Solutions Inc., Windsor, Canada) is used to acquire CBCT images and conduct synthetic experiments. It comprises multiple structures mimicking real anatomy, namely, skin, skull, brain parenchyma, ventricular system, cerebral vasculature and an inflatable tumor. A removable plug is embedded in the skull to emulate a craniotomy. Brain tissue and blood vessels are made from polyurethane, a soft tissue simulant. In order to simulate multiple stages of tumor resection surgery, 40 ml distilled water was injected into the inflatable tumor initially. The tumor was subsequently deflated to 25 ml, 15 ml, 5 ml and 0 ml. At each stage, a 10s 3D CBCT image was acquired using the Ultravist 370 contrast agent to enhance the blood vessels. The acquisitions were reconstructed on a $512 \times 512 \times 398$ grid at a voxel resolution of 0.48mm^3. The experimental setup and a typical acquisition of the phantom are shown in Fig. 1. A detailed description and visualization of the phantom is included in the supplementary material.

The clinical data used in this study was provided by our clinical partner. It comprised 3D DSA images acquired during tumor resection surgery of a glioma patient. The images were acquired preoperatively, following craniotomy, during resection, and postoperatively, to monitor blood flow within the brain during and after surgery. The surgery was performed in a hybrid operating room with Siemens Artis zeego system (Forchheim, Germany) and as with the phantom experiments, the acquisitions were reconstructed on a $512 \times 512 \times 398$ grid with voxel resolution of 0.48 mm^3. We evaluated the proposed approach using the phantom and clinical data sets. The former involved four independent registration experiments. The image acquired with the tumor in its deflated state (with 0 ml of water) was considered to be the Source, while, those acquired at each inflated state of the tumor were considered as Targets. The latter involved three independent experiments, namely, registration of the preoperative image to images acquired following craniotomy, during tumor resection, and postoperatively.

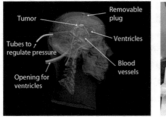 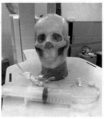 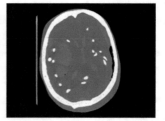

Fig. 1. The CAD model of the phantom, the experiment setting and an example slice of CBCT acquisition of the phantom are shown from left to right.

Results: We compared the performance of our registration method with CPD, using the phantom and clinical data sets. For fair comparison, we fixed the parameters associated with the non-rigid transformation, namely, the smoothing factor associated with the Tikhonov regularization and the width of the

Gaussian kernel, to 1, for both HdMM and CPD. Following preliminary investigations, we identified 0.5 to be a suitable value for the uniform distribution component weight in CPD, which remained fixed for all experiments. The maximum number of EM-iterations was set to 100 for all experiments, using both methods. The mean surface distance metric (MSD) is used to evaluate registration accuracy in all experiments conducted. As the phantom data set lacks any tumor resection/missing data, these samples are registered using just CPD and HdMM. In contrast, the clinical data set is registered using CPD, HdMM and HdMM+, to evaluate the gain in registration accuracy provided by the correspondence refinement step (in HdMM+), when dealing with missing data. We assess registration accuracy for both data sets in two ways: (1) by evaluating the MSD between the registered Source and Target sets (henceforth referred to as Error1); and (2) by evaluating the MSD between the vessel centerlines, extracted from the warped preoperative image, and each corresponding intraoperative image (henceforth referred to as Error2). Additionally, for the clinical data set, in order to evaluate the degree of overlap between the cerebral vasculature following registration of the preoperative to each intraoperative image, we also compute the Dice and Jaccard scores between their respective vessel segmentations.

The average MSD errors, Dice, and Jaccard scores for all experiments are summarized by the box plots depicted in Fig. 2. These plots indicate that, HdMM consistently outperforms CPD in all experiments conducted, and in terms of all measures used to assess registration accuracy. The initial average MSD is 5.42 ± 1.07 mm and 6.06 ± 0.68 mm for phantom and clinical data, respectively. Applying the registration pipeline, the average Error1 for the phantom data set (averaged across all four registration experiments), is 0.89 ± 0.36 mm and 0.50 ± 0.05 mm, using CPD and HdMM respectively. While, the average Error2 is 1.88 ± 0.52 mm and 1.54 ± 0.15 mm for CPD and HdMM, respectively. For the clinical data set, the average Error1 is 2.44 ± 0.28 mm and 1.15 ± 0.36 mm and average Error2 is 3.72 ± 0.46 mm and 2.24 ± 0.55 m, for CPD and HdMM, respectively. Further improvement in registration accuracy is achieved using HdMM+, which achieved average Error1 and Error2 of 0.78 ± 0.12 mm and 1.55 ± 0.22 mm, respectively. The mean Dice and Jaccard scores (refer to Fig. 2(c)) evaluated using vessels segmented from the warped preoperative image and each corresponding intraoperative image indicate that, similar to the MSD errors, HdMM+ outperformed both CPD and HdMM. To qualitatively assess the registration accuracy of our approach, vessels extracted from the warped preoperative image, are overlaid on its intraoperative counterpart (acquired following craniotomoy and tumor resection), as shown in Fig. 3. Figure 3(a) and (c) depicts the registration result of CPD, while, Fig. 3(b) and (d) depicts that of HdMM. These images summarize the superior registration accuracy of the proposed approach, relative to CPD.

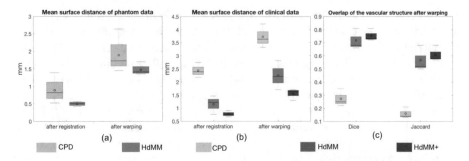

Fig. 2. MSD errors evaluated following registration of the phantom and clinical data sets are presented in (a) and (b) respectively. Average Dice and Jaccard scores evaluating the overlap between vessels segmented in the registered preoperative and corresponding intraoperative images are depicted in (c).

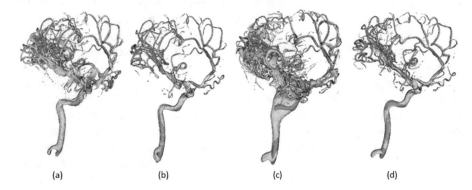

Fig. 3. Overlay of 3D cerebral vasculature segmented from the registered preoperative (yellow) DSA image and the target intraoperative image (green). Using CPD (a) and HdMM (b) prior to resection, using CPD (c) and HdMM (d) post resection.

4   Discussion and Conclusion

The presented results (refer to Figs. 2 and 3) for the phantom and clinical data experiments indicate that the proposed approach is able to preserve fine structural details, and consistently outperforms CPD in terms of registration accuracy. This is attributed to the higher discriminative capacity afforded by the hybrid representation of vessel centerlines used by HdMM, enabling it to establish correspondences with greater anatomical validity than CPD. Complex structures such as vessel bifurcations require more descriptive features for accurate registration, than afforded by spatial positions alone. Consequently, a registration framework such as HdMM that jointly models the PDF of spatial positions and centerline orientations, is better equipped for registering complex geometries such as cerebral vasculature than point matching methods that rely on spatial positions alone (such as CPD).

An additional advantage of the proposed approach is its inherent and automatic robustness to outliers that may be present in the data. This is attributed to the heavy-tailed nature of the constituent Student's t-distributions in the HdMM, and the estimation of different values for the degrees of freedom associated with each component in the HdMM. This is a significant advantage over CPD, as the latter requires manual tuning of a weight associated with the uniform distribution component in the mixture model, which regulates its robustness to outliers during registration. These advantages and the significant improvement in registration accuracy afforded by HdMM indicate that it is well-suited to applications involving registration of vascular structures. This is encouraging for its future use in intraoperative guidance applications, and specifically, for vessel-guided *brain shift* compensation.

Evaluation on a single clinical data set is a limitation of the current study. However, the proposed work-flow is not standard clinical practice, as there is a limited number of hybrid installations, equipped with CBCT capable devices in upright sitting position. Furthermore, the protocol induces a slight amount of additional X-ray and contrast agent dose which is typically not a problem for the patient population under consideration. However, prior to this study, there was no indication whether vessel-based *brain shift* compensation can be performed successfully at all, given 3D DSA images. Thus, getting a single data set posed a significant challenge. The potential of the proposed workflow to ensure high precision in surgical guidance, in the vicinity of cerebral vasculature, is particularly compelling for neurosurgery.

Disclaimer: The methods and information presented in this work are based on research and are not commercially available.

References

1. Bayer, S., Maier, A., Ostermeier, M., Fahrig, R.: Intraoperative imaging modalities and compensation for brain shift in tumor resection surgery. Int. J. Biomed. Imaging **2017**, 6028645 (2017). https://doi.org/10.1155/2017/6028645
2. Bijral, A., Breitenbach, M., Grudic, G.: Mixture of watson distributions: a generative model for hyperspherical embeddings. In: Proceedings of Machine Learning Research (2007)
3. Farnia, P., Ahmadian, A., Khoshnevisan, A., Jaberzadeh, A., Serej, N.D., Kazerooni, A.F.: An efficient point based registration of intra-operative ultrasound images with MR images for computation of brain shift; a phantom study. In: IEEE EMBC 2011, pp. 8074–8077 (2011)
4. Frangi, A.F., Niessen, W.J., Vincken, K.L., Viergever, M.A.: Multiscale vessel enhancement filtering. In: Wells, W.M., Colchester, A., Delp, S. (eds.) MICCAI 1998. LNCS, vol. 1496, pp. 130–137. Springer, Heidelberg (1998). https://doi.org/10.1007/BFb0056195
5. Smit-Ockeloen, I., Ruijters, D., Breeuwer, M., Babic, D., Brina, O., Pereira, V.M.: Accuracy assessment of CBCT-based volumetric brain shift field. In: Oyarzun Laura, C., et al. (eds.) CLIP 2015. LNCS, vol. 9401, pp. 1–9. Springer, Cham (2016). https://doi.org/10.1007/978-3-319-31808-0_1

6. Lee, T., Kashyap, R., Chu, C.: Building skeleton models via 3-D medial surface axis thinning algorithms. CVGIP **56**(6), 462–478 (1994)
7. Marreiros, F.M.M., Rossitti, S., Wang, C., Smedby, Ö.: Non-rigid deformation pipeline for compensation of superficial brain shift. In: Mori, K., Sakuma, I., Sato, Y., Barillot, C., Navab, N. (eds.) MICCAI 2013. LNCS, vol. 8150, pp. 141–148. Springer, Heidelberg (2013). https://doi.org/10.1007/978-3-642-40763-5_18
8. Myronenko, A., Song, X.: Point set registration: coherent point drift. IEEE Trans. Pattern. Anal. Mach. Intell. **32**(12), 2262–2275 (2010)
9. Ravikumar, N., Gooya, A., Çimen, S., Frangi, A.F., Taylor, Z.A.: Group-wise similarity registration of point sets using student's t-mixture model for statistical shape models. Med. Image Anal. **44**, 156–176 (2018)
10. Ravikumar, N., Gooya, A., Frangi, A.F., Taylor, Z.A.: Generalised coherent point drift for group-wise registration of multi-dimensional point sets. In: Descoteaux, M., Maier-Hein, L., Franz, A., Jannin, P., Collins, D.L., Duchesne, S. (eds.) MICCAI 2017. LNCS, vol. 10433, pp. 309–316. Springer, Cham (2017). https://doi.org/10.1007/978-3-319-66182-7_36

Video-Based Computer Aided Arthroscopy for Patient Specific Reconstruction of the Anterior Cruciate Ligament

Carolina Raposo[1,2(✉)], Cristóvão Sousa[2], Luis Ribeiro[2], Rui Melo[2], João P. Barreto[1,2], João Oliveira[3], Pedro Marques[3], and Fernando Fonseca[3]

[1] Institute of Systems and Robotics, University of Coimbra, Coimbra, Portugal
carolina.raposo@isr.uc.pt
[2] Perceive3D, Coimbra, Portugal
[3] Faculty of Medicine, Coimbra Hospital and University Centre, Coimbra, Portugal

Abstract. The Anterior Cruciate Ligament tear is a common medical condition that is treated using arthroscopy by pulling a tissue graft through a tunnel opened with a drill. The correct anatomical position and orientation of this tunnel is crucial for knee stability, and drilling an adequate bone tunnel is the most technically challenging part of the procedure. This paper presents, for the first time, a guidance system based solely on intra-operative video for guiding the drilling of the tunnel. Our solution uses small, easily recognizable visual markers that are attached to the bone and tools for estimating their relative pose. A recent registration algorithm is employed for aligning a pre-operative image of the patient's anatomy with a set of contours reconstructed by touching the bone surface with an instrumented tool. Experimental validation using ex-vivo data shows that the method enables the accurate registration of the pre-operative model with the bone, providing useful information for guiding the surgeon during the medical procedure.

Keywords: Computer-guidance · Visual tracking · 3D registration
Arthroscopy

1 Introduction

Arthroscopy is a modality of orthopeadic surgery for treatment of damaged joints in which instruments and endoscopic camera (the arthroscope) are inserted into the articular cavity through small incisions (the surgical ports). Since arthroscopy largely preserves the integrity of the articulation, it is beneficial to the patient in terms of reduction of trauma, risk of infection and recovery time [17]. However, arthroscopic approaches are more difficult to execute than the open surgery alternatives because of the indirect visualization and limited manoeuvrability inside the joint, with novices having to undergo a long training period [14] and experts often making mistakes with clinical consequences [16].

© Springer Nature Switzerland AG 2018
A. F. Frangi et al. (Eds.): MICCAI 2018, LNCS 11073, pp. 125–133, 2018.
https://doi.org/10.1007/978-3-030-00937-3_15

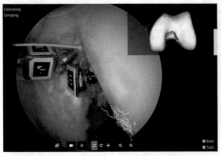 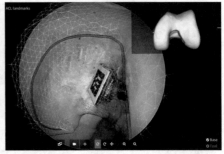

(a) Reconstruction of 3D contours   (b) Result of the 3D alignment

Fig. 1. (a) 3D digitalisation of the bone surface: the surgeon performs a random walk on the intercondylar region using a touch-probe instrumented with a visual marker with the objective of reconstructing 3D curves on the bone surface. (b) Overlay of the pre-operative MRI with highlight of intercondylar arch: The reconstructed 3D curves are used to register the pre-operative MRI with the patient anatomy.

The reconstruction of the Anterior Cruciate Ligament (ACL) illustrates well the aforementioned situation. The ACL rupture is a common medical condition with more than 200 000 annual cases in the USA alone [16]. The standard way of treatment is arthroscopic reconstruction where the torn ligament is replaced by a tissue graft that is pulled into the knee joint through tunnels opened with a drill in both femur and tibia [3]. Opening these tunnels in an anatomically correct position is crucial for knee stability and patient satisfaction, with the ideal graft being placed in the exact same position of the original ligament to maximize proprioception [1]. Unfortunately, ligament position varies significantly across individuals and substantial effort has been done to model variance and provide anatomic references to be used during surgery [5]. However, correct tunnel placement is still a matter of experience with success rates varying broadly between low and high volume surgeons [16]. Some studies reveal levels of satisfaction of only 75% with an incidence of revision surgeries of 10 to 15%, half of which caused by deficient technical execution [16].

This is a scenario where Computer-Aided Surgery (CAS) can have an impact. There are two types of navigation systems reported in literature: the ones that use intra-operative fluoroscopy [3], and the ones that rely in optical tracking to register a pre-operative CT/MRI or perform 3D bone morphing [6]. Despite being available for several years the market, penetration of these systems is residual because of their inaccuracy and inconvenience [6]. The added value of fluoroscopy based systems does not compensate the risk of radiation overdose, while optical tracking systems require additional incisions to attach markers which hinders acceptance because the purpose of arthroscopy is to minimize incisions. The ideal solution for Computer-Aided Arthroscopy (CAA) should essentially rely in processing the already existing intra-operative video. This would avoid the above mentioned issues and promote cost efficiency by not requiring additional capital equipment. Despite the intense research in CAS using endoscopic video [11], arthroscopic sequences are specially challenging because of poor texture, existence of deformable tissues, complex illumination, and very close range acquisition. In addition, the camera is hand-held, the lens scope rotates, the procedure is performed in wet medium and the surgeon often switches camera port. Our attempts of using visual SLAM pipelines reported to work in laparoscopy [10] were unfruitful and revealed the need of additional visual aids to accomplish the robustness required for real clinical uptake.

This article describes the first video-based system for CAA, where visual information is used to register a pre-operative CT/MRI with the patient anatomy such that tunnels can be opened in the position of the original ligament (patient specific surgery). The concept relates with previous works in CAS for laparoscopy that visually track a planar pattern engraved in a projector to determine its 3D pose [4]. We propose to attach similar fiducial markers to both anatomy and instruments and use the moving arthroscope to estimate the relative rigid displacements at each frame time instant. The scheme enables to perform accurate 3D reconstruction of the bone surface with a touch-probe (Fig. 1(a)) that is used to accomplish registration of the pre-operative 3D model or plan (Fig. 1(b)). The marker of the femur (or tibia) works as the world reference frame where all 3D information is stored, which enables to quickly resume navigation after switching camera port and overlay guidance information in images using augmented reality techniques. The paper describes the main modules of the real-time software pipeline and reports results in both synthetic and real *ex-vivo* experiments.

2   Video-Based Computer-Aided Arthroscopy

This section overviews the proposed concept for CAA that uses the intra-operative arthroscopic video, together with planar visual markers attached to instruments and anatomy, to perform tracking and 3D pose estimation inside the articular joint. As discussed, applying conventional SLAM/SfM algorithms [10] to arthroscopic images is extremely challenging and, in order to circumvent the difficulties, we propose to use small planar fiducial markers that can be easily detected in images and whose pose can be estimated using homography factorization [2,9]. These visual aids enable to achieve the robustness and accuracy required for deployment in real arthroscopic scenario that otherwise would be impossible. The key steps of the approach are the illustrated in Fig. 2 and described next.

The Anatomy Marker WM: The surgeon starts by rigidly attaching a screw-like object with a flat head that has an engraved known 4 mm-side square pattern. We will refer to this screw as the World Marker (WM) because the local reference frame of its pattern will define the coordinate system with respect to which all 3D information is described. The WM can be placed in an arbitrary position in the intercondylar surface, provided that it can be easily seen by the arthroscope during the procedure. The placement of the marker is accomplished using a custom made tool that can be seen in the accompanying video.

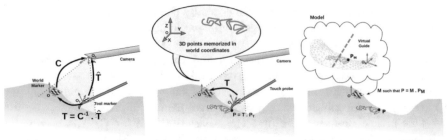

(a) Pose estimation   (b) Contour reconstruction   (c) Registration & guidance

Fig. 2. Key steps of the proposed approach: (a) 3D pose estimation inside the articular joint, (b) 3D reconstruction of points and contours on bone surface and (c) 3D registration and guidance.

3D Pose Estimation Inside the Articular Joint: The 3D pose C of the WM in camera coordinates can be determined at each time instant by detecting the WM in the image, estimating the plane-to-image homography from the 4 detected corners of its pattern and decomposing the homography to obtain the rigid transformation [2,9]. Consider a touch probe that is also instrumented with another planar pattern that can be visually read. Using a similar method, it is possible to detect and identify the tool marker (TM) in the image and compute its 3D pose $\hat{T}$ with respect to the camera. This allows the pose T of the TM in WM coordinates to be determined in a straightforward manner by $T = C^{-1}\hat{T}$.

3D Reconstruction of Points and Contours on Bone Surface: The location of the tip of the touch probe in the local TM reference frame is known, meaning that its location w.r.t. the WM can be determined using T. A point on the surface can be determined by touching it with the touch probe. A curve and/or sparse bone surface reconstruction can be accomplished in a similar manner by performing a random walk.

3D Registration and Guidance: The 3D reconstruction results are used to register the 3D pre-operative model, enabling to overlay the plan with the anatomy. We will discuss in more detail how this registration is accomplished in the next section. The tunnel can be opened using a drill guide instrumented with a distinct visual marker and whose symmetry axis's location is known in the marker's reference frame. This way, the location of the drill guide w.r.t. the pre-operative plan is known, providing real-time guidance to the surgeon, as shown in the accompanying video.

This paper will not detail the guidance process as it is more a matter of application as soon as registration is accomplished. Also note that the article will solely refer to the placement of femoral tunnel. The placement of tibial tunnel is similar, requiring the attachment of its own WM.

3   Surgical Workflow and Algorithmic Modules

The steps of the complete surgical workflow are given in Fig. 3(a). An initial camera calibration using 3 images of a checkerboard pattern with the lens scope at different rotation angles is performed. Then, the world marker is rigidly attached to the anatomy and 3D points on the bone surface are reconstructed by scratching it with an instrumented touch probe. While the points are being reconstructed and using the pre-operative model, the system performs an on-the-fly registration that allows the drilling of the tunnel to be guided. Guidance information is given using augmented reality, by overlaying the pre-operative plan with the anatomy in real time, and using virtual reality, by continuously showing the location of the drill guide in the model reference frame. As a final step, the WM must be removed. Details are given below.

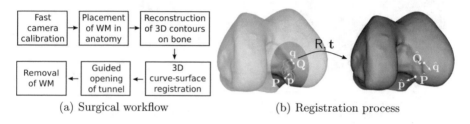

(a) Surgical workflow   (b) Registration process

Fig. 3. (a) Different steps of the surgical workflow and (b) the rigid transformation R, t is determined by searching for pairs of points $\mathbf{P}, \mathbf{Q}$ with tangents $\mathbf{p}, \mathbf{q}$ on the curve side that are a match with pairs of points $\hat{\mathbf{P}}, \hat{\mathbf{Q}}$ with normals $\hat{\mathbf{p}}, \hat{\mathbf{q}}$ on the surface side.

Calibration in the OR: Since the camera has exchangeable optics, calibration must be made in the OR. In addition, the lens scope rotates during the procedure, meaning that intrinsics must be adapted on the fly for greater accuracy. This is accomplished using an implementation of the method described in [13]. Calibration is done by collecting 3 images rotating the scope to determine intrinsics, radial distortion and center of rotation. For facilitating the process, acquisition is carried in dry environment and adaptation for wet is performed by multiplying the focal length by the ratio of the refractive indices [7].

Marker Detection and Pose Estimation: There are several publicly available libraries for augmented reality that implement the process of detection, identification and pose estimation of square markers. We opted for the ARAM library [2] and, for better accuracy, also used a photogeometric refinement step as described in [12] with the extension to accommodate radial distortion as in [8], making possible the accommodation of variable zoom in a future version.

Registration: Registration is accomplished using the method in [15] that uses a pair of points $\mathbf{P}, \mathbf{Q}$ with tangents $\mathbf{p}, \mathbf{q}$ from the curve that matches a pair of points $\hat{\mathbf{P}}, \hat{\mathbf{Q}}$ with normals $\hat{\mathbf{p}}, \hat{\mathbf{q}}$ on the surface for determining the alignment transformation (Fig. 3(b)). The search for correspondences is performed using a set of conditions that also depend on the differential information. Global registration is accomplished using an hypothesise-and-test framework.

Instruments and Hardware Setup: The software runs in a PC that is connected in-between camera tower and display. The PC is equipped with a frame grabber Datapath Limited DGC167 in an Intel Core i7 4790 and a GPU NVIDIA GeForce GTX950 that was able to run the pipeline in HD format at 60 fps with latency of 3 frames. In addition, we built the markers, custom screw removal tool, touch probe and drill guide that can be seen in the video.

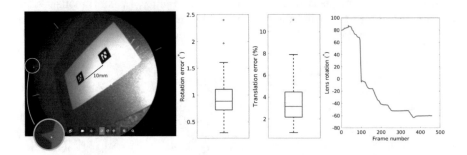

Fig. 4. Experiment on lens rotation in wet environment.

4   Experiments

This section reports experiments that assess the performance of two key features of the presented system: the compensation of the camera's intrinsics according to the rotation of the lens and the registration of the pre-operative model with the patient's anatomy. Tests on laboratory and using *ex-vivo* data are performed.

4.1   Lens Rotation

This experiment serves to assess the accuracy of the algorithm for compensating the camera's intrinsics according to the scope's rotation. We performed an initial camera calibration using 3 images of a calibration grid with the scope at 3 different rotation angles, which are represented with red lines in the image on the left of Fig. 4. We then acquired a 500-frame video sequence of a ruler with two 2.89 mm-side square markers 10 mm apart in wet environment. The rotation of the scope performed during the acquisition of the video is quantified in the plot on the right of Fig. 4 that shows that the total amount of rotation was more than 140°. The lens mark, shown in greater detail in Fig. 4, is detected in each frame for compensating the intrinsics. The accuracy of the method is evaluated by computing the relative pose between the two markers in each frame and comparing it with the ground truth pose. The low rotation and translation errors show that the algorithm properly handles lens rotation.

4.2   3D Registration

The first test regarding the registration method was performed on a dry model and consisted in reconstructing 10 different sets of curves by scratching the rear surface of the lateral condyle with an instrumented touch probe, and registering them with the virtual model shown in Fig. 5(a), providing 10 different rigid transformations. A qualitative assessment (Fig. 5(c)) of the registration accuracy is provided by representing the anatomical landmarks and the control points of Fig. 5(a) in WM coordinates using the obtained transformations. The centroid of each point cloud obtained by transforming the control points is computed and the RMS distance between each transformed point and the corresponding centroid is computed and shown in Fig. 5(f), providing a quantitative assessment of the registration accuracy. Results show that all the trials provided very similar results, with the landmarks and control points being almost perfectly aligned in Fig. 5(c) and all RMS distances being below 0.9 mm, despite the control points belonging to regions that are very distant from the reconstructed area.

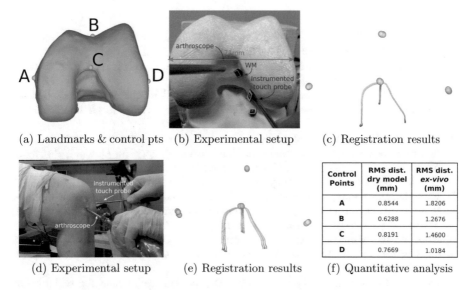

(a) Landmarks & control pts   (b) Experimental setup   (c) Registration results

(d) Experimental setup   (e) Registration results   (f) Quantitative analysis

Control Points	RMS dist. dry model (mm)	RMS dist. ex-vivo (mm)
A	0.8544	1.8206
B	0.6288	1.2676
C	0.8191	1.4600
D	0.7669	1.0184

Fig. 5. Analysis of performance of the registration algorithm in two experiments: one in the laboratory using a dry knee model and another using *ex-vivo* data.

The second experiment was performed on *ex-vivo* data and followed a similar strategy as the one on the dry model, having the difference that the total number of trials was 4. Figure 5(d) illustrates the setup of the *ex-vivo* experiment and Figs. 5(e) and (f) show the qualitative and qualitative analyses of the obtained result. Results show a slight degradation in accuracy w.r.t. the dry model test, which is expected since the latter is a more controlled environment. However, the obtained accuracy is very satisfactory, with the RMS distances of all control points being below 2 mm. This experiment demonstrates that our proposed system is very accurate in aligning the anatomy with a pre-operative model of the bone, enabling a reliable guidance of the ACL reconstruction procedure.

5   Conclusions

This paper presents the first video-based navigation system for ACL reconstruction. The software is able to handle unconstrained lens rotation and register pre-operative 3D models with the patient's anatomy with high accuracy, as demonstrated by the experiments performed both on a dry model and using *ex-vivo* data. This allows the complete medical procedure to be guided, leading not only to a significant decrease in the learning curve but also to the avoidance of technical mistakes. As future work, we will be targeting other procedures that might benefit from navigation such as resection of Femuro Acetabular Impingement during hip arthroscopy.

References

1. Barrett, D.S.: Proprioception and function after anterior cruciate reconstruction. J. Bone Joint Surg. Br. **73**(5), 833–837 (1991)
2. Belhaoua, A., Kornmann, A., Radoux, J.: Accuracy analysis of an augmented reality system. In: ICSP (2014)
3. Brown, C.H., Spalding, T., Robb, C.: Medial portal technique for single-bundle anatomical anterior cruciate ligament (ACL) reconstruction. Int. Orthop **37**, 253–269 (2013)
4. Edgcumbe, P., Pratt, P., Yang, G.-Z., Nguan, C., Rohling, R.: Pico lantern: a pick-up projector for augmented reality in laparoscopic surgery. In: Golland, P., Hata, N., Barillot, C., Hornegger, J., Howe, R. (eds.) MICCAI 2014. LNCS, vol. 8673, pp. 432–439. Springer, Cham (2014). https://doi.org/10.1007/978-3-319-10404-1_54
5. Forsythe, B., et al.: The location of femoral and tibial tunnels in anatomic double-bundle anterior cruciate ligament reconstruction analyzed by three-dimensional computed tomography models. J. Bone Joint Surg. Am. **92**, 1418–1426 (2010)
6. Kim, Y.: Registration accuracy enhancement of a surgical navigation system for anterior cruciate ligament reconstruction: a phantom and cadaveric study. Knee **24**, 329–339 (2017)
7. Lavest, J.M., Rives, G., Lapreste, J.T.: Dry camera calibration for underwater applications. MVA **13**, 245–253 (2003)
8. Lourenço, M., Barreto, J.P., Fonseca, F., Ferreira, H., Duarte, R.M., Correia-Pinto, J.: Continuous zoom calibration by tracking salient points in endoscopic video. In: Golland, P., Hata, N., Barillot, C., Hornegger, J., Howe, R. (eds.) MICCAI 2014. LNCS, vol. 8673, pp. 456–463. Springer, Cham (2014). https://doi.org/10.1007/978-3-319-10404-1_57
9. Ma, Y., Soatto, S., Kosecka, J., Sastry, S.: An Invitation to 3-D Vision: From Images to Geometric Models. Springer, Heidelberg (2004). https://doi.org/10.1007/978-0-387-21779-6
10. Mahmoud, N., et al.: ORBSLAM-based endoscope tracking and 3D reconstruction. In: Peters, T., et al. (eds.) CARE 2016. LNCS, vol. 10170, pp. 72–83. Springer, Cham (2017). https://doi.org/10.1007/978-3-319-54057-3_7

11. Maier-Hein, L., et al.: Optical techniques for 3D surface reconstruction in computer-assisted laparoscopic surgery. Med. Image Anal. **17**, 974–996 (2013)
12. Mei, C., Benhimane, S., Malis, E., Rives, P.: Efficient homography-based tracking and 3-D reconstruction for single-viewpoint sensors. T-RO **24**(6), 1352–1364 (2008)
13. Melo, R., Barreto, J.P., Falcao, G.: A new solution for camera calibration and real-time image distortion correction in medical endoscopyinitial technical evaluation. TBE **59**, 634–644 (2012)
14. Nawabi, D.H., Mehta, N.: Learning curve for hip arthroscopy steeper than expected. J. Hip. Preserv. Surg. **3**(suppl. 1) (2000)
15. Raposo, C., Barreto, J.P.: 3D registration of curves and surfaces using local differential information. In: CVPR (2018)
16. Samitier, G., Marcano, A.I., Alentorn-Geli, E., Cugat, R., Farmer, K.W., Moser, M.W.: Failure of anterior cruciate ligament reconstruction. ABJS **3**, 220–240 (2015)
17. Treuting, R.: Minimally invasive orthopedic surgery: arthroscopy. Ochsner J. **2**, 158–163 (2000)

Simultaneous Segmentation and Classification of Bone Surfaces from Ultrasound Using a Multi-feature Guided CNN

Puyang Wang[1(✉)], Vishal M. Patel[1], and Ilker Hacihaliloglu[2,3]

[1] Department of Electrical and Computer Engineering, Rutgers University,
Piscataway, NJ, USA
puyang.wang@rutgers.edu

[2] Department of Biomedical Engineering, Rutgers University, Piscataway, USA
ilker.hac@soe.rutgers.edu

[3] Department of Radiology, Rutger Robert Wood Johnson Medical School,
New Brunswick, NJ, USA

Abstract. Various imaging artifacts, low signal-to-noise ratio, and bone surfaces appearing several millimeters in thickness have hindered the success of ultrasound (US) guided computer assisted orthopedic surgery procedures. In this work, a multi-feature guided convolutional neural network (CNN) architecture is proposed for simultaneous enhancement, segmentation, and classification of bone surfaces from US data. The proposed CNN consists of two main parts: a pre-enhancing net, that takes the concatenation of B-mode US scan and three filtered image features for the enhancement of bone surfaces, and a modified U-net with a classification layer. The proposed method was validated on 650 in vivo US scans collected using two US machines, by scanning knee, femur, distal radius and tibia bones. Validation, against expert annotation, achieved statistically significant improvements in segmentation of bone surfaces compared to state-of-the-art.

1   Introduction

In order to provide a radiation-free, real-time, cost effective imaging alternative, for intra-operative fluoroscopy, special attention has been given to incorporate ultrasound (US) into computer assisted orthopedic surgery (CAOS) procedures [1]. However, problems such as high levels of noise, imaging artifacts, limited field of view and bone boundaries appearing several millimeters (mm) in thickness have hindered the wide spread adaptability of US-guided CAOS systems. This has resulted in the development of automated bone segmentation and enhancement methods [1]. Accurate and robust segmentation is important for improved guidance in US-based CAOS procedures.

In discussing state-of-the-art we will limit ourselves to approaches that fit directly within the context of the proposed deep learning-based method. A

© Springer Nature Switzerland AG 2018
A. F. Frangi et al. (Eds.): MICCAI 2018, LNCS 11073, pp. 134–142, 2018.
https://doi.org/10.1007/978-3-030-00937-3_16

detailed review of image processing methods based on the extraction of image intensity and phase information can be found in [1]. In [2], U-net architecture, originally proposed in [3], was investigated for processing in vivo femur, tibia and pelvis bone surfaces. Bone localization accuracy was not assessed but 0.87 precision and recall rates were reported. In [4], a modified version of the CNN proposed in [3] was used for localizing vertebra bone surfaces. Despite the fact that methods based on deep learning produce robust and accurate results, the success rate is dependent on: (1) number of US scans used for training, (2) quality of the collected US data for testing [4].

In this paper, we propose a novel neural network architecture for simultaneous bone surface enhancement, segmentation and classification from US data. Our proposed network accommodates a bone surface enhancement network which takes a concatenation of B-mode US scan, local phase-based enhanced bone images, and signal transmission-based bone shadow enhanced image as input and outputs a new US scan in which only bone surface is enhanced. We show that the bone surface enhancement network, referred to as pre-enhancing (*PE*), improves robustness and accuracy of bone surface localization since it creates an image where the bone surface information is more dominant. As a second contribution, a deep-learning bone surface segmentation framework for US image, named classification U-net, *cU-net* for short, is proposed. Although *cU-net* shares the same basic structure with U-net [3], it is fundamentally different in terms of designed output. Unlike U-net, *cU-net* is capable of identifying bone type and segmenting bone surface area in US image simultaneously. The bone type classification is implemented by feeding part of the features in U-net to a sequence of fully-connected layers followed by a softmax layer. To take the advantages of both *PE* and *cU-net*, we propose a framework that can adaptively balance the trade-off between accuracy and running-time by combining *PE* and *cU-net*.

2   Proposed Method

Figure 1 gives an overview of the proposed joint bone enhancement, segmentation and classification framework. Incorporating pre-enhancing net, *cU-net+PE*, into the proposed framework is expected to produce more accurate results than using only *cU-net*. However, because of the computation of the additional input features and convolution layers, *cU-net+PE* requires more running time. Therefore, the proposed framework can be configured for both (i) real-time application using only *cU-net*, and (ii) off-line application using *cU-net+PE* for different clinical purposes. In the next section, we explain how the various filtered images are extracted.

2.1   Enhancement of Bone Surface and Bone Shadow Information

Different from using only B-mode US scan as input, the proposed pre-enhancing network, that enhances bone surface, takes the concatenation of B-mode US scan ($US(x, y)$) and three filtered image features which are obtained as follows:

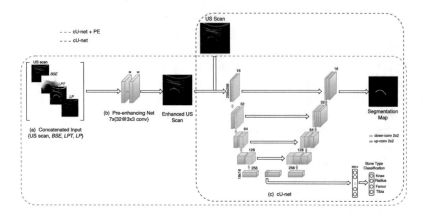

Fig. 1. Overview of the proposed simultaneous enhancement, segmentation and classification network.

Local Phase Tensor Image $(LPT(x,y))$**:** $LPT(x,y)$ image is computed by defining odd and even filter responses using [5]:

$$T_{even} = [\boldsymbol{H}(US_{DB}(x,y))]\,[\boldsymbol{H}(US_{DB}(x,y))]^{T}, \tag{1}$$

$$T_{odd} = -0.5 \times ([\nabla US_{DB}(x,y)]\,[\nabla \nabla^2 US_{DB}(x,y)]^{T} + \\ [\nabla \nabla^2 US_{DB}(x,y)]\,[\nabla US_{DB}(x,y)]^{T}).$$

Here T_{even} and T_{odd} represent the symmetric and asymmetric features of $US(x,y)$. $\boldsymbol{H}$, ∇ and ∇^2 represent the Hessian, Gradient and Laplacian operations, respectively. In order to improve the enhancement of bone surfaces located deeper in the image and mask out soft tissue interfaces close to the transducer, $US(x,y)$ image is masked with a distance map and band-pass filtered using Log-Gabor filter [5]. The resulting image, from this operation, is represented as $US_{DB}(x,y)$. The final $LPT(x,y)$ image is obtained using: $LPT(x,y) = \sqrt{T_{even}^2 + T_{odd}^2} \times cos(\phi)$, where ϕ represents instantaneous phase obtained from the symmetric and asymmetric feature responses, respectively [5].

Local Phase Bone Image $(LP(x,y))$**:** $LP(x,y)$ image is computed using: $LP(x,y) = LPT(x,y) \times LPE(x,y) \times LwPA(x,y)$, where $LPE(x,y)$ and $LwPA(x,y)$ represent the local phase energy and local weighted mean phase angle image features, respectively. These two features are computed using monogenic signal theory as [6]: $LPE(x,y) = \sum_{sc} |US_{M1}(x,y)| - \sqrt{US_{M2}^2(x,y) + US_{M2}^3(x,y)}$,

$$LwPA(x,y) = \arctan \frac{\sum_{sc} US_{M1}(x,y)}{\sqrt{\sum_{sc} US_{M1}^2 + \sum_{sc} US_{M2}^2(x,y)}}, \tag{2}$$

where $US_{M1}, US_{M2}, US_{M3}$ represent the three different components of monogenic signal image $(US_M(x,y))$ calculated from $LPT(x,y)$ image using Riesz filter [6] and sc represents the number of filter scales.

Bone Shadow Enhanced Image $(BSE(x,y))$**:** $BSE(x,y)$ image is computed by modeling the interaction of the US signal within the tissue as scattering and attenuation information using [6]:

$$BSE(x,y) = [(CM_{LP}(x,y) - \rho)/[max(US_A(x,y),\epsilon)]^{\delta}] + \rho, \qquad (3)$$

where $CM_{LP}(x,y)$ is the confidence map image obtained by modeling the propagation of US signal inside the tissue taking into account bone features present in $LP(x,y)$ image [6]. $US_A(x,y)$, maximizes the visibility of high intensity bone features inside a local region and satisfies the constraint that the mean intensity of the local region is less than the echogenicity of the tissue confining the bone [6]. Tissue attenuation coefficient is represented with δ. ρ is a constant related to tissue echogenicity confining the bone surface, and ϵ is a small constant used to avoid division by zero [6].

2.2   Pre-enhancing Network (PE)

A simple and intuitive way to view the three extracted feature images is viewing them as an input feature map of a CNN. Each feature map provides different local information of bone surface in an US scan. In deep learning, if a network is trained on a dataset of a specific distribution and is tested on a dataset that follows another distribution, the performance usually degrades significantly. In the context of bone segmentation, different US machines with different settings or different orientation of the transducer will lead to scans that have different image characteristics. The main advantage of multi-feature guided CNN is that filtered features can bring the US scan to a common domain independent of the image acquisition device. Hence, the bone surface in a US scan appears more dominant after the multi-feature guided pre-enhancing net regardless of different US image acquisition settings (Fig. 2).

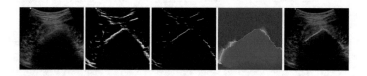

Fig. 2. From left to right: B-mode US scan, *LPT*, *LP*, *BSE*, bone-enhanced US scan.

The input data consists of a $4 \times 256 \times 256$ matrix, i.e., each channel consists of a 256×256 image. The pre-enhancing network (PE) contains seven convolutional layers with 32 feature maps and one with single feature map (Fig. 1(b)). To balance the trade-off between the large receptive field, which can acquire more semantic spatial information and the increase in the number of parameters, we set the convolution kernel size to be 3×3 with zero-padding of size 1. The batch normalization (BN) [7] and rectified linear units (ReLU) are attached to every convolutional layer except the last one for faster training and non-linearity. Finally, the last layer is a Sigmoid function that transforms the single feature map to visible image of values between $[0, 1]$. Next we explain the proposed simultaneous segmentation and classification method.

2.3 Joint Learning of Classification and Segmentation

Although U-net has been widely used in many segmentation problems in the field of biomedical imaging, it lacks the capability of classifying medical images. Inspired by the observation that the contracting path of U-net shares similar structure with many image classification networks, such as AlexNet [8]and VGG net [9], we propose a classification U-net (cU-net) that can jointly learn to classify and segment images. The network structure is shown in Fig. 1(c).

While our proposed cU-net is structurally similar to U-net, three key difference of the proposed cU-net from U-net are as follows:

1. The MaxPooling layers and the convolutional layers in the contracting path are replaced by the convolutional layers with stride two. The stride of convolution defines the step size of the kernel when traversing the image. While its default is usually 1, we use a stride of 2 for downsampling an image similar to MaxPooling. Compared to MaxPooling, strided convolution can be regarded as parameterized downsampling that preserves positional information and are easy to reverse.
2. Different from [10], for the purpose of enabling U-net to classify images, we take only part of the feature maps at the last convolution layer of the contracting path (left side) and expand it as a feature vector. The resulting feature vector is input to a classifier that consists of one fully-connected layer with a final 4-way softmax layer.
3. To further accelerate the training process and improve the generalization ability of the network, we adopt BN and add it before every ReLU layers. By reducing the internal covariance shift of features, the batch normalization can lead to faster learning and higher overall accuracy.

Apart from the above two major differences, one minor difference is the number of starting feature maps. We reduce the number of starting feature maps from 32 to 16. Overall, the proposed cU-net consists of the repeated application of one 3×3 convolution (zero-padded convolution), each followed by BN and ReLU, and a 2×2 strided convolution with stride 2 (down-conv) for downsampling. At each downsampling step, we double the number of feature maps. Every step in the expansive path consists of an upsampling of the feature map followed by a dilated 2×2 convolution (up-conv) that halves the number of feature maps, a concatenation with the corresponding feature map from the contracting path, and one 3×3 convolution followed by BN and ReLU.

2.4   Data Acquisition and Training

After obtaining the institutional review board (IRB) approval, a total of 519 different US images, from 17 healthy volunteers, were collected using SonixTouch US machine (Analogic Corporation, Peabody, MA, USA). The scanned anatomical bone surfaces included knee, femur, radius, and tibia. Additional 131 US scans were collected from two subjects using a hand-held wireless US system (Clarius C3, Clarius Mobile Health Corporation, BC, Canada). All the collected data was annotated by an expert ultrasonographer in the preprocessing stage. Local phase images and bone shadow enhanced images were obtained using the filter parameters defined in [6]. For the ground truth labels we dilated the ground truth contours to a width of 1 mm.

We apply a random split of US images from SonixTouch in training (80%) and testing (20%) sets. The training set consists of a total of 415 images obtained from SonixTouch only. The rest 104 images from SonixTouch and all 131 images from Clarius C3 were used for testing. We also made sure that during the random split of the SonixTouch dataset the training and testing data did not include the same patient scans. Experiments are carried out three times on random training-testing splits and average results are reported. For training both *cU-net* and pre-enhancing net (*PE*), we adapt a 2-step training phase. In a total of 30,000 training iterations, the first 10,000 iterations were only performed on *cU-net* and we jointly train the *cU-net* and pre-enhancing net for another 20,000 iterations. We used cross entropy loss for both segmentation and classification tasks of *cU-net*. As for the pre-enhancing net, to force the network only enhance bone surfaces, we used Euclidean distance between output and input as the loss. ADAM stochastic optimization [11] with batch size of 16 and a learning rate of 0.0002 are used for learning the weights.

For the experimental evaluation and comparison, we selected two reference methods: original U-net [3] and modified U-net for bone segmentation [4] (denoted as *TMI*). For the proposed method, we included two configurations: *cU-net+PE* and *cU-net*, where *cU-net* is the trained model without pre-enhancing net (PE). To further validate the effectiveness of *cU-net* and *PE*, *U-net+PE* (*U-net* trained with enhanced images) and *U-net* trained using same input image features as *PE* (denoted as *U-net2*) were added to the comparison. All these methods were implemented and evaluated on segmenting several bone surfaces including knee, femur, radius, and tibia. To localize the bone surface, we threshold the estimated probability segmentation map and use the center pixels along each scanline as a single bone surface. The quality of the localization was evaluated by computing average Euclidean distance (AED) between the two surfaces. Apart from AED, we also evaluated the bone segmentation methods with regards to recall, precision, and their harmonic mean, the F-score. Since manual ground truths cannot be regarded as absolute gold standard, true positive are defined as detected bone surface points that are maximum 0.9 mm away from the manual ground truth.

3   Experimental Results

The AED results (mean ± std) in Table 1 show that the proposed *cU-net+PE* outperforms other methods on test scans obtained from both US machines. Note that training set only contains images from one specific US machine (Sonix-Touch) while testing is performed on both. A further paired t-test between *cU-net+PE* and U-net at a 5% significance level with *p-value* of 0.0014 clearly indicates that the improvements of our method are statistically significant. The *p-values* for the remaining comparisons were also <0.05 proving the achieved significance. The average recall and precision rates as well as F-scores are reported in Table 1. Although our method is not performing the best in term of average precision, the more practical measurement for detection tasks, F-score, shows the superiority of our method on bone detection performance. Further experiments of *U-net+PE* and *U-net2* yield 0.949/0.876 and 0.941/0.856 in term of F-score on both US machines. From the fact that *cU-net+PE* > *U-net+PE* > *U-net2*, the proposed *cU-net* and *PE* are shown to improve the segmentation result independently. Qualitative results in Fig. 3 show that *TMI* method achieves high precision but low recall due to missing bone boundaries which is more important for our clinical application. It can be observed that quantitative results are consistent with the visual results. Average computational time for bone surface and shadow enhancement was 2 s (MATLAB implementation).

Table 1. AED, 95% confidence level (CL), recall, precision, and F-scores for the proposed and state of the art methods.

	SonixTouch				Clarius C3			
	cU-net+PE	*cU-net*	U-net[3]	TMI[4]	*cU-net+PE*	*cU-net*	U-net[3]	TMI[4]
AED	**0.246±0.101**	0.338±0.158	0.389±0.221	0.399±0.201	**0.368±0.237**	0.544±0.876	1.141±1.665	0.644±2.656
95%CL	**0.267**	0.371	0.435	0.440	**0.409**	0.696	1.429	1.103
Recall	**0.97**	0.948	0.929	0.891	**0.873**	0.795	0.673	0.758
Precision	0.965	0.943	0.930	**0.963**	0.94	0.923	0.907	**0.961**
F-score	**0.968**	0.945	0.930	0.926	**0.906**	0.855	0.773	0.847

Moreover, we evaluate the classification performance of the proposed *cU-net* by calculating classification errors on four different anatomical bone types. The proposed classification U-net, *cU-net*, is near perfect in classifying bones for US images of SonixTouch ultrasound machine with an overall classification error of 0.001. However, the classification errors increase significantly to 0.389 when *cU-net* is tested on test images of Clarius C3 machine. We believe it is because of the imbalanced dataset and dataset bias since the training set only contains 3 tibia images and no images from Clarius C3 machine. Furthermore, Clarius C3 machine is a convex array transducer and is not suitable for imaging bone surfaces located close to the transducer surface which was the case for imaging distal radius and tibia bones. Due to suboptimal transducer and imaging extracted features were not representative of the actual anatomical surfaces.

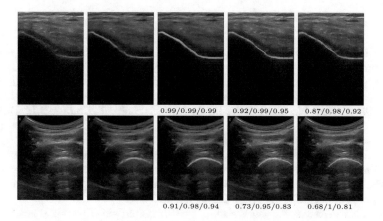

Fig. 3. From left to right column: B-mode US scans, *PE*, *cU-net+PE*, U-net [3], TMI [4]. Green represents manual expert segmentation and red is obtained using corresponding algorithms. Recall/Precision/F-score are shown under segmentation results.

4   Conclusion

We have presented a multi-feature guided CNN for simultaneous enhancement, segmentation and classification of bone surfaces from US data. To the best of our knowledge this is the first study proposing these tasks simultaneously in the context of bone US imaging. Validation studies achieve a 44% and 27% improvement in overall AED errors over the state-of-the-art methods reported in [4] and [3] respectively. In the experiments, our method yields more accurate and complete segmentation even under not only difficult imaging conditions but also different imaging settings compared to state-of-the-art. In this study the classification task involved the identification of bone types. However, this can be changed to identify US scan planes as well. Correct scan plane identification is an important task for spine imaging in the context of pedicle screw insertion and pain management. One of the main drawbacks of the proposed framework is the long computation time required to calculate the various phase image features. However, the proposed *cU-net* is independent of the *cU-net+PE*. Therefore, for real-time applications initial bone surface extraction can be performed using *cU-net* and updated during a second iteration using *cU-net+PE*. Future work will involve extensive clinical validation, real-time implementation of phase filtering, and incorporation of the extracted bone surfaces into a registration method.

Acknowledgement. This work was supported in part by 2017 North American Spine Society Young Investigator Award.

References

1. Hacihaliloglu, I.: Ultrasound imaging and segmentation of bone surfaces: a review. Technology **5**, 1–7 (2017)
2. Salehi, M., Prevost, R., Moctezuma, J.-L., Navab, N., Wein, W.: Precise ultrasound bone registration with learning-based segmentation and speed of sound calibration. In: Descoteaux, M., Maier-Hein, L., Franz, A., Jannin, P., Collins, D.L., Duchesne, S. (eds.) MICCAI 2017. LNCS, vol. 10434, pp. 682–690. Springer, Cham (2017). https://doi.org/10.1007/978-3-319-66185-8_77
3. Ronneberger, O., Fischer, P., Brox, T.: U-net: convolutional networks for biomedical image segmentation. In: Navab, N., Hornegger, J., Wells, W.M., Frangi, A.F. (eds.) MICCAI 2015. LNCS, vol. 9351, pp. 234–241. Springer, Cham (2015). https://doi.org/10.1007/978-3-319-24574-4_28
4. Baka, N., Leenstra, S., van Walsum, T.: Ultrasound aided vertebral level localization for lumbar surgery. IEEE Trans. Med. Imaging **36**(10), 2138–2147 (2017)
5. Hacihaliloglu, I., Rasoulian, A., Rohling, R.N., Abolmaesumi, P.: Local phase tensor features for 3-D ultrasound to statistical shape+ pose spine model registration. IEEE Trans. Med. Imaging **33**(11), 2167–2179 (2014)
6. Hacihaliloglu, I.: Enhancement of bone shadow region using local phase-based ultrasound transmission maps. Int. J. Comput. Assisted Radiol. Surg. **12**(6), 951–960 (2017)
7. Ioffe, S., Szegedy, C.: Batch normalization: accelerating deep network training by reducing internal covariate shift. In: Proceedings of the 32nd International Conference on Machine Learning, ICML 2015, pp. 448–456 (2015)
8. Krizhevsky, A., Sutskever, I., Hinton, G.E.: ImageNet classification with deep convolutional neural networks. In: Pereira, F., Burges, C.J.C., Bottou, L., Weinberger, K.Q. (eds.) Advances in Neural Information Processing Systems 25, pp. 1097–1105. Curran Associates, Inc. (2012)
9. Simonyan, K., Zisserman, A.: Very deep convolutional networks for large-scale image recognition. arXiv preprint arXiv:1409.1556 (2014)
10. Kurmann, T., et al.: Simultaneous recognition and pose estimation of instruments in minimally invasive surgery. In: Descoteaux, M., Maier-Hein, L., Franz, A., Jannin, P., Collins, D.L., Duchesne, S. (eds.) MICCAI 2017. LNCS, vol. 10434, pp. 505–513. Springer, Cham (2017). https://doi.org/10.1007/978-3-319-66185-8_57
11. Kingma, D., Ba, J.: Adam: a method for stochastic optimization. In: Proceedings of the International Conference on Learning Representations (ICLR) (2015)

Endoscopic Laser Surface Scanner for Minimally Invasive Abdominal Surgeries

Jordan Geurten[1], Wenyao Xia[2,3], Uditha Jayarathne[2,3], Terry M. Peters[2,3], and Elvis C. S. Chen[2,3(✉)] (iD)

[1] University of Waterloo, Waterloo, ON, Canada
[2] Western University, London, ON, Canada
[3] Robarts Research Institute, London, ON, Canada
{tpeters,chene}@robarts.ca

Abstract. Minimally invasive surgery performed under endoscopic video is a viable alternative to several types of open abdominal surgeries. Advanced visualization techniques require accurate patient registration, often facilitated by reconstruction of the organ surface in situ. We present an active system for intraoperative surface reconstruction of internal organs, comprising a single-plane laser as the structured light source and a surgical endoscope camera as the imaging system. Both surgical instruments are spatially calibrated and tracked, after which the surface reconstruction is formulated as the intersection problem between line-of-sight rays (from the surgical camera) and the laser beam. Surface target registration error after a rigid-body surface registration between the scanned 3D points to the ground truth obtained via CT is reported. When tested on an *ex vivo* porcine liver and kidney, root-mean-squared surface target registration error of 1.28 mm was achieved. Accurate endoscopic surface reconstruction is possible by using two separately calibrated and tracked surgical instruments, where the trigonometry between the structured light, imaging system, and organ surface can be optimized. Our novelty is the accurate calibration technique for the tracked laser beam, and the design and the construction of laser apparatus designed for robotic-assisted surgery.

Keywords: Surface reconstruction · Scanning · Calibration
Surgical navigation · Minimally invasive abdominal surgery

1 Introduction

Minimally invasive surgery (MIS) is a viable surgical approach for many abdominal intervention including liver resection and partial nephrectomy [8]. In these interventions, the multi-port approach is the current standard of care, where multiple incisions are created to allow access of surgical instruments into the abdominal cavity. An endoscopic camera is used as a surrogate for direct human vision. Advanced visualization, such as overlaying of subsurface anatomical details onto endoscopic video is only possible if both surgical camera and patient anatomy

© Springer Nature Switzerland AG 2018
A. F. Frangi et al. (Eds.): MICCAI 2018, LNCS 11073, pp. 143–150, 2018.
https://doi.org/10.1007/978-3-030-00937-3_17

are spatially tracked in a common coordinate system, and accurate camera calibration [7] and patient registration [2] can be achieved *in vivo*.

As an intraoperative imaging modality, the surgical camera can be used as a localizer to facilitate patient registration. Three dimensional (3D) surface reconstruction techniques in the current literature [4,5] can be categorized as either passive or active [6]. Passive methods employ only the acquired images to detect anatomical features to reconstruct a dense surface of the surgical scene. However, such approaches are computationally intensive and suffer from feature-less surfaces with specular highlights. Active methods project structured light into the abdominal cavity, replacing natural features with light patterns. These patterns serve as the basis for surface reconstruction using trigonometry.

We present the 'EndoScan', an active system for endoscopically performing 3D surface reconstruction of abdominal organs. The system comprises two optically tracked surgical instruments: a surgical endoscope camera and a plane laser source, each with a 13 mm to 15 mm outer diameter form factor. We envision this system being integrated into existing endoscopic surgical navigation systems where the surgical camera and plane laser source enter the abdomen via separate ports. Once the target organ is scanned, it can be used for rigid-body registration [1] with preoperative patient data, or serve to initialize subsequent deformable registration [2]. The proposed system was validated by means of CT registration with 3D surface scans obtained from the EndoScan, where the surface Target Registration Error [3] (surface TRE) is reported.

2   Methods and Materials

The proposed 3D scanner employs a laser projection system as a means of introducing structured light into the abdominal cavity, and an imaging system for the acquisition of the projected laser pattern. Both subsystems are spatially tracked by an optical tracking system (Spectra, Northern Digital Inc., Canada) and are designed to be compatible with the da Vinci robotic system (Intuitive Surgical Inc., USA).

A stereo laparoscope (Surgical laparoscope, Olympus) was used as the imaging subsystem (Fig. 2a). An optical dynamic reference frame (DRF), denoted by (C), was rigidly attached at the handle of the laparoscope (Fig. 2a). The hand-eye calibration between the optical axis of the right channel camera (O) and its DRF (C) was performed [7] and denoted as $^{C}T_{O}$ (Fig. 1b). Video was captured as 800×600 pixel image and image distortions were removed prior to any subsequent image processing.

A red laser diode (5 mW, 650 nm) with a diffractive lens (plane divergence: 120°) was integrated into the tip of a medical grade stainless steel tube (outer diameter: 15 mm, length: 38 cm) as part of the laser projection subsystem (Fig. 2b). The laser diode is controlled by a commercial microcontroller (Atmel, USA), capable of outputting 40 mA at 5 V. All electronic components were housed at the distal end of the stainless steel tube, to which a DRF (L) is rigidly attached (Fig. 2b). Serial communication and power to the laser instrument is provided via a standard USB connection from the host computer.

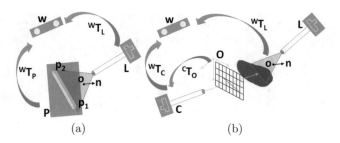

Fig. 1. Coordinate systems: optical DRFs are rigidly attached to the laser apparatus (**L**) and surgical camera (**C**) and the tracker is used as the world coordinate system (**W**). (a) The objective of laser apparatus calibration is to determine the laser plane origin and normal pair (**o**, **n**) in **L** using the tracked line-phantom **P**, and (b) Surface reconstruction is formulated as the intersections between light-of-sight ray and laser plane: the hand-eye calibration of the surgical camera is denoted as $^{C}\mathbf{T_O}$.

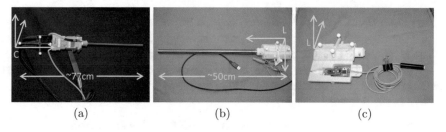

Fig. 2. (a) A stereo surgical endoscopic (Olympus), (b) A custom laser instrument. Both instruments are spatially tracked using an optical DRF rigidly attached at the handle, and (c) A custom housing was designed for the laser instrument which houses the microcontroller. In addition, a magnetic tracker sensor was integrated into the laser instrument but not used for this study.

2.1   Laser Beam Calibration

The optical tracker records the location and orientation of the DRF directly, therefore, the relationship between the laser beam and the laser DRF (**L**) must be calibrated. The laser beam can be represented by a point on the beam (**o**) and its plane normal (**n**). The laser beam calibration determines the pair (**o**, **n**) in the DRF coordinate system (**L**) (Fig. 1).

A calibration phantom, a raised metal block with a thin engraved line attached to a DRF **P**, was developed (Fig. 3a). The end points of the engraved line, (**p₁**, **p₂**), are known in **P** by manufacturing. To calibrate the orientation of the plane laser beam, it must be aligned with the engraved line (Fig. 3b). Once aligned, the paired points (**p₁**, **p₂**) must lie on the plane of the laser beam (Fig. 1a):

$$\begin{bmatrix} \mathbf{p_1'} & \mathbf{p_2'} \\ 1 & 1 \end{bmatrix} = (^{\mathbf{W}}\mathbf{T_L})^{-1}(^{\mathbf{W}}\mathbf{T_P})\begin{bmatrix} \mathbf{p_1} & \mathbf{p_2} \\ 1 & 1 \end{bmatrix} \tag{1}$$

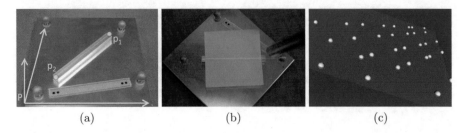

(a)   (b)   (c)

Fig. 3. Laser plane calibration: (a) A custom "line" calibration phantom was designed. The geometry of the line, *i.e.* ($\mathbf{p_1}$, $\mathbf{p_2}$), is known at the local coordinate of its DRF $\mathbf{P}$ by design, (b) The calibration is performed by aligning the laser beam projection to the engraved line from various distances and angles. A white sheet was overlaid to the line to provide better visibility, and (c) Laser plane calibration is formulated as a plane-fitting to a set of 3D points problem.

where the points ($\mathbf{p_1'}$, $\mathbf{p_2'}$) are the end points of the engraved line specified in $\mathbf{L}$ (Fig. 1a), while $^\mathbf{W}\mathbf{T_P}$ and $^\mathbf{W}\mathbf{T_L}$ are the rigid body tracking poses of the DRFs attached to the line phantom and the laser instrument, respectively. After n acquisitions, a set of $2n$ points is measured via Eq. (1) and the laser beam geometry ($\mathbf{o}$, $\mathbf{n}$) can be computed using any plane fitting algorithm.

2.2   Surface Reconstruction as Line-to-Plane Intersection

Using the ideal pinhole camera model, for a given camera intrinsic matrix A, a point $Q = (X, Y, Z)^T$ in the 3D optical axis $\mathbf{O}$ can be projected onto the image:

$$q = AQ \tag{2}$$

where $q = (u, v, w)^T$. Given a pixel location, the corresponding ray (emanating from the camera center) can be computed by:

$$Q = A^{-1}q \tag{3}$$

where a pixel is represented in the canonical camera coordinate system of $q = (u, v, 1)^T$. For each pixel in the image coinciding with the laser projection, a line-of-sight ray can be projected by Eq. (3), and

$$\begin{bmatrix} Q' & C' \\ 0 & 1 \end{bmatrix} = (^\mathbf{W}\mathbf{T_C})(^\mathbf{C}\mathbf{T_O}) \begin{bmatrix} Q & C \\ 0 & 1 \end{bmatrix} \tag{4}$$

where Q' is the normalized line-of-sight ray specified in the world coordinate system, and $C = [0, 0, 0]^T$ is the camera origin and C' is the camera center specified in the world coordinate system of the tracker ($\mathbf{W}$). Simultaneously, the pose of the laser beam is known via tracking:

$$\begin{bmatrix} \mathbf{n'} & \mathbf{o'} \\ 0 & 1 \end{bmatrix} = (^\mathbf{W}\mathbf{T_L}) \begin{bmatrix} \mathbf{n} & \mathbf{o} \\ 0 & 1 \end{bmatrix} \tag{5}$$

where the pair $(\mathbf{n}', \mathbf{o}')$ specifies the pose of the laser beam in $\mathbf{W}$. Assuming Q' and $\mathbf{n}'$ are not perpendicular, the intersection between the line-of-sight ray and the laser beam can be computed:

$$^{W}q = \frac{(\mathbf{o}' - C') \cdot \mathbf{n}'}{Q' \cdot \mathbf{n}'} Q' + C' \tag{6}$$

where ^{W}q is a point on organ surface intersected by the laser beam specified in $\mathbf{W}$. The intrinsic matrix A is determined as part of the hand-eye calibration [7].

2.3   Validation

To assess the proposed surface scanning system, a validation setup similar to that described in [5] was constructed. An *ex vivo* phantom with a porcine kidney and a lobe of porcine liver rigidly secured in a torso box was constructed (Fig. 4c). A CT scan of the torso phantom was acquired using an O-Arm (Medtronic, Ireland) (Fig. 4a), serving as the ground truth for subsequent analysis.

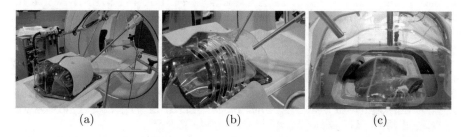

(a)   (b)   (c)

Fig. 4. *Ex vivo* experimental setup: the experiment was performed in a simulated operating room equipped with an O-arm CT scanner (Medtronic, Ireland), by which the CT of the torso phantom was acquired and used as the ground truth, (a) The proposed surface scanning system is comprised of two surgical instruments: an endoscope camera (left) and a single-plane laser (right), (b) A porcine kidney and a lobe of porcine liver were rigidly secured in the torso phantom, and (c) a close-up of laser surface scanning procedure. The laser instrument is on the left.

Two entry ports were made on the torso phantom: one close to the umbilicus for the endoscope camera, and the other at the lower abdominal region for the laser system (Fig. 4b). These locations were chosen to mimic a typical MIS abdominal surgical approach. During the scanning procedure, the endoscope camera was held rigidly using a stabilizer, while the laser apparatus was swept free-hand by an operator. The distances from the organ surface to endoscope camera and the laser instrument were roughly 10 cm and 15 to 20 cm, respectively (Fig. 4c), while the angle between the instruments was roughly 40° (Fig. 4d). Total scan time was approximately 3 min.

3   Results

The spatial calibration between the laser beam to its DRF was achieved using 18 measurements (Fig. 3b), acquired under 5 min. The RMS distance between these 36 acquired points to the fitted plane equation was 0.83 mm.

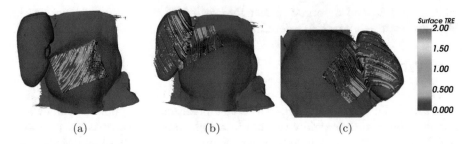

(a)   (b)   (c)

Fig. 5. Surface reconstruction of the (a) liver, and (b, c) the kidney/liver lobes using two camera views. By optimizing the geometry between the camera, laser and organ surface, sub-mm surface reconstruction was achieved. Edges of the liver where the surface normals are oblique to the camera and laser exhibit large reconstruction error.

Two scans of the organ surface were acquired. First, the camera was rigidly mounted with the viewing axis of the camera centered over the liver (Fig. 4b). The laser beam projection image was segmented and reconstructed in 3D using methods described in Sect. 2.2. Once reconstructed in $\mathbf{W}$, the 3D surface was registered to the CT organ scan via rigid-body ICP [1].

Accuracy of the liver surface reconstruction is visualized in Fig. 5a. The position of the laser scan line area corresponds approximately to the fixed viewing area of the camera. 127 images (scanlines) were acquired, resulting in 33571 points in the laser scan of the liver. After the rigid-body ICP registration, the Euclidean distance between each vertex on the scanline and the surface was computed, and summarized in Table 1.

Table 1. Accuracy of the laser surface scanning system evaluated using *ex vivo* porcine model, where the mean, standard deviation (std), root mean square (RMS), maximum (max) errors, and percentages of STRE under 1 mm and 2 mm are reported.

Surface TRE	Mean (mm)	Std Dev (mm)	RMS (mm)	Max (mm)	<1 mm	<2 mm
Liver	0.74	1.04	1.28	13.18	78.20%	92.11%
Kidney/Liver	0.23	0.31	0.39	7.80	98.38%	99.44%

A subsequent scan was performed where the kidney and the liver were positioned in the camera view. First, the center of the kidney is centered in the camera viewing area, followed by the junction between the kidney and liver being centered in the camera viewing area. In our torso phantom, the junction between the kidney and liver exhibits high surface curvature. 97 images were acquired, resulting in a total of 43910 vertices on the laser scanlines. The Euclidean distance error between the laser scanlines and the CT surface after rigid-body ICP registration is summarized in Table 1. Similar to the previous experiment, vertices with surface normals perpendicular to the camera viewing axis and those at the edge of the camera viewing area, tend to exhibit higher than average registration error (Fig. 5). By repositioning the camera and optimizing the laser beam orientation, a surface reconstruction with sub-millimeter accuracy was achieved (Table 1).

The results of the ICP registration between the laser scanlines and CT surface is shown in Table 1. More than 90% of the vertices exhibit surface TRE of less than 2 mm, resulting in a submillimeter mean surface TRE. The surface reconstruction generated by our proposed system provides an accurate means of performing registration of multi-modal patient-specific data. These data can be used to enhance the visualization of the surgical scene (Fig. 6).

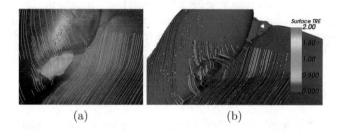

(a)   (b)

Fig. 6. Endoscopic image overlay: (a) the 3D reconstructed point overlaid on the endoscopic image after the rigid-body registration, and (b) corresponding view in CT.

4   Discussion and Conclusion

A 3D surface scanning system for multi-port MIS abdominal surgeries is presented. Based on a novel calibration framework, the dynamic spatial relationship between the camera and the laser instruments are known via preoperative calibration and intraoperative tracking. This allows us to formulate the surface scanning as the intersection problem between line-of-sight rays and the laser beam, and to optimize the trigonometry between the organ surface, the structured light, and the imaging system. In *ex vivo* experiments, our system achieves sub-millimeter surface reconstruction that is competitive to other systems [4,5].

A commercial clinical endoscope was integrated to minimize impact on surgical work-flow. Both camera and laser calibrations require minimal image acquisition (typically 10 to 12) and user interaction [7]. Our proposed system can be readily applied to other surgical scenarios such as neuro and orthopaedic surgery, and is designed to be compatible with the da Vinci surgical robotic systems.

In contrast to single-shot methods [5], our system requires multiple images to reconstruct a surface, and cannot account for motion of the organ during the scan (such as those due to breathing and cardiac motion). Using a single-beam laser allows us to reconstruct a 3D scanline in real-time since the segmentation of a single laser projection is trivial, the computational requirement for our system is extremely low. Accurate segmentation of the laser projection from endoscopy image is crucial for surface reconstruction. Laser planes perpendicular to the organ surface, result in thin and accurate segmentation. Conversely, if the incident angle is oblique, the laser projection is diffused in appearance and the true incident pixels are ambiguous to locate. Lower surface TRE was achieved in the second validation experiment where both organs were scanned, possibly since the laser beam was carefully adjusted to produce thin projections.

In our approach, we explored the efficacy of using two separately tracked devices in the context of multi-port MIS, where the binocular disparity is known via intraoperative tracking and preoperative calibration. Since the mathematical principle governing the system is trigonometry, there exists a strong angular dependence between the surgical camera and laser plane source and the system accuracy. If the two subsystems were integrated into a single device, the minimal angle between the light projection and optical axis would limit the surface reconstruction accuracy [4]. This study demonstrated the proposed system's ability to accurately reconstruct organ surfaces.

References

1. Besl, P.J., McKay, N.D.: A method for registration of 3-D shapes. IEEE Trans. Pattern Anal. Mach. Intell. **14**(2), 239–256 (1992)
2. Hill, D.L.G., Batchelor, P.G., Holden, M., Hawkes, D.J.: Medical image registration. Phys. Med. Biol. **46**(3), R1–R45 (2001)
3. Ma, B., Ellis, R.E.: Analytic expressions for fiducial and surface target registration error. In: Larsen, R., Nielsen, M., Sporring, J. (eds.) MICCAI 2006. LNCS, vol. 4191, pp. 637–644. Springer, Heidelberg (2006). https://doi.org/10.1007/11866763_78
4. Maier-Hein, L., et al.: Optical techniques for 3D surface reconstruction in computer-assisted laparoscopic surgery. Med. Image Anal. **17**(8), 974–996 (2013)
5. Maier-Hein, L., et al.: Comparative validation of single-shot optical techniques for laparoscopic 3-D surface reconstruction. IEEE Trans. Med. Imaging **33**(10), 1913–1930 (2014)
6. Mirota, D.J., Ishii, M., Hager, G.D.: Vision-based navigation in image-guided interventions. Ann. Rev. Biomed. Eng. **13**(1), 297–319 (2011)
7. Morgan, I., Jayarathne, U., Rankin, A., Peters, T.M., Chen, E.C.S.: Hand-eye calibration for surgical cameras: a procrustean perspective-n-point solution. Int. J. Comput. Assisted Radiol. Surg. **12**(7), 1141–1149 (2017)
8. Vibert, E., Perniceni, T., Levard, H., Denet, C., Shahri, N.K., Gayet, B.: Laparoscopic liver resection. Br. J. Surg. **93**(1), 67–72 (2006)

Deep Adversarial Context-Aware Landmark Detection for Ultrasound Imaging

Ahmet Tuysuzoglu[1]([✉]), Jeremy Tan[2], Kareem Eissa[1], Atilla P. Kiraly[1], Mamadou Diallo[1], and Ali Kamen[1]

[1] Siemens Healthineers, Medical Imaging Technologies, Princeton, NJ, USA
ahmet.tuysuzoglu@siemens-healthineers.com
[2] Imperial College London, London, UK

Abstract. Real-time prostate gland localization in trans-rectal ultrasound images is required for automated ultrasound guided prostate biopsy procedures. We propose a new deep learning based approach aimed at localizing several prostate landmarks efficiently and robustly. Our multitask learning approach primarily makes the overall algorithm more contextually aware. In this approach, we not only consider the explicit learning of landmark locations, but also build-in a mechanism to learn the contour of the prostate. This multitask learning is further coupled with an adversarial arm to promote the generation of feasible structures. We have trained this network using ~4000 labeled trans-rectal ultrasound images and tested on an independent set of images with ground truth landmark locations. We have achieved an overall Dice score of 92.6% for the adversarially trained multitask approach, which is significantly better than the Dice score of 88.3% obtained by only learning of landmark locations. The overall mean distance error using the adversarial multitask approach has also improved by 20% while reducing the standard deviation of the error compared to learning landmark locations only. In terms of computational complexity both approaches can process the images in real-time using a standard computer with a CUDA enabled GPU.

1 Introduction

Multi-parametric MRI can greatly improve prostate cancer detection and can also lead to a more accurate biopsy verdict by highlighting areas of suspicion [1]. Unfortunately, MR-guided procedures are costly and restrictive, whereas ultrasound guidance offers more flexibility and can exploit added MR information through fusion [9]. A key step in diagnostic MR and live trans-rectal ultrasound registration is the real-time, automated prostate gland localization within the

---

A. Tuysuzoglu and J. Tan—Equal contribution.

Disclaimer: This feature is based on research, and is not commercially available. Due to regulatory reasons its future availability cannot be guaranteed.

© Springer Nature Switzerland AG 2018
A. F. Frangi et al. (Eds.): MICCAI 2018, LNCS 11073, pp. 151–158, 2018.
https://doi.org/10.1007/978-3-030-00937-3_18

ultrasound image. This localization could be achieved by automatically identifying image landmarks on the border of the prostate. This task by itself is in general challenging due to low tissue contrast leading to fuzzy boundaries and varying prostate gland sizes in the population. Furthermore, prostate calcifications cause shadowing within the ultrasound image hindering the observation of the gland boundary. An example of this case is shown in Fig. 1(a). Learning these landmark locations is further complicated by inherent label noise as these landmarks are not defined with absolute certainty. A small inter-slice variability in prostate shape could result in rather larger deviation in the landmark locations, which are placed by expert annotators. Our analysis of this uncertainty is further explained in Sect. 2.

Through an initial set of experiments we observed that individual landmark detection/regression does not yield satisfactory results as the global context in terms of how the landmarks are connected is not properly utilized. Even for expert annotators, context is essential to place the challenging landmarks, specifically ones in regions with little signal or cues. Incorporating topological/spatial priors into landmark detection tasks is an active area of research with broad applications. Conditional Random Fields incorporating priors have been used with deep learning to improve delineation tasks in computer vision [3,11]. In medical imaging, improving landmark and contour localization tasks through the use of novel deep learning architectures has been presented in [6,10]. In particular in [10], the authors considered the sequential detection of prostate boundary through the use of recurrent neural networks in polar coordinate transformed images; however, their method assumes that the prostate is already localized and cropped.

In this work we propose a deep adversarial multitask learning approach to address the challenges associated with robust prostate landmark localization. Our design aims to improve performance in regions, where the boundary is ambiguous, by using the spatial context to inform landmark placement. Multitask learning provides an effective way to bias a network to learn additional information that can be useful for the original task through the use of auxiliary tasks [2]. In particular, to bring in the global context, we learn to predict the complete boundary contour in addition to each landmark location to enforce the overall algorithm in being contextually aware. This multitasking network is further coupled by a discriminator network that provides feedback regarding the predicted contour feasibility. Our work shares similarities with [4], where the authors used multitasking with adversarial regularization in human pose estimation in an extensive network. Unlike the method in [4], our approach is easily trainable and can perform at high frame rates and compared to [10], it does not require prior prostate gland localization.

2   Methods

This study includes data from trans-rectal ultrasound examinations of 32 patients, resulting in 4799 images. Six landmarks distributed on the prostate boundary are marked by expert annotators. In particular, the landmark locations are chosen to cover the anterior section of the gland (close to bladder), posterior section (close to rectum), and left and right extent of the gland considering the shape of the probe pressing into the prostate. Examples of annotations can be seen in Fig. 1(a). Nonetheless the landmarks cannot be placed with complete certainty due to poor boundaries, missing defining features, shadowing and other physiological occurrences such as calcifications. We characterized this landmark annotation uncertainty by measuring the change in landmark position in successive frames. The mean and standard deviation for each landmark position is given in Table 1. It is understood that part of this positional difference is due to probe and patient movement but nevertheless they can be treated as a lower bound for the localization error that can be achieved.

Each image is acquired as part of a 2D sweep across the prostate and all images were resampled to have a resolution of 0.169 mm/pixel and then padded or cropped so that the resulting image size is 512×512. Training data is tripled via augmentation with translation ($\pm$30–70 pixels) plus noise ($\sigma = 0.05$) and rotation ($\pm$4–7°) plus noise ($\sigma = 0.05$). We split the data into 3 sets: 23 patients for training (3717 images, 77%), 6 patients for validation (853 images, 18%), and 3 patients for testing (229 images, 5%). For all methods explained below the ultrasound data is given to the network as 2-D images.

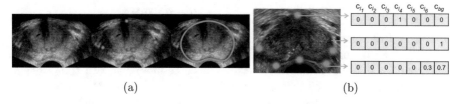

(a)   (b)

Fig. 1. (a) Ultrasound images with target labels: 2D Gaussian landmarks (center, green) and contours (right, green). (b) Each pixel has a distribution over 7 classes: 6 landmark classes and the background class. Moving away from the center of a landmark, the landmark probability decreases and the background probability increases.

2.1 Baseline Approach for Landmark Detection

Given the landmark locations, our approach takes a classification approach through the use of a shared background in locating the landmarks rather than the classical regression approach. The network has a 5 layer convolutional encoder and a corresponding decoder with 5×5 kernels, padding of 2, stride of 1, and a pooling factor of 2 at each layer. The number of filters in the first layer is 32; this doubles with every convolutional layer in the encoder to a maximum of 512. The decoder halves the number of filters with each convolutional layer. The final output is convolved with a 1×1 kernel into 7 channels (one for each landmark and a background class). The configuration of the convolutional, batch normalizing, rectifying, and pooling layers can be seen in Fig. 2.

We model each landmark as a 2D Gaussian function centered on the land-mark. The standard deviation of this Gaussian can in part incorporate the uncertainty involved in the landmark locations. In contrast to the regression approaches that regress locations or probability maps independently for each landmark, here we take a classification approach which couples the estimation through a shared background. For each pixel in the ultrasound image, we assign a probability distribution over 7 classes, where we treat each landmark and the background as separate classes. For a pixel that is at the center of a Gaussian for a landmark, the probability for that landmark class is 1 whereas rest of the probabilities are set to zero. These probabilities are obtained by independently normalizing each Gaussian distribution so that the maximum of the Gaussian is 1. Similarly for a pixel that does not overlap with any of the Gaussian functions, the background class has probability 1 and rest of the classes are set to zero. For a pixel that overlaps with one of the landmarks but not necessarily at the center, the probability distribution over the classes is shared between the corresponding landmark class and the background class. This is illustrated in Fig. 1(b). This framework can be trivially extended to scenarios where the Gaussian functions for the landmarks overlap. We learn a mapping of training images $\mathbf{x}$ in train-ing set $\mathbf{X}$ that represents the probability distribution of every pixel in $\mathbf{x}$ over the classes. This mapping, $S_{\mathrm{lm}}(\mathbf{x})$, is learnt through the minimization of the following supervised loss where $\mathbf{Y}_{\mathrm{lm}}$ denotes the training set labels:

$$\mathcal{L}_{\mathrm{lm}} = -\mathbb{E}_{(\mathbf{x},\mathbf{y}_{\mathrm{lm}})\sim(\mathbf{X},\mathbf{Y}_{\mathrm{lm}})}[\log S_{\mathrm{lm}}(\mathbf{x})]. \qquad (1)$$

During test time the landmark locations are obtained by processing the out-put maps, i.e., by extracting the maxima. The joint prediction of landmark and background classes could help the network become more aware of the positions of each landmark relative to one another. However, this background class encom-passes the entire space wherever a landmark does not exist. As such, it does not explicitly relate the points or highlight specific image features that are relevant to the connections between points (e.g. organ contour).

2.2 Multitask Learning for Joint Landmark and Contour Detection

When deciding a landmark location, expert annotators/clinicians are equipped with the prior knowledge that the landmarks exist along the prostate boundary which is a smooth, closed contour. Motivated by this intuition we identify two distinct priors: First, the points lie along the prostate boundary, and then this boundary must form a smooth, closed contour despite occlusions. We incorpo-rate these priors through multitask learning and the use of an adversarial cost function.

In multitask learning, the network must identify a set of auxiliary labels in addition to the main labels. The main labels (in this case landmarks) help the network to learn the appearance of the landmarks; meanwhile the auxiliary labels should promote learning of complementary cues that the network may otherwise ignore. A fuzzy contour following the prostate boundary is obtained by Gaussian

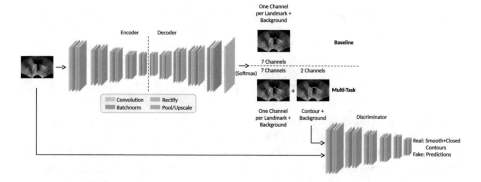

Fig. 2. Our baseline network has an encoder-decoder architecture where the receptive field size is large enough to contain the entire prostate. The multitask network outputs a boundary contour along with the landmarks which is then fed to a discriminator network to evaluate its similarity to training set samples.

blurring the spline generated by the main landmark labels. The boundary is used as an auxiliary label to incorporate the first spatial prior, that all landmarks lie on the prostate boundary. The goal of the multitask addition is to bias the network's features such that prostate boundary detection is enhanced. Since the boundary overlaps directly with the landmarks, the auxiliary task lends itself well to exploitation in the shared parameter representation. Figure 2 displays the addition of the auxiliary label for the multitask framework. Note that the network size does not increase, except for the final layer, because the parameters are shared between both tasks.

Similar to the landmark setup, we learn a mapping of training images, $S_{\mathrm{cnt}}(\mathbf{x})$, representing the likelihood of being a contour pixel by minimizing the following supervised loss, where $\mathbf{Y}_{\mathrm{cnt}}$ denotes the training set labels associated with the contour:

$$\mathcal{L}_{\mathrm{cnt}} = -\mathbb{E}_{(\mathbf{x},\mathbf{y}_{\mathrm{cnt}})\sim(\mathbf{X},\mathbf{Y}_{\mathrm{cnt}})}[\log S_{\mathrm{cnt}}(\mathbf{x})]. \tag{2}$$

Discriminator Network

While the multitask framework aims to increase the network's awareness of the prostate boundary features, it does not enforce any constraint on the predicted contour shape. As such, a discriminator network is added to motivate fulfillment of the second prior, that the boundary is a smooth closed shape. This is helpful because the low tissue contrast can make it challenging for the boundary detection (learned by the multitask network) to give clean estimates without false positives. The discriminator network is trained in a conditional style where the input training image is provided together with the network generated or the real contour. The design is similar to the encoder in the main encoder-decoder network with the difference being the discriminator network is extended one layer further and the first 3 layers have a pooling factor of 4 instead of 2. These changes are made to rapidly discard high resolution details and focus the discriminator's evaluation on the large scale appearance. We then define the discriminator loss as follows:

$$\mathcal{L}_{\text{adv}_D} = -\mathbb{E}_{(\mathbf{x},\mathbf{y}_{\text{cnt}})\sim(\mathbf{X},\mathbf{Y}_{\text{cnt}})}[\log D\,(\mathbf{x},\mathbf{y}_{\text{cnt}})]$$
$$-\mathbb{E}_{(\mathbf{x}\sim\mathbf{X})}[\log\,(1-D\,(\mathbf{x},S_{\text{cnt}}(\mathbf{x})))]. \tag{3}$$

In [5], the authors defined the generator loss as the negative of the discriminator loss defined in Eq. 3, resulting in a min-max problem over the generator and discriminator parameters. The authors in [5] (and several others [7,8]) have also stated the difficulty with the min-max optimization problem and suggested maximizing the log probability of the discriminator being mistaken as the generator loss. This corresponds to the following adversarial loss for the landmark and contour network S:

$$\mathcal{L}_{\text{adv}_S} = -\mathbb{E}_{(\mathbf{x}\sim\mathbf{X})}[\log D\,(\mathbf{x},S_{\text{cnt}}(\mathbf{x}))]. \tag{4}$$

Adversarial Landmark and Contour Detection Framework
The landmark and contour detection network is trained by minimizing the following functional with respect to its parameters θ_S:

$$\underset{\theta_S}{\arg\min}\ \mathcal{L}_{\text{total}} = \mathcal{L}_{\text{lm}} + \lambda_1\mathcal{L}_{\text{cnt}} + \lambda_2\mathcal{L}_{\text{adv}_S} \tag{5}$$

The discriminator is trained by minimizing $\mathcal{L}_{\text{adv}_D}$ with respect to its parameters θ_D. We optimize these two losses in an alternating manner by keeping θ_S fixed in the optimization of the discriminator and θ_D fixed in the optimization of the detector network. In our experiments, we picked $\lambda_1 = 1$ and $\lambda_2 = 0.02$ using cross validation.

3   Results and Discussion

Landmark location has a range of acceptable solutions on the prostate boundary that is also visible in the noise of the annotated labels. As such, the Dice score between the spline interpolated prostate masks is used as the primary evaluation metric. In addition, the Euclidean distance between predictions and targets and the 80th percentile of this distance are calculated. Baseline Dice score and average landmark error are 88.3% and 3.56 mm respectively. The multitask approach improves these scores to 90.2% and 3.12 mm. Adversarial training further improves the results to 92.6% and 2.88 mm. In particular, note the large improvement for landmark 4 (Table 1). This is the most anterior landmark (close to bladder) which generally has the highest error due to shadowing. Also, the improvement in the standard deviation of the Dice score indicates that the adversarially regulated multitask framework produces the most robust predictions.

Figure 3 displays prediction examples given by each method. In the top row, the plain multitask approach is able to improve the right-most landmark placement, but the most anterior landmark location is still inaccurate. In such cases,

Table 1. Landmark annotation error together with error for baseline, multitask, and adversarial multitask methods in units of mm.

Metric	Noise	Baseline	Multitask	Multitask GAN
Mean landmark error $\pm$ S.D.	0.98 ± 0.28	2.11 ± 1.41	1.94 ± 1.36	1.77 ± 1.43
	1.45 ± 0.44	2.33 ± 1.28	1.90 ± 1.13	1.97 ± 0.96
	2.17 ± 0.60	4.03 ± 5.13	3.38 ± 3.68	3.41 ± 3.17
	1.99 ± 0.47	6.29 ± 6.13	6.72 ± 5.59	5.01 ± 3.90
	2.19 ± 0.74	3.44 ± 2.77	2.73 ± 1.94	3.09 ± 2.43
	1.43 ± 0.54	3.21 ± 4.05	2.02 ± 1.85	2.01 ± 1.57
Overall avg.	1.70 ± 0.51	3.56 ± 3.46	3.12 ± 2.60	2.88 ± 2.24
80th percentile	1.42	3.19	3.04	2.75
	2.05	3.44	2.85	2.72
	3.17	4.59	4.41	5.08
	2.87	8.31	9.09	7.75
	3.14	4.83	4.27	4.68
	2.03	3.71	2.75	2.90
Overall avg.	2.45	4.68	4.42	4.32
Avg. dice $\pm$ S.D.	-	$88.3\% \pm 7.3\%$	$90.2\% \pm 7.2\%$	$92.6\% \pm 3.6\%$

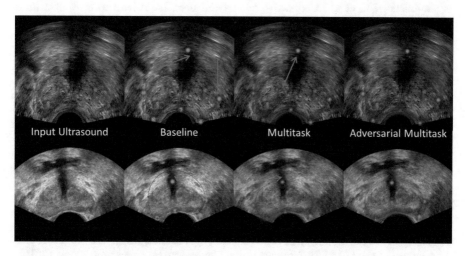

Fig. 3. Adversarially regulated multitask learning produces more complete contours resulting in better landmark placement compared to its plain counterpart. Ultrasound images with target (green) and prediction (blue diamonds, connected by spline) overlays. Red arrows indicate corrections of gross errors. Multitask predictions include an overlay of the contour prediction (blue heatmap).

features learned for boundary detection can mistakenly highlight areas with high contrast, e.g. calcification within the prostate. The adversarially trained detector improves the landmark placement significantly. In the bottom row, the boundary prediction is also hindered by shadowing, but the proposed framework still improves the overall shape of the contour along with the landmark placements.

The multitask learning framework helps biasing the landmark placement toward the prostate boundary through shared weights of two tasks, namely landmark detection and boundary estimation. As the predicted contour is not always of high quality especially when there is signal dropouts, an adversarial regularization is used to enhance boundary estimations and subsequently provide more accurate landmark detection.

References

1. Boesen, L.: Multiparametric MRI in detection and staging of prostate cancer. Scand. J. Urol. **49**, 25–34 (2015)
2. Caruana, R.: Multitask learning. In: Thrun, S., Pratt, L. (eds.) Learning to Learn, pp. 95–113. Springer, Boston (1998). https://doi.org/10.1007/978-1-4615-5529-2_5
3. Chen, L., Papandreou, G., Kokkinos, I., Murphy, K., Yuille, A.L.: Semantic image segmentation with deep convolutional nets and fully connected CRFs. CoRR (2014)
4. Chen, Y., Shen, C., Wei, X.S., Liu, L., Yang, J.: Adversarial posenet: a structure-aware convolutional network for human pose estimation. CoRR 2 (2017)
5. Goodfellow, I., et al.: Generative adversarial nets. In: Advances in Neural Information Processing Systems (2014)
6. Payer, C., Štern, D., Bischof, H., Urschler, M.: Regressing heatmaps for multiple landmark localization using CNNs. In: Ourselin, S., Joskowicz, L., Sabuncu, M.R., Unal, G., Wells, W. (eds.) MICCAI 2016. LNCS, vol. 9901, pp. 230–238. Springer, Cham (2016). https://doi.org/10.1007/978-3-319-46723-8_27
7. Tzeng, E., Hoffman, J., Saenko, K., Darrell, T.: Adversarial discriminative domain adaptation. In: Computer Vision and Pattern Recognition (CVPR) (2017)
8. Usman, B., Saenko, K., Kulis, B.: Stable distribution alignment using the dual of the adversarial distance. arXiv preprint arXiv:1707.04046 (2017)
9. Yacoub, J.H., Verma, S., Moulton, J.S., Eggener, S., Oto, A.: Imaging-guided prostate biopsy: conventional and emerging techniques. Radiographics **32**, 819–837 (2012)
10. Yang, X., et al.: Fine-grained recurrent neural networks for automatic prostate segmentation in ultrasound images. In: Proceedings of the Thirty-First AAAI Conference on Artificial Intelligence (2017)
11. Zheng, S., et al.: Conditional random fields as recurrent neural networks. In: Proceedings of the 2015 IEEE International Conference on Computer Vision (2015)

Towards a Fast and Safe LED-Based Photoacoustic Imaging Using Deep Convolutional Neural Network

Emran Mohammad Abu Anas[1(✉)], Haichong K. Zhang[1], Jin Kang[1], and Emad M. Boctor[1,2]

[1] Electrical and Computer Engineering,
Johns Hopkins University, Baltimore, MD, USA
eanas1@jhmi.edu
[2] Radiology and Radiological Science,
Johns Hopkins University, Baltimore, MD, USA

Abstract. The current standard photoacoustic (PA) technology is based on heavy, expensive and hazardous laser system for excitation of a tissue sample. As an alternative, light emitting diode (LED) offers safe, compact and inexpensive light source. However, the PA images of an LED-based system significantly suffer from low signal-to-noise-ratio due to limited LED-power. With an aim to improve the quality of PA images, in this work we propose to use deep convolutional neural networks that is built upon a previous state-of-the-art image enhancement approach. The key contribution is to improve the optimization of the network by guiding its feature extraction at different layers of the architecture. In addition to using a high quality target image at the output of the network, multiple target images with intermediate qualities are employed at in-betweens layers of the architecture to guide the feature extraction. We perform an end-to-end training of the network using a set of 4,536 low quality PA images from 24 experiments. On the test set from 15 experiments, we achieve a mean peak signal-to-noise ratio of 34.5 dB and a mean structural similarity index of 0.86 with a gain in the frame rate of 6 times compared to the conventional approach.

Keywords: Photoacoustic · LED · Laser
Convolutional neural networks · Densenet · Super-resoluton

1 Introduction

Photoacoustic (PA) is an emerging interventional imaging modality based on the photoacoustic phenomenon of generation of acoustic waves following light absorption in a soft-tissue sample. The primary applications of the PA technique include imaging of tissue chromophore (e.g. blood vessel) and exogenous contrast agents [3,6]. The standard work-flow of PA imaging starts with excitation of a sample using an intense short light pulse, followed by local thermo-elastic expansion due to sudden temperature rise. As a consequence of thermal expansion,

© Springer Nature Switzerland AG 2018
A. F. Frangi et al. (Eds.): MICCAI 2018, LNCS 11073, pp. 159–167, 2018.
https://doi.org/10.1007/978-3-030-00937-3_19

wideband acoustic signals are generated, and an ultrasound receiver is then used to collect the signal, which is usually known as PA signal.

For sources of PA imaging, the commercially available systems usually prefer Nd:YAG, Ti:Sapphire or dye laser [1], and they are capable to generate high energy laser pulse at biologically relevant wavelengths. Due to the high intense light source, a laser enclosure is recommended to install in the system to prevent the operator from incident irradiation. In addition to expensive and bulky laser system, such enclosure makes the system more cumbersome and does not allow the operator directly contacting with the sample [3].

Light emitting diode (LED) is a potential alternative that offers compact, safe and inexpensive illumination system in contrast to the conventional laser source. However, due to the limited output power, the PA signal of an LED-based system significantly suffers from low signal-to-noise-ratio (SNR) which in turn degrades the quality of the reconstructed PA images. To improve the SNR with LED-based system, the currently available technology acquires multiple (e.g. a few thousands) frames for the same sample and performs an averaging over them. In fact, the quality of a PA image is proportional to the number of frames used for averaging; an example is shown in Fig. 1(a) for two phantom PA images. Though a simple averaging over thousand of frames improves the image quality, it reduces the effective frame rate of PA images and more importantly, it often makes the PA images prone to motion artifact in *in vivo* applications (marked by circles in Fig. 1(b)). Therefore, it is recommended to use a less number of frames for averaging and perform standard signal processing to improve the SNR. The signal processing approach could be based on adaptive denoising, empirical mode decomposition or wavelet transform [2,3].

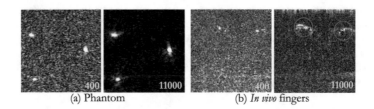

(a) Phantom   (b) *In vivo* fingers

Fig. 1. Effect of averaging number (400 vs. 11000) on (a) a phantom and (b) an *in vivo* (proper digital arteries of fingers) examples. For the *in vivo* example, higher number of averaging frames introduces motion artifact (marked by circles).

In recent years, deep neural networks based approaches have shown promising performance in various applications compared to the previous state-of-the-art signal and image processing techniques. In addition to image classification, deep networks have been successfully used for image denoising [9] and image resolution improvement [7,8] that closely fit to our problem of image quality improvement.

Inspired from the success of neural networks, in this work, we present a deep convolutional neural networks (CNN)-based approach to improve the quality of reconstructed PA images. Our architecture is built on a previous state-of-the-art image enhancement approach [8] that uses a series of dense convolutional layers to improve the quality of a 2D image. In addition, we propose to improve the optimization of the network by guiding its feature extraction using a sequence of target images. The target images are maintained to have an increasing order of image quality, and they are employed at different layers of the architecture to guide the feature extraction for an improved prediction of the image quality.

2 Methods

2.1 Architecture

Figure 2 shows our CNN-based architecture to improve the quality of reconstructed PA images; it takes a low quality PA image as input and at the end it generates an improved version of the given PA image. For convenience, in Fig. 2 we indicate the number of feature maps (or channels) for each convolutional layer as 'xx' in 'Conv xx'. In addition, the successively increasing feature

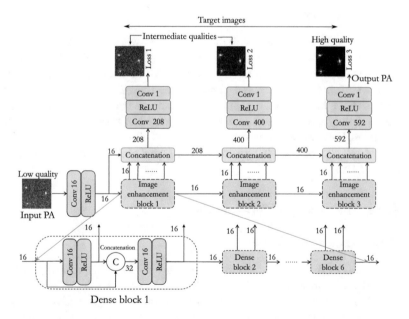

Fig. 2. The proposed architecture to improve the quality of a PA image. The input image is processed through three image enhancement networks, where each unit consists of six dense blocks. Furthermore, each dense block includes two dense 3×3 convolutional layers followed by rectified linear units. To generate an output image for each image enhancement block, all the features from the dense blocks are concatenated. Finally, a sequence of three target images with an increasing order of image quality are used to compute the mean square losses for three image enhancement blocks and these losses contribute equally to the total loss function.

maps are mentioned in the figure. The proposed architecture consists of three sequentially connected image enhancement blocks; for each block we use the architecture in [8] that was primarily proposed to improve the resolution of 2D images. Note that unlike [8] we do not use any upsamling layers in the network since both input and target images are of the same sizes (224×224 pixels) in our case. Following the architecture pattern in [8], we use six dense blocks to build each image enhancement network. Furthermore, each dense block includes two densely connected 3×3 convolutional layers followed by rectified linear units (ReLU). In principle, a dense convoluional layer uses all the features from its previous layers as inputs, as a result, it allows feature propagation more effectively and eliminates the vanishing gradient problem [5]. Note that instead of exactly using the same hyper-parameters (i.e. number of dense blocks and number of convoluional layers in each dense block) suggested in [8], we utilize the validation set to determine them (more about the validation set in Sect. 3.3 (Materials)). To produce an output image for each image enhancement block, all the generated features from the dense blocks are concatenated as shown in Fig. 2, and finally a convolution with one feature map is performed.

2.2   Loss Function

As mentioned earlier, the key contribution in this work is to guide the feature extraction of the network using a target sequence for an improved optimization. The sequence consists of three target images with an increasing order of image quality. As shown in Fig. 2, these three target images are sequentially fed to successive deeper layers. We compute the mean square losses corresponding to three target images, and subsequently we optimize the total loss function that is the average of these three individual losses. A detail description of generating a sequence of target images with an increasing order of image quality is provided in Sect. 3.4 (Training).

3   Experiments and Materials

3.1   LED Excitation Source

Our LED-based PA excitation source consisted of two LED matrices attached on both sides of the ultrasound probe. Each LED matrix included 144 LEDs arranged in four rows. The pulse repetition frequency of the LED was 1 kHz, i.e., the naive frame rate was 1 kHz. A synchronizer was employed to synchronize between LED excitation and PA signal reception.

3.2   Data Acquisition

We performed an experimental study using our LED-based PA system on 48 samples; 45 from blood mimicking phantoms and the rest 3 from volunteer fingers. For each sample, we acquired pre-beamformed PA signals for 11 s that led to a collection of 11,000 frames of PA signals. Note that only for the phantom experiments, we could manage minimal vibration during the scanning period. After acquisition of the raw PA signals, an arithmetic averaging was performed over a number of frames (say, N). Then delay-and-sum method was used for beam-forming, followed by envelope detection to reconstruct the PA intensity image PA_N, where the subscript N indicates the number of frames used in averaging the PA signals before reconstruction.

3.3 Materials

To train, validate and test the proposed approach, we divide all of our experimentally acquired data into three groups. As mentioned earlier, for *in vivo* experiments, we could not be able to manage a steady condition during the scanning period. Therefore, the reconstructed images with high averaging frame number are affected by the motion artifacts (examples in Fig. 1(b)), subsequently, they are not used in any quantitative analysis. The training and validation sets consist of only of phantom data from 24 phantoms and 6 phantoms, respectively. And, the test set consists of 15 phantoms and 3 sets of *in vivo* data, where the latter one is used only for qualitative evaluation.

3.4 Training

To generate low quality input and high quality target PA images for the training, we exploit the positive effect of the averaging frame number (N) on the reconstructed image quality. For low quality inputs, we choose lower values of N in range of 200–4000, with a step of 200. For each chosen value of N, we divide the large set of 11,000 frames into a number of subsets, where each subset consists of N frames of PA signals. Next, within each subset of N frames, the raw PA signals are averaged, followed by reconstruction to obtain one PA image. For an example of $N = 200$, therefore, we obtain a total of 55 PA images from each sample. Calculating in the same way for all N in 200–4000 with a step of 200, we obtain a total of 189 input PA images from each experiment, subsequently 4,536 input training images from 24 experiments.

In contrast, for the target sequence, we use successive higher values of N to generate three target images with an increasing order of image quality. The values of N are, therefore, chosen from 5000–7000, 8000–10000, 11000 to generate three target images with an increasing order of image quality, where the latter one indicates the possible highest quality. Since we need higher values of N for the target images, it leads to less number of target images than input images. Therefore, it may be possible to have one target sequence correspond to more than one input images. We also perform random cropping of input (similarly for output too) images for a data augmentation in training. For the validation and test sets, we also generate input images using N in range of 200–4000 with a step of 200. However, intermediate (for N in 5000–7000 and 8000–10000) target images are not required in those cases, because we use only the final output of our network to compare with the highest quality target image PA_{11000}.

4 Evaluation and Results

4.1 Peak Signal-to-Noise-Ratio and Structural Similarity Index

For a quantitative evaluation of the proposed approach based on the test set, we use peak signal-to-noise-ratio (PSNR) and structural similarity index (SSIM) as evaluation indices [4] that compare the output of our network with the highest quality target image PA_{11000}. In addition, we compare our results with those from simple averaging and densenet [8]-based techniques. In the simple averaging technique, we do not perform any further processing on the PA images that are reconstructed from the already averaged PA signal. In contrast, for the densenet-based technique, we process the PA images using their reported architecture that

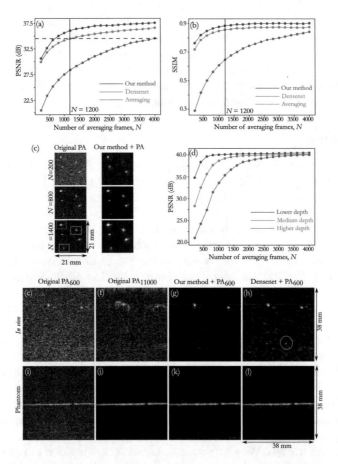

Fig. 3. Evaluation of the proposed approach. (a–b) Comparison of mean PSNR and SSIM of our method with those from simple averaging and densenet-based techniques [8] for different values of averaging frame numbers. (c–d) Effect of the imaging depth on the image quality. A qualitative comparison of our method with densenet-based technique for (e–h) an *in vivo* and (i–l) a phantom examples.

is in fact the same one shown in Fig. 2 but without using any intermediate target images during training. Note that the comparison is carried out for all values of averaging frame numbers (N) in range of 200–4000 (with a step of 200) that are used for generating low quality input images in the test set.

Figures 3(a–b) demonstrate a comparison of mean PSNR and mean SSIM (computed from 15 different experiments) of our method with those from the simple averaging and densenet-based methods for different values of N. We can notice improvement for our technique compared to two comparing methods for all values of N. In addition, we can observe comparatively higher drop in accuracy at $N < 1200$ for both of our and densenet-based methods than that at $N > 1200$. A rank-sum test is performed to measure the statistical improvement of our method with respect to two comparing methods. And we obtain p-values < 0.02 for all values of N both for PSNR and SSIM.

Another way to interpret the improvement is to compare the number of averaging frames needed to achieve a same image quality. For example, for a fixed PSNR of 34.5 dB, we achieve a gain in the frame rate of 6 times compared to the simple averaging technique ($N = 630$ vs. 4000 at dotted line in Fig. 3(a)). The corresponding mean SSIM for our method at $N = 630$ is 0.86.

4.2   Performance at Different Depths

We also investigate the performance of the proposed approach with respect to possible variations of imaging depths of targeted objects. For this purpose, we use three PA images (left column in Fig. 3(c)) of a same phantom, generated using three different values of N of 200, 800 and 1400. In addition, we present the results of our approach in the right column. To analyze the effect of imaging depth on the image quality, we select three region of interests (ROIs) around three point targets at different depths (shown in the figure). A qualitative comparison among the performance at those three ROIs indicates a successive reduced accuracy of the proposed technique for lower values of N while moving from a lower to higher depth. A corresponding quantitative analysis is presented in Fig. 3(d) that shows a comparison among the PSNRs of those ROIs for different values of N, where we can observe dependency of the performance of our method on imaging depth.

4.3   Qualitative Analysis

Figures 3(e–l) show a qualitative comparison between the proposed and densenet-based [8] methods for an *in vivo* and a phantom examples. As mentioned earlier, an averaging over a higher number of frames for the *in vivo* example (proper digital arteries of fingers) in our study leads to motion artifact in PA images. Taking the PA image with less number of averaging frames as input, our proposed method is able to improve its quality and subsequently suppresses the noise better, compared to the densenet-based technique (marked by circle in Fig. 3(h)). For the phantom example in Figs. 3(i–l), we can observe satisfactory performance for both of our and densenet-based methods. Though we train the network using only the cross-sectional images of blood vessel mimicking phantoms, we can notice its satisfactory performance on unseen 'along the axis' image.

4.4   Computation Time

The computation time obtained using NVIDIA GeForce GTX 1080 Ti is 0.05 sec for both of our and densenet-based methods.

5   Discussion and Conclusion

In this work, we have presented a real-time approach to improve the imaging quality of LED-based PA imaging technique. The key contribution in our CNN-based method is to guide its feature extraction by using a sequence of target images employed at successive layers in the architecture. We have trained the network using a set of 4,536 low quality PA images from 24 phantom experiments. On the test set from 15 experiments, we could achieve a gain in the frame rate of 6 times compared to the conventional averaging approach, with a mean PSNR of 34.5 dB and a mean SSIM of 0.86. In addition, we have demonstrated a statistical significant improvement of the proposed method compared to the state-of-the-art CNN-based image enhancement approach [8] that in turn indicates the effectiveness of our contribution of guiding the feature extraction during training.

Though we have trained the network using data from blood mimicking phantoms, we have not only observed its satisfactory performance in *in vivo* example but also noticed elimination of motion artifacts resulting from a high number of averaging frames (Fig. 3(g)). In addition, we have demonstrated its promising performance on unseen imaging planes that had not been exposed during training (Fig. 3(k)).

We have observed a comparatively reduced accuracy of the proposed approach (other methods too) at lower averaging frame numbers ($N < 1200$). We can attribute its main reason to limitation of these methods at higher imaging depth (Fig. 3(d)). In fact, the PA signal from a higher depth is affected by more noise due to increased optical scattering. As a result, we need higher averaging frame numbers to achieve the desired quality.

Future works include quantitative validation of the proposed approach with *in vivo* examples. In addition to blood vessels, we aim to include other optically interested soft-tissue and exogenous contrast agents within the imaging targets. In conclusion, we have demonstrated the potential of the proposed technique to be included in a real-time LED-based PA imaging work-flow to improve the image quality as well as to achieve a gain in the imaging speed.

Acknowledgements. We would like to thank the National Institute of Health for funding this project.

References

1. Allen, T.J., Beard, P.C.: High power visible light emitting diodes as pulsed excitation sources for biomedical photoacoustics. Biomed. Opt. Express **7**(4), 1260–1270 (2016)
2. Hariri, A., Hosseinzadeh, M., Noei, S., Nasiriavanaki, M.: Photoacoustic signal enhancement: towards utilization of very low-cost laser diodes in photoacoustic imaging. In: Photons Plus Ultrasound: Imaging and Sensing 2017, vol. 10064, p. 100645L. International Society for Optics and Photonics (2017)
3. Hariri, A., Lemaster, J., Wang, J., Jeevarathinam, A.S., Chao, D.L., Jokerst, J.V.: The characterization of an economic and portable LED-based photoacoustic imaging system to facilitate molecular imaging. Photoacoustics **9**, 10–20 (2018)
4. Hore, A., Ziou, D.: Image quality metrics: PSNR vs. SSIM. In: 2010 20th International Conference on Pattern Recognition (ICPR), pp. 2366–2369. IEEE (2010)
5. Huang, G., Liu, Z., Weinberger, K.Q., van der Maaten, L.: Densely connected convolutional networks. In: Proceedings of the IEEE CVPR, vol. 1, p. 3 (2017)
6. Jeon, M., et al.: Methylene blue microbubbles as a model dual-modality contrast agent for ultrasound and activatable photoacoustic imaging. J. Biomed. Opt. **19**(1), 016005 (2014)
7. Johnson, J., Alahi, A., Fei-Fei, L.: Perceptual losses for real-time style transfer and super-resolution. In: Leibe, B., Matas, J., Sebe, N., Welling, M. (eds.) ECCV 2016. LNCS, vol. 9906, pp. 694–711. Springer, Cham (2016). https://doi.org/10.1007/978-3-319-46475-6_43
8. Tong, T., Li, G., Liu, X., Gao, Q.: Image super-resolution using dense skip connections. In: 2017 IEEE ICCV, pp. 4809–4817. IEEE (2017)
9. Xie, J., Xu, L., Chen, E.: Image denoising and inpainting with deep neural networks. In: Advances in Neural Information Processing Systems, pp. 341–349 (2012)

An Open Framework Enabling Electromagnetic Tracking in Image-Guided Interventions

Herman Alexander Jaeger[1(✉)], Stephen Hinds[1],
and Pádraig Cantillon-Murphy[1,2,3]

[1] University College Cork, Cork, Ireland
h.jaeger@umail.ucc.ie
[2] Tyndall National Institute, Cork, Ireland
[3] Institute of Image Guided Surgery, Strasbourg, France

Abstract. Electromagnetic tracking (EMT) is a core platform technology in the navigation and visualisation of image-guided procedures. The technology provides high tracking accuracy in non-line-of-sight environments, allowing instrument navigation in locations where optical tracking is not feasible. Integration of EMT in complex procedures, often coupled with multi-modal imaging, is on the rise, yet the lack of flexibility in the available hardware platforms has been noted by many researchers and system designers. Advances in the field of EMT include novel methods of improving tracking system accuracy, precision and error compensation capabilities, though such system-level improvements cannot be readily incorporated in current therapy applications due to the 'blackbox' nature of commercial tracking solving algorithms. This paper defines a software framework to allow novel EMT designs and improvements become part of the global design process for image-guided interventions. In an effort to standardise EMT development, we define a generalised cross-platform software framework in terms of the four system functions common to all EMT systems; *acquisition, filtering, modelling* and *solving*. The interfaces between each software component are defined in terms of their input and output data structures. An exemplary framework is implemented in the Python programming language and demonstrated with the open-source Anser EMT system. Performance metrics are gathered from both Matlab and Python implementations of Anser EMT considering the host operating system, hardware configuration and acquisition settings used. Results show indicative system latencies of 5 ms can be achieved using the framework on a Windows operating system, with decreased system performance observed on UNIX-like platforms.

1 Introduction

The development of new image guided therapies relies heavily on intelligently combining data from multiple hardware sources. New techniques combining ultrasound and electromagnetic tracking (EMT) [1,2] are among techniques which combine multiple data sources to enhance the safety and accuracy of

© Springer Nature Switzerland AG 2018
A. F. Frangi et al. (Eds.): MICCAI 2018, LNCS 11073, pp. 168–175, 2018.
https://doi.org/10.1007/978-3-030-00937-3_20

procedures. Progress in these areas is made possible by the standardised open protocols [3,4] that govern how hardware and software should interact with one another. Figure 1 shows the generalised design flow of many image guided interventions (IGI). IGI applications interact with hardware through vendor authored application programming interfaces (APIs) or interface toolkits such as PLUS and IGSTK [5]. Such toolkits provide standardised methods through which IGI applications and hardware can interact. From a software perspective, this standardised approach enables developers to prototype and apply their work in a manner that can be distributed and replicated. That said, IGI application development typically falls short of incorporating custom innovations in tracking hardware. Electromagnetic tracking systems in particular are very much considered 'blackboxes' from the perspective of IGI research.

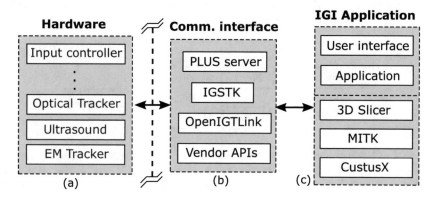

Fig. 1. A standard approach for developing cross-platform IGI applications. (a) Proprietary hardware is interfaced using an API or open communications interface (b). (c) Guided therapy applications use this interface to ensure cross-platform compatibility.

This paper outlines a framework to encourage integration of new electromagnetic tracking hardware into the current IGI design flow. The resulting framework was implemented in the Python programming language and applied to the open-source Anser EMT system [6] shown in Fig. 2. Preliminary cross-platform functionality of the framework is demonstrated with important performance metrics reported.

2   Framework Design

Electromagnetic tracking systems are complex electronic systems that incorporate advanced analog circuit design, signal processing and optimisation techniques. While the precise topology of such systems will vary depending on the core design and manufacturer, all EMT systems can be distinguished by four common processing steps outlined in Fig. 3: *acquisition, filtering, modelling,* and

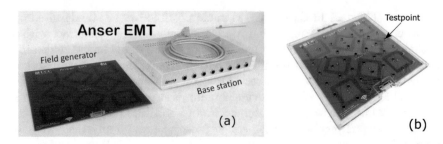

Fig. 2. (a) The Anser EMT system v1.0. (b) Field generator enclosure.

solving. Each of these processing steps can be treated as a discrete, independent stage in the tracking system software pipeline. The designed framework is structured according to these stages.

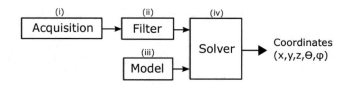

Fig. 3. The basic components which comprise all electromagnetic tracking systems are shown. The 5 degree-of-freedom sensor coordinate $[x, y, z, \theta, \varphi]$ is the most basic case for a symmetrical sensor coil, where θ and φ correspond to yaw and pitch angles respectively.

(i) Acquisition. The most fundamental step in any measurement system is data acquisition. It is the process by which physical signals are digitised into forms suitable for computation. In the case of EMT systems, the signals being measured are typically electric voltages. Such signals are induced on a tracking sensor coil when it is placed in the tracking volume of an EMT system. Acquisition hardware in the form of an analogue-to-digital converter (ADC) converts the electrical signal into a digital data stream by sampling at fixed periodic intervals. Manufacturers of acquisition systems include National Instruments (Austin, TX, U.S.A.) and Measurement Computing Corp. (Norton, MA, U.S.A).

(ii) Filtering. The sampled sensor signal contains all the necessary physical information required to resolve the sensor's position in space. EMT systems typically operate using multiple transmitters operating at distinct frequencies, thus the sampled sensor signal is a linear sum of the individual frequency components generated by each transmitting coil, as well as noise from the surrounding environment. The filter extracts the relevant signal content. A combination of digital filtering and Fourier methods are typically employed.

(iii) Model. An accurate model of the tracking system's generated magnetic field is a necessary component in all system designs. Models are typically defined as analytical expressions which define the spacial distribution of magnetic fields in the volume around the field transmitter. Each constituent transmitting coil can be characterised by a vector equation relating the magnetic flux density vector $\boldsymbol{B}$ to a point in space, $\boldsymbol{p}$:

$$\boldsymbol{B}(\boldsymbol{p}) = [B_x^p, B_y^p, B_z^p] \tag{1}$$

Commonly used models include variations of the magnetic dipole approximation [7], Biot-Savart law [8,9] and mutual inductance models [10]. Numerical models may also be used in cases where no accurate closed-form solution for the magnetic field exists.

(iv) Solver. Magnetic tracking systems resolve sensor positions through a process of non-linear optimisation in which a cost function is minimised to yield the best-fit solution for the position and orientation of the tracking sensor. The cost function is generally formulated such that the squared difference between the magnetic model of the sensor coil and acquired sensor measurements are minimised. Full formulations of the sensor model can be found in [8]. A non-linear least-squares approach is usually required to yield accurate results. Examples of general solving methods include the well known Levenburg-Marquard [11] and trust-region algorithms [12]. The general form of the optimisation problem is shown in (2):

$$\begin{aligned}
\underset{\mathbf{p}}{\text{minimise}} \quad & \sum f_i(\mathbf{p})^2 \\
\text{subject to} \quad & lb \leq \mathbf{p} \leq ub, i = 1, \ldots, n
\end{aligned} \tag{2}$$

where f_i is the ith cost function relating a single frequency component of the tracking sensor signal to the field model of the corresponding transmission coil, lb and ub are upper and lower bound constraints for the solving algorithm (if applicable) and $\mathbf{p}$ is the vector argument representing the position and orientation of the tracking sensor.

3   Framework Implementation

The proposed EMT framework is composed of four Python modules representing each of the signal processing steps shown in Fig. 1. An expansion of this design showing the data-flow between modules is shown in Fig. 4. The framework is divided into four modules labelled (i) to (iv). Analog signals from the EMT sensing electronics are acquired through a data acquisition module *daq.py*. This module provides facilities to abstract the acquisition hardware's specific API into a standard interface. The acquired digital samples are fed into the filter module *filter.py* where the frequency components of interest are conditioned and extracted from the digital waveform. The filter module allows easy configuration of filter parameters while providing routines for efficient matrix multiplications required during filtering operations. The extracted signal information is then fed to the solver module *solver.py*. Simultaneously the magnetic model of the system *model.py* is compared with the extracted signal data to minimise the system cost function. The solver module provides access to the tolerance and parameter settings for the minimisation process. The resulting sensor coordinates from the solver can be streamed to the user application using OpenIGTLink [4].

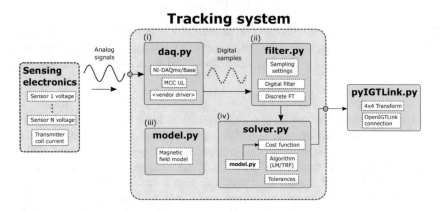

Fig. 4. (i) Analogue signals are sampled by the data acquisition module. (ii) The samples are filtered in software with relevant frequency components extracted. (iii)–(iv) A cost function utilises the component magnitudes to yield a position vector which can be transmitted using OpenIGTLink as a 4×4 transformation matrix.

The proposed framework was applied to the Anser EMT project [6]. The original open-source codebase, which was originally implemented in Matlab[1], was fully converted to Python in order to conform with the framework. The PyDAQmx driver [13] was used to provide a cross-platform interface with the NI-DAQmx driver acquisition system (National Instruments, Austin, Texas). Filtering and solving operations were performed using NumPy and SciPy libraries [14]. OpenIGTLink connectivity was achieved using PyIGTLink [15].

4   Experiments and Results

EMT framework's performance and accuracy were tested relative to the original Windows-only Matlab implementation. Testing of the framework was performed on three operating systems: Windows 10, MacOS 10.13 and Cent-OS 7.0 Linux. All reported metrics result from tests performed on a laptop PC configured with an Intel i7 4810HQ 3.5 GHz CPU and 16 GB of RAM, utilising both a Windows 10 and CentOS 7.0 installation. Compatibility with the MacOS 10.13 operating system was confirmed using a separate machine, but comparative results were

---

[1] Available at https://openemt.org.

not possible due to significant differences in the laptop hardware configuration. The variable sampling frequency of the acquisition system was set at $100\,kHz$ for all experiments.

4.1   Performance Benchmark

Performance testing measured the framework's ability to stream position measurements as quickly as possible with minimal latency over an OpenIGTLink connection to CustusX and 3DSlicer. Acquisition latency, maximum update frequency (with both a stationary and moving sensor) were recorded for multiple acquisition frame sizes shown in Tables 1 and 2. An acquisition frame constitutes the number of samples gathered by the acquisition system per single resolved position. A finite acquisition time for each frame puts a limit on the minimum latency figure. Static refers to a slow moving sensor speeds of $<5\,cm$ per second while 'Dynamic' refers to speeds $>50\,cm$ per second.

Table 1. Performance measurements using Matlab on Windows.

Matlab	Frame size	Acq. latency (ms)	Max. static (Hz)	Max. dynamic (Hz)
-	250	2.5	72	64
-	500	5	70	61
-	1000	10	65	62
-	2000	20	50	50
-	5000	50	20	20

Table 2. Performance measurements using Python framework (Windows/Linux).

Python	Frame size	Acq. latency (ms)	Max. static (Hz)	Max. dynamic (Hz)
-	250	2.5/5000+*	138/120	84/70
-	500	5/2000+	142/115	95/83
-	1000	10/1000+	102/80	66/62
-	2000	20/100	51/45	52/45
-	5000	50/50	20/21	20/20

*Due to operating system driver, see discussion.

4.2   Accuracy Benchmark

Accuracy testing consisted of comparing errors between sensor positions obtained from a 7×7 plane test x-y grid providing a total of 49 points. 150 position acquisitions at a height of $z = 70\,mm$ from the transmitter board (Fig. 2 (b)) were recorded per grid point from which the mean x, y and z coordinate of each point was calculated. Measurements were obtained from both Matlab and Python implementations. Maximum, minimum and root-mean-square (RMS) errors were calculated between the two obtained point grids. The grid obtained using the Matlab implementation was used as the reference since its performance has already been characterised in [6]. Maximum and minimum grid errors were measured as 3.1 mm and 0.1 mm respectively with an RMS error of 0.9 mm with a standard deviation of 0.75 mm.

5   Discussion

Table 2 shows how performance of the Anser EMT system varies with acquisition sample size over Windows and Linux operating systems. Benchmark results on Windows are clearly favourable to Linux particularly at low sample sizes. The high latencies in Linux were found to be caused by a low-level buffer issue caused by limitations in the NI-DAQmx Base kernel driver for Linux. Forcing the acquisition time to be greater than the solving time prevents this latency issue occurring. Empirically setting the acquisition frame to 2000 (i.e. a frame acquisition time of 20 ms) mitigates the issue, although this limits the maximum effective position update rate.

It can also be seen that the update speeds vary significantly depending on the movement speed of the sensor. This is due to the previous sensor position being used as the initial condition for the solver during each position update. A moving sensor causes previous sensor positions to lie further from the current true sensor position, resulting in the solver requiring more iterations to converge to the global minimum. Artificially forcing periodicity by limiting the update rate of the system prevents this issue from occurring. This approach must be implemented with care in order to avoid increasing the overall system latency.

The purpose of the accuracy benchmark is to showcase any significant differences between the two EMT software implementations. The benchmark is limited since it uses the Matlab implementation results as the reference standard, since no gold standard was available for the experiment. The reported mean error value of 0.9 mm falls within the mean error value of the Matlab implementation of 1.14 mm [6]. From this we can conclude that the Python implementation is of similar accuracy to the original implementation. Characterisation of this system according to the Hummel protocol [16, 17] is necessary in order to fully validate the accuracy of the system under the new framework.

6   Conclusion

An open source framework for designing electromagnetic tracking systems has been proposed. The framework was applied to a previously characterised tracking system with performance results reported. It is hoped that this work will assist in the translation of new EMT modules and platforms from research into the clinical setting.

References

1. Franz, A.M., et al.: First clinical use of the EchoTrack guidance approach for radiofrequency ablation of thyroid gland nodules. Int. J. Comput. Assisted Radiol. Surg. **12**(6), 931–940 (2017)
2. Paolucci, I., et al.: Design and implementation of an electromagnetic ultrasound-based navigation technique for laparoscopic ablation of liver tumors. Surg. Endosc. **32**(7), 3410–3419 (2018)
3. Lasso, A., Heffter, T., Rankin, A., Pinter, C., Ungi, T., Fichtinger, G.: PLUS: open-source toolkit for ultrasound-guided intervention systems. IEEE Trans. Biomed. Eng. **61**(10), 2527–2537 (2014)
4. Tokuda, J., et al.: OpenIGTLink: an open network protocol for image-guided therapy environment. Int. J. Med. Robot. Comput. Assisted Surg. **5**(4), 423–434 (2009)
5. Enquobahrie, A., et al.: The image-guided surgery toolkit IGSTK: an open source C++ software toolkit. J. Digit. Imaging **20**(Suppl. 1), 21–33 (2007)
6. Jaeger, H.A., et al.: Anser EMT: the first open-source electromagnetic tracking platform for image-guided interventions. Int. J. Comput. Assisted Radiol. Surg. **12**(6), 1059–1067 (2017)
7. Li, M., Bien, T., Rose, G.: FPGA based electromagnetic tracking system for fast catheter navigation. Int. J. Sci. Eng. Res. **4**(9), 2566–2570 (2013)
8. O'Donoghue, K., et al.: Catheter position tracking system using planar magnetics and closed loop current control. IEEE Trans. Magn. **50**(7), 1–9 (2014)
9. Sonntag, C.L.W., Sprée, M., Lomonova, E.A., Duarte, J.L., Vandenput, A.J.A.: Accurate magnetic field intensity calculations for contactless energy transfer coils. In: Proceedings of the 16th International Conference on the Computation of Electromagnetic Fields, Achen, Germany, pp. 1–4 (2007)
10. Bien, T., Li, M., Salah, Z., Rose, G.: Electromagnetic tracking system with reduced distortion using quadratic excitation. Int. J. Comput. Assisted Radiol. Surg. **9**(2), 323–332 (2014)
11. Levenberg, K.: A method for the solution of certain non-linear problems in least squares. Q. Appl. Math. **2**, 164–168 (1944)
12. Byrd, R., Schnabel, R., Shultz, G.: A trust region algorithm for nonlinearly constrained optimization. SIAM J. Numer. Anal. **24**(5), 1152–1170 (1987)
13. Cladé, P.: PyDAQmx : a Python interface to the National Instruments DAQmx driver. http://pythonhosted.org/PyDAQmx/. Accessed 1 Sept 2018
14. Oliphant, T.E.: Python for scientific computing. Comput. Sci. Eng. **9**(3), 10–20 (2007). https://doi.org/10.1109/MCSE.2007.58
15. Hiversen, D.: PyIGTLink: A Python implementation of OpenIGTLink (2016)
16. Hummel, J., et al.: Evaluation of a new electromagnetic tracking system using a standardized assessment protocol. Phys. Med. Biol. **51**(10), N205–N210 (2006)
17. Franz, A.M., Haidegger, T., Birkfellner, W., Cleary, K., Peters, T.M., Maier-Hein, L.: Electromagnetic tracking in medicine - a review of technology, validation, and applications. IEEE Trans. Med. Imaging **33**(8), 1702–1725 (2014)

Colon Shape Estimation Method for Colonoscope Tracking Using Recurrent Neural Networks

Masahiro Oda[1(✉)], Holger R. Roth[1], Takayuki Kitasaka[2], Kasuhiro Furukawa[3],
Ryoji Miyahara[4], Yoshiki Hirooka[3], Hidemi Goto[4], Nassir Navab[5],
and Kensaku Mori[1,6]

[1] Graduate School of Informatics, Nagoya University, Nagoya, Japan
moda@mori.m.is.nagoya-u.ac.jp
[2] School of Information Science, Aichi Institute of Technology, Toyota, Japan
[3] Department of Endoscopy, Nagoya University Hospital, Nagoya, Japan
[4] Department of Gastroenterology and Hepatology,
Nagoya University Graduate School of Medicine, Nagoya, Japan
[5] Technical University of Munich, München, Germany
[6] Research Center for Medical Bigdata,
National Institute of Informatics, Tokyo, Japan

Abstract. We propose an estimation method using a recurrent neural network (RNN) of the colon's shape where deformation was occurred by a colonoscope insertion. Colonoscope tracking or a navigation system that navigates physician to polyp positions is needed to reduce such complications as colon perforation. Previous tracking methods caused large tracking errors at the transverse and sigmoid colons because these areas largely deform during colonoscope insertion. Colon deformation should be taken into account in tracking processes. We propose a colon deformation estimation method using RNN and obtain the colonoscope shape from electromagnetic sensors during its insertion into the colon. This method obtains positional, directional, and an insertion length from the colonoscope shape. From its shape, we also calculate the relative features that represent the positional and directional relationships between two points on a colonoscope. Long short-term memory is used to estimate the current colon shape from the past transition of the features of the colonoscope shape. We performed colon shape estimation in a phantom study and correctly estimated the colon shapes during colonoscope insertion with 12.39 (mm) estimation error.

Keywords: Colon · Shape estimation · Recurrent neural network
LSTM

1 Introduction

CT colonography (CTC) is currently performed as one of methods to find colonic polyps from CT images. If colonic polyps or early-stage cancers are found in a

© Springer Nature Switzerland AG 2018
A. F. Frangi et al. (Eds.): MICCAI 2018, LNCS 11073, pp. 176–184, 2018.
https://doi.org/10.1007/978-3-030-00937-3_21

CTC, a colonoscopic examination or polypectomy is performed to endoscopically remove them. During a colonoscopic examination, a physician controls the colonoscope based on its camera view. However, its viewing field is unclear because the camera is often covered by fluid or the colonic wall. Furthermore, the colon changes shape significantly during colonoscope insertion. Physicians require great experience and skill to estimate how the colonoscope is traveling inside the colon. Inexperienced physicians overlook polyps or such complications as colon perforation. A colonoscope navigation system is needed that leads a physician to the polyp position. To develop a colonoscope navigation system, a colonoscope tracking method must be developed.

Endoscope tracking methods have been proposed by several research groups [1–10]. For bronchoscope tracking, image- and sensor-based methods exist. Image-based methods estimate the camera positions and movements based on 2D/3D image registrations. Registrations between temporally continuous bronchoscopic images [1] or between real and virtualized bronchoscopic images [2–4] are used for tracking. Sensor-based tracking methods use small position and direction sensors attached to a bronchoscope [5,6]. For colonoscope tracking, image- and sensor-based methods also exist. The image-based method [7] has difficulty continuing to track when unclear colonoscopic views are obtained. Electromagnetic (EM) sensors are used to obtain colonoscope shapes [8,9]. Unfortunately, they cannot guide physicians to polyp positions because they cannot map the colonoscope shape to a colon in a CT volume, which may contain polyp detection results. A colonoscope tracking method that uses CT volume and EM sensors was reported [10]. It obtains two curved lines that representing the colon and colonoscope shapes to estimate the colonoscope position on a CT volume coordinate system. This method enables real-time tracking regardless of the colonoscopic image quality. However, this method does not consider the colon deformations caused by colonoscope insertions. Large tracking errors were observed at the transverse and sigmoid colons, which are significantly deformed by a colonoscope insertion. To improve the tracking accuracy, we need to develop a method that estimates the colon shape during colonoscope insertions.

We propose a method that estimates the colon shape with the deformations caused by colonoscope insertion. The shape of the colonoscope, which is inserted into the colon, affects the colon's deformation. We propose a shape estimation network (SEN) to model the relationships between the colon and colonoscope shapes by a deep learning framework. After training, SEN estimates the colon shape from the colonoscope shape. SEN has a long short-term memory (LSTM) layer [11], which is a recurrent neural network (RNN), to perform estimations based on temporal transitions. To make maximum use of the colonoscope shape information, we developed a relative feature of the shape. Relative, positional, and directional features are given to SEN for the estimations. We performed a phantom study to confirm the performance of the proposed method.

The followings are the contributions of this paper: (1) it propose a new deep learning framework that models the relationships between the organ shape and the forces that cause organ deformations and (2) it introduce a new relative

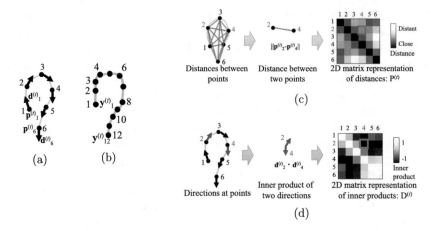

Fig. 1. (a) Green curved line represents colonoscope fiber shape. (b) shows $\mathbf{y}_m^{(t)}$ on colon centerline. (c) shows positional relation feature. Distances between two points are stored in 2D-matrix $P^{(t)}$. (d) shows directional relation feature. Inner products of two directions are stored in 2D-matrix $D^{(t)}$.

feature that represents 3D shape information as a 2D matrix shape. The feature can be processed by convolutional neural networks (CNNs) to extract features.

2   Colon Shape Estimation Method

2.1   Overview

We estimate the colon shape from the colonoscope shape. These shapes are the temporal information that was observed during the colonoscope insertions. The estimation is performed using a SEN with CNN and LSTM layers. We extract the relative features of the colonoscope shape using CNN layers and combine them with other features that are processed by a LSTM layer. LSTM performs regression based on the temporal transition of the feature values.

2.2   Colon and Colonoscope Shape Representation

We used a point-set representation to describe the colonoscope and colon shapes. Both are represented as sets of points aligned along the colonoscope and colon centerlines. The colonoscope shape of time t ($t = 1, \ldots, T$) is a set of points and directions $\mathbf{X}^{(t)} = \{\mathbf{p}_n^{(t)}, \mathbf{d}_n^{(t)}; \ n = 1, \ldots, N\}$ related to the colonoscope (Fig. 1(a)). $\mathbf{p}_n^{(t)}$ is a point aligned along the colonoscope. $\mathbf{d}_n^{(t)}$ is a tangent direction of the colonoscope fiber at $\mathbf{p}_n^{(t)}$. T is the total number of time frames and N is the total number of the points in the colonoscope shape. The colon shape is a set of points $\mathbf{Y}^{(t)} = \{\mathbf{y}_m^{(t)}; \ m = 1, \ldots, M\}$ aligned along a colon centerline (Fig. 1(b)). M is the total number of points in the colon shape.

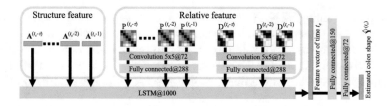

Fig. 2. Structure of shape estimation network (SEN). Input is colonoscope shape features in past time period $t = t_c - \tau, \ldots, t_c - 1$. Output is estimated colon shape of current time t_c. Numbers written after @ are kernel or unit numbers.

2.3 Colonoscope Shape Features

From $\mathbf{X}^{(t)}$, we calculate the features that related to the colonoscope shape.

Structure Features. Structure feature $\mathbf{A}^{(t)}$ includes $\mathbf{p}_n^{(t)}$, $\mathbf{d}_n^{(t)}$, and the insertion length of colonoscope $l^{(t)}$, calculated as follows. We applied the Hermite spline interpolation [12] to generate a curved line that is connected to $\mathbf{p}_n^{(t)}$. The curved line's length is used as the insertion length of colonoscope $l^{(t)}$. A structure feature is a set of these values $\mathbf{A}^{(t)} = \{\mathbf{p}_n^{(t)}, \mathbf{d}_n^{(t)}, l^{(t)}\}$.

Relative Features. Relative features include the positional relations between pairs of $\mathbf{p}_n^{(t)}$ and the directional relations between pairs of $\mathbf{d}_n^{(t)}$. Positional relation feature $\mathrm{P}^{(t)}$ is a $N \times N$ matrix with the distances between $\mathbf{p}_i^{(t)}$ and $\mathbf{p}_j^{(t)}$ ($i, j = 1, \ldots, N$) as (i, j) elements (Fig. 1(c)). Directional relation feature $\mathrm{D}^{(t)}$ is a $N \times N$ matrix with inner products $\mathbf{d}_i^{(t)} \cdot \mathbf{d}_j^{(t)}$ as (i, j) elements (Fig. 1(d)). $\mathrm{P}^{(t)}$ and $\mathrm{D}^{(t)}$ contain positional and directional relationship information.

2.4 Shape Estimation Network

We designed SEN with colonoscope shape feature input paths and the output of colon shape parameters (Fig. 2). Among the shape features, the relative features are processed by convolutional layers, which analyze the positional and directional relationship of the points on the colonoscope shape. The features extracted by the convolutional layers are combined with the structure features and given to a LSTM layer, which considers the temporal transition of all the features. To perform estimation utilizing temporal information, the SEN input is the features in a past time period $t = t_c - \tau, \ldots, t_c - 1$ until current time t_c. The LSTM layer's output is processed by fully connected layers. The final layer outputs estimated colon shape $\hat{\mathbf{Y}}^{(t_c)}$.

3 Experimental Setup

We confirmed the colon shape estimation performance of our method in phantom-based experiments. Our method needs pairs of $\mathbf{X}^{(t)}$ and $\mathbf{Y}^{(t)}$ at every time step for training SEN. $\mathbf{X}^{(t)}$ and $\mathbf{Y}^{(t)}$ were measured using an EM and distance sensors. We used a colon phantom (colonoscopy training model type I-B, Koken, Tokyo, Japan), a CT volume of the phantom, a colonoscope (CF-Q260AI, Olympus, Tokyo, Japan), an EM sensor (Aurora 5/6DOF Shape Tool Type 1, NDI, Ontario, Canada), and a distance image sensor (Kinect v2, Microsoft, WA, USA).

In colonoscopic examinations, physicians observe and treat the colon while retracting the colonoscope after its insertion up to the cecum. We assume the colonoscope tip is inserted up to the cecum when the colonoscope tracking starts. The proposed colon shape estimation method is also used during colonoscope tracking. The colonoscope was moved from the cecum to the anus.

3.1   Colonoscope Shape Measurement

The EM sensor is strap-shaped with six sensors at its tip and points along its strap-shaped body. Each sensor gives the 3D position and the 3D/2D direction along the colonoscope by inserting the sensor into the colonoscope working channel. The measured data are a set of points and directions $\mathbf{X}^{(t)} = \{\mathbf{p}_n^{(t)}, \mathbf{d}_n^{(t)};\ n = 1, \ldots, 6\}$ at time t. They are used as the colonoscope shape.

3.2   Colon Shape Measurement

We used a 3D printer to make 12 position markers to detect the surface position of the colon phantom, which has an easy-to-detect color and shape. The blue marker gives good color contrast to the orange colon phantom. The marker has a spherical shape, which enables detection from all directions. The position markers are attached to the surface of the colon phantom.

The distance image sensor is mounted to measure the surface shape of the colon phantom (Fig. 3). We obtained both distance and color images from the sensor. We applied an automated marker position extraction process to these images to obtain 12 three-dimensional points of the markers. The measured points of the markers were aligned along the colon centerline and numbered. The colon centerline was extracted from the CT volume of the colon phantom. The numbered markers are described as $\mathbf{Y}^{(t)} = \{\mathbf{y}_m^{(t)};\ m = 1, \ldots, 12\}$ at time t. $\mathbf{y}_1^{(t)}$ and $\mathbf{y}_{12}^{(t)}$ respectively correspond to markers near the cecum and the anus. $\mathbf{Y}^{(t)}$ is the colon shape.

3.3   Shape Estimation Network Training

We simultaneously recorded both $\mathbf{X}^{(t)}$ and $\mathbf{Y}^{(t)}$ during colonoscope insertions to the phantom. The measurements were performed using the experimental setup shown in Fig. 3. The shapes were recorded six times per second. Inaccurate measurement results caused by the mis-detection were manually corrected.

$\mathbf{X}^{(t)}$ and $\mathbf{Y}^{(t)}$ belong to the EM and distance image sensor coordinate systems. We registered them in the CT coordinate system using the iterative closest point (ICP) algorithm [13] and manual registrations. Registered $\mathbf{X}^{(t)}$ and $\mathbf{Y}^{(t)}$ in the CT coordinate system were used to train the SEN under these conditions: $\tau = 20$ past frames used by the LSTM layer, 50% dropout of fully connected layers, 50 mini batch size, and 480 training epochs.

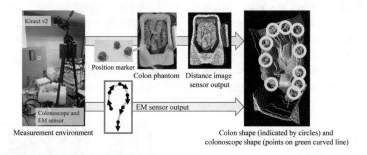

Fig. 3. Colonoscope and colon shapes measurement setup: colon phantom and sensors are mounted, as shown on the left.

3.4 Colon Shape Estimation

We measured the colonoscope shapes in a past time period, $\mathbf{X}^{(t_c-\tau)}, \ldots, \mathbf{X}^{(t_c-1)}$, during a colonoscope insertion. These colonoscope shapes were registered to the CT coordinate system using the ICP algorithm and input to the SEN to obtain estimated colon shape $\hat{\mathbf{Y}}^{(t_c)}$ of current time t_c.

3.5 Evaluation Metric

We use the mean distance (MD) (mm) between $\mathbf{Y}^{(t)}$ and $\hat{\mathbf{Y}}^{(t)}$ as an evaluation metric. The MD of one colonoscope insertion is described as

$$E = \frac{1}{12(T-\tau)} \sum_{t=\tau+1}^{T} \sum_{m=1}^{12} |\hat{\mathbf{y}}_m^{(t)} - \mathbf{y}_m^{(t)}|. \tag{1}$$

This metric indicates how an estimated colon shape is close to a ground truth.

4 Experimental Results

We evaluated the following three colon shape estimation methods: (1) our proposed method, (2) the proposed method without a relative feature, and (3) the previous method [14]. The method [14] estimates the colon shape from the colonoscope shape using regression forests and without temporal information. We recorded colonoscope and colon shapes during seven colonoscope insertions and recorded 1,179 shapes. An engineering researcher operated the colonoscope.

Shapes of six colonoscope insertions were used as training data, and the remaining colonoscope insertion was used as testing data. We performed a leave-one-colonoscope-insertion-out cross validation in our evaluation. The following are the MDs of the methods: (1) 12.39, (2) 12.61, and (3) 21.41 (mm). The proposed method performed estimation with less error than the previous method (comparing (1) and (3)). Also, using the relative feature reduced the errors (comparing (1) and (2)). For methods (1) and (3), we compared distances between the ground truth (measured) and estimated colon shapes in each frame in Fig. 4(a). Estimation results of the proposed method were close to the ground truth in most of the frames. Estimated colon shapes are shown in Figs. 4(b) and (c). The shape obtained from the proposed method was similar to the ground truth.

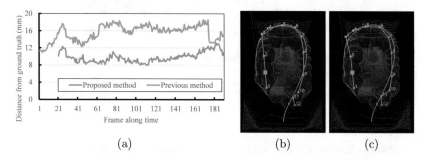

(a)   (b)   (c)

Fig. 4. (a) is distances between ground truth and estimated colon shapes in each frame for proposed and previous [14] methods. Proposed method starts estimation after $\tau = 20$ frames given. (b) and (c) show colonoscope shapes (points on green curved lines), estimated colon shapes (blue numbered points), and surface shapes of colon phantom (small dots). (b) and (c) are results of proposed and previous [14] methods.

5   Discussion

The proposed SEN accurately and stably estimated the colon shape during colonoscope insertion. SEN utilizes not only sensor information but also relative information and temporal transition for its estimation. These features contributed to the improvement of the estimation accuracy. Estimation results can be used to improve the colonoscope tracking accuracy [10]. The results of the proposed methods are important to achieve practical colonoscope tracking methods and will also contribute to the assistance of endoscopic procedures.

Our experimental result showed one application of the proposed method, which can be used as a soft organ shape estimation method of the forces that affect organ deformation. For example, bronchus shape estimation during a bronchoscopic insertion and estimation of the organ deformation were caused by contact with surgical tools. The proposed method models the relationships between the forces and organ deformations caused by the forces. This modeling framework is applicable for many computer-assisted intervention topics. The proposed method has a potential to work on phantom and real colons, even on colonoscope operations made by different operators.

The proposed SEN can be applied to estimate human colon shapes. To do this, we need pairs of colon and colonoscope shapes during colonoscope insertions into human colons. Taking X-ray images of the abdominal region is one candidate to observe these shapes, which we believe that we can extract from such X-ray images. Once SEN is trained using human data, it estimates the colon shape. This will enable colonoscope navigation during polypectomy.

This paper proposed a colon shape estimation method using an RNN technique. SEN models the relationships between the colonoscope and colon shapes during colonoscope insertions. SEN input includes the structure and relative features of colonoscope shapes. SEN was trained to output a colon shape from these features. We applied the proposed method to estimate colon phantom shapes. The proposed method achieved more accurate and stable estimation results than the previous method. Future work includes applications to a colonoscope tracking method and estimations of the human colon shape.

Acknowledgments. Parts of this research were supported by the MEXT, the JSPS KAKENHI Grant Numbers 26108006, 17H00867, the JSPS Bilateral International Collaboration Grants, and the JST ACT-I (JPMJPR16U9).

References

1. Peters, T., Cleary, K.: Image-Guided Interventions: Technology and Applications. Springer, Germany (2008). https://doi.org/10.1007/978-0-387-73858-1
2. Deligianni, F., Chung, A., Zhong, G.: Predictive camera tracking for bronchoscope simulation with CONDensation. In: Duncan, J.S., Gerig, G. (eds.) MICCAI 2005. LNCS, vol. 3749, pp. 910–916. Springer, Heidelberg (2005). https://doi.org/10.1007/11566465_112
3. Rai, L., Helferty, J.P., Higgins, W.E.: Combined video tracking and image-video registration for continuous bronchoscopic guidance. Int. J. CARS **3**, 3–4 (2008)
4. Deguchi, D., et al.: Selective image similarity measure for bronchoscope tracking based on image registration. MedIA **3**(14), 621–633 (2009)
5. Gildea, T.R., Mazzone, P.J., Karnak, D., Meziane, M., Mehta, A.: Electromagnetic navigation diagnostic bronchoscopy: a prospective study. Am. J Respir. Crit. Care Med. **174**(9), 982–989 (2006)
6. Schwarz, Y., et al.: Real-time electromagnetic navigation bronchoscopy to peripheral lung lesions using overlaid CT images: the first human study. Chest **129**(4), 988–994 (2006)
7. Liu, J., Subramanian, K.R., Yoo, T.S.: An optical flow approach to tracking colonoscopy video. Comput. Med. Imag. Graph. **37**(3), 207–223 (2013)
8. Ching, L.Y., Moller, K., Suthakorn, J.: Non-radiological colonoscope tracking image guided colonoscopy using commercially available electromagnetic tracking system. In: 2010 IEEE Conference on Robotics, Automation and Mechatronics (2010)
9. Fukuzawa, M., et al.: Clinical impact of endoscopy position detection unit (UCP-3) for a non-sedated colonoscopy. World J. Gastroenterol. **21**(16), 4903–4910 (2015)

10. Oda, M., et al.: Robust colonoscope tracking method for colon deformations utilizing coarse-to-fine correspondence findings. Int. J. CARS **12**(1), 39–50 (2017)
11. Hochreiter, S., Schmidhuber, J.: Long short-term memory. Neural Comput. **9**(8), 1735–1780 (1997)
12. Chen, E.C.S., Fowler, S.A., Hookey, L.C., Ellis, R.E.: Representing flexible endoscope shapes with Hermite splines. In: SPIE Medical Imaging, vol. 7625, 76251D (2010)
13. Besl, P.J., McKay, N.D.: A method for registration of 3-D shapes. IEEE PAMI **14**, 239–256 (1992)
14. Oda, M., et al.: Machine learning-based colon deformation estimation method for colonscope tracking. In: SPIE Medical Imaging, vol. 10576, p. 1057619 (2018)

Towards Automatic Report Generation in Spine Radiology Using Weakly Supervised Framework

Zhongyi Han[1,2], Benzheng Wei[1,2(✉)], Stephanie Leung[3,4], Jonathan Chung[3,4], and Shuo Li[3,4(✉)]

[1] College of Science and Technology, Shandong University of Traditional Chinese Medicine, Jinan, Shandong, China
wbz99@sina.com
[2] Computational Medicine Lab (CML), Shandong University of Traditional Chinese Medicine, Jinan, Shandong, China
[3] Department of Medical Imaging, Western Univeristy, London, ON, Canada
slishuo@gmail.com
[4] Digital Imaging Group (DIG), London, ON, Canada

Abstract. The objective of this work is to automatically generate unified reports of lumbar spinal MRIs in the field of radiology, i.e., given an MRI of a lumbar spine, directly generate a radiologist-level report to support clinical decision making. We show that this can be achieved via a weakly supervised framework that combines deep learning and symbolic program synthesis theory to overcome four inevitable tasks: semantic segmentation, radiological classification, positional labeling, and structural captioning. The weakly supervised framework using object level annotations without requiring radiologist-level report annotations to generate unified reports. Each generated report covers almost type lumbar structures comprised of six intervertebral discs, six neural foramina, and five lumbar vertebrae. The contents of each report contain the exact locations and pathological correlations of these lumbar structures as well as their normalities in terms of three type relevant spinal diseases: intervertebral disc degeneration, neural foraminal stenosis, and lumbar vertebrae deformities. This framework is applied to a large corpus of T1/T2-weighted sagittal MRIs of 253 subjects acquired from multiple vendors. Extensive experiments demonstrate that the framework is able to generate unified radiological reports, which reveals its effectiveness and potential as a clinical tool to relieve spinal radiologists from laborious workloads to a certain extent, such that contributes to relevant time savings and expedites the initiation of many specific therapies.

1 Introduction

Automated report generation is a worthwhile work to expedite the initiation of many specific therapies and contribute to relevant time savings in spine radiology. Nowadays, multiple lumbar spinal diseases not only have deteriorated the quality of life but have high morbidity rates worldwide. For instance, Lumbar Neural

© Springer Nature Switzerland AG 2018
A. F. Frangi et al. (Eds.): MICCAI 2018, LNCS 11073, pp. 185–193, 2018.
https://doi.org/10.1007/978-3-030-00937-3_22

Foraminal Stenosis (LNFS) has attacked about 80% of the elderly population [7]. In daily radiological practice, time-consuming report generation leads to the problem of the delay of a patient's stay in the hospital and increases the costs of hospital treatment [11]. Automatic report generation systems would offer the potential for faster and more efficient delivery of radiological reports and thus would accelerate the diagnostic process [9]. However, to date, most so-called Computer-Aided Detection (CADe) and Computer-Aided Diagnosis (CADx) techniques cannot generate radiological reports in the medical image analysis domain, let alone the spinal image analysis. In addition, MRI is widely used in clinical diagnosis of spinal diseases as is better to demonstrate the spinal anatomy [4]. Therefore, this work is devoted to the radiological report generation of lumbar MRIs to support clinical decision making.

Proposed Framework. Our proposed weakly supervised framework combines deep learning and symbolic program synthesis theory, achieving fully-automatic radiological report generation through semantic segmentation, radiological classification, positional labeling, and structural captioning. Firstly, we propose a novel Recurrent Generative Adversarial Network (RGAN) for semantic segmentation and radiological classification of intervertebral discs, neural foramina, and lumbar vertebrae. The RGAN is constituted by (1) an atrous convolution autoencoder module for fine-grained feature embedding of spinal structures; (2) a followed spatial long short-term memory based Recurrent Neural Network (RNN) module for spatial dynamic modeling; and (3) an adversarial module for correcting predicted errors and global contiguity. Secondly, we propose a strong prior knowledge based unsupervised symbolic program synthesis approach for positional labeling of multiple spinal structures. Finally, we propose a symbolic template based structural captioning method for generating unified radiological reports. The generated radiological reports contain the exact locations and pathological correlations of three spinal diseases: LNFS, Intervertebral Disc Degeneration (IDD), and Lumbar Vertebrae Deformities (LVD).

Why Weak Supervision? In this paper weakly supervised learning refers to using object level annotations (i.e., segmentation and class annotations) without requiring radiologist-level report annotations (i.e., whole text reports) to generate unified reports. To date, the weakly supervised learning manner is supposedly the one and only resolution. Because if it was possible to have a large amount of data, like natural image captioning dataset Visual Genome [5], we would directly use text report annotations to train end-to-end report generation modules as the natural image captioning technology [6]. Such technology needs a large amount of descriptive annotations (i.e., sentences, paragraphs) to train fully supervised learning model and generate coarse descriptions only. However, in daily radiological practice, different radiologists always write radiological reports in different styles and different structures, which cannot be learned with a little amount dataset. Clinical-radiological reports also contain exactly important clinical concerns, such as locations, normalities, and gradings. Since clinical concerns inside few words decide the correctness of a radiological report, it is also impossible to judge the correctness of computer-made reports compared with radiologist-made

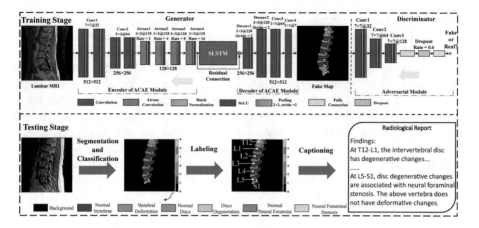

Fig. 1. The workflow of the proposed weakly supervised framework.

reports using Natural Language Processing (NLP) technologies. On contrary, it is possible to use weakly supervised learning manner decomposing the task into multiple procedures, i.e., detect clinical concerns using object level annotations first and then fill these concerns in a universal template to generate unified radiological reports.

Related Works. To the best of our knowledge, neither CADe nor CADx work has achieved spinal report generation. Existing works include but are limited to detection [1], segmentation or classification [3] of one type spinal structure. In other fields, a few works devoted to automated report generation. [13] uses a large amount of data and NLP based image captioning to study the report generation of pathology bladder cancer images. [12] uses chest X-rays data to study the report generation of thorax diseases.

2   The Proposed Framework for Report Generation

The workflow of the weakly supervised framework is illustrated in Fig. 1. The framework combines two type theories. The first type is our proposed learning-based methods RGAN for segmentation and classification (see Sect. 2.1). The second type is a strong prior knowledge based unsupervised symbolic program synthesis for labeling and captioning (see Sect. 2.2). The framework thus can concentrate on intuitive perceptual thinking while focuses on rule-based thinking.

2.1   Recurrent Generative Adversarial Network

RGAN comprises two sub-networks: a generative network and a discriminative network. The generative network is designed to generate pixel-level predicted maps, i.e., each pixel in a generated map has the possibility of seven classes comprised of normal/abnormal neural foramina, normal/abnormal intervertebral discs, normal/abnormal vertebrae, and background. The discriminative network is designed to supervise and encourage the generative network. When training, inspired by [2], the generative network aims at fooling the discriminative network, while the discriminative network makes great efforts to discriminate its inputs whether are fake maps generated by the generative network or real maps from ground truth. When a strong confrontation occurs, the discriminative network eagerly prompts the generative network to look out mismatches in a wide range of higher-order statistics. The generative network comprises of a deep Atrous Convolution Autoencoder (ACAE) module and a Spatial Long Short-Term Memory (SLSTM) based RNN module, while the discriminative network comprises of an adversarial module.

ACAE Module. The ACAE module comprises of four standard convolution layers, four atrous convolution layers as an encoder, and two deconvolution layers as a decoder. For each location i on the output feature map y and each kernel k on the weight w and bias b, atrous convolution are applied over the input feature map x as $y[i] = f(\sum_k x[i + r \cdot k] * w[k] + b[k])$. The $r \cdot k$ is equivalent to convolving the input x with upsampled kernels, which is produced by inserting zeros between two consecutive values of each kernel along each spatial dimension. Progressive rates r of $\{2, 4, 8, 16\}$ is adopted after cross-validation, which modifies kernel's receptive fields adaptively. The ACAE module practically produces semantic task-aware features using fewer parameters and larger receptive fields. The ACAE module also has little-stacked downsampling operations, so that avoids severely reducing the feature resolution among low-dimensional manifold. The ACAE module thus enables RGAN to not only address the high variability and complexity of spinal appearances in MRI explicitly but also effectively preserve fine-grained differences between normal and abnormal structures.

RLSTM Based RNN Module. This module is to memorize the spatial pathological correlations between neighboring structures. For instance, current neural foramen has a high probability of being abnormal when neighboring discs or vertebra are abnormal. The module has a spatial top-down structure. Assuming $M \in \mathbb{R}^{n \times n \times c}$ represents a set of deep convolutional feature maps generated by the encoder of ACAE module with widths of n, heights of n, and channels of c. Firstly, the module downsamples its input feature maps to $M' \in \mathbb{R}^{\frac{n}{i} \times \frac{n}{i} \times c}$, where i is the size of 4 according to the receptive fields of spinal structures. Secondly, the module patch-wisely unstacks these downsampled feature maps M' to a set of spatial sequences $M'' \in \mathbb{R}^{(\frac{n}{i})^2 \times c}$. Thirdly, the module recurrently memorizes long-period context information between spatial sequences and generates outputs $S \in \mathbb{R}^{(\frac{n}{i})^2 \times c}$. Finally, the module adaptively upsamples the outputs S into $S' \in \mathbb{R}^{n \times n \times c}$ using two deconvolution layers. Accordingly, the module has $(\frac{n}{i})^2$ LSTM units and c-dimensions cell state. The module is capable of selectively memorizing and forgetting semantic information of previous spinal structures when transforming the high-level semantic features into sequential inputs of LSTM units.

Adversarial Module. The adversarial module of the discriminative network comprises of three convolutional layers with large kernels, three batch normalizations, three average pooling layers, and two fully connected layers with dropout. When training, the adversarial module first receives the predicted maps from the generative network and manual maps from ground truth and then outputs a single scalar. The adversarial processes substantially correct predicted errors and break through small dataset limitation, so as to achieve continued gains on global-level contiguity and avoidable over-fitting.

2.2   Prior Knowledge-Based Symbolic Program Synthesis

In this paper, unsupervised symbolic program synthesis refers to leveraging prior human knowledge to discover inherent patterns in spinal structures. This study assumed that human knowledge representation is symbolic and that reasoning, language, planning, and vision could be understood in terms of symbolic operations. Therefore, we can design a model-free symbolic programing to realize labeling and captioning.

Unsupervised Labeling. The input of the unsupervised labeling process is the predicted maps generated by RGAN, and the output is three dictionaries comprised of locations and normalities of three spinal structures. The keys of each dictionary are the locations of one type structure, while the values of the dictionary are the normality conditions at the locations of one type structure in a lumbar spine. The first step of the unsupervised labeling process is to discover patterns for location assignment of each pixel. According to our observations, locations, surrounding correlations are the inherent patterns inside lumbar spinal structures, i.e., in a lumbar spine, all intervertebral discs are separated by vertebrae that like the blank of a piano. Let intervertebral disc as an example, we first calculate out the minimal height of vertebral in the training set and then let the height divided by four be the margin between pixels of intervertebral discs. We thus get the margined pixels of intervertebral discs into lists. Since generated maps have a few spots, the second step is to decide the true label of margined pixels. For instance, at the L5-S1 intervertebral disc, we compare the pixel amounts between normal and abnormal labels and then choose the one that has the most amount pixels as the final label. We collect the final results into dictionary for the next captioning process.

Template-Based Captioning. The input of this captioning process is three dictionaries and the output is a fully structural radiological report. Although reports wrote by different radiologists always have different styles and different patterns, the focus is still the clinical concern. After summarizing common patterns inside radiological reports as a decision problem, we can use If-Then symbolic operations to create a unified template. For instance, at L5-S1 if the neural foramen is abnormal, intervertebral disc and vertebra are normal, then the output would be *"At L5-S1, the neural foramen has obvious stenosis, the intervertebral disc does not have obvious degenerative changes, and the above vertebra*

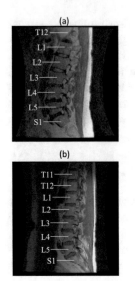

(a) Radiological Report

At T12-L1, the intervertebral disc has obvious degenerative changes. The neural foramen does not have stenosis.

At L1-L2, the above vertebra has deformative changes. The intervertebral disc does not have obvious degenerative changes. The neural foramen does not have obvious stenosis.

At L2-L3, the neural foramen has obvious stenosis. The intervertebral disc does not have obvious degenerative changes. The above vertebra does not have deformative changes.

At L3-L4, disc degenerative changes are associated with neural foraminal stenosis.

At L4-L5, disc degenerative changes are associated with neural foraminal stenosis.

At L5-S1, the intervertebral disc has obvious degenerative changes. The above vertebra also has deformative changes. They lead to the neural foraminal stenosis.

(b) Radiological Report

At T12-L1, the intervertebral disc has obvious degenerative changes. The neural foramen does not have stenosis.

At L1-L2, the above vertebra does not have deformative changes. The intervertebral disc does not have degenerative changes. The neural foramen also does not have stenosis.

At L2-L3, the above vertebra does not have deformative changes. The intervertebral disc does not have degenerative changes. The neural foramen also does not have stenosis.

At L3-L4, the neural foramen has obvious stenosis. The intervertebral disc does not have obvious degenerative changes. The above vertebra does not have deformative changes.

At L4-L5, disc degenerative changes are associated with neural foraminal stenosis.

At L5-S1, the intervertebral disc has obvious degenerative changes. The above vertebra also has deformative changes. They lead to neural foraminal stenosis to a certain extent.

Fig. 2. The generated radiological reports. The text in purple color represents that our framework is helpful for building comprehensive pathological analysis.

does not have deformative changes.". It is noteworthy that this process can significantly promote clinical pathogenesis-based diagnosis. While the SLSTM-based RNN module can memorize the spatial pathological correlations between neighboring structures, LVD and LDD are substantially crucial pathogenic factors and vital predictors of LNFS. Accordingly, for instance, if the neural foramen, disc, and vertebra are abnormal at L3-L4, the captioning process can output *"At L3-L4, the intervertebral disc has obvious degenerative changes. The above vertebra also has deformative changes. They lead to the neural foraminal stenosis to a certain extent."*. If the neural foramen is normal but disc or vertebra is abnormal, one can predict that the neural foramen has a great possibility to be stenosis. Therefore, this captioning process promotes early diagnosis when the pathogenic factor is solely occurring. This process is also helpful for building comprehensive pathological analysis and benefits to clinical surgery planning.

3   Results

Dataset. Our dataset is collected from multicenter and different models of vendors including 253 multicenter clinical patients. Average years of patient age is 53 ± 38 with 147 females and 106 males. Among sequential T1/T2-weighted MRI scans of each patient, one lumbar middle scan was selected to better present neural foramina, discs, and vertebra simultaneously in the sagittal direction. The segmentation ground truth is easily labeled by our lab tool according to the clinical criterion. The ground truth of classification was annotated as normal or

Table 1. Performance comparisons between RGAN and other models.

Method	Pixel accuracy	Dice coefficient	Specificity	Sensitivity
FCN [10]	0.917 ± 0.004	0.754 ± 0.033	0.754 ± 0.035	0.712 ± 0.032
U-Net [8]	0.920 ± 0.004	0.797 ± 0.013	0.816 ± 0.027	0.770 ± 0.026
ACAE	0.958 ± 0.002	0.841 ± 0.013	0.862 ± 0.018	0.823 ± 0.024
ACAE+SLSTM	0.959 ± 0.002	0.848 ± 0.009	0.865 ± 0.021	0.837 ± 0.025
ACAE+Adversarial	0.960 ± 0.004	0.863 ± 0.006	0.873 ± 0.015	0.855 ± 0.027
RGAN	$\mathbf{0.962 \pm 0.003}$	$\mathbf{0.871 \pm 0.004}$	$\mathbf{0.891 \pm 0.017}$	$\mathbf{0.860 \pm 0.025}$

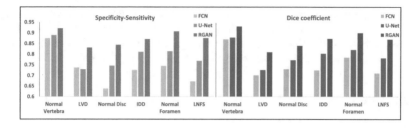

Fig. 3. Specificity-sensitivity and dice coefficient of three type models.

abnormal by extracting from clinical reports, which are double-checked by board-certified radiologists. Five-fold cross-validation is employed for the performance evaluation and comparison.

Performance of Radiological Report Generation. The representative radiological reports generated by our proposed framework are illustrated in Fig. 2. The framework can produce pathological correlations between LNFS, LVD, and IDD as shown in the text in purple color. Representative results demonstrate the advantages of the framework, which efficiently combines deep learning that is robust to noisy data and symbolic program synthesis that is easier to interpret and requires less training data. Generated unified reports also demonstrate that the weakly supervision is robust and efficient, and endows our framework an potential as a clinical tool to relieve spinal radiologists from laborious workloads to a certain extent.

Performance Inter- and Intra-comparison of RGAN. As illustrated in Table 1 and Fig. 3, RGAN achieves more higher performance than Fully Convolutional Network (FCN) [10] and U-Net [8] in the segmentation and classification of three type spinal structures. FCN and U-Net are implemented strictly upon public resources. After removing the SLSTM based RNN module and the adversarial module, RGAN also achieves higher performance than its ablated versions as shown in the third-sixth rows of Table 1. Since no existing works achieved simultaneous segmentation and classification of multiple spinal structures, we do not conduct extra comparisons.

4   Discussion and Conclusion

We show that using the weakly supervised framework that combines deep learning and symbolic program synthesis is very efficient and flexible to generate spinal radiological reports. The reason for using object segmentation rather than object detection is that segmentation is better to present the spatial correlations between spinal structures. The study just has a try, and further work will focus on (1) considering more uncommon spinal diseases, and (2) collecting more clinical data in order to realize end-to-end report generation.

Acknowledgment. This work was partly funded by the Natural Science Foundation of Shandong Province (No. ZR2015FM010), the Project of Shandong Province Higher Educational Science and Technology Program (No. J15LN20), the Project of Shandong Province Medical and Health Technology Development Program (No. 2016WS0577).

References

1. Cai, Y., Osman, S., Sharma, M., Landis, M., Li, S.: Multi-modality vertebra recognition in arbitrary views using 3D deformable hierarchical model. IEEE Trans. Med. Imaging **34**(8), 1676–1693 (2015)
2. Goodfellow, I., et al.: Generative adversarial nets. In: Advances in Neural Information Processing Systems, pp. 2672–2680 (2014)
3. He, X., Yin, Y., Sharma, M., Brahm, G., Mercado, A., Li, S.: Automated diagnosis of neural foraminal stenosis using synchronized superpixels representation. In: Ourselin, S., Joskowicz, L., Sabuncu, M.R., Unal, G., Wells, W. (eds.) MICCAI 2016. LNCS, vol. 9901, pp. 335–343. Springer, Cham (2016). https://doi.org/10.1007/978-3-319-46723-8_39
4. Kim, S., et al.: A new MRI grading system for cervical foraminal stenosis based on axial T2-weighted images. Korean J. Radiol. **16**(6), 1294–1302 (2015)
5. Krishna, R., et al.: Visual genome: connecting language and vision using crowd-sourced dense image annotations. Int. J. Comput. Vis. **123**(1), 32–73 (2017)
6. Kulkarni, G., et al.: Baby talk: understanding and generating image descriptions. In: Proceedings of the 24th CVPR. Citeseer (2011)
7. Rajaee, S.S., Bae, H.W., Kanim, L.E., Delamarter, R.B.: Spinal fusion in the united states: analysis of trends from 1998 to 2008. Spine **37**(1), 67–76 (2012)
8. Ronneberger, O., Fischer, P., Brox, T.: U-Net: convolutional networks for biomedical image segmentation. In: Navab, N., Hornegger, J., Wells, W.M., Frangi, A.F. (eds.) MICCAI 2015. LNCS, vol. 9351, pp. 234–241. Springer, Cham (2015). https://doi.org/10.1007/978-3-319-24574-4_28
9. Rosenthal, D.F., et al.: A voice-enabled, structured medical reporting system. J. Am. Med. Inform. Assoc. **4**(6), 436–441 (1997)
10. Shelhamer, E., Long, J., Darrell, T.: Fully convolutional networks for semantic segmentation. IEEE Trans. Pattern Anal. Mach. Intell. **39**(4), 640–651 (2017)
11. Vorbeck, F., Ba-Ssalamah, A., Kettenbach, J., Huebsch, P.: Report generation using digital speech recognition in radiology. Eur. Radiol. **10**(12), 1976–1982 (2000). https://doi.org/10.1007/s003300000459

12. Wang, X., Peng, Y., Lu, L., Lu, Z., Summers, R.M.: TieNet: text-image embedding network for common thorax disease classification and reporting in chest X-rays. arXiv preprint arXiv:1801.04334 (2018)
13. Zhang, Z., Xie, Y., Xing, F., McGough, M., Yang, L.: MDNet: a semantically and visually interpretable medical image diagnosis network. In: 2017 IEEE Conference on Computer Vision and Pattern Recognition (CVPR), pp. 3549–3557, July 2017

Computer Assisted Interventions: Surgical Planning, Simulation and Work Flow Analysis

A Natural Language Interface for Dissemination of Reproducible Biomedical Data Science

Rogers Jeffrey Leo John$^{(\boxtimes)}$, Jignesh M. Patel, Andrew L. Alexander,
Vikas Singh, and Nagesh Adluru

University of Wisconsin-Madison, Madison, USA
rl@cs.wisc.edu

Abstract. Computational tools in the form of software packages are
burgeoning in the field of medical imaging and biomedical research.
These tools enable biomedical researchers to analyze a variety of data
using modern machine learning and statistical analysis techniques. While
these publicly available software packages are a great step towards a mul-
tiplicative increase in the biomedical research productivity, there are still
many open issues related to validation and reproducibility of the results.
A key gap is that while scientists can validate domain insights that are
implicit in the analysis, the analysis itself is coded in a programming language and that domain scientist may not be a programmer. Thus, there
is no/limited direct validation of the program that carries out the desired
analysis. We propose a novel solution, building upon recent successes in
natural language understanding, to address this problem. Our platform
allows researchers to perform, share, reproduce and interpret the analysis pipelines and results via natural language. While this approach still
requires users to have a conceptual understanding of the techniques, it
removes the burden of programming syntax and thus lowers the barriers
to advanced and reproducible neuroimaging and biomedical research.

Keywords: Natural language user interface · Systems
Reproducibility · Provenance tracking · Neuro/medical image analysis
Surgical data science

1 Introduction

Large amounts of complex data are available in neuroimaging and biomedical
imaging domains. Advances in machine learning and data science have set the
stage for a new generation of analytics that will support improved decision-
making by leveraging insights from data [1,2]. However, obtaining insights from
data is often non-trivial. The researcher, who sifts through the data, must
develop and adopt sophisticated computational pipelines to arrive at meaningful
insights. These pipelines involve several complex stages such as data cleaning,
data merging, data exploration, machine learning model estimation, statistical
testing, and visualization, in addition to sophisticated image processing [1,3,4].

© Springer Nature Switzerland AG 2018
A. F. Frangi et al. (Eds.): MICCAI 2018, LNCS 11073, pp. 197–205, 2018.
https://doi.org/10.1007/978-3-030-00937-3_23

This necessarily complex nature of the modern medical imaging methods challenges adoptability, reproducibility and ultimately their translational impact.

Furthermore, each stage in the analysis may involve using various software packages, and require that the researchers be proficient in using these packages (e.g., SQL to filter, slice and dice the data and R for data analysis). These diverse requirements for constructing data science pipelines place a significant cognitive overhead on the researcher, and increase the barriers for entry and reproducibility. We note that many researchers publish code repositories, but it is well-recognized that such an approach does not fully address the core issue of sharing and reproducing analysis pipelines [5]. This current situation holds back progress in the field as testing of new hypotheses and models can take much longer. Recent emerging research suggests that conversational interfaces can reduce some of the barriers in reproducibility and adaptability of advanced computational methods [6,7]. In this paper, we present a conversational interface that allows dissemination and use of advanced neuroimaging and general biomedical data analysis pipelines such as those in [1,3,4] with excellent reproducibility and provenance tracking. We believe that such an interface is a key step towards democratizing biomedical data analysis.

Provenance Tracking and Reproducibility. One of the key aspects that distinguishes our system from GUI-based pipeline tools is the ability to easily construct shareable and reproducible pipelines. Also, as described later in Sect. 3, the system records all the natural language conversations, and these records/logs not only serve as documentation of the thought processes of the researcher but also provide a rich source for learning and improving the analyses themselves.

Our system has a replay mechanism through which entire pipelines can be re-created from the conversation logs. Researchers can also create variants of their pipelines by modifying the conversation logs and feeding it through the replay mechanism. For example, in our Scenario-2, Daisy – a researcher in the surgery department of a hospital – receives additional data on surgeries. She wants to retrain her model on the new data with modifications to the hyper-parameters. Retraining the model requires Daisy to reproduce all the steps that she took previously to prepare the data for training. In addition to that, Daisy wants to add more visualizations. She can recreate the

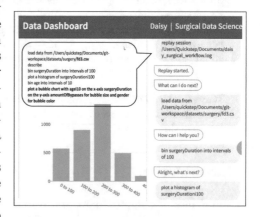

Fig. 1. Replay of an analysis. A sample of the conversational log is shown in the callout (modifications are highlighted). Researchers can also replay by modifying some parameters selected in the original analysis. This capability can enable researchers to test the robustness of the pipeline and its dependence on the choice of parameters.

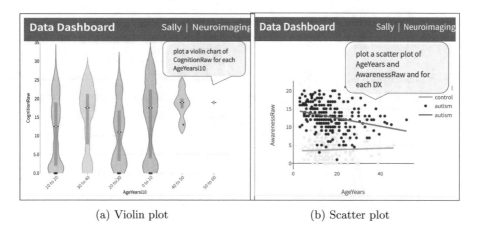

(a) Violin plot   (b) Scatter plot

Fig. 2. Exploratory data visualization by the neuroscientist in Sect. 2 to choose the variables of interest for performing advanced deformation analysis of longitudinal MRI data [4].

complete pipeline with the necessary modifications by editing the conversation logs of the original pipeline (in Sect. 2) and replaying the conversations. As shown in Fig. 1, Daisy recreates the complete pipeline by asking the system to replay the conversation log. Sharing a pipeline created in our system now is as simple as sharing the conversation that was used to create the pipeline.

Related Work and Core Contributions. There is a large body of research aimed at simplifying data access for non-programmers through the use of natural language [8,9]. Recent advances in natural language understanding has seen the emergence of bot frameworks such as Microsoft LUIS [10], Watson Conversation [11] and Amazon Lex [12] that are used for general purpose and simpler tasks such as ordering pizza or navigating maps. Our core technical innovation is to disseminate biomedical data science pipelines using a finite state machine (FSM)-based Natural Language (NL) interface that allows the researcher to compose complex, domain-specific image processing and data analysis tasks using dialogues that can be translated in appropriate analysis action(s). We note that our interface is complementary and targets a significantly broader set of researchers than the alternative methods to disseminate neuroimaging pipelines, such as Nipype, Dipy, C-PAC, PyMVPA, DLTK or NiftyNet. With these existing approaches, a typical researcher is still left with the time-consuming steps of learning how to code using the various tools (each with its own pros and cons) and gluing together tasks performed using these tools into a workflow, all the while taking on the challenge of making decisions to navigate the search space of possible pipelines. Our natural language interface is a layer over programming language interfaces, which makes building workflows easier and provides a general architecture that can amplify the translational impact of advanced computational methodologies and software tools such as the ones listed above.

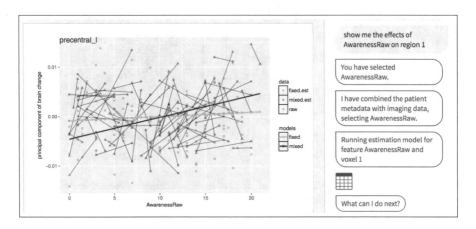

Fig. 3. Visualization of relationship between a cognitive score and brain deformations generated using advanced longitudinal analysis of neuroimaging data using mixed effects models on manifolds [4]. The conversation used is shown on the right panel.

2   Archetypal Analysis Scenarios

Our system is implemented as an intelligent chatbot agent that lets users assemble complex data analysis pipelines through conversations. While the precise interpretation of general natural language continues to be challenging, *controlled natural language* (CNL) [13] methods are starting to become practical as natural interfaces in complex decision-making domains [14]. This observation is the crucial insight and foundation for our system. In addition, data science pipeline components can often be abstracted into "templates of code". These two features enable us to develop a system that uses CNL to create and share reproducible biomedical data science pipelines. We demonstrate our system using two archetypal examples, one in neuroimaging and the other in surgical data science.

Scenario-1: A Neuroimaging Data Science Pipeline. Imagine that a neuroscientist, Sally, is interested in observing the effects of age on one of the cognitive measures. She is an expert in neuroscience. While conversant in neuroimaging methods, she is not an expert in that area. She has conducted a longitudinal study and collected various cognitive features and MRI data at several time points. She is interested in performing mixed-effects analysis using both the imaging and cognitive data. One of her goals is to visualize the effects of a cognitive measure on longitudinal change in a brain region. This task is conceptually simple. However, to perform this analysis, Sally needs to carry out significant amount of longitudinal image processing, derive appropriate deformation representations and estimate the mixed effects models [4]. Our system

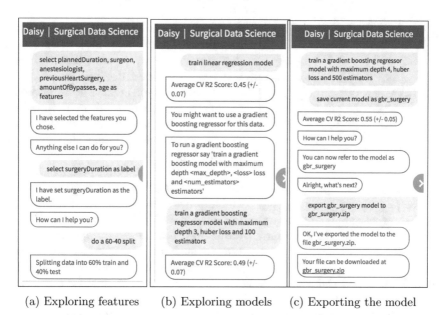

(a) Exploring features   (b) Exploring models   (c) Exporting the model

Fig. 4. Sample interactions of Daisy. She can iteratively explore the model space and the feature space until she finds the right combination of model and features that give her the best results. She can then save, export and share the model with other researchers which can enhance the translational impact and reproducibility of her work.

can abstract all such processing, with provenance tracking should she want to dive into the actual steps, and avail the longitudinal model parameters for her to explore. In addition to image processing, she also needs to combine/join imaging and the cognitive information. Our system offers simple-to-use data join features with interactions such as "combine the longitudinal imaging features with the cognitive measures". Sally can explore (Fig. 2) the data to find various measures of interest. For example, to pick measures that are correlated with age, Sally can visualize scatter plots of various cognitive measures against age (Fig. 2b). She can then estimate a statistical model to see the effects of the measure on a specific region of the brain. Once Sally estimates the model she can explore the various parameters of the statistical model (Fig. 3). Internally, the system loads data from a database or file into a Pandas [15] dataframe, visualizes data using Plotly [16] and uses scikit-learn [17] for machine learning. For neuroimaging, the statistical model is built in Matlab whereas the visualizations are build using R. The system seamlessly orchestrates all these tools and libraries without requiring any such knowledge on the part of the user.

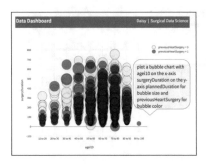

Fig. 5. Exploratory visualization of features (e.g. age, surgical duration and history) using bubble charts. The conversation by Daisy is shown in the call-out.

Scenario 2: A Surgical Data Science Pipeline. Daisy is a researcher in the department of surgery at a hospital. Daisy has years of experience in surgical procedures and fundamentals. She is interested in identifying patterns from accumulated data on existing surgical case durations and developing models to predict the duration of a new surgery. Such a model would enable the operating room (OR) planners in making efficient OR schedules, decrease the cost and improve patient care, while maintaining the current OR utilization rate. While she has conceptual understanding of the importance of such models she is less familiar with which features to use and what model to build. A sample of Daisy's interactions with our system to analyze the surgical dataset is presented in Figs. 4 and 5.

At each stage, Daisy issues commands in natural language. Daisy begins by creating exploratory visualizations to explore the data and gain intuition into the relevant feature representations that can be used in the model. Daisy proceeds to carve out training and validation datasets and builds a regression model. The system also *proactively* reports metrics such as cross-validation accuracy after training (Fig. 4b) that may help Daisy take the next set of actions. The system also interactively guides her towards constructing a pipeline by providing hints and recommending further actions to the user. As seen in Fig. 4b, the system currently uses simple heuristics built into its knowledge base to recommend a gradient boosting regression model for the task.

Deep Learning (DL) via Dialogue. Daisy is excited about the recent developments of DL and its impact on biomedical science. However, due to lack of background in programming, Daisy does not have a comfortable place to begin exploring such models for her work.

Her journey into DL-based analysis can begin with a simple conversation with our system such as "show me what you can do with deep learning". Figure 6 shows Daisy creating a simple DL pipeline to predict surgical case duration. The system employs a simple but intuitive

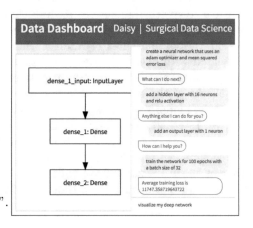

Fig. 6. Sample conversation to design and train a deep learning model.

vocabulary to build deep networks. Internally the system uses Keras [18] to construct DL pipelines. The DL capabilities of the system are currently limited to the deployment of deep networks on a single machine. Future extensions will include support to build complex DL pipelines and the capabilities to deploy and monitor DL pipelines in the cloud. We note that such capabilities augment (not replace) already publicly available tools such as `Matlab`, `DLTK` and `NiftyNet` for applying deep learning in neuroimaging and other biomedical imaging domains.

3   The Core System Architecture

Next, we describe the various components of our conversational interface and the underlying system that powers the interface.

Client-Server Design. The conversational nature of the system naturally lends itself to using a `Jupyter` [19] notebook style of interactive computing, where a Programming Language (PL)-specific kernel controls code executions triggered by the client. The chat server parses the messages, extracting semantic information about the task to be performed, disambiguating whenever required, and finally generating the executable code. The chat server triggers code generation from the code templates. A dynamic repository of code templates is maintained, along with a mapping from specific task to the corresponding code template. These templates are specific to the underlying libraries and can be automatically learned by employing techniques from PL research.

Control Flow Architecture. The control flow in the system is shown in Fig. 7. The user chats with the **conversational agent** in a Controlled Natural Language (CNL). The conversation agent is responsible for steering the conversation towards a full task specification. The chat client sends the natural language conversations to the chat server. If the chat server determines that it needs more information to complete the task, it prompts the user until it has a complete task specification. The system then signals the **task code generator** to identify the template that best matches the

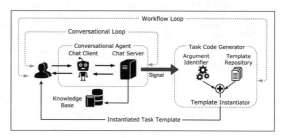

Fig. 7. Control flow in the system. The chat client sends the natural language conversations typed by the user to a web server. The web server forwards the conversation to a Natural Language Understanding (NLU) unit which is also a part of the chat server. The argument identifier extracts the template parameters from the task specification, and the template instantiator completes the chosen template with the user specified parameter values.

specification. The chat server also consults the knowledge base if necessary, to guide the user during data analysis.

Controlled Natural Language and Storyboard. While commonly used natural language is expressive and capable of representing arbitrary concepts, it poses a challenge for automatic semantic inference. CNLs offer a balance between the expressiveness and ease of semantic inference by restricting the vocabulary and grammar. The conversations between the user and our system are guided through a "storyboard". The storyboard describes the dialogue between the user and the system, and the actions that the system must take in response. It is essentially a finite state machine (FSM) implemented in `Python`. The FSM framework is crucial to the system to unambiguously extract information from conversations and map the extracted information to executable code. The FSM transitions allow the system to drive the conversation towards a complete task specification. Finally, the task templates allow the system to generate and execute the code, decoupling underlying libraries from the conversational agent.

4 Conclusion

We present a framework for performing biomedical data analysis using a natural language (NL) interface. Our system, the first of its kind for the medical imaging community, provides a novel framework for combining domain-specific NL and domain-specific computational methods to orchestrate complex analysis tasks using easy conversations. We believe this framework will significantly lower the burden of provenance tracking and barriers to complicated setups of software packages and programming syntax required in advanced statistical and machine learning based analysis methods. The ultimate outcome would be increased productivity, rigor, reproducibility and the translational impact of advanced analysis workflows in neuro and biomedical imaging domains. In the future, we plan to perform rigorous user studies to study the benefits of using such a conversational approach with appropriate IRB approvals and randomized user selection.

Acknowledgments. This work was supported in part by the NIH grants CPCP U54-AI117924, BRAIN Initiative R01-EB022883 and Waisman IDDRC U54-HD090256.

References

1. Kim, H.J., Adluru, N., et al.: Multivariate GLMS on Riemannian manifolds with applications to statistical analysis of DWI. In: CVPR, pp. 2705–2712 (2014)
2. Maier-Hein, L., Vedula, S.S., et al.: Surgical data science for next-generation interventions. Nat. Biomed. Eng. **1**(9), 691 (2017)
3. Kim, H.J., Adluru, N., Bendlin, B.B., Johnson, S.C., Vemuri, B.C., Singh, V.: Canonical correlation analysis on Riemannian manifolds and its applications. In: Fleet, D., Pajdla, T., Schiele, B., Tuytelaars, T. (eds.) ECCV 2014. LNCS, vol. 8690, pp. 251–267. Springer, Cham (2014). https://doi.org/10.1007/978-3-319-10605-2_17
4. Kim, H.J., Adluru, N., et al.: Riemannian nonlinear mixed effects models: analyzing longitudinal deformations in neuroimaging. In: CVPR (2017)

5. Halchenko, Y.O., Hanke, M.: Open is not enough. An integrated, community-driven computing platform for neuroscience. Front. Neuroinform. **6**, 22 (2012)
6. John, R.J.L., Potti, N., Patel, J.M.: Ava: from data to insights through conversations. In: CIDR (2017)
7. John, R.J.L., Adluru, N., et al.: Image analysis through conversations: reducing barriers and improving provenance tracking in AD research. AAIC **13**(7), P1484–P1485 (2017)
8. Androutsopoulos, I., Ritchie, G.D., Thanisch, P.: Natural language interfaces to databases - an introduction. Nat. Lang. Eng. **1**(1), 29–81 (1995)
9. Weizenbaum, J.: Eliza - a computer program for the study of natural language communication between man and machine. CACM **9**(1), 36–45 (1966)
10. Williams, J., Kamal, E., et al.: Fast and easy language understanding for dialog systems with Microsoft LUIS. In: SIGDIAL, pp. 159–161 (2015)
11. IBM: Watson conversation (2016)
12. Amazon: Lex (2016). https://aws.amazon.com/lex
13. Kuhn, T.: A survey and classification of controlled natural languages. Comput. Linguist. **40**(1), 121–170 (2014)
14. Troegner, D.: Grammer for NL recognition: adaptation to air traffic phraseology. Technical report, Institute of Flight Control, German Aerospace Center (2011)
15. McKinney, W.: Pandas: a foundational python lib for data analysis and statistics (2010)
16. Plotly: Collaborative data science (2015)
17. Pedregosa, F., Varoquaux, G., et al.: Scikit-learn: ML in Python. JMLR **12**, 2825–2830 (2011)
18. Chollet, F., et al.: Keras (2015). https://keras.io
19. Kluyver, T., Ragan-Kelley, B., Pérez, F., et al.: Jupyter notebooks - a publishing format for reproducible computational workflows (2016)

Spatiotemporal Manifold Prediction Model for Anterior Vertebral Body Growth Modulation Surgery in Idiopathic Scoliosis

William Mandel[1], Olivier Turcot[2], Dejan Knez[3], Stefan Parent[2], and Samuel Kadoury[1,2(✉)]

[1] MedICAL, Polytechnique Montreal, Montreal, QC, Canada
samuel.kadoury@polymtl.ca
[2] Sainte-Justine Hospital Research Center, Montreal, QC, Canada
[3] Faculty of Electrical Engineering, University of Ljubljana, Ljubljana, Slovenia

Abstract. Anterior Vertebral Body Growth Modulation (AVBGM) is a minimally invasive surgical technique that gradually corrects spine deformities while preserving lumbar motion. However the selection of potential surgical patients is currently based on clinical judgment and would be facilitated by the identification of patients responding to AVBGM prior to surgery. We introduce a statistical framework for predicting the surgical outcomes following AVBGM in adolescents with idiopathic scoliosis. A discriminant manifold is first constructed to maximize the separation between responsive and non-responsive groups of patients treated with AVBGM for scoliosis. The model then uses subject-specific correction trajectories based on articulated transformations in order to map spine correction profiles to a group-average piecewise-geodesic path. Spine correction trajectories are described in a piecewise-geodesic fashion to account for varying times at follow-up exams, regressing the curve via a quadratic optimization process. To predict the evolution of correction, a baseline reconstruction is projected onto the manifold, from which a spatiotemporal regression model is built from parallel transport curves inferred from neighboring exemplars. The model was trained on 438 reconstructions and tested on 56 subjects using 3D spine reconstructions from follow-up exams, with the probabilistic framework yielding accurate results with differences of $2.1 \pm 0.6°$ in main curve angulation, and generating models similar to biomechanical simulations.

1 Introduction

Spinal morphology and more particularly 3D morphometric parameters, have demonstrated significant potential in assessing the risk of spinal disease progression. For spinal deformities such as adolescent idiopathic scoliosis (AIS), personalized 3D reconstructions generated from radiographs allows surgeons to assess the severity and decide on efficient treatment options. A recently introduced

Supported by the Canada Research Chairs and NSERC Discovery Grants.

© Springer Nature Switzerland AG 2018
A. F. Frangi et al. (Eds.): MICCAI 2018, LNCS 11073, pp. 206–213, 2018.
https://doi.org/10.1007/978-3-030-00937-3_24

minimally invasive surgical technique called Anterior Vertebral Body Growth Modulation (AVBGM) consists of instrumenting the spine with traditional vertebral implants to link a segment of vertebrae together by a flexible polypropylene cable applied to the spine anteriorly. The fusion-less technique applies compressive forces on the convex side of the spinal curve, thereby modulating the distribution of pressure on the vertebral growth plates. In combination with natural bone growth, this allows to retain spine flexibility [1]. While this new surgical technique showed promising results for skeletally immature patients [2], difficulties were reported to predict short and long-term post-operative correction [3]. Biomechanical models were shown to reproduce surgical outcomes, but are not adapted for real-time surgical applications [4].

A recent study evaluated differences in hand-crafted 3D parameters in progressive AIS groups using images from the patient's first visit [5] to predict progression, by manually selecting the best features that can characterize the intrinsic nature of 3D spines. On the other hand, dimensionally-reduced growth trajectories of various anatomical sites have been investigated in neurodevelopment studies for newborns, based on geodesic shape regression to compute the diffeomorphisms based on image time series of a population [6]. These regression models were also used to estimate spatio-temporal evolution of the cerebral cortex, by automatically identifying the points of interest and inertia between the first and follow-up images based on non-rigid transformations [7]. The concept of parallel transport curves in the tangent space from low-dimensional manifolds proposed by Schiratti et al. [8] was used to analyze shape morphology [9] and adapted for radiotherapy response [10], but lacks the capability to predict correction from applied forces following surgery.

This paper presents a prediction model for patient response to AVBGM from pre-operative 3D spine models reconstructed from biplanar X-ray images (Fig. 1). The method first trains a piecewise-geodesic manifold using a collection of pre-operative and longitudinal 3D reconstructions of the spine acquired during follow-up evaluations of patients treated with AVBGM for AIS. A discriminant adjacency matrix is constructed to separate responding and non-responding patients. During testing, an unseen baseline spine model is projected onto the manifold, where a piecewise-geodesic curve describing spatiotemporal evolution is regressed using discrete approximations, from which the curvature evolution is inferred, yielding a prediction of the intervertebral displacements and shape morphology describing deformation correction. The main contribution of this paper is the introduction of a piecewise-geodesic transport curve in the tangent space from low-dimensional samples designed for the correction of spinal deformities, where a new time-warping function controlling the rate of correction is obtained from clinical parameters.

2   Method

2.1   Discriminant Embedding of Longitudinal Spine Models

A sample spine reconstruction is represented by $\mathbf{S} = \{\mathbf{s}_1, \ldots, \mathbf{s}_m\}$, modelling a series of $m = 17$ vertebral shapes. For each $\mathbf{s}_i$ vertebra, template-based models

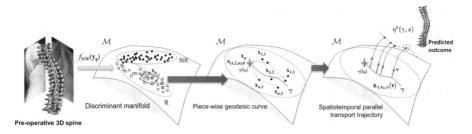

Fig. 1. Proposed prediction framework for spine surgery outcomes. In the training phase, a dataset of spine models are embedded in a spatio-temporal manifold $\mathcal{M}$, into responsive (R) or non-responsive (NR) groups. During testing, an unseen baseline 3D spine reconstruction $\mathbf{y}_q$ is projected on $\mathcal{M}$ using f_{NW} based on Nadaraya-Watson kernels. The closest samples to the projected point $\mathbf{x}$ are selected to regress the spatiotemporal curve γ used for predicting the correction due with AVBGM.

are obtained where vertex coordinates have one-to-one correspondences between samples. In addition to the mesh-based representation, each model $\mathbf{s}_i$ possesses a list of annotated landmarks to compute local intervertebral rigid transformations, such that $A = [T_1, T_2, \ldots, T_m]$, with $T_i = \{R, t\}$ a rigid inter-vertebral transform. Hence, the overall shape of the spine is described as a vector of sequential registrations assigned to each vertebral level, whereby considering the ensemble of transformations, we obtain a combination of previous transforms:

$$\mathbf{y}_i = [T_1, \mathbf{s}_1; T_1 \circ T_2, \mathbf{s}_2, \ldots, T_1 \circ T_2 \circ \ldots \circ T_m, \mathbf{s}_m] \tag{1}$$

using recursive compositions. The feature array $\mathbf{y}_i$ dictates the location and rotation of the object constellation, while procuring the morphology of the vertebrae $\mathbf{S}$. The model is deformed by applying displacements to the inter-vertebral parameters. By extending this to the entire absolute vector representing the spine model, this then achieves a global deformation. In this case, registrations are described in the reference coordinate system of the lower vertebra, corresponding to it's principal axes of the cuneiform shape with the origin positioned at the center of mass of the vertebra. The rigid transformations are the combination of a rotation matrix R and a translation vector t. We formulate the rigid transformation $T = \{R, t\}$ of a vertebra mesh $\mathbf{s}_i$ as $y = Rx + t$ where $x, y, t \in \Re^3$. Composition is given by $T_1 \circ T_2 = \{R_1 R_2, R_1 t_2 + t_1\}$.

We propose to embed a collection of non-responsive (NR) and (2) responsive (R) patients to AVBGM which will offer a maximal separation between the classes, by using a discriminant graph-embedding. Here, n labelled points $\mathbb{Y} = \{(\mathbf{y}_i, l_i, t_i)\}_{i=1}^n$ defined in $\mathbb{R}^D$ are embedded in the low-dimensional manifold $\mathcal{M}$, where l_i describes the label (NR or R) and t_i defines the time of follow-up. We assume that for the sampled data, an underlying manifold of the high-dimensional data exists such that $\mathbb{X} = \{(\mathbf{x}_i, l_i, t_i)\}_{i=1}^n$ defined in $\mathbb{R}^d$. We rely on the assumption that a locally linear mapping $\mathbf{M}_i \in \mathbb{R}^{D \times d}$ exists, where local neighbourhoods are defined as tangent planes estimated with $\mathbf{y}_j - \mathbf{y}_i$ and

$\mathbf{x}_j - \mathbf{x}_i$, describing the paired distances between linked neighbours i, j. Hence, the relationship can be established as $\mathbf{y}_j - \mathbf{y}_i \approx \mathbf{M}_i(\mathbf{x}_j - \mathbf{x}_i)$.

Because the discriminant manifold structure in $\mathbb{R}^d$ requires to maintain the local structure of the underlying data, a undirected similarity graph $\mathcal{G} = (\boldsymbol{V}, \boldsymbol{W})$ is built, where each node $\boldsymbol{V}$ are connected to each other with edges that are weighted with the graph $\boldsymbol{W}$. The overall structure of $\mathcal{M}$ is therefore defined with $\boldsymbol{W}_w$ for feature vectors belonging to the same class and $\boldsymbol{W}_b$, which separate features from both classes. During the embedding of the discriminant locally linear latent manifold, data samples are divided between $\boldsymbol{W}_w$ and $\boldsymbol{W}_b$.

2.2 Piecewise-Geodesic Spatiotemporal Manifold

Once sample points $\mathbf{x}_i$ are in manifold space, the objective is to regress a regular and smooth piecewise-geodesic curve $\gamma : [t_1, t_N]$ that accurately fits the embedded data describing the spatiotemporal correction following AVBGM within a 2 year period. For each sample data $\mathbf{x}_i$, the K closest individuals demonstrating similar baseline features are identified from the embedded data, creating neighborhoods $\mathcal{N}(\mathbf{x}_q)$ with measurements at different time points, thus creating a low-dimensional Riemannian manifold where data points $\mathbf{x}_{i,j}$, with i denoting a particular individual, j the time-point measurement and $j = 0$ the pre-operative model. By assuming the manifold domain is complete and piecewise-geodesic curves are defined for each time trajectories, time-labelled data can be regressed continuously in $\mathbb{R}^D$, thereby creating smooth curves in time intervals described by samples in $\mathbb{R}^d$.

However, due to the fact the representation of the continuous curve is a variational problem of infinite dimensional space, the implementation follows a discretization process which is derived from the procedure in [11], such that:

$$E(\gamma) = \frac{1}{K_d} \sum_{i=1}^{K_d} \sum_{j=0}^{t_N} w_i \|\gamma(t_{i,j}) - (\mathbf{x}_{i,j} - (\mathbf{x}_{i,0} - \mathbf{x}_q))\|^2$$

$$+ \frac{\lambda}{2} \sum_{i=1}^{K_d} \alpha_i \|v_i\|^2 + \frac{\mu}{2} \sum_{i=1}^{K_d} \beta_i \|a_i\|^2. \tag{2}$$

This minimization process simplifies the problem to a quadratic optimization, solved with LU decomposition. The piecewise nature is represented by the term $K_d \in \mathcal{N}(\mathbf{x}_q)$, defined as samples along γ. The 1st component of Eq. (2) is a penalty term to minimize the geodesic distance between samples $\mathbf{x}_{i,j}$ and the regressed curve, where w_i are weight variables based on sample distances. This helps regress a curve that will lie close to $\mathbf{x}_{i,j}$, shifted by $\mathbf{x}_q$ in order to have the initial reconstructions co-registered. The 2nd term represents the velocity of the curve (defined by v_i, approximating $\dot{\gamma}(t_i)$), minimizing the L_2 distance of the 1st derivative of γ. By minimizing the value of the curve's first derivatives, this prohibits any discontinuities or rapid transitions of the curve's direction, and is modulated by α_i. Finally, an acceleration penalty term (defined by a_i) focuses on the 2nd derivative of γ with respect to t_i by minimizing the L_2 norm. The acceleration is modulated by β_i. Estimates for v_i and a_i (weighted by $\{\lambda, \mu\}$, respectively), are generated using geometric finite differences. These estimates dictates the forward and backward step-size on the regressed curve, leading to directional vectors in $\mathcal{M}$ as shown in [11]. In order to minimize $E(\gamma)$, a non-linear conjugate gradient technique defined in the low-dimensional space $\mathbb{R}^d$ is used, thus avoiding convergence and speed issues. The regressed curve γ is therefore defined for all time points, originating at t_0. The curve creates a group average of spatiotemporal transformations based on individual correction trajectories.

2.3   Prediction of Spine Correction

Finally, to predict the evolution of spine correction from an unseen pre-operative spine model, we use the geodesic curve $\gamma : \mathbb{R}^D \to \mathcal{M}$ modelling the spatiotemporal changes of the spine, where each point $\mathbf{x} \in \mathcal{M}$ is associated to a speed vector $\mathbf{v}$ defined with a tangent plane on the manifold such that $\mathbf{v} \in T_{\mathbf{x}}\mathcal{M}$.

Based on Riemannian theory, an exponential mapping function at $\mathbf{x}$ with velocity $\mathbf{v}$ can be defined from the geodesics such that $e_{\mathbf{x}}^{\mathcal{M}}(\mathbf{v})$. Using this concept, parallel transport curves defined in $T_{\mathbf{x}}$ can help define a series of time-index vectors along γ as proposed by [8]. The collection of parallel transport curves allows to generate an average trajectory in ambient space $\mathbb{R}^D$, describing the spine changes due to the corrective forces of tethering. The general goal is to begin the process at the pre-operative sample, and navigate the piecewise-geodesic curve describing correction evolution in time, where one can extract the appearance at any point (time) in $\mathbb{R}^D$ using the exponential mapping. For implementation purposes, the parallel transport curve are constrained within a smooth tubular boundary perpendicular to the curve (from an ICA) to generate the spatiotemporal evolution in the coordinate system of the pre-operative model.

Hence, given the manifold at time t_0 with $\mathbf{v}$ defined in the tangent plane and the regressed piecewise-geodesic curve γ, the parallel curve is obtained as:

$$\eta^{\mathbf{v}}(\gamma, s) = e_{\gamma(s)}^{\mathcal{M}}(\mathbf{x}_{\gamma, t_0, s}(\mathbf{v})), \quad s \in \mathbb{R}^d. \tag{3}$$

Therefore by repeating this mapping for manifold points seen as samples of individual progression trajectories along $\gamma(s)$, an evolution model can be generated. Whenever a new sample is embedded, new samples points along $\gamma(s)$, denoted as $\eta^{\mathbf{v}}(\gamma, \cdot)$ can be generated parallel to the regressed piecewise curve in $\mathcal{M}$, capturing the spatiotemporal changes in correction.

A time warp function allowing s to vary along the geodesic curve is described as $\phi_i(t) = \theta_i(t - t_0 - \tau_i) + t_0$. Here, we propose to incorporate a personalized acceleration factor based on the spine maturity and flexibility derived from the spine bending radiographs and Risser grade. A coefficient $\theta_i = C_i \times R_i$ describing the change in Cobb angle C_i between poses, and modulated by the Risser grade R_i. This coefficient regulates the rate of correction based on the K neighbouring samples. Finally, to take under account the relative differences between the group-wise samples and the query model once mapped onto the regressed curve, a time-shift parameter τ_i is incorporated in the warp function.

For spine correction evolution, displacement vectors $\mathbf{v}_i$ are obtained by a PCA of the hyperplane crossing $T_{\mathbf{x}_i}\mathcal{M}$ in manifold $\mathcal{M}$ [8]. Hence, for any query sample $\mathbf{x}_q$ which represents the mapped pre-operative 3D reconstruction (prior to surgery), the predicted model at time t_k can be regressed from the piecewise-geodesic curve generated from embedded samples $\mathbf{x}$ in $\mathcal{N}(\mathbf{x}_q)$ such that:

$$\mathbf{y}_{q,t_k} = \eta^{\mathbf{v}_q}(\gamma, \phi_i(t_k)) + \epsilon_{q,t_k} \tag{4}$$

which yields a predicted post-operative model $\mathbf{y}_{q,t_k}$ in high-dimensional space $\mathbb{R}^D$, and ϵ_{q,t_k} a zero-mean Gaussian distribution. The generated model offers a complete constellation of inter-connected vertebral models composing the spine shape $\mathbf{S}$, at first-erect (FE), 1 or 2-year visits, including landmarks on vertebral endplates and pedicle extremities, which can be used to capture the local shape morphology with the correction process.

3   Experiments

The discriminant manifold was trained from a database of 438 3D spine reconstructions generated from biplanar images [12], originating from 131 patients demonstrating several types of deformities with immediate follow-up (FE), 1 year and 2 year visits. Patients were recruited from a single center prospective study, with the inclusion criteria being evaluated by an orthopaedic surgeon and a main curvature angle between $30°$ and $60°$. Patients were divided in two groups, with the first group composed of 94 responsive patients showing a reduction in Cobb angle over or equal to $10°$ between the FE and follow-up visit. The second group was composed of 37 non-responsive (NP) patients with a reduction of less than $10°$. Each vertebra model of the spine were annotated with 4 pedicle tips and 2 center points placed on the vertebral endplates, and validated by an experienced radiologist. These expert-selected landmarks were used to establish the local coordinate system for each vertebra, describing the orientation and location (known pose), and used as control points to warp triangulated shape models generated from CT images of a cadaveric spine.

We evaluated the geometrical accuracy of the predictive manifold for 56 unseen surgical patients with AVBGM (mean age 12 ± 3, average main Cobb angle on the frontal plane at the first visit was $47° \pm 10°$), with predictions at $t = 0$ (FE), $t = 12$ and $t = 24$ months. For the predicted models, we evaluated the 3D root-mean-square difference of the vertebral landmarks generated, the Dice coefficients of the vertebral shapes and in the main Cobb angle. The results are shown in Table 1. Results were confronted to other techniques such as biomechanical simulations performed on each subject using finite element modelling with ex-vivo parameters [4], a locally linear latent variable model [13] and a deep auto-encoder network [14]. Figure 2 shows a sample prediction result for an 11 y.o. patients at FE, 12 and 24-months for a patient with right-thoracic deformity, which are more common in the scoliotic population. Results from

Table 1. 3D RMS errors (mm), Dice (%) and Cobb angles (°) for the proposed method, and compared with biomechanical simulations, locally linear latent variable models (LL-LVM) and deep auto-encoders (AE). Predictions are evaluated at FE, 1 and 2-yrs.

	FE visit			1-year visit			2-year visit		
	3D RMS	Dice	Cobb	3D RMS	Dice	Cobb	3D RMS	Dice	Cobb
Biomec. sim	3.3 ± 1.1	85 ± 3.4	2.8 ± 0.8	3.6 ± 1.2	84 ± 3.6	3.2 ± 0.9	4.1 ± 2.3	82 ± 3.9	3.6 ± 1.0
LL-LVM [13]	3.6 ± 1.4	83 ± 4.0	3.8 ± 1.5	4.7 ± 3.3	79 ± 4.4	5.5 ± 2.6	6.6 ± 4.4	71 ± 5.9	7.0 ± 3.9
Deep AE [14]	4.1 ± 1.5	80 ± 4.4	5.1 ± 2.7	5.0 ± 1.9	77 ± 4.9	5.8 ± 3.0	6.3 ± 4.6	72 ± 5.7	6.6 ± 4.2
Proposed	2.4 ± 0.8	92 ± 2.7	1.8 ± 0.5	2.9 ± 0.9	90 ± 2.8	2.0 ± 0.7	3.2 ± 1.3	87 ± 3.1	2.1 ± 0.6

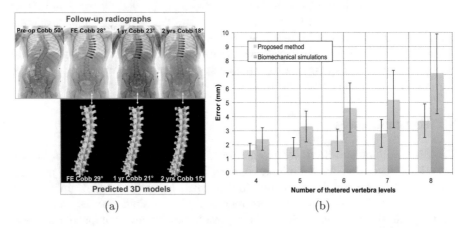

(a)   (b)

Fig. 2. (a) Comparison in actual and predicted Cobb angles in a 11 y.o. patient at the first-erect visit, at 1-yr and at 2-yrs postop. Top row depicts the actual X-rays, while the bottom row presents the predicted 3D spine geometry. (b) Errors with 5 different tethering levels, comparing results with biomechanical simulations at 2 yrs.

the predicted geometrical models show the regressed spatio-temporal geodesic curve yields anatomically coherent structures, with accurate local vertebral morphology.

To evaluate robustness with respect to varying instrumented levels, we measured the accuracy of the predicted models for tethering between 4 and 8 vertebrae at 2 yrs, ranging from thoracic to lumbar regions. Figure 2(b) shows the improvement of the spatiotemporal geodesic curve in comparison to traditional biomechanical models, particularly when the number of levels are higher.

4   Conclusion

In this paper, we proposed an accurate predictive model of spine morphology and Cobb angle correction obtained at the first-erect, 1-year and 2-year visits, following anterior vertebral body growth modulation. The piecewise-geodesic curve capturing spatio-temporal changes could be used for patient selection of AVBGM as a decision-sharing tool prior to surgery. Our approach is based on smooth and regular trajectories embedded in a discriminant manifold, which enable an efficient navigation on a low-dimensional domain trained from operative cases, yielding results similar to actual surgical outcomes. Future work will include a multi-center evaluation before it can be used in clinical practice.

References

1. Skaggs, D.L., Akbarnia, B.A., Flynn, J.M., Myung, K., Sponseller, P., Vitale, M.: A classification of growth friendly spine implants. J. Pediatr. Orthop. **34**(3), 260–274 (2014)
2. Crawford III, C.H., Lenke, L.G.: Growth modulation by means of anterior tethering resulting in progressive correction of juvenile idiopathic scoliosis: a case report. JBJS **92**(1), 202–209 (2010)
3. Samdani, A.F., et al.: Anterior vertebral body tethering for immature adolescent idiopathic scoliosis: one-year results on the first 32 patients. Eur. Spine J. **24**(7), 1533–1539 (2015)
4. Cobetto, N., Parent, S., Aubin, C.E.: 3D correction over 2 years with anterior vertebral body growth modulation: a finite element analysis of screw positioning, cable tensioning and postop functional activities. Clin. Biome. **51**, 26–33 (2018)
5. Nault, M.L., Mac-Thiong, J.M., Roy-Beaudry, M., Turgeon, I., Parent, S.: Three-dimensional spinal morphology can differentiate between progressive and nonprogressive patients with adolescent idiopathic scoliosis at the initial presentation: a prospective study. Spine **39**(10), E601 (2014)
6. Singh, N., Hinkle, J., Joshi, S., Fletcher, P.T.: A hierarchical geodesic model for diffeomorphic longitudinal shape analysis. In: Gee, J.C., Joshi, S., Pohl, K.M., Wells, W.M., Zöllei, L. (eds.) IPMI 2013. LNCS, vol. 7917, pp. 560–571. Springer, Heidelberg (2013). https://doi.org/10.1007/978-3-642-38868-2_47
7. Fishbaugh, J., Prastawa, M., Gerig, G., Durrleman, S.: Geodesic regression of image and shape data for improved modeling of 4D trajectories. In: IEEE ISBI, pp. 385–388. IEEE (2014)
8. Schiratti, J.B., Allassonniere, S., Colliot, O., Durrleman, S.: Learning spatiotemporal trajectories from manifold-valued longitudinal data. In: Advances in Neural Information Processing Systems, pp. 2404–2412 (2015)
9. Kadoury, S., Mandel, W., Roy-Beaudry, M., Nault, M.L., Parent, S.: 3-D morphology prediction of progressive spinal deformities from probabilistic modeling of discriminant manifolds. IEEE Trans. Med. Imag. **36**(5), 1194–1204 (2017)
10. Chevallier, J., Oudard, S., Allassonnière, S.: Learning spatiotemporal piecewise-geodesic trajectories from longitudinal manifold-valued data. In: 31st Conference on Neural Information Processing Systems (NIPS 2017) (2017)
11. Boumal, N., Absil, P.A.: A discrete regression method on manifolds and its application to data on SO (n). IFAC Proc. Vol. **44**(1), 2284–2289 (2011)
12. Humbert, L., de Guise, J., Aubert, B., Godbout, B., Skalli, W.: 3D reconstruction of the spine from biplanar X-rays using parametric models based on transversal and longitudinal inferences. Med. Eng. Phy. **31**(6), 681–687 (2009)
13. Park, M., Jitkrittum, W., Qamar, A., Szabó, Z., Buesing, L., Sahani, M.: Bayesian manifold learning: the locally linear latent variable model (LL-LVM). In: Advances in Neural Information Processing Systems, pp. 154–162 (2015)
14. Thong, W., Parent, S., Wu, J., Aubin, C.E., Labelle, H., Kadoury, S.: Three-dimensional morphology study of surgical adolescent idiopathic scoliosis patient from encoded geometric models. Eur. Spine J. **25**(10), 3104–3113 (2016)

Evaluating Surgical Skills from Kinematic Data Using Convolutional Neural Networks

Hassan Ismail Fawaz[✉], Germain Forestier, Jonathan Weber,
Lhassane Idoumghar, and Pierre-Alain Muller

IRIMAS, Université de Haute-Alsace,
2 rue des Frères Lumière, 68093 Mulhouse, France
{hassan.ismail-fawaz,germain.forestier,jonathan.weber,
lhassane.idoumghar,pierre-alain.muller}@uha.fr

Abstract. The need for automatic surgical skills assessment is increasing, especially because manual feedback from senior surgeons observing junior surgeons is prone to subjectivity and time consuming. Thus, automating surgical skills evaluation is a very important step towards improving surgical practice. In this paper, we designed a Convolutional Neural Network (CNN) to evaluate surgeon skills by extracting patterns in the surgeon motions performed in robotic surgery. The proposed method is validated on the JIGSAWS dataset and achieved very competitive results with 100% accuracy on the suturing and needle passing tasks. While we leveraged from the CNNs efficiency, we also managed to mitigate its black-box effect using class activation map. This feature allows our method to automatically highlight which parts of the surgical task influenced the skill prediction and can be used to explain the classification and to provide personalized feedback to the trainee.

Keywords: Kinematic data · RMIS · Deep learning · CNN

1 Introduction

Over the past one hundred years, the classical training program of Dr. William Halsted has governed surgical training in different parts of the world [15]. His teaching philosophy of "see one, do one, teach one" is still one of the most practiced methods to this day [1]. The idea is that the trainee could become an expert surgeon by watching and assisting in mentored surgeries [15]. These training methods, although broadly used, lack of an objective surgical skill evaluation technique [9]. Conventional surgical skill assessment is currently based on checklists that are filled by an expert surgeon observing the surgery [14]. In an attempt to evaluate surgical skills without relying on an expert's opinion, Objective Structured Assessment of Technical Skills (OSATS) has been proposed and is used in clinical practice [12]. Unfortunately, this type of observational evaluation is still prone to several external and subjective variables: the checklists' development process, the inter-rater reliability and the evaluator bias [7].

© Springer Nature Switzerland AG 2018
A. F. Frangi et al. (Eds.): MICCAI 2018, LNCS 11073, pp. 214–221, 2018.
https://doi.org/10.1007/978-3-030-00937-3_25

Other studies showed that a strong relationship exists between the postoperative outcomes and the technical skill of a surgeon [2]. This type of approach suffers from the fact that a surgery's outcome also depends on the patient's physiological characteristics [9]. In addition, acquiring such type of data is very difficult, which makes these skill evaluation methods difficult to apply for surgical training. Recent advances in surgical robotics such as the *da Vinci* surgical robot (Intuitive Surgical Inc. Sunnyvale, CA) enabled the collection of motion and video data from different surgical activities. Hence, an alternative for checklists and outcome-based methods is to extract, from these motion data, global movement features such as the surgical task's time completion, speed, curvature, motion smoothness and other holistic features [3,9,19]. Although most of these methods are efficient, it is not clear how they could be used to provide a detailed and constructive feedback for the trainee to go beyond the simple classification into a category (i.e. novice, expert, etc.). This is problematic as studies [8] showed that feedback on medical practice allows surgeons to improve their performance and reach higher skill levels.

Recently, a new field named *Surgical Data Science* [11] has emerged thanks to the increasing access to large amounts of complex data which pertain to the patient, the staff and sensors for perceiving the patient and procedure related data such as videos and kinematic variables [5]. As an alternative to extracting global movement features, recent studies tend to break down surgical tasks into smaller segments called surgical gestures, manually before the training phase, and assess the performance of the surgical task based on the assessment of these gestures [13]. Although these methods obtained very accurate and promising results in terms of surgical skill evaluation, they require a huge amount of labeled gestures for the training phase [13]. We have identified two main limits in the existing approaches that classify a surgeon's skill level based on the kinematic data. First is the lack of an interpretable result of skill evaluation usable by the trainee to achieve higher skill levels. Additionally current state of the art Hidden Markov Models require gesture boundaries that are pre-defined by human annotators which is time consuming and prone to inter-annotator reliability [16].

In this paper, we propose a new architecture of Convolutional Neural Networks (CNN) dedicated to surgical skill evaluation (Fig. 1). By using one dimensional filters over the kinematic data, we mitigate the need to pre-define sensitive and unreliable gesture boundaries. The original hierarchical structure of our deep learning model enables us to represent the gestures in latent low-level variables (first and second layers), as well as capturing global information related to the surgical skill level (third layer). To provide interpretable feedback, instead of using a final fully-connected layer like most traditional approaches [18], we place a Global Average Pooling (GAP) layer which enables us to benefit from the Class Activation Map [18] (CAM) to visualize which parts of the surgical task contributed the most to the surgical skill classification (Fig. 2). We demonstrate the accuracy of our approach using a standardized experimental setup on the largest publicly available dataset for surgical data analysis: the JHU-ISI Gesture and Skill Assessment Working Set (JIGSAWS) [5]. The main contribution of our work is to show that deep learning can be used to understand the latent and

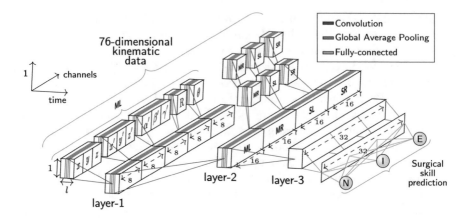

Fig. 1. The network architecture whose input is a surgical task with variable length l recorded by the four manipulators (**ML**: master left, **MR**: master right, **SL**: slave left, **SR**: slave right) of the da Vinci surgical system. The output is a surgical skill prediction (**N**: Novice, **I**: Intermediate and **E**: Expert)

complex structures of what constitutes a surgical skill, especially that there is still much to be learned on what is exactly a surgical skill [9].

2 Method

2.1 Dataset

We first present briefly the dataset used in this paper as we rely on features definition to describe our method. The JIGSAWS [5] dataset has been collected from eight right-handed subjects with three different skill levels (Novice (N), Intermediate (I) and Expert (E)) performing three different surgical tasks (suturing, needle passing and knot tying) using the *da Vinci* surgical system. Each subject performed five trials of each task. For each trial the kinematic and video data were recorded.

In our work, we only focused on kinematic data which are numeric variables of four manipulators: left and right masters (controlled directly by the subject's hands) and left and right slaves (controlled indirectly by the subject via the master manipulators). These kinematic variables (76 in total) are captured at a frequency equal to 30 frames per second for each trial. We considered each trial as a multivariate time series (MTS) and designed a one dimensional CNN dedicated to learn automatically useful features for surgical skill classification.

2.2 Architecture

Our approach takes inspiration of the recent success of CNN for time series classification [17]. The proposed architecture (Fig. 1) has been specifically designed to classify surgical skills using kinematic data. The input of the CNN is a MTS with variable length l and 76 channels. The output layer contains the surgical skill level (N, I, E). Comparing to CNNs for image classification, where usually the network's input has two dimensions (width and height) and 3 channels (RGB), our network's input is a time series with one dimension (length l of the surgical task) and 76 channels (the kinematic variables x, y, z, x', etc.).

The main challenge we encountered when designing our network was the huge number of input channels (76) compared to the RGB channels (3) for the image classification task. Therefore, instead of applying the convolutions over the 76 channels, we proposed to carry out different convolutions for each cluster and sub-cluster of channels. In order to decide which channels should be grouped together, we used domain knowledge when clustering the channels.

First we divide the 76 variables into four different clusters, such as each cluster contains the variables from one of the four manipulators: the $1^{st}, 2^{nd}, 3^{rd}$ and 4th clusters correspond respectively to the four manipulators (ML: master left, MR: master right, SL: slave left and SR: slave right) of the *da Vinci* surgical system. Thus, each cluster contains 19 of the 76 total kinematic variables.

Next, each cluster of 19 variables is split into five different sub-clusters such as each sub-cluster contains variables that we hypothesize are highly correlated. For each cluster, the variables are grouped into five sub-clusters: 1st sub-cluster with 3 variables for the Cartesian coordinates (x, y, z); 2nd sub-cluster with 3 variables for the linear velocity (x', y', z'); 3rd sub-cluster with 3 variables for the rotational velocity $(\alpha', \beta', \gamma')$; 4th sub-cluster with 9 variables for the rotation matrix R; 5th sub-cluster with 1 variable for the gripper angular velocity (θ).

Figure 1 shows how the convolutions in the first layer are different for each sub-cluster of channels. Following the same reasoning, the convolutions in the second layer are different for each cluster of channels (ML, MR, SL and SR). However, in the third layer, the same convolutions are applied for all channels.

In order to reduce the number of parameters in our model and benefit from the CAM method [18], we replaced the fully-connected layer with a GAP operation after the third convolutional layer. This results in a summarized MTS that shrinks from a length l to 1, while preserving the same number of channels in the third layer. As for the output layer, we use a fully-connected softmax layer with three neurons, one for each class (N, I, E).

Without any cross-validation, we choose to use 8 filters at the first convolutional layer, then we increase the number of filters (by a factor of 2), thus balancing the number of parameters for each layer while going deeper into the network. The Rectified Linear Unit (ReLU) activation function is employed for the three convolutional layers with a filter size of 3 and a stride of 1.

2.3   Training and Testing

To train the network, we used the multinomial cross-entropy as our objective cost function. The network's parameters were optimized using Adam [10]. Following [17], without any fine-tuning, the learning rate was set to 0.001 and the exponential decay rates of the first and second moment estimates were set to 0.9 and 0.999 respectively. Each trial was used in a forward-pass followed by a back-propagation update of the weights which were initialized using Glorot's uniform initialization [6]. Before each training epoch, the train set was randomly shuffled. We trained the network for 1000 epochs, then by saving the model at each training epoch, we chose the one that minimized the objective cost function on a random (non-seen) split from the training set. Thus, we only validate the number of epochs since no extra-computation is needed to perform this step. Finally, to avoid overfitting, we added a $l2$ regularization parameter equal to 10^{-5}. Since we did not fine-tune the model's hyper-parameters, the same network architecture with the same hyper-parameters was trained on each surgical task resulting in three different models[1].

To evaluate our approach we adopted the standard benchmark configuration, Leave One Super Trial Out (LOSO) [1]: for each iteration of cross-validation (five in total), one trial of each subject was left out for the test and the remaining trials were used for training.

2.4   Class Activation Map

By employing a GAP layer, we benefit from the CAM [18] method, which makes it possible to identify which regions of the surgical task contributed the most to a certain class identification. Let $A_k(t)$ be the result of the third convolutional layer which is a MTS with K channels (in our case K is equal to 32 filters and t denotes the time dimension). Let w_k^c be the weight between the output neuron of class c and the kth filter. Since a GAP layer is used, the input to the output neuron of class c (z_c) and the CAM $(M_c(t))$ can be defined as:

$$z_c = \sum_k w_k^c \sum_t A_k(t) = \sum_t \sum_k w_k^c A_k(t); \quad M_c(t) = \sum_k w_k^c A_k(t) \qquad (1)$$

In order to avoid upsampling the CAM, we padded the input of each convolution with zeros, thus preserving the initial MTS length l throughout the convolutions.

3   Results

3.1   Surgical Skill Classification

Table 1 reports the micro and macro measures (defined in [1]) of four different methods for the surgeons' skill classification of the three surgical tasks. For our approach (CNN), we report the average of 40 runs to eliminate any bias due to the random seed. From these results, it appears that the CNN method is much more accurate than the other approaches with 100% accuracy for the suturing and needle passing tasks. As for the knot tying task, we report 92.1% and 93.2% respectively for the micro and macro configurations. Indeed, for knot tying, the model is less accurate compared to the other two. This is due to the complexity of this task, which is in compliance with the results of the other approaches.

---

[1] Our source code is available on https://germain-forestier.info/src/miccai2018/.

In [13], the authors designed Sparse Hidden Markov Models (S-HMM) to evaluate the surgical skills. Although the latter method utilizes the gesture boundaries during the training phase, our approach achieves much higher accuracy while still providing the trainee with interpretable skill evaluation.

Approximate Entropy (ApEn) is used to extract features from each trial [19], which are then fed to a nearest neighbor classifier. Although both methods (ApEn and CNN) achieve state of the art results with 100% accuracy for the suturing and needle passing surgical tasks, it is not clear how ApEn could be extended to provide feedback for the trainee. In addition, we hypothesize that by doing cross-validation and hyper-parameters fine tuning, we could squeeze higher accuracy from the CNN, especially for the knot tying task.

Finally, in [4], the authors introduce a sliding window technique with a discretization method to transform the MTS into bag of words. Then, they build a vector for each class from the frequency of the words, which is compared to vectors of the MTS in the test set to identify the nearest neighbor with a cosine similarity metric. The authors emphasized the need to obtain *interpretable* surgical skill evaluation, which justified their relatively low accuracy. On contrast, our

Table 1. Surgical skill classification results (%)

Method	Suturing		Needle passing		Knot tying	
	Micro	Macro	Micro	Macro	Micro	Macro
S-HMM [13]	97.4	n/a	96.2	n/a	94.4	n/a
ApEn [19]	**100**	n/a	**100**	n/a	**99.9**	n/a
Sax-Vsm [4]	89.7	86.7	96.3	95.8	61.1	53.3
CNN (proposed)	**100**	**100**	**100**	**100**	92.1	**93.2**

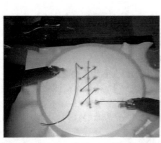
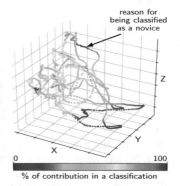

(a) The last frame of subject (Novice) H's fourth trial of the suturing task.

(b) Trial's corresponding trajectory for the left master manipulator (best viewed in color).

Fig. 2. Example of feedback using Class Activation Map (a video illustrating this feedback is available on https://germain-forestier.info/src/miccai2018/).

approach does not trade off accuracy for feedback: CNN is much more *accurate* and equally *interpretable*.

3.2   Feedback Visualization

The CAM technique allows us to visualize which parts of the trial contributes the most to a certain skill classification. Patterns in movements could be understood by identifying for example discriminative behaviors specific to a novice or an expert. We can also pinpoint to the trainees their good/bad movements in order to improve themselves and achieve potentially higher skill levels.

Figure 2 gives an example on how to visualize the feedback for the trainee by constructing a heatmap from the CAM. A trial of a novice subject is studied: its last frame is shown in Fig. 2a and its corresponding heatmap is illustrated in Fig. 2b. In the latter, the model was able to detect which movements (red area) were the main reason behind subject H's classification (as a novice). This feedback could be used to explain to a young surgeon which movements are classifying him/her as a novice and which ones are classifying another subject as an expert. Thus, the feedback could guide the novices into becoming experts.

4   Conclusion

In this paper, we presented a new method for classifying surgical skills. By designing a specific CNN, we achieved 100% accuracy, while providing interpretability that justifies a certain skill evaluation, which reduces the CNN's black-box effect.

In our future work, due to the natural extension of CNNs to image classification, we aim at developing a unified CNN framework that uses both video and kinematic data to classify surgical skills accurately and to provide highly interpretable feedback for the trainee.

References

1. Ahmidi, N., et al.: A dataset and benchmarks for segmentation and recognition of gestures in robotic surgery. IEEE Trans. Biomed. Eng. **64**(9), 2025–2041 (2017)
2. Bridgewater, B., et al.: Surgeon specific mortality in adult cardiac surgery: comparison between crude and risk stratified data. Br. Med. J. **327**(7405), 13–17 (2003)
3. Fard, M.J., Ameri, S., Darin Ellis, R., Chinnam, R.B., Pandya, A.K., Klein, M.D.: Automated robot-assisted surgical skill evaluation: predictive analytics approach. Int. J. Med. Robot. Comput. Assist. Surg. **14**, e1850 (2018)
4. Forestier, G., Petitjean, F., Senin, P., Despinoy, F., Jannin, P.: Discovering discriminative and interpretable patterns for surgical motion analysis. In: Artificial Intelligence in Medicine, pp. 136–145 (2017)
5. Gao, Y., et al.: The JHU-ISI gesture and skill assessment working set (JIGSAWS): a surgical activity dataset for human motion modeling. In: Modeling and Monitoring of Computer Assisted Interventions, MICCAI Workshop (2014)
6. Glorot, X., Bengio, Y.: Understanding the difficulty of training deep feedforward neural networks. Int. Conf. Artif. Intell. Stat. **9**, 249–256 (2010)

7. Hatala, R., Cook, D.A., Brydges, R., Hawkins, R.: Constructing a validity argument for the objective structured assessment of technical skills (OSATS): a systematic review of validity evidence. Adv. Health Sci. Educ. **20**(5), 1149–1175 (2015)
8. Islam, G., Kahol, K., Li, B., Smith, M., Patel, V.L.: Affordable, web-based surgical skill training and evaluation tool. J. Biomed. Inform. **59**, 102–114 (2016)
9. Kassahun, Y., et al.: Surgical robotics beyond enhanced dexterity instrumentation: a survey of machine learning techniques and their role in intelligent and autonomous surgical actions. Int. J. Comput. Assist. Radiol. Surg. **11**(4), 553–568 (2016)
10. Kingma, D.P., Ba, J.: Adam: a method for stochastic optimization. In: International Conference on Learning Representations (2015)
11. Maier-Hein, L., et al.: Surgical data science for next-generation interventions. Nat. Biomed. Eng. **1**(9), 691–696 (2017)
12. Niitsu, H., et al.: Using the objective structured assessment of technical skills (OSATS) global rating scale to evaluate the skills of surgical trainees in the operating room. Surg. Today **43**(3), 271–275 (2013)
13. Tao, L., et al.: Sparse hidden Markov models for surgical gesture classification and skill evaluation. In: Abolmaesumi, P., Joskowicz, L., Navab, N., Jannin, P. (eds.) IPCAI 2012. LNCS, vol. 7330, pp. 167–177. Springer, Heidelberg (2012). https://doi.org/10.1007/978-3-642-30618-1_17
14. Tedesco, M.M., Pak, J.J., Harris, E.J., Krummel, T.M., Dalman, R.L., Lee, J.T.: Simulation-based endovascular skills assessment: the future of credentialing? J. Vasc. Surg. **47**(5), 1008–1014 (2008)
15. Polavarapu, V.: H., Kulaylat, A., Sun, S., Hamed, O.: 100 years of surgical education: the past, present, and future. Bull. Am. Coll. Surg. **98**(7), 22–27 (2013)
16. Vedula, S.S., et al.: Analysis of the structure of surgical activity for a suturing and knot-tying task. Public Libr. Sci. One **11**(3), 1–14 (2016)
17. Wang, Z., Yan, W., Oates, T.: Time series classification from scratch with deep neural networks: a strong baseline. In: International Joint Conference on Neural Networks, pp. 1578–1585 (2017)
18. Zhou, B., Khosla, A., Lapedriza, A., Oliva, A., Torralba, A.: Learning deep features for discriminative localization. In: IEEE Conference on Computer Vision and Pattern Recognition, pp. 2921–2929 (2016)
19. Zia, A., Essa, I.: Automated Surgical Skill Assessment in RMIS Training. ArXiv e-prints (2017)

Needle Tip Force Estimation Using an OCT Fiber and a Fused convGRU-CNN Architecture

Nils Gessert[1]($\boxtimes$), Torben Priegnitz[1], Thore Saathoff[1], Sven-Thomas Antoni[1], David Meyer[2], Moritz Franz Hamann[2], Klaus-Peter Jünemann[2], Christoph Otte[1], and Alexander Schlaefer[1]

[1] Institute of Medical Technology, Hamburg University of Technology, Hamburg, Germany
nils.gessert@tuhh.de
[2] Department of Urology, University Hospital Schleswig-Holstein, Kiel, Germany

Abstract. Needle insertion is common during minimally invasive interventions such as biopsy or brachytherapy. During soft tissue needle insertion, forces acting at the needle tip cause tissue deformation and needle deflection. Accurate needle tip force measurement provides information on needle-tissue interaction and helps detecting and compensating potential misplacement. For this purpose we introduce an image-based needle tip force estimation method using an optical fiber imaging the deformation of an epoxy layer below the needle tip over time. For calibration and force estimation, we introduce a novel deep learning-based fused convolutional GRU-CNN model which effectively exploits the spatio-temporal data structure. The needle is easy to manufacture and our model achieves a mean absolute error of 1.76 ± 1.5 mN with a cross-correlation coefficient of 0.9996, clearly outperforming other methods. We test needles with different materials to demonstrate that the approach can be adapted for different sensitivities and force ranges. Furthermore, we validate our approach in an ex-vivo prostate needle insertion scenario.

Keywords: Force estimation · Optical coherence tomography
Convolutional GRU · Convolution Neural Network · Needle placement

1 Introduction

Needle insertion is widely used in minimally invasive procedures, e.g., for biopsies or brachytherapy. Automated needle insertion is challenging and includes aspects like image guidance, needle steering, and force measurement [14]. Precise estimation of the forces acting on the needle tip is particularly interesting, e.g., for monitoring the needle-tissue interaction and detecting tissue ruptures, or to generate feedback during an intervention [10]. One approach is to measure the forces at the needle shaft. While this allows for simple integration of conventional force-torque sensors, the measurements do not reflect the actual

© Springer Nature Switzerland AG 2018
A. F. Frangi et al. (Eds.): MICCAI 2018, LNCS 11073, pp. 222–229, 2018.
https://doi.org/10.1007/978-3-030-00937-3_26

forces acting on the needle tip. As large frictional forces act on the needle shaft during insertion, force sensors need to be decoupled or located close to the tip in order to obtain accurate needle tip force estimates [6]. The small diameter of the needles complicates the integration of sensors [12], which is particularly challenging for conventional mechatronic force sensors [4,6]. In contrast, fiber optical force sensors are small, largely biocompatible, and not affected by electromagnetic interference, i.e., they are MRI-compatible [2]. Therefore, sensors based on Fabry-Pérot interferometry [2] or Fiber Bragg Gratings [8] have been proposed. Although these approaches have shown promising calibration results, they are rarely validated with tissue experiments [9] and manufacturing and signal processing can be difficult, e.g., when the fibers are subjected to varying temperatures or lateral forces. Yet another approach is based on optical coherence tomography (OCT), where A-scan images of a cylindric instrument tip have been used to estimate the deformation and hence the strain acting on a translucent silicone layer [7].

We consider force sensing using OCT and a sharp needle with a cone tip mounted on a needle using epoxy resin. The axial force acting on the tip is inferred from the epoxy layer's deformation observed in a series of A-scans. We can tailor our method to specific application scenarios by using softer epoxy resin for higher sensitivity, as required for microsurgery, or stiffer epoxy resin for larger forces, e.g., as occurring during biopsies [2]. Generally, our approach is flexible and easy to manufacture as the epoxy material is interchangeable, the cone shape can be varied, and no accurate fiber placement is required. However, this imposes some challenges for calibration and force estimation, namely the robust identification of the deformation of the epoxy layer and a non-linear mapping of the measured deformations to forces. To this end we propose a force estimation method based on a novel convolutional gated recurrent unit-convolutional neural network (convGRU-CNN) architecture. Considering the high temporal sampling rate of OCT, we use a sequence of subsequent A-scans as an input to our model. In this way, we can take advantage of a rich spatio-temporal signal space for precise force estimates.

First, we present a detailed description of the force sensing needle and our convGRU-CNN architecture. Second, we describe our setups for calibration and evaluation of the needles. Third, we study the repeatability of force estimation for three different needles with different epoxy resin types. Finally, we present results for needle insertion into actual ex-vivo prostate tissue illustrating the feasibility of the approach and the importance of measurements at the needle tip.

2   Materials and Methods

2.1   Needle Design and Experimental Setup

A schematic drawing of our needle and the needle driver is shown in Fig. 1. The needle has a diameter of 1.25 mm. An epoxy resin layer of approximately 0.5 mm connects the cone shaped tip to the needle shaft. An optical fiber is embedded

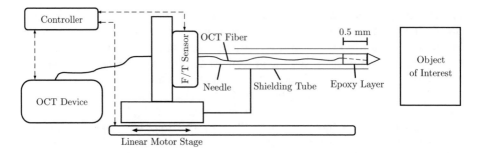

Fig. 1. Schematic drawing of the needle and the experimental setup. Not to scale. The needle contains an OCT fiber that images a deformable epoxy layer at the needle tip. Forces are measured by the force sensor at the base. A shielding tube is decoupled from the needle and the force sensor and prevents shaft friction measurements for tissue insertion experiments. The setup is moved with a linear stage.

into the shaft and glued to the epoxy. The fiber is connected to an OCT device (Thorlabs Telesto I). A linear motion stage is used to drive the needle along its axial direction. For calibration and evaluation, a force sensor (ATI Nano43) is mounted between the needle shaft and the motion stage. To study how the sensitivity of the sensor can be varied by using different epoxy resin, the resin was mixed with Norland Optical Adhesive (NOA) 1625 in different concentrations. The layer and the needle tip on top are attached using NOA 63. For calibration, the needle was driven against a metal plate. A large set of data was acquired by deforming the tip with random magnitude and velocity. For evaluation, the needle was inserted into a freshly resected human prostate at constant velocity. As the force sensor at the base measures the total force including friction, we consider a second setup using a shielding tube decoupled from the needle and the force sensor. In this way, we can measure the actual axial tip forces. Note, that this would be impractical for actual application as the tube is not flexible and would increase trauma. A photograph of the experimental setup is shown in Fig. 2. We provide a video and ultrasound recording of two insertion procedures with pork liver and a human ex-vivo prostate in our supplementary material.

2.2 Model Architecture

For our model input, we consider a series of A-scans prior to the current observation, as the current force estimate likely depends on prior deformation [1]. Furthermore, we do not extract the epoxy surface as an explicit deformation feature but instead let our model learn relevant features. In this way, we avoid inconsistencies when extracting features for different materials and tips and we exploit information captured in the deformed epoxy layer itself. Prior approaches for spatio-temporal data used CNNs to extract features from image data which are fed into a recurrent model [3]. Alternatively, the temporal dimension can also be handled by a convolution operation [13]. Also, convolutional long-short

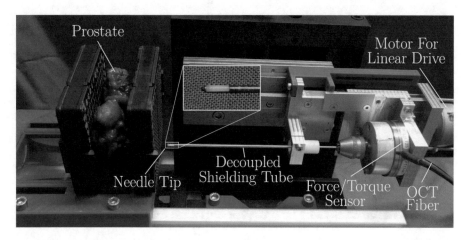

Fig. 2. Photograph of the experimental setup for the prostate insertion experiment. Note, that for calibration the needle is driven against a metal plate.

term memory (convLSTM) cells have been introduced which allow for temporal processing of high dimensional structured data [15]. Based on these approaches, we propose a novel convGRU-CNN architecture, as shown in Fig. 3. First, convGRU units take care of the temporal processing which results in a set of 1D feature maps. Then, a ResNet inspired [5] 1D CNN takes care of spatial processing. Compared to LSTMs, GRUs merge the input and forget gate and they merge the cell and hidden state for higher efficiency. We use a combination of convLSTMs and GRUs by replacing the matrix multiplications with convolutions. The proposed architecture is compared to other approaches that have been introduced for spatio-temporal data processing. We consider a 2D CNN that processes both the temporal and the spatial dimension with convolutions. Its structure is the same as the CNN part in the convGRU-CNN model. Moreover, we consider a CNN-GRU model where the 1D CNN first processes the A-scans at each time step separately. Then, the CNN feature vector is fed into two standard GRUs. Next, we consider a pure 1D CNN that does not consider prior A-scans for the current force prediction. Last, we consider a pure 3-layer GRU model. All networks are trained end-to-end in a single optimization run. We use the Adam algorithm for mini-batch gradient descent with a batch size of $B = 100$. We implement our models using the Tensorflow environment.

2.3 Data Acquisition and Datasets

OCT is an interferometry-based image modality using near infrared light to create 1D depth scans (A-scans) of up to 3 mm reflecting the inner structure of materials. We acquired A-scans at a rate of 5500 Hz and force measurements at 500 Hz. We match the two data streams with nearest-neighbor interpolation, using the streams' timestamps. Our dataset consists of sequences of t_s subsequent A-scans, each labled with a force measurement. Given that we do not need the

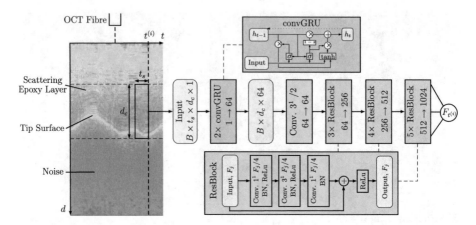

Fig. 3. The convGRU-CNN model we employ. A series t_s of cropped A-scans of size d_c is fed into the model. The metal tip's lower surface cannot be penetrated by infrared light which is why this signal part is considered noise. The first block in a series of ResBlocks uses a stride of 2 for the convolutions with kernel 3^1 and increases the number of feature maps. Subsequent blocks have a stride of 1 and keep the same feature map amount. The change in the number of feature maps is denoted in each group of ResBlocks. F_j denotes the number of feature maps of ResBlock j.

full imaging depth of the OCT, image data beyond the maximum depth of the cone tip surface is cropped.

We consider calibration datasets for three needles with different epoxy resin types for evaluation with our convGRU-CNN model. Each dataset contains approximately 90000 sequences of A-scans, each labeled with an axial force. By default we use a window of $t_s = 50$ with a crop size $d_c = 70$ pixels. We use 80% of the data for training and validation sets, which we use to optimize hyper-paramters, e.g., t_s, d_c, l_r, and network depth. The remaining 20% of the data are used for testing. Sequences from the three sets are non-overlapping. Furthermore, one of the needles was evaluated in an ex-vivo experiment in a human prostate. We evaluate our proposed architecture by comparing it to the models mentioned in Sect. 2.2, reporting the mean absolute error (MAE), relative MAE (rMAE) and correlation coefficient (CC) between predictions and targets. All errors are given for the test set.

3   Results

First, we report the results for different needles with a different stiffness of the epoxy layer. The results with the corresponding force magnitudes are shown in Table 1. The absolute error values vary, as the corresponding force ranges differ, however, the relative measures rMAE and CC show that models perform overall similar. Next, we present results for alternative model architectures. The results are shown in Table 2. The results show, that models that take prior A-scans into

Table 1. Comparison of needles with different epoxy layer stiffnesses. The MAE in mN and rMAE (with standard deviation), the CC and the maximum force range in mN are shown. The convGRU-CNN model was used for this experiment.

	MAE	rMAE	CC	Max
Needle 1	1.76 ± 1.5	0.0213 ± 0.0180	0.9996	379
Needle 2	7.46 ± 6.2	0.0275 ± 0.0231	0.9994	974
Needle 3	24.26 ± 22.4	0.0369 ± 0.0322	0.9989	3202

Table 2. Comparison of different models. The MAE in mN and rMAE (with standard deviation) and the CC are shown. Needle 1 was used for this experiment.

	MAE	rMAE	CC
convGRU-CNN	$\mathbf{1.76 \pm 1.5}$	$\mathbf{0.0213 \pm 0.0180}$	**0.9996**
CNN-GRU	2.06 ± 3.4	0.0249 ± 0.0419	0.9988
2D CNN	2.09 ± 3.6	0.0252 ± 0.0440	0.9987
1D CNN	3.24 ± 4.0	0.0392 ± 0.0488	0.9980
GRU	3.22 ± 4.1	0.0389 ± 0.0490	0.9980

account perform better. Moreover, our proposed model outperforms previously introduced approaches for our application. Last, we show results for a needle insertion experiment for two different scenarios in Fig. 4. One experiment was conducted with the shielding tube and one without. With the tube, predicted values closely match the measured values. Without, there are large deviations as the sensor also measures friction forces.

4   Discussion

We introduce a novel technique for needle tip force estimation using an OCT fiber that images the deformation of an epoxy layer. As OCT has been used for needle-based tissue analysis [11], it may become more widely available in clinical settings. Our method comes with the typical advantages of optical methods, such as MRI-compatibility and bio-compatibility, while also being flexible and easy to manufacture. This is highlighted by the results for three different needles with epoxy layers of different stiffness. All needles show similar relative calibration errors with a CC in the range of 0.9996 to 0.9989, indicating that our method generalizes well for different epoxy resins. This allows for easy adaptation of our method to different scenarios with different requirements for force sensitivity and range.

Moreover, we propose a novel method for processing the spatio-temporal OCT data. Previously, time series of A-scans have been processed using recurrent architectures [11]. The approach shares parameters over time, however, it lacks effective spatial exploitation with parameter sharing over space through convolutions. As our convGRU model takes care of efficient processing of both temporal

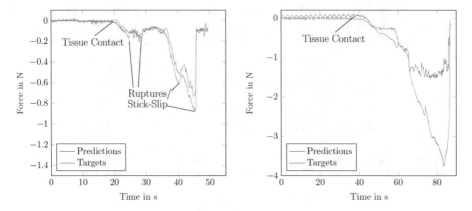

Fig. 4. Predicted and measured force values are shown for an insertion with the shielding tube (left) and without (right). Note, that differences between predictions and targets are caused by friction during target measurements, not inaccurate model calibration. Needle 2 and the model convGRU-CNN are used for this experiment.

and spatial information, it outperforms the pure temporal GRU and pure spatial 1D CNN with an MAE of 1.76 ± 1.5 compared to an MAE of 3.24 ± 4.0 and 3.22 ± 4.1, respectively. Furthermore, we adopted a CNN-GRU and 2D CNN model from non-medical domains for comparison of spatio-temporal processing architectures [3,15]. Compared to the other models, the convGRU units in our model enable temporal processing first while keeping the data structure intact for subsequent CNN processing. This leads to superior performance for the problem at hand.

Lastly, we tested our needle in an ex-vivo experiment with a human prostate. Several other needle tip force estimation methods have been proposed, however, they often lack validation in tissue experiments [9]. One of the reasons for this is the difficulty to measure pure tip forces inside tissue as large friction forces will also be captured by external force sensors [6]. Therefore, we use a shielding tube that decouples friction forces from the needle. Although the decoupling is not perfect due to deformations, we can show that our method accurately captures events such as ruptures. Without the mechanism, in-tissue evaluation is not possible as frictional forces overlap with tip forces. The results indicate that our method is usable for actual force estimation in soft tissue.

5   Conclusion

We propose a novel method for needle tip force estimation. Our approach uses an OCT fiber imaging the deformation of an epoxy layer to infer the force that acted on the needle tip. The concept is easy to realize and allows flexibility by using different materials for different force sensitivity and maximum range requirements. In order to process the spatio-temporal OCT data we propose a novel convGRU-CNN architecture. For our problem, the method outperforms prior approaches for similar problems and also methods from other domains. Experimental results for force estimation in human prostate tissue underline the method's potential for practical application.

Acknowledgments. This work was partially supported by DFG grants SCHL 1844/2-1 and SCHL 1844/2-2.

References

1. Aviles, A.I., Alsaleh, S.M., Hahn, J.K., Casals, A.: Towards retrieving force feedback in robotic-assisted surgery: a supervised neuro-recurrent-vision approach. IEEE Trans. Haptics **10**(3), 431–443 (2017)
2. Beekmans, S., Lembrechts, T., van den Dobbelsteen, J., van Gerwen, D.: Fiber-optic fabry-Pérot interferometers for axial force sensing on the tip of a needle. Sensors **17**(1), 38 (2016)
3. Donahue, J., et al.: Long-term recurrent convolutional networks for visual recognition and description. In: CVPR, pp. 2625–2634 (2015)
4. Hatzfeld, C., Wismath, S., Hessinger, M., Werthschtzky, R., Schlaefer, A., Kupnik, M.: A miniaturized sensor for needle tip force measurements. Biomed. Eng. **62**(1), 109–115 (2017)
5. He, K., Zhang, X., Ren, S., Sun, J.: Deep residual learning for image recognition. In: CVPR, pp. 770–778 (2016)
6. Kataoka, H., Washio, T., Chinzei, K., Mizuhara, K., Simone, C., Okamura, A.M.: Measurement of the tip and friction force acting on a needle during penetration. In: Dohi, T., Kikinis, R. (eds.) MICCAI 2002. LNCS, vol. 2488, pp. 216–223. Springer, Heidelberg (2002). https://doi.org/10.1007/3-540-45786-0_27
7. Kennedy, K.M., et al.: Quantitative micro-elastography: imaging of tissue elasticity using compression optical coherence elastography. Sci. Rep. **5**(15), 538 (2015)
8. Kumar, S., Shrikanth, V., Amrutur, B., Asokan, S., Bobji, M.S.: Detecting stages of needle penetration into tissues through force estimation at needle tip using fiber bragg grating sensors. J. Biomed. Opt. **21**(12), 127009 (2016)
9. Mo, Z., Xu, W., Broderick, N.G.: Capability characterization via ex-vivo experiments of a fiber optical tip force sensing needle for tissue identification. IEEE Sens. J. **18**, 1195–1202 (2017)
10. Okamura, A.M., Simone, C., O'leary, M.D.: Force modeling for needle insertion into soft tissue. IEEE Trans. Biomed. Eng. **51**(10), 1707–1716 (2004)
11. Otte, C., et al.: Investigating recurrent neural networks for OCT a-scan based tissue analysis. Methods Inf. Med. **53**(4), 245–249 (2014)
12. Rodrigues, S., Horeman, T., Sam, P., Dankelman, J., van den Dobbelsteen, J., Jansen, F.W.: Influence of visual force feedback on tissue handling in minimally invasive surgery. Br. J. Surg. **101**(13), 1766–1773 (2014)
13. Sun, L., Jia, K., Yeung, D.Y., Shi, B.E.: Human action recognition using factorized spatio-temporal convolutional networks. In: CVPR, pp. 4597–4605 (2015)
14. Taylor, R.H., Menciassi, A., Fichtinger, G., Fiorini, P., Dario, P.: Medical robotics and computer-integrated surgery. In: Siciliano, B., Khatib, O. (eds.) Springer Handbook of Robotics, pp. 1657–1684. Springer, Cham (2016). https://doi.org/10.1007/978-3-319-32552-1_63
15. Xingjian, S., Chen, Z., Wang, H., Yeung, D.Y., Wong, W.K., Woo, W.C.: Convolutional LSTM network: a machine learning approach for precipitation nowcasting. In: Advances in Neural Information Processing Systems, pp. 802–810 (2015)

Fast GPU Computation of 3D Isothermal Volumes in the Vicinity of Major Blood Vessels for Multiprobe Cryoablation Simulation

Ehsan Golkar[1]([⊠]), Pramod P. Rao[2], Leo Joskowicz[3], Afshin Gangi[2], and Caroline Essert[1]

[1] ICube, Université de Strasbourg, Strasbourg, France
golkar@unistra.fr
[2] Department of Radiology, University Hospital of Strasbourg, Strasbourg, France
[3] CASMIP Laboratory, The Hebrew University of Jerusalem, Jerusalem, Israel

Abstract. Percutaneous cryoablation is a minimally invasive procedure of hypothermia for the treatment of tumors. Several needles are inserted in the tumor through the skin, to create an iceball and kill the malignant cells. The procedure consists of several cycles alternating extreme freezing and thawing. This procedure is very complex to plan, as the iceball is formed from multiple needles and influenced by major blood vessels nearby, making its final shape very difficult to anticipate. For computer assistance to cryoablation planning, it is essential to predict accurately the final volume of necrosis. In this paper, a fast GPU implementation of 3D thermal propagation is presented based on heat transfer equation. Our approach accounts for the presence of major blood vessels in the vicinity of the iceball. The method is validated first in gel conditions, then on an actual retrospective patient case of renal cryoablation with complex vascular structure close to the tumor. The results show that the accuracy of our simulated iceball can help surgeons in surgical planning.

1 Introduction

Cryosurgery is a treatment of tumors using hypothermia introduced in the 1960s [7]. The percutaneous ablation of a tumor consist of percutaneously inserting one or more cryoprobes under CT, MR or ultrasound guidance to kill cancerous cells by extreme cold. The process generates alternating cycles of freezing and thawing by decompressing a gas through the needle tip, forming an iceball around it [5]. The recommended lethal freezing temperature is between $0\,°C$ to $-50\,°C$ [10].

Percutaneous cryoablation has become popular, as it shortens the hospital stay and is reproducible. However, the uncertainty of its final result is a limitation in many applications [9]. The volume of iceball should cover the entire tumor shape with an additional margin to ensure the complete ablation of the lesion. In the context of cryoablation planning, an accurate simulation of the iceball formation is essential. However, simulating an iceball generated from multiple needles and taking into account various factors, i.e., the surrounding anatomy or

© Springer Nature Switzerland AG 2018
A. F. Frangi et al. (Eds.): MICCAI 2018, LNCS 11073, pp. 230–237, 2018.
https://doi.org/10.1007/978-3-030-00937-3_27

the injection of protective heated fluid, is very complex and difficult to anticipate accurately. In addition, the synergistic effect created by several probes depends on their actual location and influences the final shape of the iceball [1].

Previous papers described representations of iceballs in gel, either based on simplified computational models [9] or measurements [12]. Ge et al. described a soft tissue parametrization model of the iceball without validating it on real data [6]. Talbot et al. describes a GPU-based algorithm to model iceballs [14]. None of these models take into account the heating effect of large blood vessels. More recent papers describe more elaborated methods that account for the influence of blood vessels in radio-frequency ablation (RFA), which is another type of hypothermia [8,13]. In [11], Rieder et al. proposed a GPU-based algorithm using a simplified approximated model based on a weighted distance field to compute RFA. This approach allows for real-time computation of the thermal ablation volume. These models proposed in the three cited works are limited to a single active needle and have not been validated on actual cryoablation data.

In this paper, we present a three dimensional (3D) finite difference model and simulation of heat transfer for cryoablation. The novelty of our approach is that it simulates the iceball creation taking into account large blood vessels and multiple cryoablation needles using a fast GPU-based algorithm. To validate our approach, we compared our results to two kinds of ground truth: temperature measurements reported in [12] for a gel with known properties, and retrospective images of the cryoablation of a renal tumor close to large blood vessels. Our simulation uses parameters of the human tissues and includes metabolic heat.

2   Materials and Methods

2.1   General Formulation

The general heat equation describes the distribution of heat over time t in a region defined in an x, y and z Cartesian coordinate system [3]. The heat propagation is described by a partial differential equation:

$$C\frac{\partial T}{\partial t} = \frac{\partial}{\partial x}(K_x \frac{\partial T}{\partial x}) + \frac{\partial}{\partial y}(K_y \frac{\partial T}{\partial y}) + \frac{\partial}{\partial x}(K_z \frac{\partial T}{\partial z}) + I(x, y, z, t) \qquad (1)$$

where I is the internal heat generation function, t is the time, constants K denote the spatial thermal conductivities in x, y, z, and C denotes the heat capacity.

This formulation can be approximated by a discretization in which $\Delta x = \Delta y = \Delta z$ are the spacings between a cell (i, j, k) and its neighbours in the x, y, z directions, respectively. This discrete approximation of heat conduction is then:

$$T_{i,j,k}^{new} = T_{i,j,k} + \frac{\Delta t.\beta}{C_{i,j,k}(\Delta x)^3}.H_{i,j,k} \qquad (2)$$

where $C_{i,j,k}$ is the volumetric heat capacity. The new temperature $T_{i,j,k}^{new}$ after a time step Δt is computed by adding its previous temperature $T_{i,j,k}$ and the coefficient of heat flow $H_{i,j,k}$. The relaxation factor β should be chosen within the range $[1, 2]$. In this study β was set to 1.95.

The resulting heat flow $H_{i,j,k}$ is computed from six neighbouring cells:

$$H_{i,j,k} = \kappa_{i-\frac{1}{2},j,k}.(T_{i-1,j,k} - T_{i,j,k}) + \kappa_{i+\frac{1}{2},j,k}.(T_{i+1,j,k} - T_{i,j,k})$$
$$+\kappa_{i,j-\frac{1}{2},k}.(T_{i,j-1,k} - T_{i,j,k}) + \kappa_{i,j+\frac{1}{2},k}.(T_{i,j+1,k} - T_{i,j,k}) \tag{3}$$
$$+\kappa_{i,j,k-\frac{1}{2}}.(T_{i,j,k-1} - T_{i,j,k}) + \kappa_{i,j,k+\frac{1}{2}}.(T_{i,j,k+1} - T_{i,j,k})$$

The $\kappa_{i-\frac{1}{2},j,k}$, $\kappa_{i,j-\frac{1}{2},k}$, $\kappa_{i,j,k-\frac{1}{2}}$ are the thermal conductances between cell (i,j,k) and the prior adjacent cells in the x, y, z directions, respectively. Similarly, $\kappa_{i+\frac{1}{2},j,k}$, $\kappa_{i,j+\frac{1}{2},k}$, $\kappa_{i,j,k+\frac{1}{2}}$ are the conductances between cell (i,j,k) and posterior adjacent cells as in [3]. Thermal conductance of $\kappa_{i,j,k+\frac{1}{2}}$ is defined by:

$$\kappa_{i,j,k+\frac{1}{2}} = \frac{\Delta x}{1/(2K_{i,j,k}) + 1/(2K_{i,j,k+1}) + R_{i,j,k+\frac{1}{2}}} \tag{4}$$

where $K_{i,j,k}$ and $K_{i,j,k+1}$ are the thermal conductivities of the current cell (i,j,k) and its adjacent cell $(i,j,k+1)$. The other five κ values in Eq. (3) are obtained similarly. The thermal resistance between these cells is denoted by $R_{i,j,k+\frac{1}{2}}$. Since the thermal resistance has a very small impact on heating flows, we do not take it into account any further.

To avoid the numerical instability in heat transform equation, the time step Δt is set to 0.05 s which satisfies the following stability criterion:

$$\Delta t < \frac{C_{i,j,k}(\Delta x)^3}{\Sigma \kappa}, \forall i, j, k \tag{5}$$

$$\Sigma \kappa = \kappa_{i-\frac{1}{2},j,k} + \kappa_{i+\frac{1}{2},j,k} + \kappa_{i,j-\frac{1}{2},k} + \kappa_{i,j+\frac{1}{2},k} + \kappa_{i,j,k-\frac{1}{2}} + \kappa_{i,j,k+\frac{1}{2}} \tag{6}$$

To simulate the growth of the iceball, the 3D heat propagation is computed iteratively within a grid of voxels centered at the needle tip inside a $10 \times 10 \times 10$ cm cube. To obtain accurate results, a very fine grid is required, but this sharply increases the computation time. In this study, we use a grid resolution of $\Delta x = \Delta y = \Delta z = 1$ mm, which is smaller than the diameter of the thinnest needle (*IceRod* by Galil Medical, diameter 1.5 mm).

Voxels located in the active part of the cryoablation needles are labeled as the source of cold; their temperature is kept constant during the freezing cycles. Boundary conditions are represented by the voxels at the border of the cube, which are forced to the temperature of the environment. The algorithm was implemented on a GPU to reduce computation time incurred by a finely discretized cube. We use CUDA toolkit for NVidia's GPUs and the method described in [2] to optimally use the parallelization capabilities of the GPU processing units and to avoid the repeated computation by two threads on the same heat cell.

2.2   Propagation of Cold in the Human Body Near Heating Sources

When the iceball is created inside the human body, the metabolic heat influences its creation and final shape. To account for metabolic heat, Pennes bioheat equation as described in Eq.(1), can be expressed as:

$$C\frac{\partial T}{\partial t} = \frac{\partial}{\partial x}(K_x\frac{\partial T}{\partial x}) + \frac{\partial}{\partial y}(K_y\frac{\partial T}{\partial y}) + \frac{\partial}{\partial x}(K_z\frac{\partial T}{\partial z}) + C_b\omega_b(T_a - T_t) + Q_m \quad (7)$$

where C_b denotes the heat capacity of blood, ω_b is the blood perfusion rate, T_a is the arterial temperature, T_t is the temperature at time t, and Q_m is the metabolic heat rate of tissue. When a major vessel or any heating source, e.g., injected warm protective liquid, is inside the cube, their associated voxels are labeled and their temperature is kept constant and equal to the source temperature. In this study we consider all sources of heat as constant and homogeneous.

2.3   Validation in Silico

We first validated the simulation with an in silico study using gel properties. The goal was to measure the performance of our simulation approach in terms of accuracy and computation times in theoretical conditions. We simulated the propagation of cold with 1 to 4 evenly spaced cryoprobes arranged in parallel at 20 mm intervals. The experiment was done using two types of cryoprobes from Galil Medical: *IceEdge* 2.4 mm (10G) and *IceRod* 1.5 mm (17G).

Each experiment consists in simulating 3 cycles: 10 min of freezing, followed by 5 min of passive thaw, and 10 min of freezing. We used the parameters provided by the manufacturer to model the action of the probes. For *IceEdge*, the freezing temperature at probe's tip was set to $-138.0\,°C$. The length of the active freezing part of the probe was set to 28 mm at 5.2 mm from the tip. For *IceRod*, we used a freezing temperature of $-119.4\,°C$. We set the active freezing part to 31 mm at 4.2 mm from the tip.

For all settings, we measured the diameter of the resulting $0\,°C$, $-20\,°C$ and $-40\,°C$ isotherm surfaces at their largest sections. We then compared our simulation results with the dimensions of the isotherm surfaces measured in a recent study [12], where a thermocouple matrix structure was designed to measure the iceball temperatures in ultrasound (US) gel at $37\,°C$. To obtain the same conditions, we used the thermophysical properties of a similar gel described in [4].

2.4   Validation on Intraoperative MRI Images

We performed a second experiment on retrospective MR images of an actual renal cryoablation procedure where the tumor was located close to major vessels. During the procedure, warm saline solution was injected to protect sensitive structures nearby from being frozen.

The tumor was located on the upper right part of the kidney, close to major blood vessels. Four *IceRod* needles were inserted. This time, cryoablation was performed in four cycles: 10 min of active freezing, followed by 9 min of passive thawing and 1 min of active thawing and again 10 min active freezing. The 10 mn active freezing temperature of IceRod was set to $-138.0\,°C$ while 1 mn active thawing temperature was set to $58.0\,°C$. During the whole process, dissection water at $37.0\,°C$ was continuously injected around the kidney.

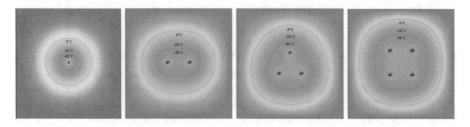

Fig. 1. Heat propagation simulation after complete process for 1 to 4 IceEdge probes evenly spaced by 20 mm. The largest sections of the iceballs in probe's axis are represented. The colormap is within the range $[-138.0\,^{\circ}\mathrm{C}, 37\,^{\circ}\mathrm{C}]$

MR images of $256 \times 232 \times 25$ voxels with a $1.5 \times 1.5 \times 5$ mm^3 voxel size were acquired during the procedure at three stages: (1) before cryoablation, (2) after 10 min of freezing, and (3) at the end of the cryosurgery. The segmentation of all structures of interest was particularly challenging, due to the injection of saline solution between preoperative and intraoperative images, that cause a deformation of the internal organs.

We first registered the preoperative MR image to the intraoperative MR image using interactive deformable point-based registration. Then, on the registered preoperative MR image, we interactively segmented the kidney and the tumor. On the intraoperative MR images, we segmented the injected saline solution, the renal vessels (vein and artery), and the iceballs at different stages, i.e. after the first and the second freezing cycles as a ground truth. Note that during a cryoablation procedure, the iceball (less than $0\,^{\circ}\mathrm{C}$) appears as a black hole in the MR image. We also segmented the four probes, and used their position as an input to reproduce the same setup in our simulation. Both segmentation and registration were performed under the supervision of an experienced radiologist.

Next, a simulation was performed with commonly used soft tissue parameters accounting for frozen/unfrozen state [6]. To measure the accuracy of our modeling, the Hausdorff distance and the Dice coefficient were computed to compare the similarity of the segmented and simulated iceballs.

3　Results

The results of our experiment with gel parameters are shown on Fig. 1. Table 1 summarizes the maximum diameters of ground truth isotherm surfaces at $0\,^{\circ}\mathrm{C}$, $-20\,^{\circ}\mathrm{C}$ and $-40\,^{\circ}\mathrm{C}$ (from [12]) and our simulated iceballs, for both the *IceRod* and the *IceEdge* probe models. The results of the simulation are very close to the measurements, with a mean error of 0.28 mm, i.e. 5.8% of the diameter of the reference iceball. This has to be put into perspective with the configuration of the multi-needle thermocouple matrix structure used in [12], which was designed with a minimum spacing of 0.5 cm between measuring thermocouples, being a potential source of a slight inaccuracy.

Table 1. Maximum diameters (cm) of ground truth and simulated iceballs

Needle type	# of needles	Ground truth [12]			Simulation		
		0 °C	−20 °C	−40 °C	0 °C	−20 °C	−40 °C
IceEdge	1	4.3	3.3	2.4	4.0	2.9	2.1
	2	6.2	5.2	4.2	6.1	5.1	4.2
	3	6.9	5.9	4.9	6.4	5.3	4.4
	4	7.5	6.6	5.6	7.1	6.1	5.0
IceRod	1	3.6	2.6	1.8	3.9	2.7	1.8
	2	5.7	4.7	3.7	6.0	4.8	3.9
	3	6.2	5.2	4.4	6.1	5.0	4.0
	4	6.9	5.9	5.0	6.7	5.7	4.7

The results were obtained using a desktop computer equipped with a core-i7 3.40 GHz CPU with 16 Gb RAM and a GeForce GTX-1060 GPU with 6 GB memory. The computation times of the simulation in CPU single thread and GPU implementations were 540 s and 84 s for a computation within a $10 \times 10 \times 10$ cm cube. GPU implementation was 6.4× faster than with the CPU.

The results of the second experimentation are presented in Figs. 2 and 3, where the segmented iceball is in white, and our simulated iceball is in red. The dark blue mesh is a portion of the vascular structure, and the light blue mesh is the segmented saline solution. As we can see, the simulated iceball nicely fits around the vessels and is also deformed by the saline solution.

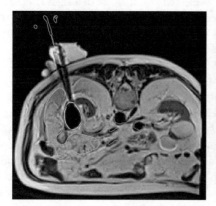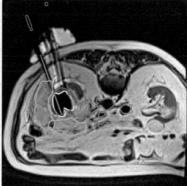

Fig. 2. Simulation of the iceball after the first freezing cycle displayed on 2 slices of a preoperative MRI. The segmented iceball is in white, simulated iceball is in red, vascular structure is in dark blue, segmented saline solution is in light blue.

On Fig. 3 right, we show the simulated iceball in red, compared to the theoretical ellipsoidal iceballs in yellow. We can observe that the synergistic effect and the influence of the vessels and saline solution provide a completely different shape. This emphasizes the essential interest of such a simulation for cryoablation planning. The actual iceball differs significantly from theoretical ellipsoids and is smaller, which could lead to an insufficient ablation of cancerous cells.

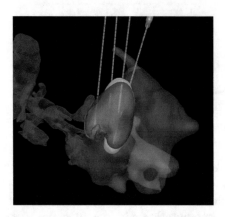 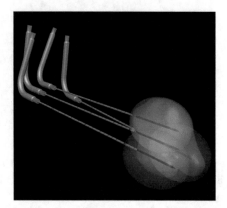

Fig. 3. Left: 3D mesh of the segmented (white) and simulated (red) iceballs after the first freezing cycle. Vessels are in dark blue, saline solution in light blue. Right: simulated iceball (red) and theoretical ellipsoids (yellow).

In terms of accuracy, we obtained a Hausdorff distance of 7.98 mm between segmented and simulated iceball meshes, and a Dice coefficient of 0.83 after the first freezing cycle. At the end of the process, the Hausdorff distance is 8.12 mm and Dice coefficient is 0.82. These measurements show a promising similarity between the two shapes. However, this comparison is subjected to the possible errors in the manual segmentations which can introduce inaccuracies.

Finally, the computation times were for the first freezing cycle 205 s. for CPU and 38 s. for GPU respectively, and for the complete process 664 s. for CPU and 110 s. for GPU. As for the first experiment, the GPU implementation sped up the computation by approximately 6 times. Let us note that the computation time does not depend on the complexity of the scene or the number of heating structures. It only depends on the size of the cube and the duration of the simulated process. When using a small number of needles, or needle models producing small iceballs, it is possible to reduce significantly the computation times by reducing the size of the cube. As an example, a cube of $7 \times 7 \times 7$ cm would use only 1/3 of the time to compute (around 40 s).

4   Conclusion

We presented a fast computation approach for the simulation of iceballs created from multiple needles during cryosurgery in presence of heating sources such as blood vessels. These preliminary validation results on real patient images showed that it was possible to reach a good accuracy within a time compatible with preoperative planning, either interactive or automatic. Such a simulation coupled with a planner could help to find the best number of required probes. In the future, we plan to extend these results by experimenting on larger datasets, even if this kind of validation is quite challenging, as it demands quite a lot of efforts and manipulations to obtain validation data.

Acknowledgments. This work was supported in part by a grant from the Mamonide France-Israel Research in Biomedical Robotics, 2016–18.

References

1. Young, J.L., et al.: Are multiple cryoprobes additive or synergistic in renal cryotherapy? Urology **79**(2), 484.e1–484.e6 (2012)
2. Allard, J., Courtecuisse, H., Faure, F.: Implicit FEM solver on GPU for interactive deformation simulation. In: GPU Computing Gems Jade Edition, pp. 281–294. Elsevier (2011)
3. Blomberg, T.: Heat conduction in two and three dimensions: computer modelling of building physics applications. Ph.D. thesis, Department of Building Physics, Lund University, Sweden (1996). Report TVBH1008, ISBN 91-88722-05-8
4. Choi, J., Bischof, J.C.: Review of biomaterial thermal property measurements in the cryogenic regime and their use for prediction of equilibrium and non-equilibrium freezing applications in cryobiology. Cryobiology **60**(1), 52–70 (2010)
5. Gage, A.A., Baust, J.: Mechanisms of tissue injury in cryosurgery. Cryobiology **37**(3), 171–186 (1998)
6. Ge, M., Chua, K., Shu, C., Yang, W.: Analytical and numerical study of tissue cryofreezing via the immersed boundary method. Int. J. Heat and Mass Transf. **83**, 1–10 (2015)
7. Gonder, M.J., Soanes, W.A., Smith, V.: Experimental prostate cryosurgery. Investig. Urol. **1**, 610 (1964)
8. Huang, H.W.: Influence of blood vessel on the thermal lesion formation during radiofrequency ablation for liver tumors. Med. Phy. **40**(7), 073303 (2013)
9. Magalov, Z., Shitzer, A., Degani, D.: Isothermal volume contours generated in a freezing gel by embedded cryo-needles with applications to cryo-surgery. Cryobiology **55**(2), 127–137 (2007)
10. Mazur, P.: Physical-chemical factors underlying cell injury in cryosurgical freezing. Technical report, Oak Ridge National Laboratory, Tennessee (1967)
11. Rieder, C., Kroeger, T., Schumann, C., Hahn, H.K.: GPU-based real-time approximation of the ablation zone for radiofrequency ablation. IEEE Trans. Vis. Comput. Graph. **17**(12), 1812–1821 (2011)
12. Shah, T.T., et al.: Modeling cryotherapy ice ball dimensions and isotherms in a novel gel-based model to determine optimal cryo-needle configurations and settings for potential use in clinical practice. Urology **91**, 234–240 (2016)
13. Shao, Y., Arjun, B., Leo, H., Chua, K.: A computational theoretical model for radiofrequency ablation of tumor with complex vascularization. Comput. Biol. Med. **89**, 282–292 (2017)
14. Talbot, H., Lekkal, M., Bessard-Duparc, R., Cotin, S.: Interactive planning of cryotherapy using physics-based simulation. In: proceedings of Medicine Meets Virtual Reality (MMVR), pp. 423–429 (2014)

A Machine Learning Approach to Predict Instrument Bending in Stereotactic Neurosurgery

Alejandro Granados[1]([✉]), Matteo Mancini[1], Sjoerd B. Vos[1,3], Oeslle Lucena[6],
Vejay Vakharia[1,2,3], Roman Rodionov[2,3], Anna Miserocchi[2],
Andrew W. McEvoy[2], John S. Duncan[2,3], Rachel Sparks[1],
and Sébastien Ourselin[1,4,5]

[1] Wellcome/EPSRC Centre for Interventional and Surgical Sciences,
UCL, London, UK
alejandro.granados@ucl.ac.uk
[2] National Hospital of Neurology and Neurosurgery, London, UK
[3] Department of Clinical and Experimental Epilepsy,
Institute of Neurology, National Hospital for Neurology and Neurosurgery,
London, UK
[4] Dementia Research Centre, UCL Institute Neurology, London, UK
[5] School of Biomedical Engineering and Imaging Sciences,
St Thomas Hospital, Kings College London, London, UK
[6] Medical Imaging Computing Lab, State University of Campinas,
Campinas, Brazil

Abstract. The accurate implantation of stereo-electroencephalography (SEEG) electrodes is crucial for localising the seizure onset zone in patients with refractory epilepsy. Electrode placement may differ from planning due to instrument deflection during surgical insertion. We present a regression-based model to predict instrument bending using image features extracted from structural and diffusion images. We compare three machine learning approaches: *Random Forest, Feed-Forward Neural Network* and *Long Short-Term Memory* on accuracy in predicting global instrument bending in the context of SEEG implantation. We segment electrodes from post-implantation CT scans and interpolate position at 1 mm intervals along the trajectory. Electrodes are modelled as elastic rods to quantify 3 degree-of-freedom (DOF) bending using Darboux vectors. We train our models to predict instrument bending from image features. We then iteratively infer instrument positions from the predicted bending. In 32 SEEG post-implantation cases we were able to predict trajectory position with a MAE of 0.49 mm using RF. Comparatively a FFNN had MAE of 0.71 mm and LSTM had a MAE of 0.93 mm.

Keywords: Machine learning · Instrument bending
Neurosurgery · Trajectory prediction · Surgical planning

© Springer Nature Switzerland AG 2018
A. F. Frangi et al. (Eds.): MICCAI 2018, LNCS 11073, pp. 238–246, 2018.
https://doi.org/10.1007/978-3-030-00937-3_28

1   Introduction

Minimally-invasive surgical interventions use thin, tubular, and flexible instruments inserted through the skull to target small regions of interest with the aim of acquiring data (e.g. electroencephalography, biopsy) or delivering therapy (e.g. injection, stimulation, ablation). The accurate placement of these instruments is important for patient safety, accurate diagnosis, and treatment efficacy [1,11,22]. Preoperative trajectory planning aims to minimise target point errors whilst avoiding critical structures [9,18]. However, accurate surgical implantation may be difficult to achieve as instruments may deflect during insertion. Deflection may be caused by instrument design (mechanical properties, tip shape), tissue properties (stiffness, inhomogeneity, anisotropy), insertion forces (depth, velocity, steering) and physiological processes [11,17]. The prediction of instrument trajectories inserted into deformable tissue is a challenging problem and an active area of research [5,9,17].

Needle-Tissue Interaction Models. Modelling of trajectory deflection is mostly based on mechanical modelling of tissue-needle interaction. These methods require accurate extraction of the mechanical properties of tissue and instrument together with insertion measurements (e.g. forces, velocities) to accurately predict instrument deflection. Typically such methods use approximations or simplifications derived from hand-crafted modelling techniques to account for unknown parameters. Different instrument models have been proposed including cantilever beams [17], Finite Element Methods (FEM) [5,9], Timoshenko formulation, and Cosserat rods [12,19]. A mechanical model proposed by [17] predicts needle deflection during needle-tissue interaction by modelling forces at the tip (dependent on tissue stiffness) and friction forces along the needle shaft. A simulation-based approach for haptic radiofrequency ablation proposed by [9] iteratively computes instrument deflection during insertion using a FEM.

Machine Learning Models. Several approaches use data-driven machine learning models to predict trajectories (e.g. vehicles, rigged skeleton models) based on spatio-temporal data. These model-free approaches require large amounts of data that must be general enough to predict unseen cases. While, the application of machine learning to predict instrument bending has to the best of our knowledge not yet been presented, these approaches represent a promising avenue to learn features of bending from real world data (i.e. previous examples of instrument trajectories and medical images). Machine learning techniques have long been applied to prediction of spatio-temporal data, most recently with Deep Learning techniques [7]. Recurrent Neural Networks (RNNs), in particular Long Short-Term Memory (LSTM) and Gated Recurrent Units (GRUs), have been applied to predict trajectories by taking into account data at previous timesteps and learning in sequences. An example of this is the prediction of the direction of white matter fibre streamlines from diffusion weighted imaging (DWI) [15].

Our Contributions. We present a novel machine learning regression approach to predict global instrument bending from image features. Instruments are modelled as elastic rods with 3DOF bending and twisting. This method is applied

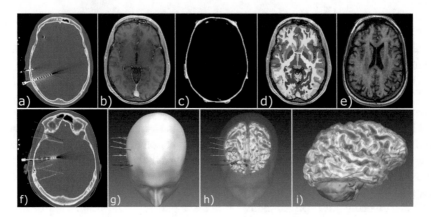

Fig. 1. *Top:* Imaging modalities: (a) post-implantation CT scan, (b) MRI, (c) probabilities from segmentation, (d) parcellation, (e) dMRI. *Bottom:* (f) SEEG electrode segmentation and interaction of electrodes with surface models including: (g) scalp, (h) cortex (in translucent pink), white matter (in white) and (i) deep grey matter (in blue).

to predicted intra-cranial electrode bending using features extracted from structural T1-weighted (T1-w) and diffusion MRI (dMRI).

2   Methods

Image Acquisition and Preprocessing. Prior to electrode implantation, MRI data was acquired either on a 3T GE Signa HDx, consisting of a 3D-T1-w and single-shell dMRI scan (as in [20]), or on a 3T GE MR750, using a T1-w MPRAGE and a multi-shell dMRI scan (as in [13]). dMRI was corrected for susceptibility-induced and eddy-current induced distortions using FSLs topup and eddy, respectively. The T1-w MRI was used to compute a brain parcellation and segmentation probabilities using geodesic information flows (GIF) [2] (Fig. 1). Smoothed 3D polygon meshes of the scalp [4] and superficial grey, white, and deep grey matter were generated from the parcellation. dMRI was modelled as a multi-tissue constrained-spherical deconvolution (MT-CSD) [10] with the Dhollander algorithm [3] implemented in MRtrix3 [21]. We characterise fibre direction and density using the 'fixel' framework [16]. Rigid registration of the CT image to the T1-w MRI was performed by minimising normalised mutual information (NMI) [14]. Similarly, dMRI images were registered by minimising the NMI between the T1-w MRI and b0 dMRI scan. A CT image was acquired immediately after electrode implantation.

Instrument Segmentation and Interpolation. Automatic segmentation of SEEG electrode contacts was performed [8] (Fig. 1). We interpolated instrument

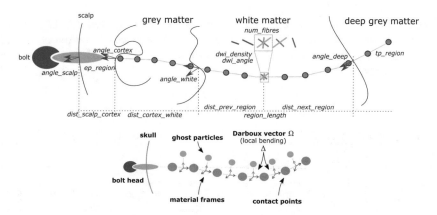

Fig. 2. *Top:* Interpolation points (red circles) along trajectory with structural, white matter fibre tracks-related and trajectory-related features. *Bottom:* Elastic rod model where interpolated points are particles. Material frames and their rate of change (Darboux vectors) are computed to characterise local/global bending.

position from the electrode contact positions at 1 mm intervals using a shape-preserving piecewise cubic Hermite interpolation (PCHIP) [6]. For each position, the following set of features were calculated (Fig. 2, top).

- **Structural:** voxel probability of being background, cerebral spin fluid, grey matter, white matter, deep grey matter and brain stem; and the brain region.
- **White matter fibre tracks:** number and direction of crossing fibres, fibre density and angle of the fibre with respect to the trajectory.
- **Trajectory:** number of regions traversed, length of region at position, angle with respect to surfaces scalp, superficial grey, white, and deep grey matter, distance to grey matter, distance to cortex, distance to previous and next region, and distance from scalp to cortex and from cortex to white matter.

Instrument Bending Model. Instruments were modelled as Cosserat elastic rods in the Position-based Dynamics library. Particles were placed at the interpolated instrument position. Ghosts particles were placed orthogonally half-way between each particle. A material frame is computed between particles with a unit vector aligned tangentially to the direction of the rod and two orthonormal vectors. The rate of change between two consecutive material frames was computed as a Darboux vector [12] (Fig. 2, bottom), where the x, y and z components indicate lateral bending, upward/downward bending and twisting, respectively. For each particle two Darboux vectors were computed: (a) *local bending* (between material frames of neighbouring particles) and (b) *global bending* (between the material frame corresponding to the first particle and the current particle).

Training Model. An Ordinary Least Squares multiple regression was executed (Statsmodels library) to determine which features have a statistically significant effect on bending. Three regression models were built and evaluated: (a) Random

Forest (RF), (b) Feed-Forward Neural Network (FFNN) and (c) LSTM (see Table 1). Global bending at the electrode tip was used as the predicted output of the regression model. Local bending and previous global bending are used as input features.

Table 1. Training model architecture

Model	ML Library	Topology	Details	Activation	Noise
RF	scikit-learn	trees: 200 max. tree depth: 50			No
FFNN	Keras with Tensorflow as a backend	layers: 3 Multiple Layer Perceptron hidden units: equal to number of features	- L2 normalisation (hyperparameter of 1e-4) - normal function to initialise weights	- hidden layer: scaled exponential linear unit (SELU) - output layer: linear	Gaussian $(\mu = 0, \sigma = 0.0025)$
LSTM		layers: - Input layer - 3 LSTM layers (200, 100, 50 units) - Dropout (0.2) between LSTM layers - Dense	sequences of data (window length of 5 interpolated points)	- output layer: linear	No

3   Experimental Design and Validation

We trained our models from 32 post-implantation SEEG cases (296 electrodes, 13107 interpolation points) comprising two different surgical approaches, placing a guiding stylet close to or far from target point. Through multiple linear regression, we found a significant effect on instrument bending of the features listed in Table 2 ($R^2 = 0.313$). The data from these features (27 in total) was normalised. We created dichotomous variables for the treating categorical variables.

A 5-fold cross validation was performed for each model (i.e. RF, FFNN and LSTM). For each fold, we split the data into three sets. A *validation set* contains a trajectory randomly selected from 15 SEEG cases (i.e. 15 trajectories in total). The remaining data is split into a *train set* containing 80% and a *test set* containing 20%. We then conducted two experiments using these three sets: (a) model validation and (b) trajectory accuracy. In experiment (a), we trained our regressor models using the train set and evaluated the inference scores against the test set. The models were trained and average prediction scores across folds are reported in Table 3.

In experiment (b), we selected 30 trajectories from the validation set across folds (15, 4, 4, 4, 3 respectively). Using the trained models of the respective folds, the insertion of an electrode was simulated iteratively starting with the first six interpolated points (sequence length for LSTM) at 1 mm intervals from the electrode bolt. Details of the simulation loop can be found in Algorithm 1.

We then evaluated the accuracy of the trajectory bending prediction (Fig. 3). Distances between true and predicted trajectories were measured. RF had the lowest MAE ($\mu = 0.49, \sigma = 0.43$), followed by FFNN ($\mu = 0.71, \sigma = 0.41$) and by LSTM ($\mu = 0.93, \sigma = 0.65$). Under the current training paradigm, we

Table 2. Features with significant effect ($p < 0.05$) on instrument bending

Positively correlated	Coefficient	Negatively correlated	Coefficient
Displacement w.r.t. planned trajectory	0.2753	x-component of previous bending	−0.0533
z-component of previous bending	0.1315	y-component of previous bending	−0.0472
Angle w.r.t. white matter	0.0379	Number of fibre tracks	−0.0157
Distance to previous region	0.0346	Length of the current traversed region	−0.0089
Distance of cortex traversed	0.0343	Using stylet	−0.0048
Probabilities of segmentation of deep grey matter	0.0328		
Probabilities of segmentation of white matter	0.0320		
Probabilities of segmentation of grey matter	0.0279		
MRI voxel intensity	0.0240		
Angle w.r.t. cortex	0.0215		
Closest distance to grey matter	0.0198		
Regions traversed	0.0135		
Target point region categories (with the exception of central and insula)			

observed that LSTMs tend to accumulate error (given the current accuracy of the 5-fold cross validation in Table 3). Further analysis and method development is required to keep predicted electrode bending within realistic values.

Table 3. Performance of bending prediction of (a) RF, FFNN and LSTM models

Model	K-Fold μ (σ)		
	MSE	MAE	R^2
RF	0.0004 (0.0001)	0.0077 (0.0007)	0.8533 (0.0260)
FFNN	0.0004 (0.0001)	0.0079 (0.0007)	0.8540 (0.0230)
LSTM	0.0007 (0.0002)	0.0126 (0.0015)	0.6583 (0.1043)

Algorithm 1. Simulation of electrode implantation based on predicted bending

1: Load images and 3D meshes
2: **do**
3:     **Generate trajectory features:** *The Medical Imaging Interaction Toolkit* (MITK)
                                            The Visualisation Toolkit (VTK)
4:         - load position of particles along trajectory
5:         - generate features from imaging along inserted trajectory and save
6:     **Predict bending:** *Keras* Python deep learning library / *Tensorflow* ML framework
7:         - load image features along trajectory of electrode
8:         - normalise and categorise features
9:         - generate sequences (only for LSTM)
10:        - load trained model for the corresponding fold
11:        - predict global bending (Darboux vector)
12:    **Compute position of electrode tip:** *Position-based dynamics* library
13:        - create an elastic rod consisting of three particles (and two ghost particles)
             in the direction of the trajectory
14:        - fix two of the particles (and one ghost particle)
15:        - apply constraints (distance, perpendicular bisector, ghost point
             edge distance, and Darboux vector)
16:        - set predicted bending as a resting Darboux vector
17:        - compute position of particle (tip of electrode) and append to trajectory
18: **while** *current insertion depth < planned insertion depth*

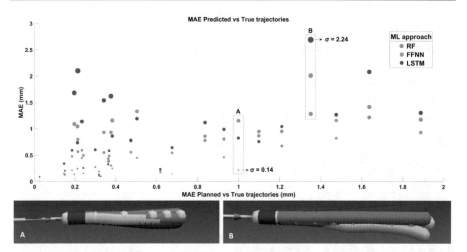

Fig. 3. Prediction accuracy. *Top:* Mean average error (MAE) of predicted trajectories (RF, FFNN, LSTM) with respect to True trajectory. X-axis indicates the MAE of True trajectory with respect to Plan (rigid) trajectory. Size of circle indicates standard deviation (see two examples for reference). *Bottom*: 3D rendering of planned (in white), true (in yellow) and predicted (RF in red, FFNN in green, LSTM in blue) electrode trajectories of two examples highlighted in scatter plot above.

4   Conclusion

We present a novel machine learning regression model to predict local instrument bending from image features. The instrument is modelled as an elastic rod, with 3DOF, that traverses soft tissue, characterised as inhomogeneous and anisotropic. Our method allows for the prediction of orientation and position along the instrument trajectory. The main limitation of our current work is that we study instrument bending in a specific application (SEEG electrode implantation). In future work, we will validate our method in other applications. Additionally, we will integrate our model into a trajectory planning algorithm with the aim of improved pre-operative planning.

Acknowledgements. This publication represents in part independent research commissioned by the Health Innovation Challenge Fund (WT106882), the Wellcome/EPSRC [203145Z/16/Z], and the National Institute for Health Research University College London Hospitals Biomedical Research Centre (NIHR BRC UCLH/UCL High Impact Initiative). We are grateful to the Wolfson Foundation and the Epilepsy Society for supporting the Epilepsy Society MRI scanner. The views expressed in this publication are those of the authors and not necessarily those of the Wellcome Trust or NIHR. Oeslle Lucena thanks FAPESP (2016/18332-8) and FAPESP (2017/23747-5).

References

1. Abolhassani, N., Patel, R., Mehrdad, M.: Needle insertion into soft tissue: a survey. Med. Eng. Phys. **29**(4), 413–431 (2007)
2. Cardoso, M.J., Modat, M., Wolz, R., et al.: Geodesic information flows: spatially-variant graphs and their application to segmentation and fusion. IEEE Trans. Med. Imag. **34**(9), 1976–1988 (2015)
3. Dhollander, T., Raffelt, D., Connelly, A.: Unsupervised 3-tissue response function estimation from single-shell or multi-shell diffusion MR data without a co-registered T1 image. In: ISMRM Workshop on Breaking the Barriers of Diffusion MRI, vol. 5 (2016)
4. Dogdas, B., Shattuck, D.W., Leahy, R.M.: Segmentation of skull and scalp in 3-D human MRI using mathematical morphology. Hum. Brain Mapp. **26**(4), 273–285 (2005)
5. Duriez, C., Guébert, C., Marchal, M., Cotin, S., Grisoni, L.: Interactive Simulation of flexible needle insertions based on constraint models. In: Yang, G.-Z., Hawkes, D., Rueckert, D., Noble, A., Taylor, C. (eds.) MICCAI 2009. LNCS, vol. 5762, pp. 291–299. Springer, Heidelberg (2009). https://doi.org/10.1007/978-3-642-04271-3_36
6. Fritsch, F.N., Carlson, R.E.: Monotone piecewise cubic interpolation. SIAM J. Numer. Anal. **17**(2), 238–246 (1980)
7. Gamboa, J.: Deep Learning for Time-Series Analysis. arXiv preprint. arXiv:1701.01887 (2017)
8. Granados, A., Vakharia, V., Rodionov, R., et al.: Int. J. CARS **13**, 935 (2018). http://doi.org/10.1007/s11548-018-1740-8
9. Hamze, N., Peterlik, I., Cotin, S., Essert, C.: Preoperative trajectory planning for percutaneous procedures in deformable environments. Comput. Med. Imaging Graph. **47**, 16–28 (2016)
10. Jeurissen, B., Tournier, J.D., Dhollander, T., Connelly, A., Sijbers, J.: Multi-tissue constrained spherical deconvolution for improved analysis of multi-shell diffusion MRI data. NeuroImage **103**, 411–426 (2014)
11. de Jong, T.: Needle deflection in tissue. Master's thesis, Delft University of Technology (2015)

12. Kugelstadt, T., Schömer, E.: Position and orientation based cosserat rods. In: Eurographics ACM SIGGRAPH Symposium on Computer Animation, pp. 1–10 (2016)
13. Mancini, M., et al.: Anatomy-constrained automated fibre tract reconstruction for surgery planning: a validation study in language-related white matter tracts. Proc. Int. Soc. Mag. Reson. Med. **26**, 075 (2018)
14. Modat, M., Cash, D.M., Daga, P., et al.: Global image registration using a symmetric block-matching approach. J. of Med. Imag. **1**(2), 024003 (2014)
15. Poulin, P., et al.: Learn to track: deep learning for tractography. In: Descoteaux, M., et al. (eds.) MICCAI 2017. LNCS, vol. 10433, pp. 540–547. Springer, Cham (2017). https://doi.org/10.1007/978-3-319-66182-7_62
16. Raffelt, D., Smith, R., Ridgway, G.R., et al.: Connectivity-based fixel enhancement: whole-brain statistical analysis of diffusion MRI measures in the presence of crossing fibres. NeuroImage. **117**, 40–55 (2015)
17. Roesthuis, R.J., van Veen, Y.R.J., Jahya, A., Misra, S.: Mechanics of needle-tissue interaction. In: IEEE International Conference Intelligent Robots and Systems, pp. 2557–2563 (2011)
18. Sparks, R., Vakharia, V.N., Rodionov, R., et al.: Anatomy-driven multiple trajectory planning (ADMTP) of intracranial electrodes for epilepsy surgery. Int. J. Comput. Assist. Radiol. Surg. **12**(8), 1–11 (2017)
19. Spillmann, J., Harders, M.: Inextensible elastic rods with torsional friction based on Lagrange multipliers. Comput. Anim. Virtual Worlds **19**, 271–281 (2010)
20. Taylor, P.N., Sinha, N., Wang, Y., et al.: The impact of epilepsy surgery on the structural connectome and its relation to outcome. NeuroImage **18**, 202–214 (2018)
21. Tournier, J.D., Calamante, F., Connelly, A.: MRtrix: diffusion tractography in crossing fiber regions. Int. J. Imag. Syst. Technol. **22**(1), 53–66 (2012)
22. Vakharia, V.N., Sparks, R., O'Keeffe, A.G., et al.: Accuracy of intracranial electrode placement for stereoencephalography: a systematic review and meta-analysis. Epilepsia. **58**(6), 921–932 (2017)

Deep Reinforcement Learning for Surgical Gesture Segmentation and Classification

Daochang Liu and Tingting Jiang$^{(\boxtimes)}$

National Engineering Lab for Video Technology,
Cooperative Medianet Innovation Center, School of EECS,
Peking University, Beijing 100871, China
{daochang,ttjiang}@pku.edu.cn

Abstract. Recognition of surgical gesture is crucial for surgical skill assessment and efficient surgery training. Prior works on this task are based on either variant graphical models such as HMMs and CRFs, or deep learning models such as Recurrent Neural Networks and Temporal Convolutional Networks. Most of the current approaches usually suffer from over-segmentation and therefore low segment-level edit scores. In contrast, we present an essentially different methodology by modeling the task as a sequential decision-making process. An intelligent agent is trained using reinforcement learning with hierarchical features from a deep model. Temporal consistency is integrated into our action design and reward mechanism to reduce over-segmentation errors. Experiments on JIGSAWS dataset demonstrate that the proposed method performs better than state-of-the-art methods in terms of the edit score and on par in frame-wise accuracy. Our code will be released later.

Keywords: Surgical gesture segmentation
Surgical gesture classification · Deep reinforcement learning
Time series analysis

1 Introduction

Joint surgical gesture segmentation and classification is fundamental for objective surgical skill assessment and for improving efficiency and quality of surgery training [1]. The goal is to segment robotic kinematic data or video sequence and to classify segmented pieces into surgical gestures, such as *reaching for the needle*, *orienting needle* and *pushing needle through the tissue*, etc.

Variant temporal models have been exploited in prior works on surgical gesture segmentation and classification. One branch of works has been based on hidden Markov models (HMMs) [2–4], differing from each other in how the emission probability is modeled. HMM-based methods assume that gesture label at frame t is only conditioned on previous frame $t-1$, leaving long-term dependency unconsidered. Another branch has been based on conditional random fields (CRFs) [5–7] and their extensions, which obtains the gesture sequence by minimizing an overall energy function. Although these methods capture

© Springer Nature Switzerland AG 2018
A. F. Frangi et al. (Eds.): MICCAI 2018, LNCS 11073, pp. 247–255, 2018.
https://doi.org/10.1007/978-3-030-00937-3_29

temporal patterns by the pairwise potentials in their energy functions, they produce severe over-segmentation and therefore suboptimal segmental edit scores. In recent years, a third branch using deep learning has set new benchmarks for this task. Recurrent neural networks, in particular LSTMs, were applied in [8]. A memory cell is maintained in LSTM to remember and forget action changes over time. [9] proposed a spatiotemporal CNN, in which the spatial component described relationships of objects in the scene, and a long temporal convolutional filter captured how the relationships change temporally. Thereupon, [10, 11] went further and built a hierarchical encoder-decoder network called Temporal Convolutional Network (TCN) composed of long temporal convolutional filters, upsampling/downsampling layers, and normalization layers. In spite of the promising performance improvement achieved, these methods are only driven by frame-wise accuracy due to their cross-entropy training loss.

Unlike prior works, we propose an essentially different deep reinforcement learning approach for joint surgical gesture segmentation and classification, which is driven by both frame-wise accuracy and segment-level edit score. Reinforcement learning has gained remarkable success recently in domains like playing Go [12], Atari games [13], and anatomical landmark detection in medical images [14], etc. However, reinforcement learning has not been applied in surgery gesture segmentation in existing works. We formulate the task as a sequential decision-making process and train an agent to operate in a human-like manner. The agent looks through the surgical data sequence from the beginning, segment the sequence step by step and classify frames simultaneously. To highlight, our agent learns a strategical policy—skim fast in the middle of segments and examine attentively at segment boundaries, which resembles human intelligence. Additionally, current deep learning methods like RNN and TCN handle temporal consistency *implicitly* by memory cells or temporal convolutions. On the contrary, we enforce temporal consistency *explicitly* by the design of action and reward. The reward consists of two terms that guide the agent to high accuracy and high edit score respectively. To combine reinforcement learning with the hierarchical representation learned by deep neural networks, features extracted by TCN are utilized as powerful state representation for the agent. The proposed method is tested on the suturing task of the JIGSAWS dataset [1, 15]. Experiments show that our method outperforms state-of-the-art methods in terms of edit score. In summary, our contributions are three-fold:

- Joint surgical gesture segmentation and classification is formulated, to our best knowledge for the first time, as a sequential decision-making problem using deep reinforcement learning.
- The two evaluation metrics of frame-level accuracy and segment-level edit score are both incorporated into the rewarding mechanism.
- Our method outperforms state-of-the-art methods in terms of edit score while retaining comparable frame-wise accuracy.

2   Preliminary

Reinforcement learning (RL) is a computational approach to decision-making problems with definite goals [16], where an artificial agent learns its policy from

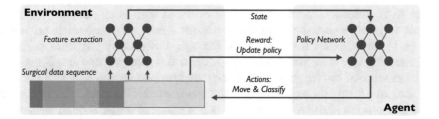

Fig. 1. Overview diagram of the proposed method. An agent perceives the environment, selects an action, and update its policy to maximize future rewards.

interactions with the environment. At each time step, the agent observes the state of environment and selects an action accordingly, which in turn affects the environment. The agent earns a numerical reward for each action and updates its policy to maximize future reward. This sequential decision-making process is formalized as a Markov Decision Process (MDP) [16] $\mathcal{M} := (\mathcal{S}, \mathcal{A}, \mathcal{P}, \mathcal{R}, \gamma)$, where $\mathcal{S}$ is a finite set of states, $\mathcal{A}$ is a finite set of actions, $\mathcal{P} : \mathcal{S} \times \mathcal{A} \times \mathcal{S} \to [0, 1]$ denotes state transition probabilities, $\mathcal{R} : \mathcal{S} \times \mathcal{A} \to \mathbb{R}$ denotes a reward function for each action performed in certain state, and $\gamma \in [0, 1]$ is the discount factor balancing between immediate and long-term reward. The agent learns from experience to optimize its policy $\pi : \mathcal{S} \times \mathcal{A} \to [0, 1]$, which is stochastic in general. The goal is to maximize discounted future reward accumulated from current time step to the end of learning episode.

3   Proposed Method

The input to our model is a data sequence $\{x_t\}$, which can be either visual features extracted from surgery video frames or kinematic data frames collected from surgical robots, together with its ground truth gesture label sequence $\{y_t\}$. Each $x_t \in \mathbb{R}^{n_x}$ and each $y_t \in \{1, 2, \ldots, n_y\}$, where n_x is the dimensions of features, n_y is the number of gesture classes, and $1 \leq t \leq n_t$. Note that the number of frames n_t may differ between each data sequence.

We propose to model joint surgical gesture segmentation and classification as a sequential decision-making problem, illustrated in Fig. 1. An agent is built to interact with the visual or kinematic data sequence, i.e., the environment. Initially positioned at the beginning of data sequence, the agent selects a proper step size and moves forward at each time step, concurrently classifying frames stepped over. Following the standard paradigm of reinforcement learning, we formalize the task as a Markov Decision Process. The action, the state and the reward of our proposed MDP model are detailed as follows.

Action. The action of the proposed model includes two subactions, which are to decide how far to move forward and to choose which class label to give. The action set is defined as:

$$\mathcal{A} := \mathcal{K} \times \mathcal{C} \tag{1}$$

where $\mathcal{K}$ represents a predefined set of optional step sizes, and $\mathcal{C}$ represents the set of gesture classes. From the start, the agent keeps selecting an action pair (k, c) from action set $\mathcal{A}$ to walk through and classify the data sequence until reaching the end. Step size set $\mathcal{K}$ is defined to contain one small step and one large step: $\mathcal{K} := \{k_s, k_l\}$. This binary design enables the agent to alter its step size based on the confidence in the gesture label to give. The agent can adopt the smaller step when the state is not discriminative enough such as at the boundaries between gestures, and adopt the larger step otherwise. At each action, the k frames stepped over by the agent are labeled with the same class c, explicitly enforcing temporal consistency.

State. Raw features $\{x_t\}$ are challenging for the agent to fully understand the surgical activity. Therefore we define the state to be a combination of high-level representation and other auxiliary information, which assists the agent to make a better decision. We utilize TCN [10, 11] to extract such high-level representation from raw features.

The state observed at frame t is the concatenation of current and future feature vectors extracted by TCN, gesture transition probabilities from a language and duration model [17], and a one-hot vector, which is formalized below:

$$s^t := (s_{tcn}^t, s_{tcn}^{t+k_s}, s_{tcn}^{t+k_l}, s_{trans}, s_{hot}) \tag{2}$$

where $s_{tcn}^t, s_{tcn}^{t+k_s}, s_{tcn}^{t+k_l}$ are respectively TCN features at the current frame, k_s frames later and k_l frames later, s_{trans} are probabilities of transition into each gesture computed from a statistical language model, $s_{hot} \in \{0, 1\}^{n_y}$ is a one-hot vector such that the gesture class given by last action is 1 and all others are 0.

Statistical Language and Duration Model. Similar to [17], we use a statistical model to describe the length and contextual pattern of gestures. Specifically, we use Gaussian distributions for gesture durations and a bigram language model for gesture transitions, assuming the gesture class depends only on one previous class. The statistical model is formalized as:

$$p(i \mid j, l) := \begin{cases} \frac{N(j,i)}{N(j)} \cdot CDF_j(l) & \text{if } i \neq j \\ 1 - CDF_j(l) & \text{if } i = j \end{cases} \tag{3}$$

where $p(i \mid j, l)$ is the probability of transition from gesture j to gesture i given l—how many frames the agent has stayed in gesture j, $N(j, i)$ and $N(j)$ are respectively occurrence counts of ordered gesture pair (j, i) and gesture j alone in training data, CDF_j stands for the cumulative distribution function of a Gaussian distribution modeling the length of gesture j. The Gaussian distributions are parameterized by maximum likelihood estimation using training data. Then s_{trans} is set as the probabilities of transition to each gesture, given the gesture class of last action and how long the agent has stayed in this gesture.

Reward. The reward is numerical feedback for each action performed by the agent. Given action pair (k, c) performed at frame t, the reward in our MDP model is designed as:

$$r(s^t, (k, c)) := \alpha k - \sum_{t'=t}^{t+k-1} \mathbb{1}(y_{t'} \neq c) \qquad (4)$$

where the first term encourages the agent to adopt the larger step, the second term penalizes the errors caused by this action, and α is a weight parameter balancing the two terms. The two evaluation metrics of accuracy and edit score are both incorporated in this reward inherently. While the second term serves as straightforward guidance for the agent to achieve high frame-wise accuracy, the first term is crucial for a good edit score at segment-level. Preference for the larger step can mitigate the jittering between gestures and therefore can reduce over-segmentation errors, which is validated in our experiments section.

Policy Learning. We use a multilayer perceptron (MLP) to model the policy, whose input layer has the same number of units as the dimensions of the state, and output layer has the same number of units as the dimensions of action space. The policy network takes environment state as input and output a distribution over action space. With the MDP process well defined, any standard reinforcement learning method can be applied to policy learning. We choose Trust Region Policy Optimization (TRPO) [18] since it is theoretically guaranteed to improve the policy monotonically.

4   Experiments

We evaluate the proposed method on JIGSAWS [1,15], a public benchmark dataset recorded using the *da Vinci* surgical system. We use the video and kinematic data from the suturing task, which contains 39 sequences performed by eight subjects with varying skill levels. For video data, we use features extracted from each frame image by a spatial CNN [9], which is consistent with TCN [11]. As for kinematic data, we pick the same subset of features as in [11], which are position, velocity and gripper angle for both slave manipulators.

Experiments Setup. The standardized leave-one-user-out (LOUO) evaluation setup of JIGSAWS is followed in our experiments. Trials performed by a single user are left out as testing set while all remaining trials are used as training set, resulting in 8-fold cross-validation. Since our RL based method is inherently stochastic, we train the TCN for state feature extraction five times, train the agent using TRPO three times, and test on each data sequence ten times, with $5 * 3 * 10 = 150$ runs in total. Results are averaged over these 150 runs. We also include an ablation study to measure the impact of each component of the state.

We include three evaluation metrics: accuracy, edit score, and F1 score. Accuracy is the percentage of correctly labeled frames, measuring the performance at the frame level. Edit score is the normalized Levenshtein distance between predicted gesture sequence and ground truth, measuring the performance at the segment level, which is between 0 and 100 (the higher the better). F1 score is introduced for this task in [10]. Each predicted gesture segment is considered to be true or false positive according to whether its Intersection over Union (IoU) with

Table 1. Results on the suturing task of JIGSAWS. F1@{10,25,50} stands for F1 score with the IoU threshold set to 10%, 25% and 50%. TCN* stands for our re-implemented version of TCN with several minor changes for state feature extraction. The four entries at the bottom are results of our RL method with partial state or full state.

Method	Video			Kinematic		
	Acc	Edit	F1@{10,25,50}	Acc	Edit	F1@{10,25,50}
SD-SDL [3]	-	-	-	78.6	83.3	-
Bidir LSTM [8]	-	-	-	83.3	81.1	-
LC-SC-CRF [7]	-	-	-	**83.4**	76.8	-
Seg-ST-CNN [9]	74.7	66.6	-	-	-	-
TCN [11]	81.4	83.1	-	79.6	85.8	-
TCN*	**81.71**	86.63	91.0, 89.5, 82.0	82.57	86.58	90.5, 89.3, **82.4**
RL (no tcn)	32.35	15.04	13.1, 6.1, 3.4	32.90	17.21	14.8, 7.5, 4.6
RL (no future)	80.84	81.58	87.5, 85.6, 77.4	81.48	81.07	86.5, 84.6, 77.4
RL (no trans)	81.32	87.30	91.5, 90.1, 81.8	82.06	87.12	90.7, 89.1, 81.8
RL (full)	81.43	**87.96**	**92.0**, **90.5**, **82.2**	82.07	**87.86**	**91.1**, **89.5**, 82.3

respect to the corresponding ground truth segment is above a threshold. Then F1 score is the harmonic mean of the precision and recall: $F1 = \frac{2*precision*recall}{precision+recall}$.

Implementation Details. The proposed model is implemented with Python and *OpenAI Baselines* library [19]. The policy network is of one hidden layer and 64 hidden units. We set k_s to be the minimum gesture length in training set, and k_l to be the minimum of mean gesture lengths for each class, which are 4 and 21 frames for example. The discount factor γ and the reward weight α are set to 0.9 and 0.1 respectively in experiments. Besides, we re-implement the TCN for state feature extraction using PyTorch with several minor changes, which can be regarded as a baseline for our RL method. The convolutional layers in the decoder of TCN are replaced with transposed convolutional layers. And due to the data is highly imbalanced, we use weighted cross-entropy as the training loss of TCN instead. Activations before the last fully-connected layer are used as state features, which is of 32 dimensions. Our code will be released later.

Result. Experiment results on both video and kinematic data are shown in Table 1. Our RL based approach is compared to the original TCN, the modified TCN and several other recent works. All results of prior works are excerpted from [11]. Compared to existing works, the proposed method achieves higher edit score and F1 score at a negligible cost of accuracy. We present the result of ablation study on the state design as well. Each of following components is removed from the state to justify its necessity: (1) all TCN features (2) TCN features at future frames (3) transition probabilities from the statistical model. Results show that all these components are required to achieve the best performance. And the high-level representation extracted by TCN is the most important one.

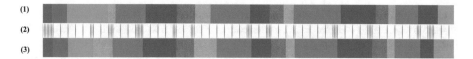

Fig. 2. Prediction example: (1) ground truth sequence (2) step history of the agent (3) predicted sequence. Each color corresponds to a gesture. Our agent learns to skim fast in the middle of gestures and examine cautiously at the boundaries.

Table 2. Experiments on step size

Step Size	Video		Kinematic	
	Acc	Edit	Acc	Edit
1	81.65	80.09	82.31	80.12
2	81.67	83.46	82.24	82.47
4	81.53	86.04	82.16	85.35
8	80.95	87.56	81.91	87.27
16	79.12	88.28	79.81	88.13
32	72.94	84.05	72.86	84.04
4 & 21	81.43	87.96	82.07	87.86

A prediction example produced by our agent is provided in Fig. 2. We plot the history of steps of the agent, finding it interesting that the agent tends to select the larger step in the middle of gestures and the smaller step at the boundaries. Such behavior pattern verifies our intuitions on the action and reward design.

Does the Larger Step Really Benefit? To further validate our reward design that encourages the larger step, we complete a comparative experiment on the step size. We set the step size set $\mathcal{K}$ to contain only a single option, and set this option to 1, 2, 4, 8, 16, 32 frames. From the result in Table 2, the larger step the agent can take, the higher edit score is achieved unless the step is excessively large. But larger steps such as 8, 16 and 32 degrade the accuracy considerably. Our binary design of step sizes achieves the promising result on both metrics.

5 Conclusion and Future Work

In this work, we proposed a novel method based on deep reinforcement learning for joint surgical gesture segmentation and classification. An artificial agent is trained to act in a human-like manner. By the state, the action and the reward formulation, temporal consistency is explicitly stressed and over-segmentation errors are reduced. The proposed method outperforms the state-of-the-art on JIGSAWS dataset in terms of edit score, while retaining comparable frame-wise accuracy. Future work can be made in following two aspects: (1) developing the step size options into a continuous set (2) combining the state feature extraction network and the policy network for an end-to-end model.

Acknowledgement. This work was partially supported by National Basic Research Program of China (973 Program) under contract 2015CB351803 and the Natural Science Foundation of China under contracts 61572042, 61390514, 61527804. We also acknowledge the high-performance computing platform of Peking University for providing computational resources. Thanks to Dingquan Li for his valuable comments and inspiration.

References

1. Ahmidi, N., et al.: A dataset and benchmarks for segmentation and recognition of gestures in robotic surgery. IEEE Trans. Biomed. Eng. **64**(9), 2025–2041 (2017)
2. Tao, L., Elhamifar, E., Khudanpur, S., Hager, G.D., Vidal, R.: Sparse hidden Markov Models for Surgical gesture classification and skill evaluation. In: Abolmaesumi, P., Joskowicz, L., Navab, N., Jannin, P. (eds.) IPCAI 2012. LNCS, vol. 7330, pp. 167–177. Springer, Heidelberg (2012). https://doi.org/10.1007/978-3-642-30618-1_17
3. Sefati, S., Cowan, N.J., Vidal, R.: Learning shared, discriminative dictionaries for surgical gesture segmentation and classification. In: MICCAI Workshop: M2CAI, vol. 4 (2015)
4. Varadarajan, B., Reiley, C., Lin, H., Khudanpur, S., Hager, G.: Data-derived models for segmentation with application to surgical assessment and training. In: Yang, G.-Z., Hawkes, D., Rueckert, D., Noble, A., Taylor, C. (eds.) MICCAI 2009. LNCS, vol. 5761, pp. 426–434. Springer, Heidelberg (2009). https://doi.org/10.1007/978-3-642-04268-3_53
5. Tao, L., Zappella, L., Hager, G.D., Vidal, R.: Surgical gesture segmentation and recognition. In: Mori, K., Sakuma, I., Sato, Y., Barillot, C., Navab, N. (eds.) MICCAI 2013. LNCS, vol. 8151, pp. 339–346. Springer, Heidelberg (2013). https://doi.org/10.1007/978-3-642-40760-4_43
6. Lea, C., Hager, G.D., Vidal, R.: An improved model for segmentation and recognition of fine-grained activities with application to surgical training tasks. In: WACV, pp. 1123–1129. IEEE (2015)
7. Lea, C., Vidal, R., Hager, G.D.: Learning convolutional action primitives for fine-grained action recognition. In: ICRA, pp. 1642–1649. IEEE (2016)
8. DiPietro, R., et al.: Recognizing surgical activities with recurrent neural networks. In: Ourselin, S., Joskowicz, L., Sabuncu, M.R., Unal, G., Wells, W. (eds.) MICCAI 2016. LNCS, vol. 9900, pp. 551–558. Springer, Cham (2016). https://doi.org/10.1007/978-3-319-46720-7_64
9. Lea, C., Reiter, A., Vidal, R., Hager, G.D.: Segmental spatiotemporal CNNs for fine-grained action segmentation. In: Leibe, B., Matas, J., Sebe, N., Welling, M. (eds.) ECCV 2016. LNCS, vol. 9907, pp. 36–52. Springer, Cham (2016). https://doi.org/10.1007/978-3-319-46487-9_3
10. Lea, C., Flynn, M.D., Vidal, R., Reiter, A., Hager, G.D.: Temporal convolutional networks for action segmentation and detection. In: CVPR (2017)
11. Lea, C., Vidal, R., Reiter, A., Hager, G.D.: Temporal convolutional networks: a unified approach to action segmentation. In: Hua, G., Jégou, H. (eds.) ECCV 2016. LNCS, vol. 9915, pp. 47–54. Springer, Cham (2016). https://doi.org/10.1007/978-3-319-49409-8_7
12. Silver, D., et al.: Mastering the game of go with deep neural networks and tree search. Nature **529**(7587), 484–489 (2016)

13. Mnih, V., et al.: Human-level control through deep reinforcement learning. Nature **518**(7540), 529 (2015)
14. Ghesu, F.C., Georgescu, B., Mansi, T., Neumann, D., Hornegger, J., Comaniciu, D.: An artificial agent for anatomical landmark detection in medical images. In: Ourselin, S., Joskowicz, L., Sabuncu, M.R., Unal, G., Wells, W. (eds.) MICCAI 2016. LNCS, vol. 9902, pp. 229–237. Springer, Cham (2016). https://doi.org/10. 1007/978-3-319-46726-9_27
15. Gao, Y., et al.: JHU-ISI gesture and skill assessment working set (JIGSAWS): a surgical activity dataset for human motion modeling. In: MICCAI Workshop: M2CAI, vol. 3, p. 3 (2014)
16. Sutton, R.S., Barto, A.G.: Reinforcement learning: An introduction. MIT press, Cambridge (1998)
17. Richard, A., Gall, J.: Temporal action detection using a statistical language model. In: CVPR, pp. 3131–3140 (2016)
18. Schulman, J., Levine, S., Abbeel, P., Jordan, M., Moritz, P.: Trust region policy optimization. In: International Conference on Machine Learning, pp. 1889–1897 (2015)
19. Dhariwal, P., et al.: OpenAI Baselines (2017). https://github.com/openai/ baselines

Automated Performance Assessment in Transoesophageal Echocardiography with Convolutional Neural Networks

Evangelos B. Mazomenos[1]([✉]), Kamakshi Bansal[1], Bruce Martin[3], Andrew Smith[3], Susan Wright[2], and Danail Stoyanov[1]([✉])

[1] UCL Wellcome/EPSRC Centre for Interventional and Surgical Sciences, Department of Computer Science, University College London, London, UK
{e.mazomenos,danail.stoyanov}@ucl.ac.uk
[2] St George's University Hospitals, NHS Foundation Trust, London, UK
[3] St Bartholomew's Hospital, NHS Foundation Trust, London, UK

Abstract. Transoesophageal echocardiography (TEE) is a valuable diagnostic and monitoring imaging modality. Proper image acquisition is essential for diagnosis, yet current assessment techniques are solely based on manual expert review. This paper presents a supervised deep learning framework for automatically evaluating and grading the quality of TEE images. To obtain the necessary dataset, 38 participants of varied experience performed TEE exams with a high-fidelity virtual reality (VR) platform. Two Convolutional Neural Network (CNN) architectures, AlexNet and VGG, structured to perform regression, were finetuned and validated on manually graded images from three evaluators. Two different scoring strategies, a criteria-based percentage and an overall general impression, were used. The developed CNN models estimate the average score with a root mean square accuracy ranging between $84\% - 93\%$, indicating the ability to replicate expert valuation. Proposed strategies for automated TEE assessment can have a significant impact on the training process of new TEE operators, providing direct feedback and facilitating the development of the necessary dexterous skills.

Keywords: Automated skill assessment
Transoesophageal echocardiography · Convolutional Neural Networks

1 Introduction

Transoesophageal echocardiography (TEE) is the standard for anaesthesia management and outcome evaluation in cardiovascular interventions. It is also used extensively for monitoring critically ill patients in intensive care. The success of the procedure is chiefly dependent on the acquisition of appropriate US views

© Springer Nature Switzerland AG 2018
A. F. Frangi et al. (Eds.): MICCAI 2018, LNCS 11073, pp. 256–264, 2018.
https://doi.org/10.1007/978-3-030-00937-3_30

that allow for a thorough hemodynamic evaluation to be conducted. To capture high-quality TEE images, practitioners must possess refined psychomotor abilities and advanced hand-eye coordination. Both require rigorous training and practice.

To facilitate the education of new interventionalists, standardize reporting and quality, accreditation organisations have defined a set of practice guidelines, for performing a comprehensive TEE exam [5,6]. Nevertheless, training is hindered because performance evaluation is, almost exclusively, carried out through expert supervision. Typically, senior medical personnel grade TEE exams and review logbooks, a laborious process that requires significant amount of time. As a result, trainees rarely receive immediate feedback. Performance evaluation is a key element in interventional medicine and alternative, preferably automated, methods for evaluating TEE competency are necessary [14]. So far, objective assessment in TEE is focused exclusively on the kinematic analysis of the US probe with various motion parameters found to be indicative of the level of operational expertise [9,10]. Although these are important findings, probe kinematic information is not available in clinical settings and only captured in simulation systems. Recent studies emphasise the benefits of virtual reality (VR) simulators that offer a risk-free environment where trainees can practice repeatedly at the their own convenience [2]. Evidence of performance improvement after training on VR systems, as well as skill retention and transferability have been reported [1,3,4,11,13]. Incorporating performance evaluation and structured feedback, will allow further use of VR platforms for training and assessment.

In this work, we introduce the use of Convolutional Neural Networks (CNNs) for the automated evaluation of acquired TEE images. CNNs have found many applications in medical imaging and computer-assisted surgery [8], but this is the first time they are applied to skills assessment. We aim to generate high-level features in order to develop a system capable of assigning TEE performance scores, essentially replicating expert evaluation. We generated a dataset of 16060 simulated TEE images from participants of varied experience and use it to retrain two CNN architectures (Alexnet, VGG), converted to perform regression. Three reviewers provided ground truth labels by blindly grading the images with two different manual scores. Tested on a set of 2596 images, the developed CNN architectures estimated the average reviewers' score with a root mean square error (RMSE) ranging from $7\% - 14\%$. This level of accuracy, which is near the resolution of the average scores from the three evaluators, highlights the potential of CNN algorithms for refined performance evaluation.

2 Methods

2.1 Dataset Generation

We experimented using the HeartWorks TEE simulation platform, (Inventive Medical, Ltd, London, U.K.) a high-fidelity VR simulator that emulates realistic exam settings (Fig. 1). Synthetic US images are generated based on an anatomically accurate cardiac model, illustrated in Fig. 1b, that is deformable to mimic a

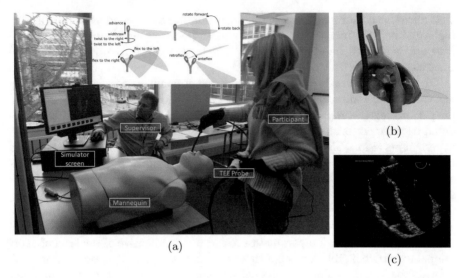

(a)

(b)

(c)

Fig. 1. (a) The HeartWorks simulator, inset the US probe movements; (b) The heart model, the probe and US scanning field; (c) The simulated TEE image

beating heart. A detector on the probe's tip extracts the position and orientation of the US scanning field which are then used to graphically render the 2D US slice (Fig. 1c) from the 3D model. The data collection study consisted of a single TEE exam in which participants had to capture 10 US views, shown in Fig. 2 in a specific sequence. The selected views are a subset of the 20 suggested views recommended by ASE/SCA [6] and include planes from every depth window of the TEE exam (mid-esophageal, transgastric and deep-transgastric)). Experiments were performed under supervision by a consultant anaesthetist that introduced the study and relayed the sequence of views. For capturing and storing data the participant used a foot-pedal to generate a full-HD image and a short video ($\sim 1.5s$) of the imaged US plane. Each video contained 44 frames.

In total, 38 participants of varied experience performed the experiments. The population included accredited anaesthetists having performed more than 500 exams, less experienced practitioners and trainees in the early stage of their residency. Participants were allowed time to familiarise themselves with the setup and the simulator. Manual scoring was blindly performed by three expert anaesthetists based solely on the acquired videos/images. Each view was assessed with two distinct image quality metrics. The first metric is a criteria-based score evaluated on a predetermined checklist, of which each item was assigned a binary value (0-not met, 1-met). The checklists for two of the views are depicted in Table 1 and are derived following the latest ASE/SCA imaging guidelines for each view [6]. This technique broadly evaluates three attributes, the correct angulation of the US probe in each view, the presence/visibility of specific heart tissue and the proper positioning of the probe in the oesophageal lumen. The number of items varied for different views so did the maximum score. The percentage of

1: ME4C (TV)   2: ME2C   3: ME AV SAX   4: TG mid SAX   5: ME RV inflow-outflow

6:ME AV LAX   7: TG2C   8: ME4C (LV)   9:dTG LAX   10: ME MV commis

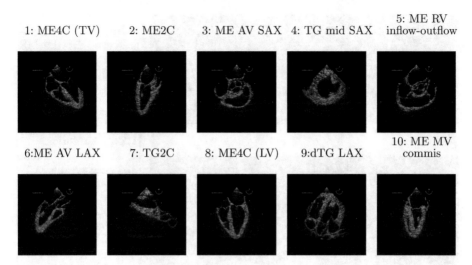

Fig. 2. The sequence of the 10 TEE views used in the study: 1: Mid-Esophageal 4-Chamber (centred at tricuspid valve), 2: Mid-Esophageal 2-Chamber, 3: Mid-Esophageal Aortic Valve Short-Axis, 4: Transgastric Mid-Short-Axis, 5: Mid-Esophageal Right Ventricle inflow-outflow, 6: Mid-Esophageal Aortic Valve Long-Axis, 7: Transgastric 2-Chamber, 8: Mid-Esophageal 4-Chamber (centred at left ventricle), 9: Deep Transgastric Long-Axis, 10: Mid-Esophageal Mitral Commissural.

criteria (CP) met over the total number was used to provide a uniform measure among all views. The second score is a general impression (GI) assessment of the US video/image scored on a 0–4 scale, which assess the overall quality of the acquired image. Grades from the three evaluators were averaged to obtain a single mean score per US view for each volunteer. As expected the two scores are highly correlated ($\rho \sim 0.93$). Inter-rater variability was independently evaluated for each view, using the interclass correlation coefficient (ICC) and Krippendorff's Alpha (KA). Both metrics show very good agreement between the three evaluators with ICC ~ 0.9 and KA ~ 0.8 for all views.

Figure 3 illustrates two examples in the opposite ends of the quality spectrum from views 3 and 7. The average quality scores are given inset and we annotated the elements in the images that satisfy the criteria in the checklist of each view, provided in Table 1. The images on the left are of poor quality and only meet a small number of the checklists' items. For example the top left ME AV SAX image has the correct probe rotation and visualises the three cusps of the aortic valve. It fails to meet the rest of the criteria. The bottom left image of the TG2C view, only achieved correct probe angulation, but because of inadequate positioning fails to satisfy the rest of the criteria. Consequently, both CP and GI scores are low, since both images on the left side are of unacceptable quality. Images on the right side are examples of ideally imaged views fully satisfying the respective checklists and achieving full marks in both metrics.

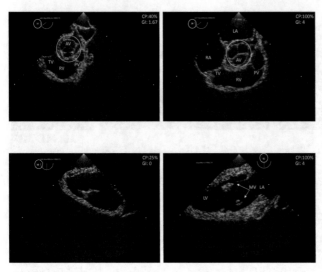

Table 1. The checklists used for the ME AV SAX (View 3) and TG 2C (View 7) TEE views.

ME AV SAX (3)
1) 30°-45°rotation
2) AV centred in screen
3) 3 cusps visible
4) Imaging plane at level of leaflet tips
5) Probe tip appropriately behind LA

TG 2C (7)
1) 85°-95°rotation
2) LA and LV both visible
3) MV visible on right side of screen
4) Post. and Ant. MV leaflets seen

Fig. 3. Scoring examples for Views 3 and 7, from different participants, with annotated structures of importance. Left images are scored poorly whereas right images obtain excellent marks. **Top row, View 3** - LA: left atrium, RA: right atrium, TV: tricuspid valve, RV: right ventricle, AV: aortic valve, PV: pulmonary valve, circle indicates visibility of AV cusps; **Bottom row, View 7** - LV: left ventricle, LA: left atrium, MV: mitral valve and arrows showing leaflets

We recorded 365 video sequences from the 38 participants with 15 views failing to store properly. For our investigation, we extracted all 16060 (i.e. 365×44) frames from the stored videos and used the mean manual scores as labels. All frames from a given video were labelled with the average score of that view on the premise that reviewers assigned their grades after watching the short videos so we consider that the mark equally represents all frames. No probe movement takes place in the videos, only the simulated beating of the heart model. Therefore the qualitative attributes of the stored view are the same in all frames. We divide the dataset using the $80\% - 20\%$ rule for training and testing, considering the total number of volunteers. Frames from 32 participants were designated for training (13464) and from 6 for testing (2596).

2.2 CNN Architectures

We opted to develop CNN models for performing a regression task and train them to learn to estimate the performance score as a single continuous variable; $CP \in \{0, \ldots, 100\}$, $GI \in \{0, \ldots 4\}$. Since the checklists' criteria and their number are different among views, it was not feasible to structure and train a single model for evaluating individual criteria for all views. This would require

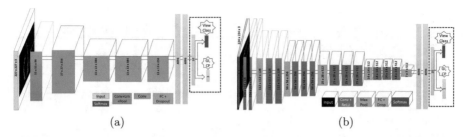

(a)   (b)

Fig. 4. The two networks (a) Alexnet, (b) VGG, developed for the TEE score estimation task. The customized output stage with the added FC layers and the softmax activation for classification is enclosed in the boxes.

a non-efficient approach with separate sub-models per view. Hence a single CP score per view was computed and estimated. We experimented with two established CNN architectures namely, Alexnet and VGG, originally built to perform image classification tasks [7,12]. We repurpose them by restructuring their output stage and consider 10 available classes, one for each TEE view. The final fully-connected (FC) layer of both CNNs is resized with a dimension of 10. One additional FC layer with output size $d = 1$ and linear activation is added to complete the regression operation and estimate the score. For classifying the input to one of the TEE views, softmax activation is applied after the FC layer with $d = 10$. Effectively we structure our network so that it can be trained to both estimate the performance scores and recognize the corresponding view of the input. Figure 4 illustrates the two customised architectures with the added layers.

3   Experimentation and Results

CNN models were implemented with the TensorFlow framework. The training dataset was randomized and images were resized from 1200×1000, to 227×227 for Alexnet and 224×224 for VGG. Batches of 128 (Alexnet) and 64 (VGG) were used. The mean square error was set as the loss function and gradient descent optimization with adaptive moment estimation was performed with a learning rate of 0.001. Both networks were initialized with publicly available weights from the ILSVRC challenge [7,12], apart from the additional dense layers we introduced, which were assigned random weights and trained from scratch. Backpropagation was used to update the weights. The two architectures were independently trained for each performance metric and convergence was achieved after 2 K iterations for Alexnet and after 12 K for VGG. The models were also trained to classify images to their respective view, achieving over 98% accuracy. Table 2 lists overall RMSE results and the RMSE on score intervals, from estimating the two image quality scores on the 2596 testing images. Both models perform adequately but, owing to its denser structure, VGG outperforms Alexnet significantly and has smaller error variability, providing excellent accuracy for

Table 2. Overall and interval RMSE results of the developed networks.

Criteria percentage score (CP)

Network	$CP < 55\%$	$55\% \le CP < 75\%$	$75\% \le CP < 90\%$	$CP \ge 90\%$	Total
Alexnet	20.38	14.59	18.9	12.1	16.23
VGG	5.55	5	11.8	5.34	7.28

General impression score (GI)

Network	$GI < 1.8$	$1.8 \le GI < 2.8$	$2.8 \le GI < 3.8$	$GI > 3.8$	Total
Alexnet	0.65	0.44	0.84	1.13	0.83
VGG	0.42	0.31	0.46	0.45	0.42

both metrics. To obtain a single score per video, similarly to the three evaluators, we grouped the predictions of the frames from the same video and averaged them. The per video results, for 59 videos from the 6 testing participants (one video was not captured) are shown in Fig. 5. The RMSE of the grouped results is lower for both networks, that also give consistent estimations in frames from the same video, indicated by low standard deviation values ($\sigma_{CP} \simeq 3.5$, $\sigma_{GI} \simeq 0.2$).

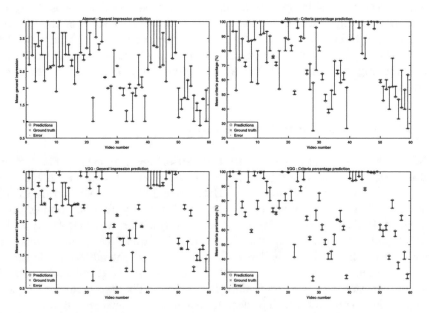

Fig. 5. Grouped estimation results per testing video. RMSE and average σ values: (top) Alexnet − CP: 15.78 ($\sigma = 3.34$), GI: 0.8 ($\sigma = 0.22$); (bottom) VGG − CP: 5.2 ($\sigma = 3.55$), GI: 0.33 ($\sigma = 0.23$)

4   Conclusions

In this article we demonstrated the applicability of CNNs architectures for automated quality evaluation of TEE images. We collected a rich dataset of 16060 simulated images graded with two manual scores (CP, GI) assigned by three evaluators. We experimented with two established CNN models, restructured to perform regression and trained these to estimate the manual scores. Validated on 2596 images, the developed models estimate the manual scores with high accuracy. Alexnet achieved an overall RMSE of 16.23% and 0.83, while the denser VGG had better performance achieving 7.28% and 0.42 for CP and GI respectively. These very promising outcomes indicate the potential of CNN methods for automated skill assessment in image-guided surgical and diagnostic procedures. Future work will focus on augmenting the CNN models and investigating their translational ability in evaluating the quality of real TEE images.

Acknowledgements. The authors would like to thank all participants who volunteered for this study. The work was supported by funding from the EPSRC (EP/N013220/1, EP/N027078/1, NS/A000027/1) and Wellcome (NS/A000050/1).

References

1. Arntfield, R., et al.: Focused transesophageal echocardiography for emergency physicians-description and results from simulation training of a structured four-view examination. Crit. Ultrasound J. **7**(1), 27 (2015)
2. Bose, R.R., et al.: Utility of a transesophageal echocardiographic simulator as a teaching tool. J. Cardiothorac. Vasc. Anesth. **25**(2), 212–215 (2011)
3. Damp, J., et al.: Effects of transesophageal echocardiography simulator training on learning and performance in cardiovascular medicine fellows. J. Am. Soc. Echocardiogr. **26**(12), 1450–1456 (2013)
4. Ferrero, N.A., et al.: Simulator training enhances resident performance in transesophageal echocardiography. Anesthesiology **120**(1), 149–159 (2014)
5. Flachskampf, F., et al.: Recommendations for transoesophageal echocardiography: update 2010. Eur. J. Echocardiogr. **11**(7), 557–576 (2010)
6. Hahn, R.T., et al.: Guidelines for performing a comprehensive transesophageal echocardiographic examination: recommendations from the American society of echocardiography and the society of cardiovascular anesthesiologists. J. Am. Soc. Echocardiogr. **26**(9), 921–964 (2013)
7. Krizhevsky, A., et al.: Imagenet classification with deep convolutional neural networks. In: Pereira, F., Burges, C.J.C., Bottou, L., Weinberger, K.Q. (eds.) NIPS 2012, pp. 1097–1105. Curran Associates Inc., USA (2012)
8. Litjens, G., et al.: A survey on deep learning in medical image analysis. Med. Image. Anal. **42**, 60–88 (2017)
9. Matyal, R., et al.: Manual skill acquisition during transesophageal echocardiography simulator training of cardiology fellows: a kinematic assessment. J. Cardiothorac. Vasc. Anesth. **29**(6), 1504–1510 (2015)
10. Mazomenos, E.B., et al.: Motion-based technical skills assessment in transoesophageal echocardiography. In: Zheng, G., Liao, H., Jannin, P., Cattin, P., Lee, S.-L. (eds.) MIAR 2016. LNCS, vol. 9805, pp. 96–103. Springer, Cham (2016). https://doi.org/10.1007/978-3-319-43775-0_9

11. Prat, G., et al.: The use of computerized echocardiographic simulation improves the learning curve for transesophageal hemodynamic assessment in critically ill patients. Ann. Intensive Care **6**(1), 27 (2016)
12. Simonyan, K., Zisserman, A.: Very deep convolutional networks for large-scale image recognition (2014). CoRR abs/1409.1556
13. Sohmer, B., et al.: Transesophageal echocardiography simulation is an effective tool in teaching psychomotor skills to novice echocardiographers. Can. J. Anaesth. **61**(3), 235–241 (2014)
14. Song, H., et al.: Innovative transesophageal echocardiography training and competency assessment for Chinese anesthesiologists: role of transesophageal echocardiography simulation training. Curr. Opin. Anaesthesiol. **25**(6), 686–691 (2012)

DeepPhase: Surgical Phase Recognition in CATARACTS Videos

Odysseas Zisimopoulos[1]([✉]), Evangello Flouty[1], Imanol Luengo[1],
Petros Giataganas[1], Jean Nehme[1], Andre Chow[1], and Danail Stoyanov[1,2]

[1] Digital Surgery, Kinosis, Ltd., 230 City Road, EC1V 2QY London, UK
odysszis@gmail.com
[2] University College London, Gower Street, WC1E 6BT London, UK

Abstract. Automated surgical workflow analysis and understanding can assist surgeons to standardize procedures and enhance post-surgical assessment and indexing, as well as, interventional monitoring. Computer-assisted interventional (CAI) systems based on video can perform workflow estimation through surgical instruments' recognition while linking them to an ontology of procedural phases. In this work, we adopt a deep learning paradigm to detect surgical instruments in cataract surgery videos which in turn feed a surgical phase inference recurrent network that encodes temporal aspects of phase steps within the phase classification. Our models present comparable to state-of-the-art results for surgical tool detection and phase recognition with accuracies of 99 and 78% respectively.

Keywords: Surgical vision · Instrument detection
Surgical workflow · Deep learning · Surgical data science

1 Introduction

Surgical workflow analysis can potentially optimise teamwork and communication within the operating room to reduce surgical errors and improve resource usage [1]. The development of cognitive computer-assisted intervention (CAI) systems aims to provide solutions for automated workflow tasks such as procedural segmentation into surgical phases/steps allowing to predict the next steps and provide useful preparation information (*e.g.* instruments) or early warnings messages for enhanced intraoperative OR team collaboration and safety. Workflow analysis could also assist surgeons with automatic report generation and optimized scheduling as well as off-line video indexing for educational purposes. The challenge is to perform workflow recognition automatically such that it does not pose a significant burden on clinicians' time.

Early work on automated phase recognition monitored the surgeon's hands and tool presence [2,3] as it is reasonable to assume that specific tools are used to carry out specific actions during an operation. Instrument usage can be used to

© Springer Nature Switzerland AG 2018
A. F. Frangi et al. (Eds.): MICCAI 2018, LNCS 11073, pp. 265–272, 2018.
https://doi.org/10.1007/978-3-030-00937-3_31

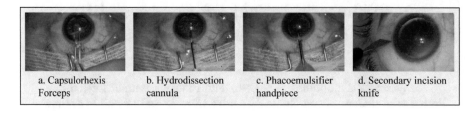

| a. Capsulorhexis | b. Hydrodissection | c. Phacoemulsifier | d. Secondary incision |
| Forceps | cannula | handpiece | knife |

Fig. 1. Examples of tools in the training set and their corresponding labels.

train random forests models [4] or conditional random fields [5] for phase recognition. More recently, visual features have been explicitly used [6,7]; however, these features were hand-crafted which limits their robustness [8]. The emergence of deep learning techniques for image classification [9] and semantic segmentation [10] provide a desirable solution for more robust systems allowing for automated feature extraction and have been applied in medical imaging tasks in domains such as laparoscopy [11] and cataract surgery [12]. EndoNet, a deep learning model for single and multi task tool and phase recognition in laparoscopic procedures was introduced in [11] relying on AlexNet as a feature extractor for tool recognition and a hierarchical Hidden Markov Model (HHMM) for inferring the phase. Similar architectures have since performed well on laparoscopic data [13] with variations of the feature predictor (e.g. ResNet-50 or Inception) and the use of LSTM instead of HHMM [14]. Such systems also won the latest MICCAI 2017 EndoVis workflow recognition challenge[1] focusing on laparoscopic procedures where video is the primary cue. Despite promising accuracy results, ranging 60–85%, in laparoscopy and the challenging environment with deformation, the domain adaptation, resilience to variation of methods and their application to other procedures has been limited.

In this work, we propose an automatic workflow recognition system for cataract surgery, the most common surgical procedure worldwide with 19 million operations performed annually [15]. The environment of the cataract procedure is controlled with few camera motions and the view of the anatomy is approximately opposite to the eye. Our approach follows the deep learning paradigm for surgical tool and phase recognition. A residual neural network (ResNet) is used to recognize the tools within the video frames and produce image features followed by a recurrent neural network (RNN) which operates on sequences of tool features and performs multi-class phase classification. For training and testing of the phase recognition models we produced phase annotations by hand-labeling the CATARACTS dataset[2]. Our results perform near the state-of-the-art for both tool and phase recognition.

---

[1] https://endovissub2017-workflow.grand-challenge.org/.

[2] https://cataracts.grand-challenge.org/.

2   Materials and Methods

2.1   Augmented CATARACT Dataset

We used the CATARACTS dataset for both tool and phase recognition. This dataset consists of 25 train and 25 test videos of cataract surgery recorded at 30 frames per second (fps) at a resolution of 1920×1080. The videos are labelled with tool presence annotations performed by assigning a presence vector to each frame indicating which tools are touching the eyeball. For the task of tool recognition we only used the 25 train CATARACTS videos as the tool annotations of the test videos are not publicly available. There is a total of 21 different tool classes, with some examples shown in Fig. 1. The 25 train videos were randomly split into train, validation (videos 4, 12 and 21) and hold-out test (2 and 20) sets. Frames were extracted with a rate of 3 fps and half of the frames without tools were discarded. As an overview, the dataset was split into a 80-10-10% split of train, validation and hold-out test sets of with 32,529, 3,666 and 2,033 frames, respectively.

For the task of phase recognition, we created surgical phase annotations for all 50 CATARACTS videos, 25 of which are part of the train/validation/hold-out test spit and were used for both tool and phase recognition, while the remaining 25 videos were solely used as an extra test set to assess the generalisation of phase recognition. Annotation was carried out by a medical doctor and an ophthalmology nurse according to the most common phases in cataract surgery, that is Extracapsular cataract extraction (ECCE) using Phacoemulsification and implantation of an intraocular lens (IOL). A timestamp was recorded for each phase transition according to the judgement of the annotators, resulting in a phase-label for each frame. A total of 14 distinct phases were annotated comprising of: (1) Access the anterior chamber (ACC): sideport incision, (2) AAC: mainport incision, (3) Implantable Contact Lenses (ICL): inject viscoelastic, (4) ICL: removal of lens, (5) Phacoemulsification (PE): inject viscoelastic, (6) PE: capsulorhexis, (7) PE: hydrodissection of lens, (8) PE: phacoemulsification, (9) PE: removal of soft lens matter, (10) Inserting of the Intraocular Lens (IIL): inject viscoelastic, (11) IIL: intraocular lens insertion, (12) IIL: aspiration of viscoelastic, (13) IIL: wound closure and (14) IIL: wound closure with suture.

2.2   Tool Recognition with CNNs

For tool recognition we trained the ResNet-152 [9] architecture towards multi-label classification in 21 tool classes. ResNet-152 is comprised of a sequence of 50 residual blocks each consisting of three convolutional layers followed by a batch-normalization layer and ReLU activation, as described in Fig. 2. The output of the third convolutional layer is added to the input of the residual block to produce the layer's output.

We trained the network towards multi-label classification using a fully connected output layer with sigmoid activations. This can essentially be seen as 21

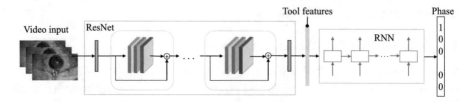

Fig. 2. Pipeline for tool and phase recognition. ResNet-152 consists of 50 residual blocks, each composed of three convolutional layers with batch-normalization layer and ReLU activations. Two pooling layers (green) are used in the input and the output of the network. The CNN receives video frames and calculates tool features which are then passed into an RNN for phase recognition.

parallel networks, each focused on single-task recognition, using shared weights. The loss function optimized was the sigmoid cross-entropy,

$$\mathcal{L}_{CNN} = -\frac{1}{N_t}\frac{1}{C_t}\sum_{i=1}^{N_t}\sum_{c=1}^{C_t} p_c^i \log \hat{p}_c^i + \left(1 - p_c^i\right)\log\left(1 - \hat{p}_c^i\right)$$

where $p_c^i \in \{0, 1\}$ is the ground-truth label for class c in input frame i, $\hat{p}_c^i = \sigma(p_c^i)$ is the corresponding prediction, N_t is the total number of frames within a mini-batch and $C_t = 21$ is the total number of tool classes.

2.3 Phase Recognition with RNNs

Since surgical phases evolve over time it is natural that the current phase depends on neighbouring phases and to capture this temporal information we focused on an RNN-based approach. We used tool information to train two RNNs towards multi-class classification. We gathered two different types of information from the CNN: tool binary presence from the output classification layer and tool features from the last pooling layer. The aim of training on tool features was to capture information (*e.g.* motion and orientation of the tools) and visual cues (*e.g.* lighting and colour) that could potentially enhance phase recognition.

Initially, we trained an LSTM consisting of one hidden layer with 256 nodes and an output fully connected layer with 14 output nodes and softmax activations. The loss function used in training was the cross-entropy loss defined as:

$$\mathcal{L}_{LSTM} = -\frac{1}{N_p}\sum_{i=1}^{N_p}\sum_{c=1}^{C_p} p_c^i \log[\phi(p_c^i)], \quad \phi(p_c) = \frac{e^{p_c}}{\sum_{c=1}^{C_p} e^{p_c}}, \tag{1}$$

where $p_c^i \in \{0, 1\}$ is the ground-truth label for class c for input vector i, N_p is the mini-batch size and $C_p = 14$ is the total number of phase classes.

We additionally trained a two-layered Gated Recurrent Unit (GRU) [16] with 128 nodes per layer and a fully connected output layer with 14 nodes and softmax activation. Similar to the LSTM, we trained the GRU on both binary tool information and tool features using the Adam optimizer and the cross-entropy loss.

3   Experimental Results

3.1   Evaluation Metrics

For the evaluation of the multi-label tool presence classification problem we calculated the area under the receiver-operating characteristic curve (ROC), or else area under the curve (AUC), which is also the official metric used in the CATARACTS challenge. Additionally, we calculated the subset (sAcc) and hamming (hAcc) accuracy. sAcc calculates the proportion of instances whose binary predictions are exactly the same as the ground-truth. The hamming accuracy between a ground-truth vector $\mathbf{g}^i$ and a prediction vector $\mathbf{p}^i$ is calculated as

$$hAcc = \frac{1}{N} \sum_{i=1}^{N} \frac{xor(\mathbf{g}^i, \mathbf{p}^i)}{C},$$

where N and C are the total number of samples and classes, respectively.

For the evaluation of phase recognition we calculated the per-frame accuracy, mean class precision and recall and the f1-score of the phase classes.

3.2   Tool Recognition

We trained ResNet-152 for multi-label tool classification into 21 classes on a training set of 32,529 frames. In our pipeline each video frame was pre-processed by re-shaping to input dimensions of 224×224 and applying random horizontal flips and rotations (within $45°$) with mirror padding. ResNet-152 was initialized with the weights trained on ImageNet [17] and the output layer was initialized with a gaussian distribution ($\mu = 0$, $\sigma = 0.01$). The model was trained using stochastic gradient descent with a mini-batch size of 8, a learning rate of 10^{-4} and a momentum of 0.9 for a total of 10,000 iterations.

Evaluated on the train and hold-out test sets, ResNet-152, achieved a hamming accuracy of 99.58% and 99.07%, respectively. The subset accuracy was calculated at 92.09% and 82.66%, which is lower because predictions that do not exactly match the ground-truth are considered to be wrong. Finally, the AUC was calculated at 99.91% and 99.59% on the train and test sets, respectively. Our model was further evaluated on the CATARACTS challenge test set achieving an AUC of 97.69%, which is close to the winning AUC of 99.71%. Qualitative results are shown in Fig. 3. The model was able to recognize the tools in most cases, with the main challenges posed by the quality of the video frames and the location of the tool with regards to the surface of the eyeball (the tools were annotated as present when touching the eyeball).

3.3   Phase Recognition

For phase recognition we trained both the LSTM and GRU models on both binary and feature inputs. The length of the input sequence was tuned at 100, which corresponds to around 33 s within the video. This is a reasonable choice

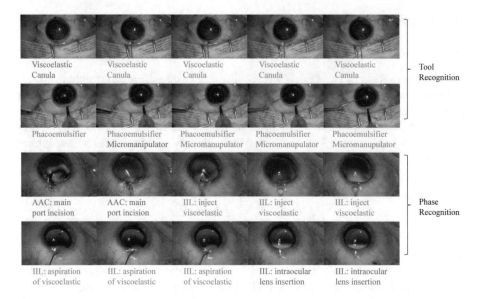

Fig. 3. Example results for the tasks of tool and phase recognition. The main challenge in recognizing tools was noisy frames. In the first row the viscoelastic canula is successfully recognized (green) in all but the first blurry frame. In the second row, the model produced a false positive (red) on the micromanipulator as it is not touching the eyeball. In the last two rows we can see the results of phase recognition. The model produced false predictions in the absence of tools, such as in phase transitions.

since most phases span a couple of minutes. For phase inference we took 100 frame batches, extracted tool-features and classified the 100-length batches in a sliding-window fashion. Both models were trained using the Adam optimizer with a learning rate of 0.001 and momentum parameters $\beta_1 = 0.9$ and $\beta_2 = 0.999$ for 4 epochs.

Tested on binary inputs the LSTM achieved an accuracy of 75.20%, 66.86% and 85.15% on the train, validation and hold-out test sets, respectively, as shown in Table 1. The discrepancy in the performance on the validation and test sets seems to occur because the test set might be easier for the model to infer. An additional challenge is class imbalance. For example, phases 3 and 4 appear only in two videos and are not "learned" adequately. These phases appear in the validation set but not in the test set, reducing the performance on the former. When trained on tool features the LSTM achieved better results across all sets. In order to further assess the ability of the LSTM to generalize, we tested on the CATARACTS test set and achieved an accuracy of 68.75% and 78.28% for binary and features input, respectively. The LSTM trained on tool features was shown to be the best model for phase recognition in our work. Similarly, we assessed the performance of the GRU model. On binary inputs the model achieved accuracies of 89.98% and 71.61% on train and test sets, which is better than the LSTM counterpart. On feature inputs, however, GRU had worse performance with a test accuracy of 68.96%. As a conclusion, tool features other than binary presence supplied important information for the LSTM but failed to increase the performance of the GRU. However, GRU performed comparably well on binary inputs despite having less parameters than the LSTM. As presented in Fig. 3, the presence of tools was essential for the inference of the phase; *e.g.* in the third row of the figure it is shown how the correct phase was maintained as long as the tool appeared in the field of view.

Table 1. Evaluation results for the task of phase recognition with LSTM and GRU: accuracy and average class f1-score (%). The models were evaluated on the train, validation and test sets which came from the 25 training CATARACTS videos. To further test the ability to generalize in a different dataset, we also evaluated the models on the 25 testing CATARACTS videos.

Model	Input	Train		Validation		Test		CATARACTS test set	
		Acc.	F1-score	Acc.	F1-score	Acc.	F1-score	Acc.	F1-score
LSTM	Binary	75.20	65.17	66.86	62.11	85.15	77.69	68.75	68.50
	Features	89.99	83.17	67.56	68.86	92.05	88.10	**78.28**	**74.92**
GRU	Binary	89.98	90.31	75.73	75.48	89.85	85.10	71.61	67.33
	Features	96.90	94.40	66.70	68.55	85.03	82.79	68.96	66.62

4   Discussion and Conclusion

In this paper, we presented a deep learning framework for surgical workflow recognition in cataract videos. We extracted tool presence information from video frames and employed it to train RNN models for surgical phase recognition. Residual learning allowed for results at the state-of-the-art performance achieving AUC of 97.69% on the CATARACTS test set and recurrent neural networks achieved phase accuracy of 78.28% showing potential in automating workflow recognition. The main challenge in our model was the scarcity of some phase classes that prohibited learning all surgical phases equally well. We could address this in future work using data augmentations and weighted loss functions or stratification sampling techniques. Additionally, in future work we could experiment with different architectures of RNNs like bidirectional networks or temporal convolutional networks (TCNs) [18] for an end-to-end approach which is appealing.

References

1. Maier-Hein, L., Vedula, S.S., et al.: Surgical data science for next-generation interventions. Nat. Biomed. Eng. **1**(9), 691–696 (2017)
2. Padoy, N., Blum, T., et al.: Statistical modeling and recognition of surgical workflow. Med. Image Anal. **16**(3), 632–641 (2012)
3. Meißner, C., Meixensberger, J., et al.: Sensor-based surgical activity recognition in unconstrained environments. Minim. Invasive Ther. Allied Technol. **23**(4), 198–205 (2014)

4. Stauder, R., et al.: Random forests for phase detection in surgical workflow analysis. In: Stoyanov, D., Collins, D.L., Sakuma, I., Abolmaesumi, P., Jannin, P. (eds.) IPCAI 2014. LNCS, vol. 8498, pp. 148–157. Springer, Cham (2014). https://doi.org/10.1007/978-3-319-07521-1_16

5. Quellec, G., Lamard, M., et al.: Real-time segmentation and recognition of surgical tasks in cataract surgery videos. IEEE Trans. Med. Imaging 33(12), 2352–2360 (2014)

6. Zappella, L., Béjar, B., et al.: Surgical gesture classification from video and kinematic data. Med. Image Anal. 17(7), 732–745 (2013)

7. Du, X., Allan, M., et al.: Combined 2D and 3D tracking of surgical instruments for minimally invasive and robotic-assisted surgery. Int. J. Comput. Assist. Radiol. Surg. 11(6), 1109–1119 (2016)

8. Bouget, D., Allan, M., et al.: Vision-based and marker-less surgical tool detection and tracking: a review of the literature. Med. Image Anal. 35, 633–654 (2017)

9. He, K., Zhang, X., et al.: Deep residual learning for image recognition. In: 2016 IEEE Conference on Computer Vision and Pattern Recognition. IEEE (2016)

10. Long, J., Shelhamer, E., Darrell, T.: Fully convolutional networks for semantic segmentation. In: 2015 IEEE Conference on Computer Vision and Pattern Recognition. IEEE (2015)

11. Twinanda, A.P., Shehata, S., et al.: EndoNet: a deep architecture for recognition tasks on laparoscopic videos. IEEE Trans. Med. Imaging 36(1), 86–97 (2017)

12. Zisimopoulos, O., Flouty, E., et al.: Can surgical simulation be used to train detection and classification of neural networks? Healthc. Technol. Lett. 4(5), 216–222 (2017)

13. Stauder, R., Ostler, D., et al.: The TUM LapChole dataset for the M2CAI 2016 workflow challenge. arXiv preprint (2016)

14. Jin, Y., Dou, Q., et al.: EndoRCN: recurrent convolutional networks for recognition of surgical workflow in cholecystectomy procedure video. IEEE Trans. Med. Imaging (2016)

15. Trikha, S., Turnbull, A.M.J., et al.: The journey to femtosecond laser-assisted cataract surgery: new beginnings or false dawn? Eye 27(4), 461–473 (2013)

16. Chung, J., Gulcehre, C., et al.: Empirical evaluation of gated recurrent neural networks on sequence modeling (2014)

17. Russakovsky, O., Deng, J., et al.: ImageNet large scale visual recognition challenge. Int. J. Comput. Vis. 115(3), 211–252 (2015)

18. Lea, C., Vidal, R., Reiter, A., Hager, G.D.: Temporal convolutional networks: a unified approach to action segmentation. In: Hua, G., Jégou, H. (eds.) ECCV 2016. LNCS, vol. 9915, pp. 47–54. Springer, Cham (2016). https://doi.org/10.1007/978-3-319-49409-8_7

Surgical Activity Recognition in Robot-Assisted Radical Prostatectomy Using Deep Learning

Aneeq Zia[1]([⊠]), Andrew Hung[2], Irfan Essa[1], and Anthony Jarc[3]

[1] Georgia Institute of Technology, Atlanta, GA, USA
aneeqzia@gatech.edu
[2] University of Southern California, Los Angeles, CA, USA
[3] Medical Research, Intuitive Surgical Inc., Norcross, GA, USA

Abstract. Adverse surgical outcomes are costly to patients and hospitals. Approaches to benchmark surgical care are often limited to gross measures across the entire procedure despite the performance of particular tasks being largely responsible for undesirable outcomes. In order to produce metrics from tasks as opposed to the whole procedure, methods to recognize automatically individual surgical tasks are needed. In this paper, we propose several approaches to recognize surgical activities in robot-assisted minimally invasive surgery using deep learning. We collected a clinical dataset of 100 robot-assisted radical prostatectomies (RARP) with 12 tasks each and propose 'RP-Net', a modified version of InceptionV3 model, for image based surgical activity recognition. We achieve an average precision of 80.9% and average recall of 76.7% across all tasks using RP-Net which out-performs all other RNN and CNN based models explored in this paper. Our results suggest that automatic surgical activity recognition during RARP is feasible and can be the foundation for advanced analytics.

1 Introduction

Adverse outcomes are costly to the patient, hospital, and surgeon. Although many factors contribute to adverse outcomes, the technical skills of surgeons are one important and addressable factor. Virtual reality simulation has played a crucial role to train and improve the technical skills of surgeons, however, intraoperative assessment has been limited to feedback from attendings and/or proctors. Aside from the qualitative feedback from experienced surgeons, quantitative feedback has remained abstract to the level of an entire procedure, such as total duration. Performance feedback for one particular task within a procedure might be more helpful to direct opportunities of improvement. Similarly, statistics from the entire surgery may not be ideal to show an impact on outcomes. For example, one might want to closely examine the performance of a single task if certain adverse outcomes are related to only that specific step of the entire procedure [1]. Scalable methods to recognize automatically when

© Springer Nature Switzerland AG 2018
A. F. Frangi et al. (Eds.): MICCAI 2018, LNCS 11073, pp. 273–280, 2018.
https://doi.org/10.1007/978-3-030-00937-3_32

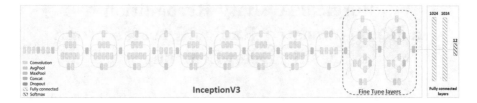

Fig. 1. RP-Net architecture. The portion shown in blue is the same as InceptionV3 architecture, whereas the green portion shows the fully connected (fc) layers we add to produce RP-Net. The number of units for each fc layers is also shown. Note the last two layers of InceptionV3 are fine-tuned in RP-Net.

particular tasks occur within a procedure are needed to generate these metrics to then provide feedback to surgeons or correlate to outcomes.

The problem of surgical activity recognition has been of interest to many researchers. Several methods have been proposed to develop algorithms that automatically recognize the phase of surgery. For laparoscopic surgeries, [2] proposed *'Endo-Net'* for recognizing surgical tools and phases in cholecystectomy using endoscopic images. In [3], RNN models were used to recognize surgical gestures and maneuvers using kinematics data. In [4], unsupervised clustering methods were used to segment training activities on a porcine model. In [5], hidden markov models were used to segment surgical workflow within laparoscopic cholecystectomy.

In this work, we developed models to detect automatically the individual steps of robot-assisted radical prostatectomies (RARP). Our models break a RARP into its individual steps, which will enable us to provide tailored feedback to residents and fellows completing only a portion of a procedure and to produce task-specific efficiency metrics to correlate to certain outcomes. By examining real-world, clinical RARP data, this work builds foundational technology that can readily translate to have direct clinical impact.

Our contributions are, (1) a detailed comparison of various deep learning models using image and robot-assisted surgical system data from clinical robot-assisted radical prostatectomies; (2) RP-Net, a modified InceptionV3 architecture that achieved the highest surgical activity recognition performance out of all models tested; (3) a simple median filter based post processing step for significantly improving procedure segmentation accuracies of different models.

2   Methodology

The rich amount of data that can be collected from the da Vinci (dV) surgical system (Intuitive Surgical, Inc., Sunnyvale, CA USA) enables multiple ways to explore recognition of the type of surgical tasks being performed during a procedure. Our development pipeline involves the following steps: (1) extraction of endoscopic video and dV surgical system data (kinematics and a subset of events), (2) design of deep learning based models for surgical task recognition, and (3) design of post-processing models to filter the initial procedure segmentation output to improve performance. We provide details on modeling below and on our dataset in the next section.

System Data Based Models: The kind of hand and instrument movements surgeons make during procedures can be very indicative of what types of task they are performing. For example, a dissection task might involve static retraction and blunt dissection through in and out trajectories, whereas a suturing task might involve a lot of curved trajectories. Therefore, models that extract motion and event based features from dV surgical system data seem appropriate for task/activity recognition. We explore multiple Recurrent Neural Network (RNN) models using only system data given the recent success of RNNs to incorporate temporal sequences. Since there are multiple data streams coming from the dV surgical system, we employ two types of RNN architectures - *single stream* (SS) and *multi-stream* (MS). For SS, all data streams are concatenated together before feeding them into a RNN. Whereas, for MS, each data stream is fed into individual RNNs after which the outputs of each RNN are merged together using a fully-connected layer to produce predictions. For training both architecture types, we divide our procedure data into windows of length W. At test time, individual windows of the procedure are classified to produce the output segmentation.

Video Based Models: Apart from the kind of motions a surgeon makes, a lot of task representative information is available in the endoscopic video stream. Tasks which are in the beginning could generally look more *'yellow'* due to the fatty tissues, whereas tasks during the later part of the surgery could look much more *'red'* due to the presence of blood after dissection steps. Moreover, the type and relative location of tools present in the image can also be very indicative of the step that the surgeon is performing. Therefore, we employ various image based convolutional neural networks (CNN) for recognizing surgical activity using video data. Within the CNNs domain, there are two type of CNN architectures that are popular and have been proved to work well for the purpose of recognition. The first type uses single images only with two-dimensional (2D) convolutions in the CNN architectures. Examples of such networks include VGG [6], ResNet [7] and InceptionV3 [8]. The second type of architecture uses a volume of images as input (e.g., 16 consecutive frames from the video) and employs three-dimensional (3D) convolutions instead of 2D. C3D is an example of such model [9]. A potential advantage of 3D models is that they can learn spatio-temporal features from video data instead of just spatial features. However, this comes at the cost of requiring more data to train as well as longer overall training times. For our task of surgical activity recognition, we employ both types of CNN models and also propose *'RP-Net'* (Radial Prostatectomy Net), which is a modified version of InceptionV3 as shown in Fig. 1.

Post-processing: Since there are parts of various tasks that are very similar visually and in terms of motions the surgeon is making, the predicted procedure segmentation can have *'spikes'* of mis-classifications. However, it can be assumed that the predicted labels would be consistent within a small window. Therefore,

Table 1. Dataset: the 12 steps of robot-assisted radical prostatectomy and general statistics.

Task no.	Task name	Mean time (sec)	Number of samples
T1	Mobilize colon/drop bladder	1063.2	100
T2	Endopelvic fascia	764.2	98
T3	Anterior bladder neck dissection	164.9	98
T4	Posterior bladder neck dissection	617.5	100
T5	Seminal vesicles	686.8	100
T6	Posterior plane/denonvilliers	171.2	99
T7	Predicles/nerve sparing	510.6	100
T8	Apical dissection	401.1	100
T9	Posterior anastomosis	403.1	100
T10	Anterior anastomosis	539.7	100
T11	Lymph node dissection left	999.6	100
T12	Lymph node dissection right	1103.6	100

in order to remove such noise from the output, we employ a simple running window median filter of length F as a post-processing step. For corner cases, we append the start and end of the predicted sequence with the median of first and last window of length F, respectively, in order to avoid mis-classifications of the corner cases by appending zeros.

3   Experimental Evaluation

Dataset: Our dataset consisted of 100 robot-assisted radical prostatectomies (RP) completed at an academic hospital. The majority of procedures were completed by a combination of residents, fellows, and attending surgeons. Each RP was broken into approximately 12 standardized tasks. The order of these 12 tasks varied slightly based on surgeon preference. The steps of each RP were annotated by one resident. A total of 1195 individual tasks were used. Table 1 shows general statistics of our dataset.

Each RP recording included one channel of endoscopic video, dV surgical system kinematic data (e.g., joint angles, endpoint pose) collected at 50 Hz, and dV surgical system event data (e.g., camera movement start/stop, energy application on/off).

The dV surgical system kinematic data originated from the surgeon console (SSC) and the patient side cart (SI). For both the SSC and SI, the joint angles for each manipulandum and the endpoint pose of the hand controller or instrument were used. In total, there were 80 feature dimensions for SSC and 90 feature dimensions for SI. The dV surgical system event data (EVT) consisted of many events relating to surgeon interactions with the dV surgical system originating at the SSC or SI. In total, there were 87 feature dimensions for EVT.

Data Preparation: Several pre-processing steps were implemented. The endo-scopic video was downsampled to 1 frame per second (fps) resulting in 1.4 million images in total. Image resizing and rescaling was model specific. All kinematic data was downsampled by a factor of 10 (from 50 Hz to 5 Hz). Different window lengths (in terms of the number of samples) W (50, 100, 200 and 300) were tried for training the models and $W = 200$ performed the best. We used zero over-lap when selecting windows for both training and testing. Mean normalization was applied to all feature dimensions for the kinematic data. All events from the dV surgical system data that occured within each window W were used as input for to our models. The events were represented as a unique integers with corresponding timestamps.

Model Training and Parameter Selection: For RNN based models, we implemented both SS and MS architectures for all possible combinations of the three data streams (SSC, SI, and EVT). Estimation of model hyperparameters was done via a grid search on the number of hidden layers (1 or 2), type of RNN unit (Vanilla, GRU or LSTM), number of hidden units per layer (8, 16, 32, 64, 128, 256, 512 or 1024) and what dropout ratio to use (0, 0.2 or 0.5). For each parameter set, we also compared forward and bi-directional RNN. The best performances were achieved using single layered bi-directional RNNs with 256 LSTM units and a dropout ratio of 0.2. Hence, all RNN based results presented were evaluated using these parameters for SS and MS architecture types.

In CNN based models, we used two approaches - training the networks from randomly initialized weights and fine-tuning the networks from pre-trained weights. For all models, we found that fine-tuning was much faster and achieved better accuracies. For single image based models, we used ImageNet [10] pre-trained weights while for C3D we used Sports-1M [11] pretrained weights. We found that fine-tuning several of the last convolutional layers led to the best per-formances across models. For the proposed RP-Net, the last two convolutional modules were fine-tuned (as shown in Fig. 1) and the last fully connected layers were trained from random initialization.

For both RNN- and CNN-based models, the dataset was split to include 70 procedures for training, 10 procedures for validation, and 20 procedures for test.

For the post-processing step, we evaluated performances of all models for values of F (median filter length) ranging from 3 to 2001, and choose a win-dow length that led to maximum increase in model performance across different methods. The final value of F was set to 301. All parameters were selected based on the validation accuracy.

Evaluation Metrics: For a given series of ground truth labels $G \in \Re^N$ and predictions $P \in \Re^N$, where N is the length of a procedure, we evaluate multiple metrics for comparing the performance of various models. These include average precision (AP), average recall (AR) and Jaccard index. Precision is evaluated using $P = \frac{tp}{tp+fp}$, recall using $R = \frac{tp}{tp+fn}$ and Jaccard index using $J = \frac{tp}{tp+fp+fn}$, where tp, fp and fn represent the true positives, false positives and false nega-tives, respectively.

Table 2. Surgical procedure segmentation results using different models. Each cell shows the average metric values across all procedures and tasks in the test set with standard deviations using the original predictions and filtered predictions in the form *original | filtered*. For LSTM models, the modalities used are given in square brackets while the architecture type used is given in parentheses.

Model Type	Average Precision	Average Recall	Average Jaccard Index
LSTM [ssc+si] (MS)	0.585±0.19 | 0.595±0.21	0.565±0.21 | 0.572±0.21	0.629±0.18 | 0.645±0.19
LSTM[ssc+si] (SS)	0.559±0.14 | 0.578±0.15	0.526±0.16 | 0.551±0.16	0.582±0.16 | 0.606±0.17
LSTM[ssc+evt] (MS)	0.625±0.13 | 0.648±0.13	0.572±0.16 | 0.593±0.17	0.633±0.18 | 0.662±0.19
LSTM[ssc+evt] (SS)	0.625±0.13 | 0.641±0.13	0.567±0.21 | 0.593±0.22	0.625±0.18 | 0.651±0.19
LSTM[ssc+si+evt] (MS)	0.437±0.29 | 0.458±0.31	0.226±0.31 | 0.471±0.32	0.552±0.15 | 0.582±0.16
LSTM[ssc+si+evt] (SS)	0.544±0.13 | 0.579±0.12	0.518±0.17 | 0.546±0.17	0.575±0.15 | 0.603±0.17
InceptionV3	0.662±0.12 | 0.782±0.14	0.642±0.15 | 0.759±0.17	0.666±0.07 | 0.786 ±0.08
VGG-19	0.549±0.16 | 0.695±0.19	0.481±0.2 | 0.573±0.22	0.529±0.08 | 0.634±0.11
ResNet	0.621±0.1 | 0.713±0.12	0.582±0.21 | 0.673±0.25	0.622±0.07 | 0.728±0.08
C3D	0.442±0.17 | 0.352±0.21	0.417±0.19 | 0.367±0.24	0.504±0.06 | 0.418±0.12
RP-Net	**0.714±0.12** | **0.809±0.13**	**0.676±0.2** | **0.767±0.23**	**0.700±0.05** | **0.808±0.07**

4   Results and Discussion

The evaluation metrics for all models are shown in Table 2. RP-Net achieved the highest scores across all evaluation metrics out of all models (see last row in Table 2). In general, we observed that the image-based CNN models (except for C3D) performed better than the RNN models. Within LSTM models, MS architecture performed slightly better than SS with the SSC+EVT combination achieving the best performance. For nearly all models, post-processing significantly improved task recognition performance.

Figure 2 shows the confusion matrix of RP-Net with post-processing. The model performed well for almost all the tasks individually except for task 9. However, we can see that most of the task 9 samples were classified as task 10. Tasks 9 and 10 are very related - they are two parts of one overall task (posterior and anterior anastomosis). Furthermore, the images from these two tasks were quite similar given they show anatomy during reconstruction after extensive dissection and energy application. Hence, one would expect that the model could be confused on these two tasks. This is also the case for tasks 3 and 4 - anterior and posterior bladder neck dissection, respectively.

Figure 3 shows several visualizations of the segmentation results as color-coded bars. Undesired spikes in the predicted surgical phase were present when using the output of RP-Net directly. This can be explained by the fact that the model has no temporal information and classifies only using a single image which can lead to mis-classifications since different tasks can look similar at certain points in time. However, using the proposed median filter for post-processing significantly remove such noise and produces a more consistent output (compare middle to bottom bars for all three sample segmentation outputs in Fig. 3).

Despite not having temporal motion information, single image-based models recognize surgical tasks quite well. One reason for this result could be due to the significantly large dataset available for single-image based models. Given the presented RNN and C3D models use a window from the overall task as input,

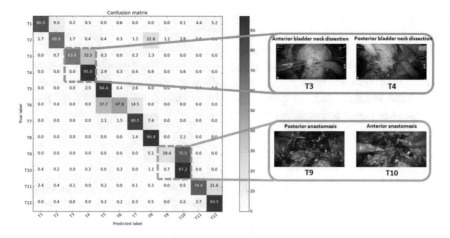

Fig. 2. Confusion matrix of results using RP-Net with post-processing. Sample images of tasks between which there is a lot of *'confusion'* are also shown.

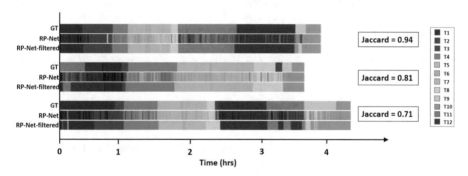

Fig. 3. Sample segmentation outputs for the best, median and lowest jaccard index achieved (from top to bottom, respectively). Within each plot, the top bar denotes the ground truth, the middle one shows the output of RP-Net, while the lowest one shows the output after applying the median filter. Please see Table 1 for task names.

the amount of training data available for such models reduces by a factor of the length of window segment. Additionally, the RNN models might not have performed as well as similar work because in this work we recognized gross tasks directly whereas prior work focused on sub-task gestures and/or maneuvers [3]. Finally, C3D models remain difficult to train. Improved training of these models could lead to better results, which aligns with the intuition that temporal windows of image frames could provide relevant information for activity recognition.

5   Conclusion

In this paper, we proposed a deep learning model called RP-Net to recognize the steps of robot-assisted radical prostatectomy (RARP). We used a clinically-relevant dataset of 100 RARPs from one academic center which enables translation of our models to directly impact real-world surgeon training and medical research. In general, we showed that image-based models outperformed models using only surgeon motion and event data. In future work, we plan to develop novel models that optimally combine motion and image features while using larger dataset and to explore how our models developed for RARP extend to other robot-assisted surgical procedures.

References

1. Hung, A.J., et al.: Utilizing machine learning and automated performance metrics to evaluate robot-assisted radical prostatectomy performance and predict outcomes. J. Endourol. **32**(5), 438–444 (2018)
2. Twinanda, A.P., Shehata, S., Mutter, D., Marescaux, J., de Mathelin, M., Padoy, N.: EndoNet: a deep architecture for recognition tasks on laparoscopic videos. IEEE Trans. Med. Imaging **36**(1), 86–97 (2017)
3. DiPietro, R., et al.: Recognizing surgical activities with recurrent neural networks. In: Ourselin, S., Joskowicz, L., Sabuncu, M.R., Unal, G., Wells, W. (eds.) MICCAI 2016. LNCS, vol. 9900, pp. 551–558. Springer, Cham (2016). https://doi.org/10.1007/978-3-319-46720-7_64
4. Zia, A., Zhang, C., Xiong, X., Jarc, A.M.: Temporal clustering of surgical activities in robot-assisted surgery. Int. J. Comput. Assist. Radiol. Surg. **12**(7), 1171–1178 (2017)
5. Padoy, N., Blum, T., Ahmadi, S.A., Feussner, H., Berger, M.O., Navab, N.: Statistical modeling and recognition of surgical workflow. Med. Image Anal. **16**(3), 632–641 (2012)
6. Simonyan, K., Zisserman, A.: Very deep convolutional networks for large-scale image recognition. CoRR abs/1409.1556 (2014)
7. He, K., Zhang, X., Ren, S., Sun, J.: Deep residual learning for image recognition. In: Proceedings of the IEEE Conference on Computer Vision and Pattern Recognition, pp. 770–778 (2016)
8. Szegedy, C., Vanhoucke, V., Ioffe, S., Shlens, J., Wojna, Z.: Rethinking the inception architecture for computer vision. In: Proceedings of the IEEE Conference on Computer Vision and Pattern Recognition, pp. 2818–2826 (2016)
9. Tran, D., Bourdev, L., Fergus, R., Torresani, L., Paluri, M.: Learning spatiotemporal features with 3D convolutional networks. In: 2015 IEEE International Conference on Computer Vision (ICCV), pp. 4489–4497. IEEE (2015)
10. Deng, J., Dong, W., Socher, R., Li, L.J., Li, K., Fei-Fei, L.: ImageNet: alarge-scale hierarchical image database. In: IEEE Conference on Computer Vision and Pattern Recognition, CVPR 2009, pp. 248–255. IEEE (2009)
11. Karpathy, A., Toderici, G., Shetty, S., Leung, T., Sukthankar, R., Fei-Fei, L.: Large-scale video classification with convolutional neural networks. In: Proceedings of the IEEE Conference on Computer Vision and Pattern Recognition, pp. 1725–1732 (2014)

Unsupervised Learning for Surgical Motion by Learning to Predict the Future

Robert DiPietro[(✉)] and Gregory D. Hager

Department of Computer Science, Johns Hopkins University, Baltimore, MD, USA
rdipietro@gmail.com

Abstract. We show that it is possible to learn meaningful representations of surgical motion, without supervision, by learning to predict the future. An architecture that combines an RNN encoder-decoder and mixture density networks (MDNs) is developed to model the conditional distribution over future motion given past motion. We show that the learned encodings naturally cluster according to high-level activities, and we demonstrate the usefulness of these learned encodings in the context of information retrieval, where a database of surgical motion is searched for suturing activity using a motion-based query. Future prediction with MDNs is found to significantly outperform simpler baselines as well as the best previously-published result for this task, advancing state-of-the-art performance from an F1 score of 0.60 ± 0.14 to 0.77 ± 0.05.

1 Introduction

Robot-assisted surgery has led to new opportunities to study human performance of surgery by enabling scalable, transparent capture of high-quality surgical-motion data in the form of surgeon hand movement and stereo surgical video. This data can be collected in simulation, benchtop training, and during live surgery, from novices in training and from experts in the operating room. This has in turn spurred new research areas such as automated skill assessment and automated feedback for trainees [1,4,16,18].

Although the ability to capture data is practically unlimited, a key barrier to progress has been the focus on supervised learning, which requires extensive manual annotations. Unlike the surgical-motion data itself, annotations are difficult to acquire, are often subjective, and may be of variable quality. In addition, many questions surrounding annotations remain open. For example, should they be collected at the low level of gestures [1], at the higher level of maneuvers [10], or at some other granularity? Do annotations transfer between surgical tasks? And how consistent are annotations among experts?

We show that it is possible to learn meaningful representations of surgery from the data itself, *without the need for explicit annotations*, by searching for representations that can reliably predict future actions, and we demonstrate the usefulness of these representations in an information-retrieval setting. The most relevant prior work is [9], which encodes short windows of kinematics

© Springer Nature Switzerland AG 2018
A. F. Frangi et al. (Eds.): MICCAI 2018, LNCS 11073, pp. 281–288, 2018.
https://doi.org/10.1007/978-3-030-00937-3_33

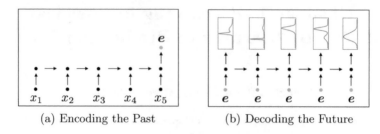

(a) Encoding the Past   (b) Decoding the Future

Fig. 1. The encoder-decoder architecture used in this work, but using only a single kinematic signal and lengths $T_p = T_f = 5$ for visualization. More accurately, each $\mathbf{x}_t \in \mathbb{R}^{n_x}$, and each time step in the future yields a multivariate mixture.

using denoising autoencoders, and which uses these representations to search a database using motion-based queries. Other unsupervised approaches include activity alignment under the assumption of identical structure [10] and activity segmentation using hand-crafted pipelines [6], structured probablistic models [14], and clustering [20].

Contrary to these approaches, we hypothesize that if a model is capable of predicting the future then it must encode contextually relevant information. Our approach is similar to prior work for learning video representations [17], however unlike [17] we leverage mixture density networks and show that they are crucial to good performance. Our contributions are (1) introducing a recurrent-neural-network (RNN) encoder-decoder architecture with MDNs for predicting future motion and (2) showing that this architecture learns encodings that perform well both qualitatively (Figs. 3 and 4) and quantitatively (Table 1).

2   Methods

To obtain meaningful representations of surgical motion without supervision, we predict future motion from past motion. More precisely, letting $\mathbf{X}_p \equiv \{\mathbf{x}_t\}_1^{T_p}$ denote a subsequence of kinematics from the past and $\mathbf{X}_f \equiv \{\mathbf{x}_t\}_{T_p+1}^{T_p+T_f}$ denote the kinematics that follow, we model the conditional distribution $p(\mathbf{X}_f \mid \mathbf{X}_p)$. This is accomplished with an architecture that combines an RNN encoder-decoder with mixture density networks, as illustrated in Fig. 1.

2.1   Recurrent Neural Networks and Long Short-Term Memory

Recurrent neural networks (RNNs) are a class of neural networks that share parameters over time, and which are naturally suited to modeling sequential data. The simplest variant is that of Elman RNNs [8], but they are rarely used because they suffer from the *vanishing gradient problem* [2]. Long short-term memory (LSTM) [11,12] was introduced to alleviate the vanishing-gradient problem, and has since become one of the most widely-used RNN

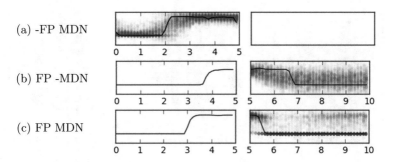

Fig. 2. Visualization of predictions. Inputs and ground truth (black) are shown along with predictions (blue). −FP MDN compresses and reconstructs the past; FP − MDN predicts one blurred future; and FP MDN predicts multiple possible futures.

architectures, achieving state-of-the-art performance in many domains, including surgical activity recognition [7]. The variant of LSTM used here is

$$\mathbf{f}_t = \sigma(\mathbf{W}_{fh}\mathbf{h}_{t-1} + \mathbf{W}_{fx}\mathbf{x}_t + \mathbf{b}_f) \qquad \mathbf{i}_t = \sigma(\mathbf{W}_{ih}\mathbf{h}_{t-1} + \mathbf{W}_{ix}\mathbf{x}_t + \mathbf{b}_i) \qquad (1)$$

$$\mathbf{o}_t = \sigma(\mathbf{W}_{oh}\mathbf{h}_{t-1} + \mathbf{W}_{ox}\mathbf{x}_t + \mathbf{b}_o) \qquad \tilde{\mathbf{c}}_t = \tanh(\mathbf{W}_{ch}\mathbf{h}_{t-1} + \mathbf{W}_{cx}\mathbf{x}_t + \mathbf{b}_c) \qquad (2)$$

$$\mathbf{c}_t = \mathbf{f}_t \odot \mathbf{c}_{t-1} + \mathbf{i}_t \odot \tilde{\mathbf{c}}_t \qquad \mathbf{h}_t = \mathbf{o}_t \odot \tanh(\mathbf{c}_t) \qquad (3)$$

where $\sigma(\cdot)$ denotes the element-wise sigmoid function and $\odot$ denotes element-wise multiplication. $\mathbf{f}_t$, $\mathbf{i}_t$, and $\mathbf{o}_t$ are known as the forget, input, and output gates, and all weight matrices $\mathbf{W}$ and all biases $\mathbf{b}$ are learned.

2.2 The RNN Encoder-Decoder

RNN encoder-decoders [5] were introduced in machine translation to encode a source sentence in one language and decode it in another language, by modeling the discrete distribution p(target sentence | source sentence). We proceed similarly, by modeling the continuous conditional distribution $p(\mathbf{X}_f \mid \mathbf{X}_p)$, using LSTM for both the encoder and the decoder, as illustrated in Fig. 1.

The encoder LSTM maps $\mathbf{X}_p$ to a series of hidden states through Eqs. 1 to 3, and the final hidden state is used as our fixed-length encoding of $\mathbf{X}_p$. Collecting the encoder's weights and biases into $\boldsymbol{\theta}^{(\text{enc})}$,

$$\mathbf{e} \equiv \mathbf{h}_{T_p}^{(\text{enc})} = f(\mathbf{X}_p; \boldsymbol{\theta}^{(\text{enc})}) \qquad (4)$$

Similarly, the LSTM decoder, with its own parameters $\boldsymbol{\theta}^{(\text{dec})}$, maps $\mathbf{e}$ to a series of hidden states, where hidden state t is used to decode the kinematics at time step t of the future. The simplest possible estimate is then $\hat{\mathbf{x}}_t = \mathbf{W}\,\mathbf{h}_t^{(\text{dec})} + \mathbf{b}$, where training equates to minimizing sum-of-squares error. However, this approach corresponds to maximizing likelihood under a unimodal Gaussian, which is insufficient because distinct futures are blurred into one (see Fig. 2).

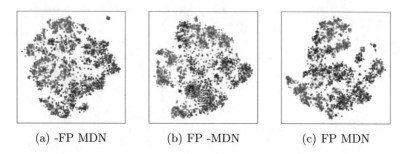

(a) -FP MDN   (b) FP -MDN   (c) FP MDN

Fig. 3. 2-D dimensionality reductions of our 64-D encodings, obtained using t-SNE, and colored according to activity: Suture Throw (green), Knot Tying (orange), Grasp Pull Run Suture (red), and Intermaneuver Segment (blue). The activity annotations are used for visualization only. Future prediction and MDNs both lead to more separation between high-level activities in the encoding space.

2.3   Mixture Density Networks

MDNs [3] use neural networks to produce conditional distributions with greater flexibility. Here, we associate each time step of the future with its own mixture of multivariate Gaussians, with parameters that depend on $\mathbf{X}_p$ through the encoder and decoder. For each time step, every component c is associated with a mixture coefficient $\pi_t^{(c)}$, a mean $\boldsymbol{\mu}_t^{(c)}$, and a diagonal covariance matrix with entries collected in $\mathbf{v}_t^{(c)}$. These parameters are computed via

$$\boldsymbol{\pi}_t(\mathbf{h}_t^{(\text{dec})}) = \text{softmax}(\mathbf{W}_\pi\, \mathbf{h}_t^{(\text{dec})} + \mathbf{b}_\pi) \tag{5}$$

$$\boldsymbol{\mu}_t^{(c)}(\mathbf{h}_t^{(\text{dec})}) = \mathbf{W}_\mu^{(c)}\, \mathbf{h}_t^{(\text{dec})} + \mathbf{b}_\mu^{(c)} \tag{6}$$

$$\mathbf{v}_t^{(c)}(\mathbf{h}_t^{(\text{dec})}) = \text{softplus}(\mathbf{W}_v^{(c)}\, \mathbf{h}_t^{(\text{dec})} + \mathbf{b}_v^{(c)}) \tag{7}$$

where the softplus is used to ensure that $\mathbf{v}_t^{(c)}$ has all positive elements and where the softmax is used to ensure that $\boldsymbol{\pi}_t$ has positive elements that sum to 1.

We emphasize that all $\pi_t^{(c)}$, $\boldsymbol{\mu}_t^{(c)}$ and $\mathbf{v}_t^{(c)}$ depend implicitly on $\mathbf{X}_p$ and on the encoder's and decoder's parameters through $\mathbf{h}_t^{(\text{dec})}$, and that the individual components of $\mathbf{x}_t$ are *not* conditionally independent under this model. However, in order to capture global context rather than local properties such as smoothness, we do not condition each $\mathbf{x}_{t+1}$ on $\mathbf{x}_t$; instead, we condition each $\mathbf{x}_t$ only on $\mathbf{X}_p$ and assume independence over time steps. Our final model is then

$$p(\mathbf{X}_f \mid \mathbf{X}_p) = \prod_{\mathbf{x}_t \in \mathbf{X}_f} \sum_c \pi_t^{(c)}(\mathbf{h}_t^{(\text{dec})}) \mathcal{N}\Big(\mathbf{x}_t;\; \boldsymbol{\mu}_t^{(c)}(\mathbf{h}_t^{(\text{dec})}), \mathbf{v}_t^{(c)}(\mathbf{h}_t^{(\text{dec})})\Big) \tag{8}$$

2.4   Training

Given past, future pairs $(\mathbf{X}_p^{(n)}, \mathbf{X}_f^{(n)})$, training is carried out by minimizing the negative log likelihood $-\sum_n \log p(\mathbf{X}_f^{(n)} \mid \mathbf{X}_p^{(n)}; \boldsymbol{\theta})$, where $\boldsymbol{\theta}$ is a collection of all

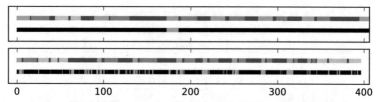

(a) Representative -FP MDN example. Precision: 0.47. Recall: 0.78. F1 Score: 0.59.

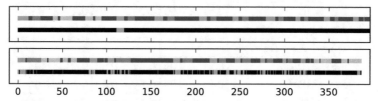

(b) Representative FP -MDN example. Precision: 0.54. Recall: 0.70. F1 Score: 0.61.

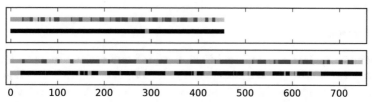

(c) Representative FP MDN example. Precision: 0.76. Recall: 0.78. F1 Score: 0.77.

Fig. 4. Qualitative results for kinematics-based suturing queries. For each example, from top to bottom, we show (1) a full activity sequence from one subject; (2) the segment used as a query; (3) a full activity sequence from a *different* subject; and (4) the retrieved frames from our query. These examples were chosen because they exhibit precisions, recalls, and F1 scores that are close to the averages reported in Table 1.

parameters from the encoder LSTM, the decoder LSTM, and the decoder outputs. This is carried out using stochastic gradient descent. We note that the encoder, the decoder, the decoder's outputs, and the negative log likelihood are all constructed within a single computation graph, and we can differentiate our loss with respect to all parameters automatically and efficiently using backpropagation through time [19]. Our implementation is based on PyTorch.

3 Experiments

Here we carry out two sets of experiments. First, we compare the predictions and encodings from our future-prediction model equipped with mixture density networks, which we refer to as FP MDN, with two baseline versions: FP − MDN, which focuses on future prediction without MDNs, and −FP MDN, which instead of predicting the future learns to compress and reconstruct the past in an autoencoder-like fashion. Second, we compare these approaches in an information-retrieval setting alongside the state-of-the-art approach [9].

Table 1. Quantitative results for kinematics-based queries.

	Precision	Recall	F1 score
Suturing			
DAE + AS − DTW [9]	0.53 ± 0.15	0.75 ± 0.16	0.60 ± 0.14
−FP MDN	0.50 ± 0.08	0.75 ± 0.07	0.59 ± 0.07
FP − MDN	0.54 ± 0.07	0.76 ± 0.08	0.62 ± 0.06
FP MDN	0.81 ± 0.06	0.74 ± 0.10	**0.77 ± 0.05**
Knot tying			
DAE + AS − DTW [9]	−	−	−
−FP MDN	0.37 ± 0.05	0.73 ± 0.02	0.49 ± 0.05
FP − MDN	0.34 ± 0.05	0.74 ± 0.02	0.46 ± 0.05
FP MDN	0.62 ± 0.08	0.74 ± 0.04	**0.67 ± 0.05**

3.1   Dataset

The Minimally Invasive Surgical Training and Innovation Center - Science of Learning (MISTIC-SL) dataset focuses on minimally-invasive, robot-assisted surgery using a *da Vinci* surgical system, in which trainees perform a structured set of tasks (see Fig. 4). We follow [9] and only use data from the 15 right-handed trainees in the study. Each trainee performed between 1 and 6 trials, for a total of 39 trials. We use 14 kinematic signals in all experiments: velocities, rotational velocities, and the gripper angle of the tooltip, all for both the left and right hands. In addition, experts manually annotated the trials so that all moments in time are associated with 1 of 4 high-level activities: Suture Throw (ST), Knot Tying (KT), Grasp Pull Run Suture (GPRS), or Intermaneuver Segment (IMS). We emphasize that these labels are not used in any way to obtain the encodings.

3.2   Future Prediction

We train our model using 5 second windows of kinematics, extracted at random during training. Adam was used for optimization with a learning rate of 0.005, with other hyperparameters fixed to their defaults [13]. We trained for 5000 steps using a batch size of 50 (approximately 50 epochs). The hyperparameters tuned in our experiments were n_h, the number of hidden units for the encoder and decoder LSTMs, and n_c, the number of mixture components. For hyperparameter selection, 4 subjects were held out for validation. We began overly simple with $n_h = 16$ and $n_c = 1$, and proceeded to double n_h or n_c whenever doing so improved the held-out likelihood. This led to final values of $n_h = 64$ and $n_c = 16$.

Results for the FP MDN and baselines are shown in Fig. 2, in which we show predictions, and in Fig. 3, in which we show 2-D representations obtained with t-SNE [15]. We can see that the addition of future prediction and MDNs leads to more separation between high-level activities in the encoding space.

3.3 Information Retrieval with Motion-Based Queries

Here we present results for retrieving kinematic frames based on a motion-based query, using the tasks of suturing and knot tying. We focus on the most difficult but most useful scenario: querying with a sequence from one subject i and retrieving frames from other subjects $j \neq i$.

In order to retrieve kinematic frames, we form encodings using *all windows* within one segment of an activity by subject i, compute the cosines between these encodings and all encodings for subject j, take the maximum (over windows) on a per-frame basis, and threshold. For evaluation, we follow [9], computing each metric (precision, recall, and F1 score) from each source subject i to each target subject $j \neq i$, and finally averaging over all target subjects.

Quantitative results are shown in Table 1, comparing the FP MDN to its baselines and the state-of-the-art approach [9], and qualitative results are shown in Fig. 4. We can see that the FP MDN significantly outperforms the two simpler baselines, as well as the state-of-the-art approach in the case of suturing, improving from an F1 score of 0.60 ± 0.14 to 0.77 ± 0.05.

4 Summary and Future Work

We showed that it is possible to learn meaningful representations of surgical motion, without supervision, by searching for representations that can reliably predict the future. The usefulness of these representations was demonstrated in the context of information retrieval, where we used future prediction equipped with mixture density networks to improve the state-of-the-art performance for motion-based suturing queries from an F1 score of 0.60 ± 0.14 to 0.77 ± 0.05.

Because we do not rely on annotations, our method is applicable to arbitrarily large databases of surgical motion. From one perspective, exploring large databases using these encodings is exciting in and of itself. From another perspective, we also expect such encodings to improve downstream tasks such skill assessment and surgical activity recognition, especially in the regime of few annotations. Finally, as illustrated in Fig. 4, we believe that these encodings can also be used to aid the annotation process itself.

Acknowledgements. This work was supported by a fellowship for modeling, simulation, and training from the Link Foundation. We would also like to thank Anand Malpani, Swaroop Vedula, Gyusung I. Lee, and Mija R. Lee for procuring the MISTIC-SL dataset.

References

1. Ahmidi, N., et al.: A dataset and benchmarks for segmentation and recognition of gestures in robotic surgery. IEEE Trans. Biomed. Eng. **64**(9), 2025–2041 (2017)
2. Bengio, Y., Simard, P., Frasconi, P.: Learning long-term dependencies with gradient descent is difficult. IEEE Trans. Neural Netw. **5**(2), 157–166 (1994)
3. Bishop, C.M.: Mixture density networks. Technical report, Aston University (1994)

4. Chen, Z., et al.: Virtual fixture assistance for needle passing and knot tying. In: Intelligent Robots and Systems (IROS), pp. 2343–2350 (2016)
5. Cho, K., et al.: Learning phrase representations using RNN encoder-decoder for statistical machine translation. In: EMNLP (2014)
6. Despinoy, F., et al.: Unsupervised trajectory segmentation for surgical gesture recognition in robotic training. IEEE Trans. Biomed. Eng. **63**(6), 1280–1291 (2016)
7. DiPietro, R., et al.: Recognizing surgical activities with recurrent neural networks. In: Ourselin, S., Joskowicz, L., Sabuncu, M.R., Unal, G., Wells, W. (eds.) MICCAI 2016 Part I. LNCS, vol. 9900, pp. 551–558. Springer, Cham (2016). https://doi.org/10.1007/978-3-319-46720-7_64
8. Elman, J.L.: Finding structure in time. Cogn. Sci. **14**(2), 179–211 (1990)
9. Gao, Y., Vedula, S.S., Lee, G.I., Lee, M.R., Khudanpur, S., Hager, G.D.: Query-by-example surgical activity detection. Int. J. Comput. Assist. Radiol. Surg. **11**(6), 987–996 (2016)
10. Gao, Y., Vedula, S., Lee, G.I., Lee, M.R., Khudanpur, S., Hager, G.D.: Unsupervised surgical data alignment with application to automatic activity annotation. In: 2016 IEEE International Conference on Robotics and Automation (ICRA) (2016)
11. Gers, F.A., Schmidhuber, J., Cummins, F.: Learning to forget: continual prediction with LSTM. Neural Comput. **12**(10), 2451–2471 (2000)
12. Hochreiter, S., Schmidhuber, J.: Long short-term memory. Neural Comput. **9**(8), 1735–1780 (1997)
13. Kingma, D.P., Ba, J.: Adam: a method for stochastic optimization. arXiv preprint arXiv:1412.6980 (2014)
14. Krishnan, S., et al.: Transition state clustering: unsupervised surgical trajectory segmentation for robot learning. Int. J. Robot. Res. **36**(13–14), 1595–1618 (2017)
15. van der Maaten, L., Hinton, G.: Visualizing data using t-SNE. J. Mach. Learn. Res. **9**(Nov), 2579–2605 (2008)
16. Reiley, C.E., Akinbiyi, T., Burschka, D., Chang, D.C., Okamura, A.M., Yuh, D.D.: Effects of visual force feedback on robot-assisted surgical task performance. J. Thorac. Cardiovasc. Surg. **135**(1), 196–202 (2008)
17. Srivastava, N., Mansimov, E., Salakhudinov, R.: Unsupervised learning of video representations using LSTMs. In: International Conference on Machine Learning, pp. 843–852 (2015)
18. Vedula, S.S., Malpani, A., Ahmidi, N., Khudanpur, S., Hager, G., Chen, C.C.G.: Task-level vs. segment-level quantitative metrics for surgical skill assessment. J. Surg. Educ. **73**(3), 482–489 (2016)
19. Werbos, P.J.: Backpropagation through time: what it does and how to do it. Proc. IEEE **78**(10), 1550–1560 (1990)
20. Zia, A., Zhang, C., Xiong, X., Jarc, A.M.: Temporal clustering of surgical activities in robot-assisted surgery. Int. J. Comput. Assist. Radiol. Surg. **12**(7), 1171–1178 (2017)

Computer Assisted Interventions:
Visualization and Augmented Reality

Volumetric Clipping Surface: Un-occluded Visualization of Structures Preserving Depth Cues into Surrounding Organs

Bhavya Ajani, Aditya Bharadwaj, and Karthik Krishnan[✉]

Samsung Research India, Bangalore, India
bhavya.ajani@samsung.com

Abstract. Anatomies of interest are often hidden within data. In this paper, we address the limitations of visualizing them with a novel dynamic non-planar clipping of volumetric data, while preserving depth cues at adjacent structures to provide a visually consistent anatomical context, with no-user interaction. An un-occluded and un-modified display of the anatomies of interest is made possible. Given a semantic segmentation of the data, our technique computes a continuous clipping surface through the depth buffer of the structures of interest and extrapolates this depth onto surrounding contextual regions in real-time. We illustrate the benefit of this technique using Monte Carlo Ray Tracing (MCRT), in the visualization of deep seated anatomies with complex geometry across two modalities: (a) Knee Cartilage from MRI and (b) bones of the feet in CT. Our novel technique furthers the state of the art by enabling turnkey immediate appreciation of the pathologies in these structures with an unmodified rendering, while still providing a *consistent* anatomical context. We envisage our technique changing the way clinical applications present 3D data, by incorporating *organ viewing presets*, similar to *transfer function presets* for volume visualization.

Keywords: Ray tracing · Focus+Context · Occlusion

1 Introduction

3D datasets present a challenge for Volume Rendering, where regions of interest (ROI) for diagnosis are often occluded. These ROIs usually cannot be discriminated from occluding anatomies by setting up a suitable transfer function. Clipping planes, Cropping and scalpel tools have been widely used to remove occluding tissue and are indispensible features of every Medical Visualization workstation.

However, none of the existing techniques render the ROIs un-occluded while maintaining depth continuity with the surrounding. In this paper we address this limitation by introducing a novel dynamic non-planar clipping of volumetric data. Matching depth between the ROIs and surrounding for improved depth perception, while still supporting an un-occluded, un-modified visualization of

© Springer Nature Switzerland AG 2018
A. F. Frangi et al. (Eds.): MICCAI 2018, LNCS 11073, pp. 291–298, 2018.
https://doi.org/10.1007/978-3-030-00937-3_34

the ROIs with no user interactions in real-time is the key contribution of this work. Additionaly, we describe our technique in the context of Cinematic rendering.

1.1 Focus+Context

Focus+Context (F+C) is well studied in visualization [1]. It uses a segmentation of the data to highlight the ROIs (*Focus*) while still displaying the surrounding anatomies (*Context*). The principle of F+C is that for the user to correctly interpret data, interact with it or orient oneself, the user simultaneously needs a detailed depiction (Focus) along with a general overview (Context). Existing F+C techniques resort to a distortion of the *visualization space*, by allocating more *space* (importance sampling, various optical properties, viewing area etc.) for the Focus [1,2]. Methods include *cut-aways* (where fragments occluding the view are removed) [3,4], rendering the context with different optical properties [3], *ghosting* of the context (where contextual fragments are made more transparent) [4] and importance sampling with several forms of sparsity [4,5] and exploded views and deformations to change the position of context fragments. Wimmer et. al [6] extended ghosting techniques to create a *virtual hole cut-away* visualization using various clipping functions such as box and sphere so as to create a vision channel for deep seated anatomies.

Humans determine spatial relationships between objects based on several depth cues [2]. In surgical planning, correct depth perception is necessary to understand the relation between vessels and tumors. State of the art ray tracing methods use various techniques including shadows to highlight foreground structures for improved depth perception. Ultimately, depth perception often necessitates interactions such as rotation.

1.2 Clinical Application

We demonstrate our technique across two different modalities: Knee cartilage in T1w MRI and complex bones of the ankle and foot in CT.

Knee MR scans are the third most common type of MRI examination [7] and Knee Osteo-arthritis is the leading cause of global disability. Lesions shows up as pot holes; varying from full-thickness going all the way through the cartilage, to a partial-thickness lesion. Subtle cartilage lesions are notoriously difficult to detect. A considerable number of chondral lesions (55%) remain undetected until arthroscopy [8]. The mean thickness of healthy cartilages in the knee varies from 1.3 to 2.7 mm [9]. Visualization of the cartilage and its texture enables better diagnosis. However, un-occluded visualization along with context to appreciate the injury and the degradation of a structure that is so thin, curved and enclosed by several muscles and bones in the knee is challenging.

Cinematic Rendering which uses MCRT has advanced state of the art in medical visualization [10]. It has been used in the clinic to generate high quality realistic images primarily with CT, but also using MR. Advances in Deep

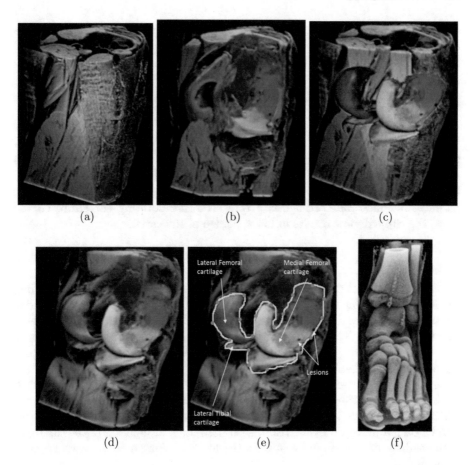

Fig. 1. Visualization of knee on a T1w 1.5T MRI (300 × 344 × 120 voxels, sagittal acquisition, resolution 0.4 × 0 × 4 × 1 mm). (a) Rendering the whole volume completely occludes the cartilage (b) Clipping plane requires manual adjustment, yet has a poor cartilage coverage due to its topology (c) Cutaway view of the cartilage, where occluding fragments are removed. Note the depth mismatch between the cartilage and surrounding anatomy causing perceptual distortion. Also note poor lighting of the focus. (d) Our proposed VCS method, with the same viewing parameters shows the cartilage with maximal coverage and smoothly extrapolates depth onto surrounding structures, allowing for improved appreciation of contextual anatomy in relation to the focus. (e) Focus (cartilage) is outlined in yellow. Boundary points of this are sampled as indicated by the control points in green to compute a clipping surface spline. It is worthwhile mentioning that an accurate cartilage segmentation is not typically necessary since the bone is hypo-intense compared to the cartilage. (f) CT foot (64 slice CT VIX, OsiriX data) using the proposed VCS method. The bones were segmented by a simple threshold at 200HU. Note that the method captures the non-planar structure of bones of the feet successfully.

Learning have made possible computation of accurate segmentations. There is a need for visualization techniques to generate high quality Focus specific F+C renderings to enable faster diagnosis.

2 Existing Techniques

2.1 Clipping Planes

Clipping planes can be used to generate an un-modified dissection view. Figure 1b shows this visualization of the knee cartilage using MCRT depicting lesions in the femoral cartilage. The placement of the clipping plane requires significant interaction. Since the cartilage is a thin structure covering the entire curved joint, the clipped view results in low coverage of the cartilage.

2.2 Cut-Aways

Cut-aways were first proposed in [4]. The idea is to cut away fragments occluding the Focus. Occluding fragments are rendered fully transparent, therefore unlike ghosting it provides an unmodified view of the cartilage. This is possible using two render passes. The Focus depths at the current view are extracted in the first pass, by checking if the ray intersects with its segmentation. A second pass renders all data. The starting locations of the rays that intersect the Focus are set to the depth extracted from the first pass so that Focus is rendered un-occluded.

A cut-away of the cartilage is shown in Fig. 1c. Note the boundaries of the cartilage where there is a clear depth mismatch resulting in *cliffs* in the visualization causing a perceptual distortion. Also note the poor lighting of the cartilage, with shadows of the context cast onto the focus, making a contralateral assessment difficult.

3 A Real-Time Depth Contiguous Clipping Surface

Similar to other F+C techniques our method requires prior semantic segmentation to define Focus and Context. Automatic segmentation of Focus (Cartilage) in T1w MRI is derived using deep learning as explained in our previous work [11].

3.1 Methodology

We extrapolate depth for Context from Focus. We use approximating Thin Plate Splines (TPS) [12] to provide a smooth, differentiable depth through the Focus onto the rest of the view frustum. Figure 1d shows the MCRT from the same viewpoint using the proposed method. The Volumetric Clipping Surface (VCS) is implicitly defined through a depth buffer in an orthographic view space or frustum.

We render the scene in two render passes. In the first render pass we compute the depth buffer that maintains depth continuity. In a second render pass we

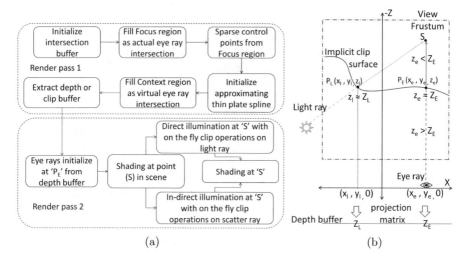

(a)   (b)

Fig. 2. (a) Overview of MCRT rendering in two render passes with a Focus specific clipping surface. Render pass 1 is done once. Render pass 2 is carried out multiple times to refine the MCRT render estimate. (b) On the fly clip operations against an implicit clip surface (marked in purple). Eye ray is marked in green and Light ray is marked in yellow. The scatter ray is not shown to avoid clutter. The clipped portion of rays are shown as a dashed line.

render the scene by clipping the eye and light rays based on this computed depth buffer (see Fig. 2b); thereby implicitly clipping them with the VCS in a warp view space. MCRT is an iterative rendering process, where several iterations are used to arrive at the estimate of the scene for a given set of viewing parameters. The first render pass is carried out once, while the second render pass is a part of each MCRT iteration.

In the first render pass, we compute an intersection buffer which stores the points of intersection (in view space) for all eye rays. The intersection buffer is conceptually divided into three distinct regions. These are regions where the eye rays (a) intersect the Focus ROI (b) intersect the Context ROI (c) do not intersect the model bounding box. The first render pass consists of two phases. In the first phase, the Focus region of the intersection buffer is filled. This contains the *actual intersection points* for all eye rays intersecting with Focus (i.e. those that intersect the segmentation texture). In the second phase, we estimate *virtual intersection points* for the Context region, from the computed *actual intersection points* in the Focus region. This provides us with a C0, C1, C2 continuous intersection buffer in view space, which we call an intersection surface.

This is done as shown in Fig. 2a. We select a sparse set of control points falling on boundary of the Focus region of the intersection buffer, by uniformly sampling the boundary contour points. In this work, we use $N = 50$ control points. Using these points, we initialize an approximating TPS taking all (x, y) co-ordinates of control points (i.e. origin of corresponding eye ray) as data sites and its z co-ordinate (i.e. intersection depth in view space) as data value. We choose a spline approximating parameter p as 0.5. The computed surface spline is used to extrapolate *virtual intersection depths* (i.e. z co-ordinate of intersection of an eye ray with origin (x, y)) maintaining continuity with intersection points on Focus region boundary. This fills the *Context region intersection buffer*. We discard the rays that do not intersect the model bounding box. The depth buffer comprises the z co-ordinates (or depths) of all intersection points.

The second render pass is carried out multiple times as part of each render estimate of the MCRT rendering pipeline. In an orthographic projection, (as is commonly used for medical visualization), as eye rays are parallel to the Z axis, an eye ray with origin $(x_e, y_e, 0)$ is clipped by moving it's origin to a point P_L (x_e, y_e, z_e) (see Fig. 2b) such that $z_e = Z_E$, where Z_E is the corresponding depth value for that eye ray. In MCRT, shading at any point S involves computation of both the direct and the indirect (scatter) illumination [13]. Hence, light rays also need to be clipped appropriately for correct illumination. As shown in Fig. 2b, a light ray is clipped at the intersection point P_L, (x_l, y_l, z_l) with the implicit clipping surface. This intersection point is computed on the fly using ray marching as a point along the light ray whose z_l co-ordinate (in view space) is closest to the corresponding clipping depth value, Z_L, in the depth buffer. To estimate the corresponding depth value for any point P (x, y, z) on the light path, the point is first mapped into screen space (using the projection matrix) to get continuous indices within the depth buffer. The depth value is than extracted using linear interpolation from the depth buffer with these continuous indices.

3.2   Computational Complexity

With the application of this technique to MCRT, the addition of the first clipping depth computation pass amounts to roughly one additional iteration, out of typically 100 iterations used to obtain a good image quality. Therefore, it comes at a low computational complexity. On a system (Win7, Intel i7 3.6 GHz dual core, 8 GB RAM, NVidia Quadro K2200) an extrapolated depth buffer for a viewing window of size 512×512 is computed in 0.1 s for the dataset in Fig. 1d.

4   Simulation

To appreciate our proposed method and to visually valdiate it, we render a simulated model. The model is a volume of size $512 \times 512 \times 512$ voxels. Its scalar values are the z indices, in the range $[-255, 255]$. The scalar values are chosen to spatially vary smoothly across the data (for simplicity along the z axis) to enable an understanding of the continuity of the clipping surface both spatially and in depth by examining the shape of the surface and the scalar values across it. The *focus* (segmentation mask) is a centered cuboid ROI of size $255 \times 255 \times 391$ voxels. The voxel spacing is such that the model scales to a unit cube. The color transfer function maps -255 to blue and 255 to red. We render this scene using a cut plane, cut-away and our method.

In the cut plane view (Fig. 3a), both Focus and Context get clipped. In the cut-away view (Fig. 3b), there is a clear depth mismatch between the Focus and

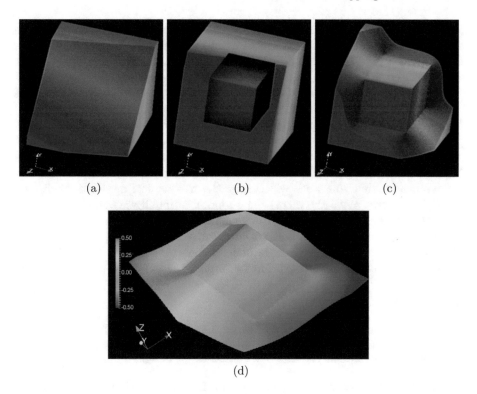

(a)   (b)   (c)

(d)

Fig. 3. Visualization of the unit cube model with a cuboid focus within it, using (a) Cut plane (b) Cut-away (c) our method. (d) Computed clipping surface (rotated by 90° for visual appreciation). Color bar indicates depth values in mm. The continuity of the surface with the object boundary and the consistency of scalar values across it indicates that the surface is smooth with continuity both spatially and in depth from the focus onto the background.

Context, which results in a perceptual distortion. In addition, the focus is poorly lit due to shadows being cast by the context. Contrast this with the visualization using our method (Fig. 3c) where the entire Focus region is made visible while keeping depth continuity with the surrounding context.

Figure 3d shows the clipping surface that was computed, (rotated by 90° as indicated by the axes legend) for purposes of visualization. Note that, in our actual rendering pipeline, we do not explicitly compute the clipping surface (this is implicity computed via the depth buffer as described in the previous section).

5   Conclusions

Advances in visualization enable better appreciation of the extent of injury/disease and its juxtaposition with surrounding anatomy. We introduce the novel idea of an on the fly computed Focus specific clipping surface.

Although we use it in the context of MCRT, these techniques are applicable to Direct Volume Rendering. We differentiate our work from other F+C works in four ways: (a) With our method, the structures of interest are rendered un-occluded and un-modified, which is essential for diagnostic interpretation, (b) The Focus transitions to the Context seamlessly by maintaining continuity of depth between the Focus and Context regions, thereby aiding interpretation, (c) There is no user interaction required to view the Focus and (d) The Focus is rendered with the same optical properties as the Context. We do not distort the visualization space or use tagged rendering and do not propagate errors in the segmentation to the visualization.

We believe that this work will change the way clinical applications display volumetric views. With the increasing adoption of intelligence in clinical appli-cations, that automatically compute semantic information, we envisage these applications incorporating *organ presets*, similar to *transfer function presets*. We envisage uses of this technique in fetal face visualization from obstretic ultrasound scans and in visualization for surgical planning and tumor resection.

References

1. Card, S.K., Mackinlay, J.D., Shneiderman, B. (eds.): Readings in Information Visu-alization: Using Vision to Think. Morgan Kaufmann, Burlington (1999)
2. Ware, C.: Information Visualization: Perception for Design. Kaufmann, Pittsburgh (2004)
3. Li, W., Ritter, L., Agrawala, M., Curless, B., Salesin, D.: Interactive cutaway illustrations of complex 3D models. ACM Trans. Graph. **26**(3) (2007)
4. Viola, I.: Importance-driven feature enhancement in volume visualization. IEEE Trans. Vis. Comput. Graph. **11**(4), 408–418 (2005)
5. Weiskopf, D., et al.: Interactive clipping techniques for texture-based volume visu-alization and volume shading. IEEE Trans. Vis. Comput. Graph. **9**(3), 298–312 (2003)
6. Wimmer, F.: Focus and context visualization for medical augmented reality. Chair for Computer Aided Medical Procedures, Technical University Munich, thesis (2007)
7. GoKnee3D RSNA 2017. www.siemens.com/press/en/pressrelease/2017/healthin eers/pr2017110085hcen.htm
8. Figueroa, D.: Knee chondral lesions: incidence and correlation between arthroscopic and magnetic resonance findings. Arthroscopy **23**(3), 312–315 (2007)
9. Hudelmaier, M., et al.: Age-related changes in the morphology and deformational behavior of knee joint cartilage. Arthritis Rheum. **44**(11), 2556–2561 (2001)
10. Comaniciu, D., et al.: Shaping the future through innovations: from medical imag-ing to precision medicine. Med. Image Anal. **33**, 19–26 (2016)
11. Raj, A., Vishwanathan, S., Ajani, B., Krishnan, K., Agarwal, H.: Automatic knee cartilage segmentation using fully volumetric convolutional neural networks for evaluation of osteoarthritis. In: IEEE International Symposium on Biomedical Imaging (2018)
12. Bookstein, F.L.: Principal warps: thin-plate splines and the decomposition of defor-mations. IEEE Trans. Pattern Anal. Mach. Intell. **11**(6), 567–585 (1989)
13. Kroes, T., Post, F.H., Botha, C.P.: Exposure render: an interactive photo-realistic volume rendering framework. PLOS one **7**(7), 1–10 (2012)

Closing the Calibration Loop:
An Inside-Out-Tracking Paradigm
for Augmented Reality in Orthopedic
Surgery

Jonas Hajek[1,2], Mathias Unberath[1(✉)], Javad Fotouhi[1], Bastian Bier[1,2],
Sing Chun Lee[1], Greg Osgood[3], Andreas Maier[2], Mehran Armand[4],
and Nassir Navab[1]

[1] Computer Aided Medical Procedures, Johns Hopkins University, Baltimore, USA
unberath@jhu.edu
[2] Pattern Recognition Lab, Friedrich-Alexander-Universität Erlangen-Nürnberg,
Erlangen, Germany
[3] Department of Orthopaedic Surgery, Johns Hopkins Hospital, Baltimore, USA
[4] Applied Physics Laboratory, Johns Hopkins University, Baltimore, USA

Abstract. In percutaneous orthopedic interventions the surgeon attempts to reduce and fixate fractures in bony structures. The complexity of these interventions arises when the surgeon performs the challenging task of navigating surgical tools percutaneously only under the guidance of 2D interventional X-ray imaging. Moreover, the intra-operatively acquired data is only visualized indirectly on external displays. In this work, we propose a flexible Augmented Reality (AR) paradigm using optical see-through head mounted displays. The key technical contribution of this work includes the marker-less and dynamic tracking concept which closes the calibration loop between patient, C-arm and the surgeon. This calibration is enabled using Simultaneous Localization and Mapping of the environment, i.e. the operating theater. In return, the proposed solution provides *in situ* visualization of pre- and intra-operative 3D medical data directly at the surgical site. We demonstrate pre-clinical evaluation of a prototype system, and report errors for calibration and target registration. Finally, we demonstrate the usefulness of the proposed inside-out tracking system in achieving "bull's eye" view for C-arm-guided punctures. This AR solution provides an intuitive visualization of the anatomy and can simplify the hand-eye coordination for the orthopedic surgeon.

Keywords: Augmented Reality · Human computer interface
Intra-operative visualization and guidance · C-arm · Cone-beam CT

J. Hajek, M. Unberath and J. Fotouhi—These authors are considered joint first authors.

© Springer Nature Switzerland AG 2018
A. F. Frangi et al. (Eds.): MICCAI 2018, LNCS 11073, pp. 299–306, 2018.
https://doi.org/10.1007/978-3-030-00937-3_35

1   Introduction

Modern orthopedic trauma surgery focuses on percutaneous alternatives to many complicated procedures [1,2]. These minimally invasive approaches are guided by intra-operative X-ray images that are acquired using mobile, non-robotic C-arm systems. It is well known that X-ray images from multiple orientations are required to warrant understanding of the 3D spatial relations since 2D fluoroscopy suffers from the effects of projective transformation. Mastering the mental mapping of tools to anatomy from 2D images is a key competence that surgeons acquire through extensive training. Yet, this task often challenges even experienced surgeons leading to longer procedure times, increased radiation dose, multiple tool insertions, and surgeon frustration [3,4].

If 3D pre- or intra-operative imaging is available, challenges due to indirect visualization can be mitigated, substantially reducing surgeon task load and fostering improved surgical outcome. Unfortunately, most of the previously proposed systems provide 3D information at the cost of integrating outside-in tracking solutions that require additional markers and intra-operative calibration that hinder clinical acceptance [3]. As an alternative, intuitive and real-time visualization of 3D data in Augmented Reality (AR) environments has recently received considerable attention [4,5]. In this work, we present a purely image-based inside-out tracking concept and prototype system that dynamically closes the calibration loop between surgeon, patient, and C-arm enabling intra-operative optical see-through head-mounted display (OST HMD)-based AR visualization overlaid with the anatomy of interest. Such *in situ* visualization could benefit residents in training that observe surgery to fully understand the actions of the lead surgeon with respect to the deep-seated anatomical targets. These applications in addition to simple task such as optimal positioning of C-arm systems, do not require the accuracy needed for surgical navigation and, therefore, could be the first target for OST HMD visualization in surgery. To the best of our knowledge, this prototype constitutes the first marker-less solution to intra-operative 3D AR on the target anatomy.

2   Materials and Methods

2.1   Calibration

The inside-out tracking paradigm, core of the proposed concept, is driven by the observation that all relevant entities (surgeon, patient, and C-arm) are positioned relative to the same environment, which we will refer to as the "world coordinate system". For intra-operative visualization of 3D volumes overlaid with the patient, we seek to dynamically recover

$$^{S}\mathbf{T}_{V}(t) = ^{S}\mathbf{T}_{W} \underbrace{\left(^{T}\mathbf{T}_{W}^{-1}(t_0) \, ^{T}\mathbf{T}_{C}(t_0) \right) \, ^{V}\mathbf{T}_{C}^{-1}}_{^{W}\mathbf{T}_{V}}, \tag{1}$$

the transformation describing the mapping from the surgeon's eyes to the 3D image volume. In Eq. 1, t_0 describes the time of pre- to intra-operative image

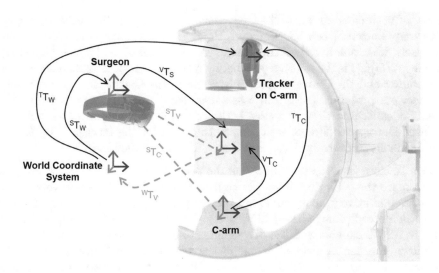

Fig. 1. Spatial relations that must be estimated dynamically to enable the proposed AR environment. Transformations shown in black are estimated directly while transformations shown in orange are derived.

registration while t is the current time point. The spatial relations that are required to dynamically estimate $^S\mathbf{T}_V$ are explained in the remainder of this section and visualized in Fig. 1.

$^W\mathbf{T}_{S/T}$: The transformations $^W\mathbf{T}_{S/T}$ are estimated using Simultaneous Localization and Mapping (SLAM) thereby incrementally constructing a map of the environment, i.e. the world coordinate system [6]. Exemplarily for the surgeon, SLAM solves

$$^W\mathbf{T}_S(t) = \underset{^W\hat{\mathbf{T}}_S}{\arg\min}\ \mathrm{d}\Big(\mathbf{f}_W\Big(\mathbf{P}\,^W\hat{\mathbf{T}}_S(t)\mathbf{x}_S(t)\Big), \mathbf{f}_S(t)\Big), \tag{2}$$

where $\mathbf{f}_S(t)$ are features in the image at time t, $\mathbf{x}_S(t)$ are the 3D locations of these feature estimates either via depth sensors or stereo, $\mathbf{P}$ is the projection operator, and $d(\cdot, \cdot)$ is the feature similarity to be optimized. A key innovation of this work is the inside-out SLAM-based tracking of the C-arm w.r.t. the *exact same* map of the environment by means of an additional tracker rigidly attached to the C-shaped gantry. This becomes possible if both trackers are operated in a master-slave configuration and observe partially overlapping parts of the environment, i.e. a feature rich and temporally stable area of the environment. This suggests, that the cameras on the C-arm tracker (in contrast to previous solutions [5,7]) need to face the room rather than the patient.

$^T\mathbf{T}_C$: The tracker is rigidly mounted on the C-arm gantry suggesting that one-time offline calibration is possible. Since the X-ray and tracker cameras have no overlap, methods based on multi-modal patterns as in [4,5,7] fail. However, if poses of both cameras w.r.t. the environment and the imaging volume, respectively, are known or can be estimated, Hand-Eye calibration is feasible [8]. Put concisely, we estimate a rigid transform $^\mathrm{T}\mathbf{T}_\mathrm{C}$ such that $\mathbf{A}(t_i)\,^\mathrm{T}\mathbf{T}_\mathrm{C} = {}^\mathrm{T}\mathbf{T}_\mathrm{C}\mathbf{B}(t_i)$, where $(\mathbf{A}/\mathbf{B})(t_i)$ is the relative pose between subsequent poses at times $i, i+1$ of the tracker and the C-arm, respectively. Poses of the C-arm $^\mathrm{V}\mathbf{T}_\mathrm{C}(t_i)$ are known because our prototype (Sect. 2.2) uses a cone-beam CT (CBCT) enabled C-arm with pre-calibrated circular source trajectory such that several poses $^\mathrm{V}\mathbf{T}_\mathrm{C}$ are known. During one sweep, we estimate the poses of the tracker $^\mathrm{W}\mathbf{T}_\mathrm{T}(t_i)$ via Eq. 1. Finally, we recover $^\mathrm{T}\mathbf{T}_\mathrm{C}$, and thus $^\mathrm{W}\mathbf{T}_\mathrm{C}$, as detailed in [8].

$^\mathrm{V}\mathbf{T}_C$: To close the loop by calibrating the patient to the environment, we need to estimate the $^\mathrm{V}\mathbf{T}_\mathrm{C}$ describing the transformation from 3D image volumes to an intra-operatively acquired X-ray image. For pre-operative data, $^\mathrm{V}\mathbf{T}_\mathrm{C}$ can be estimated via image-based 3D/2D registration, e.g. as in [9,10]. If the C-arm is CBCT capable and the 3D volume is acquired intra-procedurally, $^\mathrm{V}\mathbf{T}_\mathrm{C}$ is known and can be defined as one of the pre-calibrated C-arm poses on the source trajectory, e.g. the first one. Once $^\mathrm{V}\mathbf{T}_\mathrm{C}$ is known, the volumetric images are calibrated to the room via $^\mathrm{W}\mathbf{T}_\mathrm{V} = {}^\mathrm{W}\mathbf{T}_\mathrm{T}(t_0)\,^\mathrm{T}\mathbf{T}_\mathrm{C}\,^\mathrm{V}\mathbf{T}_\mathrm{C}^{-1}(t_0)$, where t_0 denotes the time of calibration.

2.2   Prototype

For visualization of virtual content we use the Microsoft HoloLens (Microsoft, Redmond, WA) that simultaneously serves as inside-out tracker providing $^\mathrm{W}\mathbf{T}_\mathrm{S}$ according to see Sect. 2.1. To enable a master-slave configuration and enable tracking w.r.t. the exact same map of the environment, we mount a second HoloLens device on the C-arm to track movement of the gantry $^\mathrm{W}\mathbf{T}_\mathrm{T}$. We use a CBCT enabled mobile C-arm (Siemens Arcadis Orbic 3D, Siemens Healthineers, Forchheim, Germany) and rigidly attach the tracking device to the image intensifier with the principal ray of the front facing RGB camera oriented parallel to the patient table as demonstrated in Fig. 2. $^\mathrm{T}\mathbf{T}_\mathrm{C}$ is estimated via Hand-Eye calibration from 98 (tracker, C-arm) absolute pose pairs acquired during a circular source trajectory yielding 4753 relative poses. Since the C-arm is CBCT enabled, we simplify estimation of $^\mathrm{V}\mathbf{T}_\mathrm{C}$ and define t_0 to correspond to the first C-arm pose.

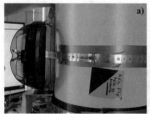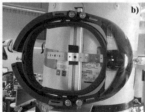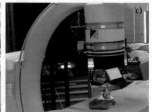

Fig. 2. The prototype uses a Microsoft Hololens as tracker which is rigidly mounted on the C-arm detector, as demonstrated in Fig. (a) and (b). In (c), the coordinate axis of the RGB tracker is shown in relation to the mobile C-arm.

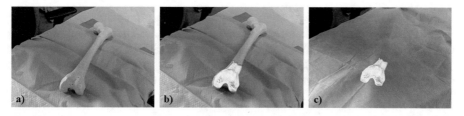

Fig. 3. Since $^S\mathbf{T}_V(t)$ is known, the real object in (a) is overlaid with the rendered volume shown in (b). Correct overlay persists even if the real object is covered in (c).

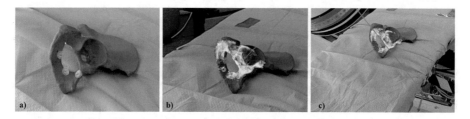

Fig. 4. (a) Pelvis phantom used for TRE assessment. (b) Lines placed during the experiment to evaluate point-to-line TRE. (c) Visualization of the X-ray source and principal ray next to the same phantom.

2.3 Virtual Content in the AR Environment

Once all spatial relations are estimated, multiple augmentations of the scene become possible. We support visualization of the following content depending on the task (see Fig. 4): Using $^S\mathbf{T}_V(t)$ we provide volume renderings of the 3D image volumes augmented on the patient's anatomy as shown in Fig. 3. In addition to the volume rendering, annotations of the 3D data (such as landmarks) can be displayed. Further and via $^S\mathbf{T}_C(t)$, the C-arm source and principal ray, seen in Fig. 4c) can be visualized as the C-arm gantry is moved to different viewing angles. Volume rendering and principal ray visualization combined are an effective solution to determine "bull's eye" views to guide punctures [11]. All rendering is performed on the HMD; therefore, the perceptual quality is limited by the computational resources of the device.

2.4 Experiments and Feasibility Study

Hand-Eye Residual Error: Following [8], we compute the rotational and translational component of $^T\mathbf{T}_C$ independently. Therefore, we state the residual of solving $\mathbf{A}(t_i)\,^T\mathbf{T}_C = \,^T\mathbf{T}_C\mathbf{B}(t_i)$ for $^T\mathbf{T}_C$ separately for rotation and translation averaged over all relative poses.

Target Registration Error: We evaluate the end-to-end target registration error (TRE) of our prototype system using a Sawbones phantom (Sawbones, Vashon, WA) with metal spheres on the surface. The spheres are annotated in a CBCT of the phantom and serve as the targets for TRE computation. Next, $M = 4$ medical experts are asked to locate the spheres in the AR environment: For every of the $N = 7$ spheres $\mathbf{p}_i$, the user j changes position in the room, and using the "air tap" gesture defines a 3D line $\mathbf{l}_i^j$ corresponding to his gaze that intersects the sphere on the phantom. The TRE is then defined as

$$\text{TRE} = \frac{1}{M \cdot N} \sum_{j=1}^{M} \sum_{i=1}^{N} \text{d}(\mathbf{p}_i, \mathbf{l}_i^j), \tag{3}$$

where $\text{d}(\mathbf{p}, \mathbf{l})$ is the 3D point-to-line distance.

Achieving "Bull's Eye" View: Complementary to the technical assessment, we conduct a clinical task-based evaluation of the prototype: Achieving "bull's eye" view for percutaneous punctures. To this end, we manufacture cubic foam phantoms and embed a radiopaque tubular structure (radius $\approx 5\,\text{mm}$) at arbitrary orientation but invisible from the outside. A CBCT is acquired and rendered in the AR environment overlaid with the physical phantom such that the tube is clearly discernible. Further, the principal ray of the C-arm system is visualized. Again, $M = 4$ medical experts are asked to move the gantry such that the principal ray pierces the tubular structure, thereby achieving the desired "bull's eye" view. Verification of the view is performed by acquiring an X-ray image. Additionally, users advance a K-wire through the tubular structure under "bull's eye" view guidance using X-rays from the view selected in the AR environment. Placement of the K-wire without breaching of the tube is verified in the guidance and a lateral X-ray view.

3   Results

Hand-Eye Residual Error: We quantified the residual error of our Hand-Eye calibration between the C-arm and tracker separately for rotational and translational component. For rotation, we found an average residual of 6.18°, 5.82°, and 5.17° around $\mathbf{e}_x$, $\mathbf{e}_y$, and $\mathbf{e}_z$, respectively, while for translation the root-mean-squared residual was 26.6 mm. It is worth mentioning that the median translational error in $\mathbf{e}_x$, $\mathbf{e}_y$, and $\mathbf{e}_z$ direction was 4.10 mm, 3.02 mm, 43.18 mm, respectively, where $\mathbf{e}_z$ corresponds to the direction of the principal ray of the tracker coordinate system, i.e. the rotation axis of the C-arm.

Target Registration Error: The point-to-line TRE averaged over all points and users was 11.46 mm.

Achieving "Bull's Eye" View: Every user successfully achieved a "bull's eye" view in the first try that allowed them to place a K-wire without breach of the tubular structure. Fig. 5 shows representative scene captures acquired from the perspective of the user. A video documenting one trial from both a bystander's and the user's perspective can be found on our homepage.[1]

---

[1] https://camp.lcsr.jhu.edu/miccai-2018-demonstration-videos/.

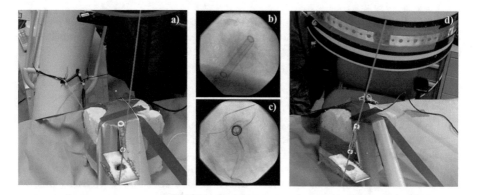

Fig. 5. Screen captures from the user's perspective attempting to achieve the "bull's eye" view. The virtual line (purple) corresponds to the principal ray of the C-arm system in the current pose while the CBCT of the phantom is volume rendered in light blue. (a) The C-arm is positioned in neutral pose with the laser cross-hair indicating that the phantom is within the field of view. The AR environment indicates misalignment for "bull's eye" view that is confirmed using an X-ray (b). After alignment of the virtual principal ray with the virtual tubular structure inside the phantom (d), an acceptable "bull's eye" view is achieved (c).

4   Discussion and Conclusion

We presented an inside-out tracking paradigm to close the transformation loop for AR in orthopedic surgery based upon the realization that surgeon, patient, and C-arm can be calibrated to their environment. Our entirely marker-less approach enables rendering of virtual content at meaningful positions, i.e. dynamically overlaid with the patient and the C-arm source. The performance of our prototype system is promising and enables effective "bull's eye" viewpoint planning for punctures.

Despite an overall positive evaluation, some limitations remain. The TRE of 11.46 mm is acceptable for viewpoint planning, but may be unacceptably high if the aim of augmentation is direct feedback on tool trajectories as in [4,5]. The TRE is compound of multiple sources of error: (1) Residual errors in Hand-Eye calibration of $^{T}\mathbf{T}_{C}$, particularly due to the fact that poses are acquired on a circular trajectory and are, thus, co-planar as supported by our quantitative results; and (2) Inaccurate estimates of $^{W}\mathbf{T}_{T}$ and $^{W}\mathbf{T}_{S}$ that indirectly affect all other transformations. We anticipate improvements in this regard when additional out-of-plane pose pairs are sampled for Hand-Eye calibration. Further, the accuracy of estimating $^{W}\mathbf{T}_{T/S}$ is currently limited by the capabilities of Microsoft's HoloLens and is expected to improve in the future.

In summary, we believe that our approach has great potential to benefit orthopedic trauma procedures particularly when pre-operative 3D imaging is available. In addition to the benefits for the surgeon discussed here, the proposed AR environment may prove beneficial in an educational context where residents must comprehend the lead surgeon's actions. Further, we envision scenarios where the proposed solution can support the X-ray technician in achieving the desired views of the target anatomy.

References

1. Gay, B., Goitz, H.T., Kahler, A.: Percutaneous CT guidance: screw fixation of acetabular fractures preliminary results of a new technique with. Am. J. Roentgenol. **158**(4), 819–822 (1992)
2. Hong, G., Cong-Feng, L., Cheng-Fang, H., Chang-Qing, Z., Bing-Fang, Z.: Percutaneous screw fixation of acetabular fractures with 2D fluoroscopy-based computerized navigation. Arch. Orthop. Trauma Surg. **130**(9), 1177–1183 (2010)
3. Markelj, P., Tomaževič, D., Likar, B., Pernuš, F.: A review of 3D/2D registration methods for image-guided interventions. Med. Image Anal. **16**(3), 642–661 (2012)
4. Andress, S., et al.: On-the-fly augmented reality for orthopedic surgery using a multimodal fiducial. J. Med. Imaging **5** (2018)
5. Tucker, E., et al.: Towards clinical translation of augmented orthopedic surgery: from pre-op CT to intra-op X-ray via RGBD sensing. In: SPIE Medical Imaging (2018)
6. Endres, F., Hess, J., Engelhard, N., Sturm, J., Cremers, D., Burgard, W.: An evaluation of the RGB-D slam system. In: 2012 IEEE International Conference on Robotics and Automation (ICRA), pp. 1691–1696. IEEE (2012)
7. Fotouhi, J., et al.: Pose-aware C-arm for automatic re-initialization of interventional 2D/3D image registration. Int. J. Comput. Assisted Radiol. Surg. **12**(7), 1221–1230 (2017)
8. Tsai, R.Y., Lenz, R.K.: A new technique for fully autonomous and efficient 3D robotics hand/eye calibration. IEEE Trans. Rob. Autom. **5**(3), 345–358 (1989)
9. Berger, M., et al.: Marker-free motion correction in weight-bearing cone-beam CT of the knee joint. Med. Phys. **43**(3), 1235–1248 (2016)
10. De Silva, T., et al.: 3D–2D image registration for target localization in spine surgery: investigation of similarity metrics providing robustness to content mismatch. Phys. Med. Biol. **61**(8), 3009 (2016)
11. Morimoto, M., et al.: C-arm cone beam CT for hepatic tumor ablation under real-time 3D imaging. Am. J. Roentgenol. **194**(5), W452–W454 (2010)

Higher Order of Motion Magnification for Vessel Localisation in Surgical Video

Mirek Janatka[1,2]([✉]), Ashwin Sridhar[1], John Kelly[1], and Danail Stoyanov[1,2]

[1] Wellcome/EPSRC Centre for Interventional and Surgical Sciences,
University College London, London, UK
[2] Department of Computer Science, University College London, London, UK
mirek.janatka@ucl.ac.uk

Abstract. Locating vessels during surgery is critical for avoiding inadvertent damage, yet vasculature can be difficult to identify. Video motion magnification can potentially highlight vessels by exaggerating subtle motion embedded within the video to become perceivable to the surgeon. In this paper, we explore a physiological model of artery distension to extend motion magnification to incorporate higher orders of motion, leveraging the difference in acceleration over time (jerk) in pulsatile motion to highlight the vascular pulse wave. Our method is compared to first and second order motion based Eulerian video magnification algorithms. Using data from a surgical video retrieved during a robotic prostatectomy, we show that our method can accentuate cardiophysiological features and produce a more succinct and clearer video for motion magnification, with more similarities in areas without motion to the source video at large magnifications. We validate the approach with a Structure Similarity (SSIM) and Peak Signal to Noise Ratio (PSNR) assessment of three videos at an increasing working distance, using three different levels of optical magnification. Spatio-temporal cross sections are presented to show the effectiveness of our proposal and video samples are provided to demonstrates qualitatively our results.

Keywords: Video motion magnification · Vessel localisation
Augmented reality · Computer assisted interventions

1 Introduction

One of the most common surgical complications is due to inadvertent damage to blood vessels. Avoiding vascular structures is particularly challenging in minimally invasive surgery (MIS) and robotic MIS (RMIS) where the tactile senses are inhibited and cannot be used to detect pulsatile motion. Vessels can be detected by using interventional imaging modalities like fluorescence or ultrasound (US) but these do not always produce a sufficient signal, or are difficult to use in practice [1]. Using video information directly is appealing because it is inherently available, but processing is required to reveal any vessel information

© Springer Nature Switzerland AG 2018
A. F. Frangi et al. (Eds.): MICCAI 2018, LNCS 11073, pp. 307–314, 2018.
https://doi.org/10.1007/978-3-030-00937-3_36

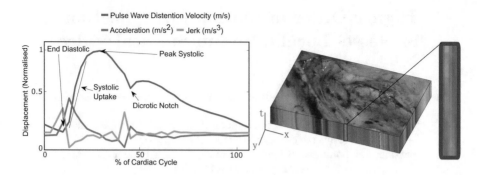

Fig. 1. (Left): The vessel distension-displacement from the pulse wave, with the higher order derivatives along with annotation of the corresponding cardio-physiological stages. Down sampled to 30 data points to reflect endoscope frame rate acquisition. (1-D Virtual Model of arterial behaviour [2]) (Right): Endoscopic video image stack. The blue box surrounds an artery with no perceivable motion, shown by the vertical white line in the cross section

hidden within the video and is not apparent to the surgeon, as can be seen in the right image of Fig. 1.

The cardiovascular system creates a pressure wave that propagates through the entire body and causes an equivalent distension-displacement profile in the arteries and veins [3]. This periodic motion has intricate characteristics, shown in Fig. 1 (left), that can be highlighted by differentiating the distension-displacement signal. The second order derivative outlines where the systolic uptake is located, whilst the third derivative highlights the end diastolic phase and the dicrotic notch. This information can be present as spatio-temporal variation between image frames and amplified using Eulerian video magnification (EVM). EVM could be applied to endoscopic video for vessel localisation by using an adaptation of an EVM algorithm and showing the output video directly to the surgeon [4]. Similarly, EVM can aid vessel segmentation for registration and overlay of pre-operative data [5], as existing linear based forms of the raw magnified video can be abstract and noisy to use directly within a dynamic scene. Magnifying the underlying video motion can exacerbate unwanted artifacts and unsought motions, and in this case regarding surgical video, of those which are not the blood vessels but due to respiration, endoscope motion or other physiological movement within the scene.

In this paper, we propose to utilise features that are apparent in the cardiac pulse wave, particularly the non-linear motion components that are emphasised by the third order of displacement, known as jerk (Green plot Fig. 1, left). We devise a custom temporal filter and use an existing technique for spatial decomposition of complex steerable pyramids [6]. The result is a more coherent magnified video compared to existing lower order of motion approaches [7,8], as the high magnitudes of jerk are prominently exclusive to the pulse wave in the surgical scene, as our method avoids amplification of residual motions due to respiration or other periodic scene activities. Quantitative results are difficult for such approaches but we report a comparison to previous work using Structure Similarity [9] and Peak Signal to Noise Ratio (PSNR) of three robotic assisted surgical videos at separate optical zoom. We provide a qualitative example of how our method achieves isolation of two cardio-physiological features over existing methods. A supplementary video of the magnifications is provided that further illustrates the results.

2   Methods

Building on previous work in video motion magnification [7,8,10] we set out to highlight the third order motion characteristics created by the cardiac cycle. In an Eulerian frame of reference, the input image signal function is taken as $I(\mathbf{x}, t)$ at position $\mathbf{x}$ ($\mathbf{x} = (x, y)$) and at time t [10]. With the linear magnification methods, $\delta(t)$ is taken as a displacement function with respect to time, giving the expression $I(\mathbf{x}, t) = f(\mathbf{x} + \delta(t))$ and is equivalent to the first-order term in the Taylor expansion:

$$I(\mathbf{x}, t) \approx f(\mathbf{x}) + \delta(t)\frac{\partial f(\mathbf{x})}{\partial \mathbf{x}} \tag{1}$$

This Taylor series expansion appropriation can be continued into higher orders of motion, as shown in [8]. Taking it to the third order, where $\hat{I}(\mathbf{x}, t)$ is the magnified pixel at point $\mathbf{x}$ and time t in the video.

$$\hat{I}(\mathbf{x}, t) \approx f(\mathbf{x}) + (1+\beta)\delta(t)\frac{\delta f(\mathbf{x})}{\delta \mathbf{x}} + (1+\beta)^2\delta(t)^2\frac{1}{2}\frac{\delta^2 f(\mathbf{x})}{\delta^2 \mathbf{x}} + (1+\beta)^3\delta(t)^3\frac{1}{6}\frac{\delta^3 f(\mathbf{x})}{\delta^3} \tag{2}$$

In a similar vein to [8], we equate a component of the expansion to an order of motion and isolate these by subtraction of the lower orders

$$I(\mathbf{x}, t) - I(\mathbf{x}, t)_{non-linear(2^{nd}order)} - I(x, t)_{linear} \approx (1+\beta)^3\delta(t)^3\frac{1}{6}\frac{\delta^3 f(x)}{\delta^3 \mathbf{x}} \tag{3}$$

assuming $(1+\beta)^3 = \alpha$, $\alpha > 0$.

$$D(\mathbf{x}, t) = \delta(t)^3\frac{1}{6}\frac{\delta^3 f(\mathbf{x})}{\delta^3 \mathbf{x}} \tag{4}$$

$$\hat{I}_{non-linear(3^{nd}order)}(\mathbf{x}, t) = I(\mathbf{x}, t) + \alpha D(\mathbf{x}, t) \tag{5}$$

This produces an approximation for for the input signal and a term that can be attenuated in order to present an augmented reality (AR) view of the original video.

2.1   Temporal Filtering

As jerk is the third temporal derivative of the signal $\hat{I}(\mathbf{x}, t)$, a filter has to be derived to reflect this. To achieve acceleration magnification, the Difference of Gaussian (DoG) filter was used [8]. This allowed for a temporal bandpass to be assigned, by subtracting two Gaussian filters, using $\sigma = \frac{r}{4\omega\sqrt{2}}$ [11] to calculate the standard deviations of them both, where r is the frame rate of the video and ω is the frequency under investigation. Taking the derivative of the second order DoG we create an approximation of the third order, which follows Hermitian polynominals [12]. Due to the linearity of the operators, the relationship between the the jerk in the signal and the third order DoG as:

$$\frac{\partial^3 I(\mathbf{x},t)}{\partial t^3} \otimes G_\sigma(t) = I(\mathbf{x},t) \otimes \frac{\partial^3 G_\sigma(t)}{\partial t^3} \tag{6}$$

2.2   Phase-Based Magnification

In the classical EVM approach, the intensity change over time is used in a pixel-wise manner [10] where a second order IIR filter detects the intensity change caused by the human pulse. An extension of this uses the difference in phase w.r.t spatial frequency [7] for linear motion, as subtle difference in phase can be detected between frames where minute motion is present. Recently, phase-based acceleration magnification has been proposed [8]. It is this methodology we utilise and amend for jerk magnification. By describing motion as phase shift, a decomposition of the signal $f(x)$ with displacement $\delta(t)$ at time t, the sum of all frequencies (ω) can be shown as:

$$f(\mathbf{x} + \delta(t)) = \sum_{\omega=-\infty}^{\infty} A_\omega e^{i\omega(\mathbf{x}+\delta(t))} \tag{7}$$

where the global phase for frequency ω for displacement $\delta(t)$ is $\phi_\omega = \omega(\mathbf{x}+\delta(t))$.

It has been shown that spatially localised phase information of a series of image over time is related to local motion [13] and has been leveraged for linear magnification [7]. This is performed by using complex steerable pyramids [14] to separate the image signal into multi-frequency bands and orientations. These pyramids contain a set of filters $\Psi_{\omega_s,\theta}$ at multiple scales, ω_s and orientations θ. The local phase information of a single 2D image $I(\mathbf{x})$ is

$$(I(\mathbf{x})) \otimes \Psi_{\omega_s,\theta}(\mathbf{x}) = A_{\omega,\theta}(\mathbf{x})e^{i\phi_{\omega_s,\theta}(\mathbf{x})} \tag{8}$$

where $A_{\omega,\theta}(\mathbf{x})$ is the amplitude at frequency ω and orientation θ, and where $\phi_{\omega_s,\theta}$ is the corresponding phase at scale (pyramid level) ω_s. The phase information is extracted ($\phi_{\omega_s,\theta}(\mathbf{x},t)$) at a given frequency ω, orientation θ and frame t. The jerk constituent part of the motion is filtered out with our third order Gaussian filter and can then be magnified and reinstated into the video ($\hat{\phi}_{\omega,\theta}(\mathbf{x},t)$) to accentuate the desired state changes in the cardiac cycle, such as the dicrotic notch and end diastolic point, shown in Fig. 1 (left).

$$D_\sigma(\phi_{\omega,\theta}(\mathbf{x},t)) = \phi_{\omega,\theta}(\mathbf{x},t) \otimes \frac{\partial^3 G_\sigma(t)}{\partial t^3} \tag{9}$$

$$\hat{\phi}_{\omega,\theta}(\mathbf{x},t) = \phi_{\omega,\theta}(\mathbf{x},t) + \alpha D_\sigma \phi_{\omega,\theta}(\mathbf{x},t) \tag{10}$$

Phase unwrapping is applied as with the acceleration methodology in order to create the full composite signal [8,15].

3   Results

To demonstrate the proposed approach, endoscopic video was captured from robotic prostatectomy using the da Vinci surgical system (Intuitive Surgical Inc, CA), where a partially occluded obturator artery could be seen. Despite being identified by the surgical team the vessel produced little perceivable motion in the video. This footage was captured at 1080p resolution at 30 Hz. For processing ease, the video was cropped to a third of the original width, which contained the motion of interest, yet still retains the spatial resolution of the endoscope. The video was motion magnified using the phase-based complex steerable pyramid technique described in [7] for first order motion and the video acceleration magnification described in [8] offline for comparison. Our method appended the video acceleration magnification method. All processes use a four level pyramid and half octave pyramid type. For the temporal processing, a bandpass was set at 1 Hz +/− 0.1 to account for a pulse around 54 to 66 bpm. From the patient's ECG reading, their pulse was stable at 60 bpm during video acquisition. This was done at three magnification factors (x2, x5, x10). Spatio-temporal slices were then taken of a site along the obturator artery for visual comparison of each temporal filter type. For a quantitative comparison, the Peak Noise to Signal Ratio (PNSR) and Structural Similarity (SSIM) index [9] was calculated on a hundred frame sample, comparing the magnified videos to their original equivalent frame.

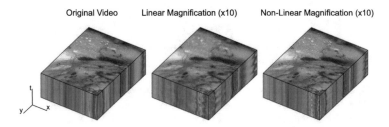

Fig. 2. Volumetric image stacks of an endoscopic scene under different types of magnification.

Figure 2 shows an apprehensible overview of our video magnification investigation. The pulse from the external iliac artery can be seen in the right corner and the obturator artery on the front face. Large distortion and blur can be observed on the linear magnification example, particularly in the front right corner, where as this is not present on the non-linear example, as change in velocity is exaggerated, where as any velocity is exaggerated in the linear case. Figure 3 displays a magnification comparison of spatio-temporal slices taken from three different for mentioned magnification methods. E and G in this figure, demonstrates the improvement in pulse wave motion granularity using jerk has in temporal processing, compared to the lower orders. The magenta in E shows a periodic saw wave, with no discerning features relating to the underlying pulse wave signal.

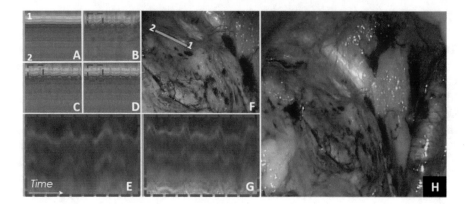

Fig. 3. Motion magnification of the obturator artery (x10). (a) Unmagnified spatio-temporal slice (STS); (b) Linear magnification [7]; (c) Acceleration magnification [8]; (d) Jerk magnification (our proposal); (e),(g) Comparative STS, blue box from (d) (jerk) in green, with (b) in magenta in (e) and (c) in magenta in (g); (f) Sample site (zoomed); (h) Overview of the surgical scene.

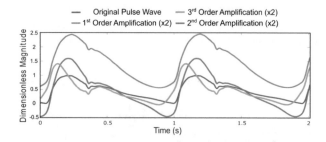

Fig. 4. 1D distension-displacement pulse wave signal amplification, using virtual data [2]. The jerk magnification shown in green creates two distinct peaks that is not present in the other two methods of lower order.

The magenta in G that depicts the use of acceleration shows a more bipolar tri-angle wave. The green in both E and G shows a consistent periodic twin peak, with the second being more diminished, which suggests that our hypothesis of a jerk temporal filter being able to detect the dicrotic notch as correct and com-parable to our model analysis shown in Fig. 4. Table 1 shows a comparison of a surgical scene at three separate working distances. This was arranged to dimin-ish the spatial resolution with the same objective in the endoscope. All three aforementioned magnification algorithms were used on each at three different motion magnification (α) factors (x2, x5, x10).

As a comparative metric, SSIM and PSNR are used as a quantitative metric, with PSNR being based on mathematical model and SSIM taking into account characteristics of the human visual system [9]. SSIM and PSNR allow for objec-tive comparisons of a processed image to a reference source, whilst it is expected that a magnified video to be altered, the residual noise generation by the process

Table 1. Results from SSIM analysis and PSNR for our surgical videos at three levels of magnification across the different temporal processing approaches.

α	Assessment	Scene level 1			Scene level 2			Scene level 3		
		Linear	Acc.	Jerk	Linear	Acc.	Jerk	Linear	Acc.	Jerk
$x2$	SSIM	34.95	34.7	35.65	33.87	34.33	35.31	34.41	35.02	35.31
	PSNR	0.94	0.95	0.96	0.93	0.94	0.96	0.95	0.96	0.96
$x5$	SSIM	30.6	31.5	33.18	28.98	31.05	33	30.32	31.88	33
	PSNR	0.88	0.9	0.93	0.85	0.89	0.92	0.9	0.92	0.92
$x10$	SSIM	27.76	28.94	30.56	25.92	28.41	30.43	27.75	29.36	30.43
	PSNR	0.82	0.85	0.88	0.78	0.83	0.87	0.85	0.86	0.88

can be seen by these proposed methods. SSIM is measured in decibels (db), where the higher the number the better the quality is. PSNR is a percentile reading, with 1 being the best possible correspondence to the reference frame. For the all surgical scene, our proposed temporal process of using jerk out performs the other low order motion magnification methods across all magnifications for SSIM and equals or outperforms the acceleration technique, particularly at $\alpha = 10$.

4   Conclusion

We have demonstrated that the use of higher order motion magnification can bring out subtle motion features that are exclusive to the pulse wave in arteries. This limits the amplification of residual signals present in surgical scenes. Our method particularly relies on the definitive cardiovascular signature characterized by the twin peaks of the end diastolic point and the dicrotic notch. Additionally, we have shown objective evidence that less noise is generated when used within laparoscopic surgery compared to other magnification technique, however, a wider sample and case specific examples would be needed to verify this claim. Further work will look at a real-time implementation of this approach as well as methods of both ground truth validation and subjective comparison within a clinical setting. Practical clinical use cases are also needed to verify the validity of using such techniques in practice and to identify the bottlenecks to translation.

Acknowledgements. The work was supported by funding from the EPSRC (EP/N013220/1, EP/N027078/1, NS/A000027/1) and Wellcome (NS/A000050/1).

References

1. Sridhar, A.N., et al.: Image-guided robotic interventions for prostate cancer. Nat. Rev. Urol. **10**(8), 452 (2013)
2. Willemet, M., Chowienczyk, P., Alastruey, J.: A database of virtual healthy subjects to assess the accuracy of foot-to-foot pulse wave velocities for estimation of aortic stiffness. Am. J. Physiol.-Heart Circ. Physiol. **309**(4), H663–H675 (2015)

3. Alastruey, J., Parker, K.H., Sherwin, S.J., et al.: Arterial pulse wave haemodynamics. In: 11th International Conference on Pressure Surges, pp. 401–442. Virtual PiE Led t/a BHR Group. Lisbon (2012)
4. McLeod, A.J., Baxter, J.S.H., de Ribaupierre, S., Peters, T.M.: Motion magnification for endoscopic surgery, vol. 9036, p. 90360C (2014)
5. Amir-Khalili, A., Hamarneh, G., Peyrat, J.-M., Abinahed, J., Al-Alao, O., Al-Ansari, A., Abugharbieh, R.: Automatic segmentation of occluded vasculature via pulsatile motion analysis in endoscopic robot-assisted partial nephrectomy video. Med. Image Anal. **25**(1), 103–110 (2015)
6. Simoncelli, E.P., Adelson, E.H.: Subband transforms. In: Woods, J.W. (ed.) Subband Image Coding. SECS, vol. 115, pp. 143–192. Springer, Boston (1991). https://doi.org/10.1007/978-1-4757-2119-5_4
7. Wadhwa, N., Rubinstein, M., Durand, F., Freeman, W.T.: Phase-based video motion processing. ACM Trans. Graph. (TOG) **32**(4), 80 (2013)
8. Zhang, Y., Pintea, S.L., van Gemert, J.C.: Video acceleration magnification. arXiv preprint arXiv:1704.04186 (2017)
9. Wang, Z., Lu, L., Bovik, A.C.: Video quality assessment based on structural distortion measurement. Sig. Process. Image Commun. **19**(2), 121–132 (2004)
10. Wu, H.-Y., Rubinstein, M., Shih, E., Guttag, J., Durand, F., Freeman, W.: Eulerian video magnification for revealing subtle changes in the world (2012)
11. Mikolajczyk, K., Schmid, C.: Indexing based on scale invariant interest points. In: 2001 Proceedings of the Eighth IEEE International Conference on Computer Vision, ICCV 2001, vol. 1, pp. 525–531. IEEE (2001)
12. Haar Romeny, B.M.: Front-End Vision and Multi-scale Image Analysis: Multi-scale Computer Vision Theory and Applications, Written in Mathematica, vol. 27. Springer Science & Business Media, Heidelberg (2003). https://doi.org/10.1007/978-1-4020-8840-7
13. Fleet, D.J., Jepson, A.D.: Computation of component image velocity from local phase information. Int. J. Comput. Vis. **5**(1), 77–104 (1990)
14. Portilla, J., Simoncelli, E.P.: A parametric texture model based on joint statistics of complex wavelet coefficients. Int. J. Comput. Vis. **40**(1), 49–70 (2000)
15. Kitahara, D., Yamada, I.: Algebraic phase unwrapping along the real axis: extensions and stabilizations. Multidimens. Syst. Sig. Process. **26**(1), 3–45 (2015)

Simultaneous Surgical Visibility Assessment, Restoration, and Augmented Stereo Surface Reconstruction for Robotic Prostatectomy

Xiongbiao Luo[1(✉)], Ying Wan[5], Hui-Qing Zeng[2(✉)], Yingying Guo[1], Henry Chidozie Ewurum[1], Xiao-Bin Zhang[2], A. Jonathan McLeod[3], and Terry M. Peters[4]

[1] Department of Computer Science, Xiamen University, Xiamen, China
xbluo@xmu.edu.cn
[2] Zhongshan Hospital, Xiamen University, Xiamen, China
13606080893@139.com
[3] Intuitive Surgical Inc., Sunnyvale, CA, USA
[4] Robarts Research Institute, Western University, London, Canada
tpeters@robarts.ca
[5] School of Electrical and Data Engineering,
University of Technology Sydney, Sydney, China
joyee.wa@gmail.com

Abstract. Endoscopic vision plays a significant role in minimally invasive surgical procedures. The maintenance and augmentation of such direct in-situ vision is paramount not only for safety by preventing inadvertent injury, but also to improve precision and reduce operating time. This work aims to quantitatively and objectively evaluate endoscopic visualization on surgical videos without employing any reference images, and simultaneously to restore such degenerated visualization and improve the performance of surgical 3-D reconstruction. An objective no-reference color image quality measure is defined in terms of sharpness, naturalness, and contrast. A retinex-driven fusion framework was proposed not only to recover the deteriorated visibility but also to augment the surface reconstruction. The approaches of surgical visibility assessment, restoration, and reconstruction were validated on clinical data. The experimental results demonstrate that the average visibility was significantly enhanced from 0.66 to 1.27. Moreover, the average density ratio of surgical 3-D reconstruction was improved from 94.8% to 99.6%.

1 Endoscopic Vision

Noninvasive and minimally invasive surgical procedures often employ endoscopes inserted inside a body cavity. Equipped with video cameras and optical fiber light sources, an endoscope provides a direct in-situ visualization of the surgical field during interventions. The quality of in-situ endoscopic vision has a critical impact on the performance of these surgical procedures.

© Springer Nature Switzerland AG 2018
A. F. Frangi et al. (Eds.): MICCAI 2018, LNCS 11073, pp. 315–323, 2018.
https://doi.org/10.1007/978-3-030-00937-3_37

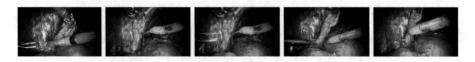

Fig. 1. Examples of degenerated surgical images due to small viewing field and very non-uniform and highly directional illumination in robotic prostatectomy

Unfortunately, the endoscope has two inherent drawbacks: (1) a relatively narrow field or small viewing angle and (2) very non-uniform and highly directional illumination of the surgical scene, due to limited optical fiber light sources (Fig. 1). These drawbacks unavoidably deteriorate the clear and high-quality visualization of both the organ being operated on and its anatomical surroundings. Furthermore, these disadvantages lead to difficultly in distinguishing many characteristics of the visualized scene (e.g., neurovascular bundle) and prevent the surgeon from clearly observing certain structures (e.g., subtle bleeding areas). Therefore, in addition to the avoidance of inadvertent injury, it is important to maintain and augment a clear field of endoscopic vision.

The objective of this work is to evaluate and augment on-site endoscopic vision or visibility of the surgical field and to simultaneously improve stereoscopic surface reconstruction. The main contributions of this work are as follows. To the best of our knowledge, this paper is the first to demonstrate objective quality assessment of surgical visualization or visibility in laparoscopic procedures, particular in robotic prostatectomy using the da Vinci surgical system. An no-reference color image quality assessment measure is defined by integrating three attributes of sharpness, naturalness, and contrast. Simultaneously, this work also presents the first study on surgical vision restoration to augment visualization in robotic prostatectomy. A retinex-driven fusion approach is proposed to restore the substantial visibility in the endoscopic imaging and on the basis of the surgical visibility restoration, this study further improves the performance of stereoscopic endoscopic field 3-D reconstruction.

2 Approaches

This section describes how to evaluate and restore the degraded endoscopic image. This restoration results not only in enhancing the visualization of the surgical scene but also improving the performance of 3-D reconstruction.

2.1 Visibility Assessment

Quantitative evaluation of surgical vision in an endoscopic video sequence is a challenging task because there are no "gold-standard" references for these surgical images in the operating room. Although no-reference color image quality evaluation methods are widely discussed in the computer vision community [1], it still remains challenging to precisely assess the visual quality of natural scene images.

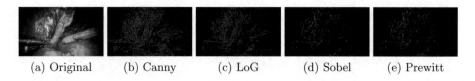

| (a) Original | (b) Canny | (c) LoG | (d) Sobel | (e) Prewitt |

Fig. 2. Comparison of different edge detection algorithms

Meanwhile, in the computer-assisted interventions community, there are no publications reporting no-reference surgical vision assessment. This work defines an no-reference objective measure to quantitatively evaluate the surgical endoscopic visibility with three characteristics of image sharpness, naturalness, and contrast related to image illumination variation and textureless regions.

Sharpness describes the structural fidelity, i.e., fine detail and edge preservation. The human visual system (HVS) is sensitive to such structural information. The sharpness ψ here is defined based on local edge gradient analysis [2]:

$$\psi = \frac{1}{M} \sum_M \sum_\Omega E(x,y), \ E(x,y) = \frac{D_{max}(x,y) + D_{min}(x,y)}{\cos \nabla(x,y)}, \quad (1)$$

where $E(x,y)$ is the computed edge width at pixel (x,y) in patch Ω on image $\mathbf{I}(x,y)$ that is divided into M patches, $D_m(x,y)$ and $D_{min}(x,y)$ indicate the distances between the edge pixel (x,y) and the maximal and minimal intensity pixels $\mathbf{I}_{max}(x,y)$ and $\mathbf{I}_{min}(x,y)$ at patch Ω, respectively, and $\nabla(x,y)$ denotes the angle between the edge gradient and the tracing direction. The computation of the edge width $E(x,y)$ should consider the impact of the edge slopes because humans perceive image contrast more than the strength of the local intensity [2]. In this work, a Canny edge detector was used as it provided a denser edge map compared to other edge detection methods (Fig. 2).

Naturalness depicts how natural surgical images appear. It is difficult to quantitatively define naturalness, which is a subjective judgment. However, by statistically analyzing thousands of images [1], the histogram shapes of natural images generally yield Gaussian and Beta probability distributions:

$$f_g(z) = \frac{1}{\sqrt{2\pi\sigma^2}} \exp(-(z-\mu)/2\sigma^2, \ f_b(z;u,v) = u^{-1}z^u \mathcal{F}(u,1-v;u+1;z), \ (2)$$

where $\mathcal{F}(\cdot)$ is the hypergeometric function that is defined in the form of a hypergeometric series. As recent work has demonstrated, since image luminance and contrast are largely independent on each other in accordance with natural image statistics and biological computation [3], the naturalness χ should be defined as a joint probability density distribution of a Gaussian and a Beta functions:

$$\chi = (\max(f_g(z), f_b(z;u,v)))^{-1} f_g(z)f_b(z;u,v). \quad (3)$$

Contrast is also an attribute important in human perception. In this work, contrast $\mathcal{C}$ is defined as the difference between a pixel $\mathbf{I}(x,y)$ and the average edge-weighted value $\omega(x, y)$ in a patch Ω (the detected edge $\phi(x, y)$) [4]:

$$C = N^{-1} \sum_N \frac{|\mathbf{I}(x, y) - \omega(x, y)|}{|\mathbf{I}(x, y) + \omega(x, y)|}, \ \omega(x, y) = \sum_{\Omega(x, y)} \phi(x, y)\mathbf{I}(x, y). \qquad (4)$$

The proposed quality index, $\mathcal{Q}$, combines the metrics defined above into a single objective measure:

$$\mathcal{Q} = a\psi^\alpha + b\chi^\beta + (1 - a - b)\log \mathcal{C} \qquad (5)$$

where a and b balance the three parts, and α and β control their sensitivities.

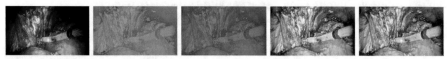

(a) Outputs at four different steps in the surgical visibility restoration approach

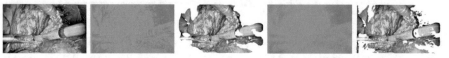

(b) Disparity maps and reconstructed surfaces at cost construction and propagation

Fig. 3. Surgical visibility restoration and augmented stereo field reconstruction

2.2   Visualization Restoration

The retinex-driven fusion framework for surgical vision restoration contains four steps (1) multiscale retinex, (2) color recovery, (3) histogram equalization, and (4) guided fusion. Figure 3(a) illustrates the output of each step in this framework.

The output $\mathbf{R}^i(x, y)$ of the multiscale retinex processing is formulated as [5]:

$$\mathbf{R}^i(x, y) = \sum_{s=1}^{S} \gamma_s \left(\log \mathbf{I}^i(x, y) - \log\left(\mathbf{I}^i(x, y) \otimes G_s(x, y)\right)\right), \ i \in \{r, g, b\}, \qquad (6)$$

where s indicates the scale level, S is set to 3, γ_s is the weight of each scale, $\otimes$ denotes the convolution operator, and $G_s(\cdot)$ is the Gaussian kernel.

A color recovery step usually follows the multiscale retinex which deteriorates the color saturation and generates a grayish image, and its output $\tilde{\mathbf{R}}^i(x, y)$ is:

$$\tilde{\mathbf{R}}^i(x, y) = \eta \mathbf{R}^i(x, y)(\log \kappa \mathbf{I}^i(x, y) - \log \sum_i \mathbf{I}^i(x, y)), \qquad (7)$$

where parameter κ determines the nonlinearity and factor η is a gain factor.

Unfortunately, the recovery step introduces the color inversion problem. To address this problem, histogram equalization processing was performed.

Although high-quality surgical visibility was achieved after the histogram equalization, it still suffers somewhat from being over-bright. A guided-filtering fusion is employed to tackle this problem. Let $\hat{\mathbf{R}}(x, y)$ be the output image after the histogram equalization processing. The guided-filtering fusion of the input image $\mathbf{I}(x, y)$ and $\tilde{\mathbf{R}}(x, y)$ first decomposes them into two-scale representation [7]: $\mathbf{M_I} = \mathcal{M}(\mathbf{I}(x, y))$, $\mathbf{M_R} = \mathcal{M}(\hat{\mathbf{R}}(x, y))$, $\mathbf{D_I} = \mathbf{I}(x, y) - \mathbf{M_I}$, $\mathbf{D_R} = \mathbf{R}(x, y) - \mathbf{M_R}$, where $\mathcal{M}$ denotes the mean-filtering operator, and then reconstructs the final output image $\check{\mathbf{R}}(x, y) = (\mathbf{w_I^M M_I} + \mathbf{w_R^M M_R} + \mathbf{w_I^D D_I}, \mathbf{w_R^D D_R})$, where the weight maps $\mathbf{w_I^M}, \mathbf{w_R^M}, \mathbf{w_I^D}$, and $\mathbf{w_R^D}$ are calculated using the guided filtering method [8].

2.3 Augmented Disparity

The surgical visibility restoration significantly corrects the illumination non-uniformity problem (Fig. 3(a)) and should be beneficial to disparity estimation.

Based on recent work on the cost-volume filtering method [9], the surgical visibility-restoration stereo endoscopic images are used to estimate the disparity in dense stereo matching. The matching cost volume can be constructed by

$$\forall \, (x, y, d) \in \mathfrak{R}^3, \mathcal{V}((x, y), d) = \mathcal{F}_\delta((x, y), (x + d, y)), \tag{8}$$

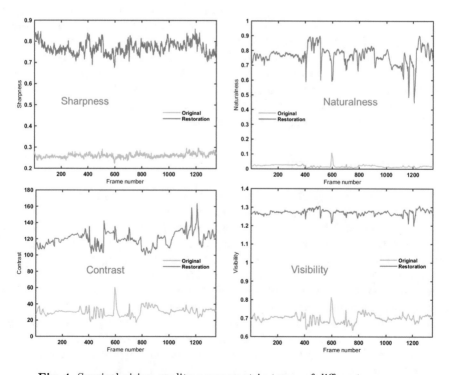

Fig. 4. Surgical vision quality assessment in terms of different measures

where $\Re^3 = \{x \in [1, W], y \in [1, H], d \in [d_{min}, d_{max}]\}$, d_{min} and d_{max} denote the disparity search range, and image size $W \times H$. The matching cost function $\mathcal{F}_\delta$ is

$$\mathcal{F}_\delta((x, y), (x + d, y)) = (1 - \delta)\mathcal{F}_c((x, y), (x + d, y)) + \delta\mathcal{F}_g((x, y), (x + d, y)), \quad (9)$$

where $\mathcal{F}_c$ and $\mathcal{F}_g$ characterize the color and gradient absolute difference between the elements of the image pair, and constant δ balances the color and gradient costs. After the cost construction, the rough disparity and the coarse recon-structed surface can be obtained (see the second and third images in Fig. 3(b)). The coarse disparity map contains image noise and artifacts. The cost propaga-tion performs a filtering procedure that aims to remove these noise and artifacts:

$$\tilde{\mathcal{V}}((x, y), d) = \sum \Psi(\mathbf{I}(x, y))\mathcal{V}((x, y), d), \quad (10)$$

where weight $\Psi(\mathbf{I}(x, y))$ is exactly calculated by using guided filtering [8]. after the cost propagation, the disparity map and the reconstructed surface become better (see the forth and the fifth images in Fig. 3(b)). Finally, the optimal disparity can be achieved by an optimization procedure (e.g., winner-takes-all).

3   Validation

Surgical stereoscopic video sequences were collected during robotic-assisted laparoscopic radical prostatectomy using the da Vinci Si surgical system (Intu-itive Surgical Inc., Sunnyvale, CA, USA). All images were acquired under a protocol approved by the Research Ethics board of Western University, London, Canada. Similar to the work [6], we set $a = 0.5$, $b = 0.4$, $\alpha = 0.3$, and $\beta = 0.7$. All the experiments were tested on a laptop installed with Windows 8.1 Professional 64-Bit Operating System, 16.0-GB Memory, and Processor Intel(R) Core(TM) i7 CPU×8 and were implemented with Microsoft Visual C++.

4   Results and Discussion

Figure 4 shows the surgical vision assessment in terms of the sharpness, natural-ness, contrast, and the proposed joint quality measures. Figure 5 compares the visibility before and after surgical vision restoration by the proposed retinex-driven fusion. The visibility was generally enhanced from 0.66 to 1.27. Figure 6 illustrates the original stereo disparity and reconstruction augmented by visibil-ity restoration. The numbers in Fig. 6 indicate the reconstructed density ratio (the number of reconstructed pixels by all the pixels on the stereo image). The average reconstructed density ratio was improved from 94.8% to 99.6%. Note that image illumination variations, low-contrast and textureless regions are sev-eral issues for accurate stereo reconstruction for which we used color and gradient (structural edges) aggregation for stereo matching. Our restoration method can improve color, contrast, and sharpness, resulting in improve the disparity.

The quality of endoscopic vision is of critical importance for minimally inva-sive surgical procedures. No-reference and objective assessment is essential for

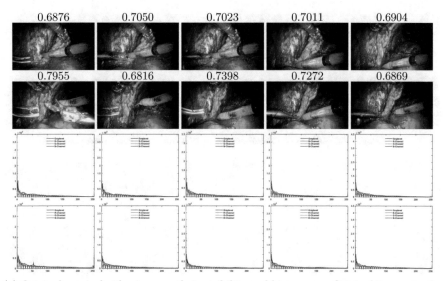

(a) Original surgical video images, their visibility and histograms: Original images in the first and second row correspond to the histograms in the third and fourth row

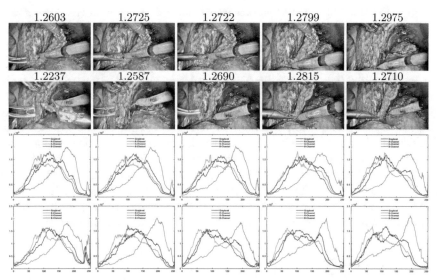

(b) Restored surgical video images, their visibility and histograms: Restored images in the first and second row correspond to the histograms in the third and fourth row

Fig. 5. Comparison of surgical endoscopic video images and their visibility and histograms before and after the restoration processing by using the proposed retinex-driven fusion framework. The numbers on the image top indicate the visibility values. The restoration greatly improved the surgical vision. In particular, the restored histograms generally yielded Gaussian and Beta functions.

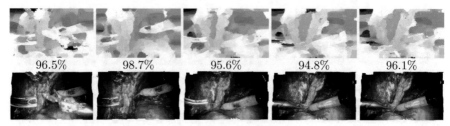

(a) Disparity and reconstruction using original surgical stereo images

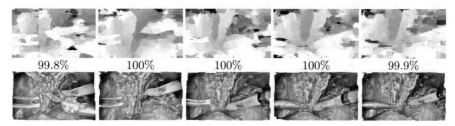

(b) Disparity and reconstruction using restored surgical stereo images

Fig. 6. Examples of disparity and reconstruction before and after the restoration

quantitatively evaluating the quality of surgical vision since references are usually unavailable in practice. Moreover, surgical vision and 3-D scene reconstruction are unavoidably deteriorated as a result of the inherent drawbacks of endoscopes. In these respects, the methods proposed above were able to quantitatively evaluate and simultaneously restore surgical vision and further improved endoscopic 3-D scene reconstruction, demonstrating that these approaches can significantly improve the visibility of visualized scenes, but also enhance 3-D scene reconstruction from stereo endoscopic images. On the other hand, the goal of surgical 3-D scene reconstruction is to fuse other imaging modalities such as ultrasound images. This fusion enables surgeons to simultaneously visualize anatomical structures on and under the organ surface. Hence, both visibility restoration and stereo reconstruction are developed to augment surgical vision.

5   Conclusions

This work developed an objective no-reference color image quality measure to quantitatively evaluate surgical vision and simultaneously explored a retinex-driven fusion method for surgical visibility restoration, which further augmented stereo reconstruction in robotic prostatectomy. The experimental results demonstrate that the average surgical visibility improved from 0.66 to 1.27 and the average reconstructed density ratio enhanced from 94.8% to 99.6%.

Acknowledgment. This work was partly supported by the Fundamental Research Funds for the Central Universities (No. 20720180062), the Canadian Institutes for Health Research, and the Canadian Foundation for Innovation.

References

1. Wang, Z., et al.: Modern Image Quality Assessment. Morgan & Claypool, San Rafael (2006)
2. Feichtenhofer, C., et al.: A perceptual image sharpness metric based on local edge gradient analysis. IEEE Sig. Process. Lett. **20**(4), 379–382 (2013)
3. Mante, V., et al.: Independence of luminance and contrast in natural scenes and in the early visual system. Nat. Neurosci. **8**(12), 1690–1697 (2005)
4. Celik, T., et al.: Automatic image equalization and contrast enhancement using Gaussian mixture modeling. IEEE Trans. Image Process. **21**(1), 145–156 (2012)
5. Rahman, Z., et al.: Retinex processing for automatic image enhancement. J. Electron. Imaging **13**(1), 100–110 (2004)
6. Yeganeh, H., et al.: Objective quality assessment of tone-mapped images. IEEE Trans. Image Process. **22**(2), 657–667 (2013)
7. Li, S., et al.: Image fusion with guided filtering. IEEE TIP **22**(7), 2864–2875 (2013)
8. He, K., et al.: Guided image filtering. IEEE Trans. Pattern Anal. Mach. Intell. **35**(6), 1397–1409 (2013)
9. Hosni, A., et al.: Fast cost-volume filtering for visual correspondence and beyond. IEEE Trans. Pattern Anal. Mach. Intell. **35**(2), 504–511 (2013)

Real-Time Augmented Reality for Ear Surgery

Raabid Hussain[1]([⊠]), Alain Lalande[1], Roberto Marroquin[1],
Kibrom Berihu Girum[1], Caroline Guigou[2], and Alexis Bozorg Grayeli[1,2]

[1] Le2i, Universite de Bourgogne Franche-Comte, Dijon, France
Raabid.Hussain@u-bourgogne.fr
[2] ENT Department, University Hospital of Dijon, Dijon, France

Abstract. Transtympanic procedures aim at accessing the middle ear structures through a puncture in the tympanic membrane. They require visualization of middle ear structures behind the eardrum. Up to now, this is provided by an oto endoscope. This work focused on implementing a real-time augmented reality based system for robotic-assisted transtympanic surgery. A preoperative computed tomography scan is combined with the surgical video of the tympanic membrane in order to visualize the ossciles and labyrinthine windows which are concealed behind the opaque tympanic membrane. The study was conducted on 5 artificial and 4 cadaveric temporal bones. Initially, a homography framework based on fiducials (6 stainless steel markers on the periphery of the tympanic membrane) was used to register a 3D reconstructed computed tomography image to the video images. Micro/endoscope movements were then tracked using Speeded-Up Robust Features. Simultaneously, a micro-surgical instrument (needle) in the frame was identified and tracked using a Kalman filter. Its 3D pose was also computed using a 3-collinear-point framework. An average initial registration accuracy of 0.21 mm was achieved with a slow propagation error during the 2-minute tracking. Similarly, a mean surgical instrument tip 3D pose estimation error of 0.33 mm was observed. This system is a crucial first step towards keyhole surgical approach to middle and inner ears.

Keywords: Augmented reality · Transtympanic procedures
Otology · Minimally invasive · Image-guided surgery

1 Introduction

During otologic procedures, when the surgeon places the endoscope inside the external auditory canal, the middle ear cleft structures, concealed behind the opaque tympanic membrane (TM), are not directly accessible. Consequently, surgeons can access these structures using the TM flap approach [1] which is both painful and exposes the patient to risk of infection and bleeding [2].

Alternatively, transtympanic procedures have been designed which aim at accessing the middle ear cleft structures through a small and deep cavity inside

A. F. Frangi et al. (Eds.): MICCAI 2018, LNCS 11073, pp. 324–331, 2018.
https://doi.org/10.1007/978-3-030-00937-3_38

the ear. These techniques have been used in different applications such as ossic-ular chain repair, drug administration and labyrinthe fistula diagnosis [3,4]. The procedures offer many advantages: faster procedure, preservation of TM and reduced bleeding. However, limited operative space, field of view and instrument manoeuvring introduce surgical complications.

Our hypothesis claims that augmented reality (AR) would improve the proce-dure of middle ear surgery by providing instrument pose information and super-imposing preoperative computed tomography (CT) image of the middle ear onto the micro/endoscopic video of TM. The key challenge is to enhance ergonomy while operating in a highly undersquared cylinderical workspace achieving sub-millimetric precision. To our knowledge, AR has not been applied to transtym-panic and otoendoscopic procedures, thus the global perspective of the work is to affirm our hypothesis.

In computer assisted surgical systems, image registration plays an integral role in the overall performance. Feature extraction methods generally do not perform well due to the presence of highly textured structures and non-linear biasing [5]. Many algorithms have been proposed specifically for endoscope-CT registration. Combinations of different intensity based schemes such as cross-correlation, squared intensity difference, mutual information and pattern inten-sity have shown promising results [6,7]. Similarly, feature based schemes involv-ing natural landmarks, contour based feature points, iterative closest point and k-means clustering have also been exploited [8,9].

Different techniques involving learned instrument models, artificial markers, pre-known kinematic and gradient information using Hough transform have been proposed to identify instruments in video frames [10]. If the target is frequently changing its appearance, gradient based tracking algorithms need continuous template updating to maintain accurate position estimation. Analogously, reli-able amount of training data is required for classifier based techniques. Although extensive research has been undertaken for identification of instruments in image plane, limited work has been accomplished to estimate 3D pose. Trained random forest classifier using instrument geometry as a prior and visual servoing tech-niques employing four marker points have been proposed [11,12]. Three point perspective framework involving collinear markers has been also suggested [13].

Our proposed approach initially registers the CT image with the microscopic video, based on fiducial markers. This is followed by a feature based motion tracking scheme to maintain synchronisation. The surgical instrument is also tracked and its pose estimated using 3-collinear-point framework.

2   Methodology

The system is composed of three main processes: initial registration, movement tracking and instrument pose estimation. The overall hierarchy is presented in Fig. 1. The proposed system has two main inputs. Firstly, the reconstructed image which is the display of the temporal bone, depicting middle ear cleft structures behind TM, obtained from preoperative CT data through OsiriX 3D endoscopy function (Pixmeo SARL, Switzerland). Secondly, the endoscopic video which is the real-time video acquired from a calibrated endoscope or surgical microscope during a surgical procedure. The camera projection matrix of the input camera was computed using [14]. The calibration parameters are later used for 3D pose estimation.

There is low similarity between the reconstructed and endoscopic images (Fig. 2), thus the performance of intensity and feature based algorithms is limited in this case. Marroquin et al. [2] established correspondence by manually identifying points in the endoscopic and CT images. However, accurately identifying natural landmarks is a tedious and time-consuming task. Thus six stainless steel fiducial markers (≈1 mm in length) were attached around TM (prior to CT acquisition).

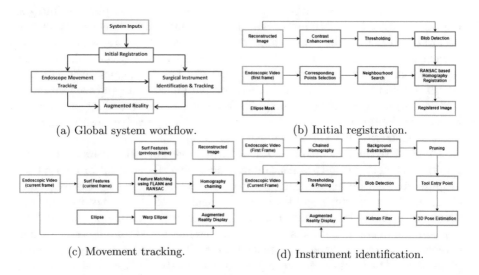

(a) Global system workflow.

(b) Initial registration.

(c) Movement tracking.

(d) Instrument identification.

Fig. 1. Overall workflow of the proposed system. A colour coding scheme, defined in (a), has been used to differentiate between different processes.

2.1   Initial Semi-automatic Endosocope-CT Registration

Since the intensity of fiducials is significantly higher than that of anatomical regions on CT images, contrast enhancement and thresholding is used to obtain fiducial regions. The centre of each fiducial is then obtained using blob detection. The user selects the corresponding fiducials in the first frame of the endoscopic video. There are very few common natural landmarks around TM, thus the fiducials ease up the process of establishing correspondence. In order to eliminate human error, similar pixels in a small neighbourhood around the selected points are also taken into account. A RANdom SAmple Consensus (RANSAC) based homography [15] registration matrix H_R, which warps the reconstructed image onto the endoscopic video, is computed using these point correspondences.

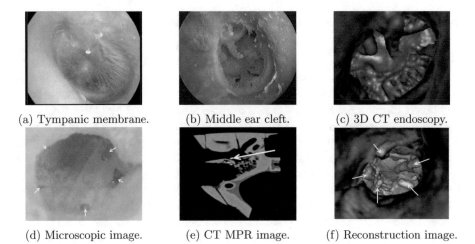

(a) Tympanic membrane.   (b) Middle ear cleft.   (c) 3D CT endoscopy.

(d) Microscopic image.   (e) CT MPR image.   (f) Reconstruction image.

Fig. 2. Problem definition. Amalgamation of a reconstructed CT image (c) with the endoscopic video (a) may be used to visualize the middle ear cleft structures (b) without undergoing a TM flap procedure. However, similarity between them is low so fiducial markers are introduced which appear (d) grey in the microscopic image, (e) white in the CT MPR image and (f) as protrusions on the CT reconstructed image.

An ellipse shaped mask is generated using the fiducial points in the endoscopic frame. Since TM does not have a well-defined boundary in the endoscopic video, this mask is used as an approximation of TM. The mask is used in the tracking process to filter out unwanted (non-planar) features.

2.2 Endoscope-Target Motion Tracking

Speeded Up Robust Features (SURF) [16] was employed in our system for tracking the movement between consecutive video frames [2]. For an accurate homography, all the feature points should lie on coplanar surfaces [15]. However, the extracted features are spread across the entire image plane comprising of the TM and auditory canal. The ellipse generated in previous step is used to filter out features that do not lie on TM (assumed planar). A robust feature matching scheme based on RANSAC and nearest neighbour (FLANN [17]) frameworks is used to determine the homography transformation H_T between consecutive frames. A chained homography framework is then used to warp the registered reconstructed image onto the endoscopic frame:

$$H^{i+1} = H_T * H^i, \tag{1}$$

where H^0 is set as identity. H^i can then be multiplied with H_R to transform the original reconstructed image to the current time step. A linear blend operator is used for warping reconstructed image onto the current endoscopic frame.

2.3 3D Pose Estimation of Surgical Instrument

In surgical microscopes, small depth of focus leads to a degradation of gradient and colour information. Thus popular approaches for instrument identification do not perform well. Consequently, three collinear ink markers were attached to the instrument (Fig. 3). The three marker regions are extracted using thresholding. Since, discrepancies are present, a pruning step followed by blob detection is carried out to extract centres of the largest three regions. A linear Kalman filter is used to refine the marker centre points to eliminate any residual degradation.

Since, the instrument may enter from any direction and protrude indefinitely, geometric priors are not valid. The proposed approach assumes that no instrument is present in the first endoscopic frame. The first frame undergoes a transformation based on H^i. Background subtraction followed by pruning (owing to discrepancies in H^i) is used to extract the tool entry point in the frame boundary. The tool entry point is then used to associate the marker centres to marker labels B, C and D. The instrument tip location can then be obtained using a set of perception based equations that lead to:

$$a = \frac{1}{3}(b + c + d + \frac{AB}{CD}(c - d) + \frac{AC}{BD}(b - d) + \frac{AD}{BC}(b - c)), \tag{2}$$

where a is projection of the surgical instrument tip A on the 2D image frame, b, c and d are projections of the markers and alphabet pairs represent the physical distance between the markers.

A three point perspective framework is then used to estimate the 3D pose of the instrument. Given focal length of the camera, known physical distance between 3 markers and their projected 2D coordinates, the position of the instrument tip can be estimated by fitting the physical geometry of the tool onto the projected lines Ob, Oc and Od (Fig. 3) [13].

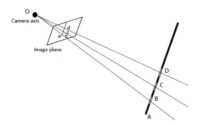

Fig. 3. Three collinear point framework for 3D pose estimation.

3   Experimental Setup and Results

The proposed system was initially evaluated on five temporal bone phantoms (corresponding patient ages: 1–55 years). All specimens underwent a preoperative CT scan (Light speed, 64 detector rows, $0.6 \times 0.6 \times 0.3$ mm^3 voxel size, General Electric Medical Systems, France). Six 1 mm fiducial markers, were attached around TM in a non-linear configuration with their combined centre coinciding with the target [18]. Real-time video was acquired using a microscope lens. Small movements were applied to the microscope in order to test the robustness of the system. The experimental setup and the augmented reality output are shown in Fig. 4. Processing speed of 12 frames per second (fps) was realized.

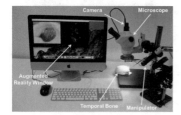

(a) Experimental setup.

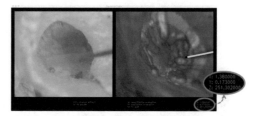

(b) Augmented Reality Window.

Fig. 4. (a) Augmented reality system. (b) Real-time video from the microscope (left) and augmented reality window (right).

The fiducial marker points in the reconstructed image were automatically detected and displayed on the screen and the user selected their corresponding fiducial points on the microscopic frame. Mean fiducial registration error (physical distance between estimated positions in microscopic and transformed reconstructed images) of 0.21 mm was observed.

During surgery, microscope will remain quasi-static. However to validate robustness of the system, combinations of translation, rotation and scaling with a speed of 0–10 mm/s were applied to the microscope. The system, evaluated at 30 s intervals, maintained synchronisation with a slow propagation error of 0.02 mm/min (Fig. 5a). Fiducial markers were used as reference points for evaluation. Template matching was used to automatically detect the fiducial points in the current frame. These were compared with the fiducial points in transformed reconstructed image to compute the tracking error.

The system was also evaluated on pre-chosen surgical target structures (incus and round window niche). TM of four temporal bone cadavers was removed and the above experiments were repeated. Similarly, a mean target registration error (computation similar to fiducial registration error) of 0.20 mm was observed with a slow propagation error of 0.05 mm/min (Fig. 5a).

For instrument pose estimation, pre-known displacements were applied in each axis and a total of 50 samples per displacement were recorded. Mean pose estimation errors of 0.20, 0.18 and 0.60 mm were observed in X, Y and Z axes respectively (Fig. 5b). The pose estimation in X and Y axes was better than in Z axis because any small deviation in instrument identification constitutes a relatively large deviation in the Z pose estimation.

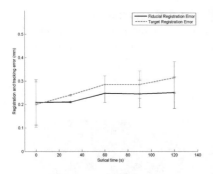 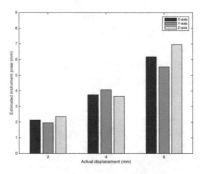

(a) Registration and tracking accuracy.   (b) 3D pose estimation accuracy.

Fig. 5. Experimental results. (a) Registration and tracking accuracy of the AR system evaluated at fiducial and surgical targets. (b) Displacement accuracy assessment of 3D pose estimation process (displayed statistics are for 50 samples).

4   Conclusion

An AR based robotic assistance system for transtympanic procedures was presented. A preoperative CT scan image of the middle ear cleft was combined with the real-time microscope video of TM using 6 fiducial markers as point correspondences in a semi-automatic RANSAC based homography framework. The system is independent of marker placement technique and is capable of functioning with endoscopes and mono/stereo microscopes. Initial registration is the most crucial stage as any error introduced during this stage will propagate throughout the procedure. Mean registration error of 0.21 mm was observed. To keep synchronisation, the relative microscope-target movements were then tracked using a SURF based robust feature matching framework. A microscopic propagation error was observed. Simultaneously, 3D pose of a needle instrument, upto 0.33 mm mean precision, was provided for assistance to the surgeon using a monovision based perspective framework. Additional geometric priors can be incorporated to compute pose of angled instruments. Initial experiments have shown promising results, achieving sub-millimetric precision, and opening new perspectives to the application of minmally invasive procedures in otology.

References

1. Gurr, A., Sudhoff, H., Hildmann, H.: Approaches to the middle ear. In: Hildmann, H., Sudhoff, H. (eds.) Middle Ear Surgery, pp. 19–23. Springer, Heidelberg (2006). https://doi.org/10.1007/978-3-540-47671-9_6
2. Marroquin, R., Lalande, A., Hussain, R., Guigou, C., Grayeli, A.B.: Augmented reality of the middle ear combining otoendoscopy and temporal bone computed tomography. Otol. Neurotol. **39**(8), 931–939 (2018). https://doi.org/10.1097/MAO.0000000000001922
3. Dean, M., Chao, W.C., Poe, D.: Eustachian tube dilation via a transtympanic approach in 6 cadaver heads: a feasibility study. Otolaryngol. Head Neck Surg. **155**(4), 654–656 (2016). https://doi.org/10.1177/0194599816655096

4. Mood, Z.A., Daniel, S.J.: Use of a microendoscope for transtympanic drug delivery to the round window membrane in chinchillas. Otol. Neurotol. **33**(8), 1292–1296 (2012). https://doi.org/10.1097/MAO.0b013e318263d33e

5. Viergever, M.A., Maintz, J.A., Klein, S., Murphy, K., Staring, M., Pluim, J.P.: A survey of medical image registration under review. Med. Image Anal. **33**, 140–144 (2016). https://doi.org/10.1016/j.media.2016.06.030

6. Hummel, J., Figl, M., Bax, M., Bergmann, H., Birkfellner, W.: 2D/3D registration of endoscopic ultrasound to CT volume data. Phys. Med. Biol. **53**(16), 4303 (2008). https://doi.org/10.1088/0031-9155/53/16/006

7. Yim, Y., Wakid, M., Kirmizibayrak, C.: Registration of 3D CT data to 2D endoscopic image using a gradient mutual information based viewpoint matching for image-guided medialization laryngoplasty. J. Comput. Sci. Eng. **4**(4), 368–387 (2010). https://doi.org/10.5626/JCSE.2010.4.4.368

8. Jun, G.X., Li, H., Yi, N.: Feature points based image registration between endoscope image and the CT image. In: IEEE International Conference on Electric Information and Control Engineering, pp. 2190–2193. IEEE Press (2011). https://doi.org/10.1109/ICEICE.2011.5778261

9. Wengert, C., Cattin, P., Du, J.M., Baur, C., Szekely, G.: Markerless endoscopic registration and referencing. In: Larsen, R., Nielsen, M., Sporring, J. (eds.) MICCAI 2006. LNCS, vol. 4190, pp. 816–823. Springer, Heidelberg (2006). https://doi.org/10.1007/11866565_100

10. Haase, S., Wasza, J., Kilgus, T., Hornegger, J.: Laparoscopic instrument localization using a 3D time of flight/RGB endoscope. In: IEEE Workshop on Applications of Computer Vision, pp. 449–454. IEEE Press (2013). https://doi.org/10.1109/WACV.2013.6475053

11. Allan, M., Ourselin, S., Thompson, S., Hawkes, D.J., Kelly, J., Stoyanov, D.: Toward detection and localization of instruments in minimally invasive surgery. IEEE Trans. Biomed. Eng. **60**(4), 1050–1058 (2013). https://doi.org/10.1109/TBME.2012.2229278

12. Nageotte, F., Zanne, P., Doignon, C., Mathelin, M.D.: Visual servoing based endoscopic path following for robot-assisted laparoscopic surgery. In: IEEE/RSJ International Conference on Intelligent Robots and Systems, pp. 2364–2369. IEEE Press (2006). https://doi.org/10.1109/IROS.2006.282647

13. Liu, S.G., Peng, K., Huang, F.S., Zhang, G.X., Li, P.: A portable 3D vision coordinate measurement system using a light pen. Key Eng. Mater. **295**, 331–336 (2005). https://doi.org/10.4028/www.scientific.net/KEM.295-296.331

14. Zhang, Z.: A flexible new technique for camera calibration. IEEE Trans. Pattern Anal. Mach. Intell. **22**(11), 1330–1334 (2000). https://doi.org/10.1109/34.888718

15. Hartley, R., Zisserman, A.: Multiple view geometry in computer vision. Cambridge University Press, Cambridge (2003)

16. Bay, A., Tuytelaars, T., Gool, L.V.: Surf: speeded up robust features. In: Leonardis, A., Bischof, H., Pinz, A. (eds.) ECCV 2006. LNCS, vol. 3951, pp. 404–417. Springer, Heidelberg (2006). https://doi.org/10.1007/11744023_32

17. Muja, M., Lowe, D.G.: Fast approximate nearest neighbors with automatic algorithm configuration. In: 4th International Conference on Computer Vision Theory and Applications, pp. 331–340, Springer, Heidelberg (2009). https://doi.org/10.5220/0001787803310340

18. West, J.B., Fitzpatrick, J.M., Toms, S.A., Maurer Jr., C.R., Maciunas, R.J.: Fiducial point placement and the accuracy of point-based, rigid body registration. Neurosurgery **48**(4), 810–817 (2001). https://doi.org/10.1097/0006123-200104000-00023

Framework for Fusion of Data- and Model-Based Approaches for Ultrasound Simulation

Christine Tanner[1(✉)], Rastislav Starkov[1], Michael Bajka[2], and Orcun Goksel[1]

[1] Computer-Assisted Applications in Medicine, ETH Zürich, Zürich, Switzerland
{tannerch,ogoksel}@vision.ee.ethz.ch
[2] Department of Gynecology, University Hospital of Zürich, Zürich, Switzerland

Abstract. Navigation, acquisition and interpretation of ultrasound (US) images relies on the skills and expertise of the performing physician. Virtual-reality based simulations offer a safe, flexible and standardized environment to train these skills. Simulations can be data-based by displaying a-priori acquired US volumes, or ray-tracing based by simulating the complex US interactions of a geometric model. Here we combine these two approaches as it is relatively easy to gather US images of normal background anatomy and attractive to cover the range of rare findings or particular clinical tasks with known ground truth geometric models. For seamless adaption and change of US content we further require stitching, texture synthesis and tissue deformation simulations. We test the proposed hybrid simulation method by replacing embryos within gestational sacs by ray-traced embryos, and by simulating an ectoptic pregnancy.

1 Introduction

Due to portability, low-costs and safety, ultrasound (US) is a widely-used medical imaging modality. A drawback of US is that its acquisition and interpretation heavily relies on the experience and skill of the sonographer. Therefore, training of sonographers in navigation, acquisition and interpretation of US images is crucial for the benefit of clinical outcomes. Training is possible with volunteers, cadavers, and phantoms, which all have associated ethical and realism issues. On the other hand, virtual-reality based simulated training offers a safe and repeatable environment. This also allows to simulate rare cases, which would otherwise be unlikely to be encountered during training in regular clinical routine [2].

Real-time US simulations can be performed using data-based approaches [1, 6,9,15,18,19] or model-based rendering approaches [4,8,13,16,17]. Data-based US simulation can provide relatively high image realism, where image slices are interpolated during simulation time from a-priori acquired US volumes, which can also incorporate interactive tissue deformations [9]. While the acquisition of a large image database for physiological cases may seem straightforward, their pre-processing, storage, and evaluation-metric definition for simulation can quickly become infeasible. Furthermore, acquisition of rare cases with representative

© Springer Nature Switzerland AG 2018
A. F. Frangi et al. (Eds.): MICCAI 2018, LNCS 11073, pp. 332–339, 2018.
https://doi.org/10.1007/978-3-030-00937-3_39

diversity, which are indeed most important for training, is a major challenge. For instance, for a comprehensive training in obstetrics, it is infeasible to collect US volumes of fetuses in all gestational ages, at different position/orientations, with different (uterus) anatomical variations, and all combinations thereof with a standardized image quality. If one wants to include cases of various imaging failures and artifact combinations, let alone rare pathological scenarios such as Siamese twins, the challenges for comprehensive training becomes apparent.

Alternatively, model-based techniques allow generating US images from a user set model, such as ray-tracing techniques through triangulated surface models of anatomy. These are then not limited by acquisition, but rather the modeling effort; i.e., any anatomical variation that can be modeled can be simulated. Nevertheless, precise modeling is a time-consuming effort and can only be afforded at small regions of discernible detail and actual clinical interest. For instance, [13] shows that a fetus (which has relatively small anatomical differences across its population) can be modeled in detail based on anatomical literature and expertise, however, it is clearly infeasible to model large volumes of surrounding background (mother's) anatomy, e.g. the intestines, and their population variability for diverse realistic US backgrounds for comprehensive training.

In this work, we propose to combine these two approaches, where a focal region of clinical interest can be modeled in detail, which is then fused with realistic image volumes forming the background. A framework (Fig. 1) and related tools are then herein introduced for synthesizing realistic US images for different simulation scenarios, where, for instance, the original images may contain content that needs to be removed ("erased") or the models may be smaller/larger than the available space for them in the images. A toolbox of hybrid US synthesis is demonstrated in this work. The proposed methods are showcased for two representative transvaginal ultrasound (TVUS) training scenarios: (i) regular fetal examination (of normal pregnancies, e.g., for controlling normative development and gestational age), and (ii) diagnosing ectopic pregnancies, which occurs when a fertilized ovum implants outside the normal uterine cavity and may lead, untreated in severe cases, to death.

2 Methods

2.1 Data-Based: Realistic Background from Images

Routine clinical images can be used to provide realistic examples for most of the anatomy. Here a mechanically-swept 3D TVUS transducer was used to collect image volumes during obstetric examination of 3 patients. Anatomical relevant structures were then manually annotated for further processing of the images and for placement and alignment of the model with the US volume. For the shown normal pregnancy scenarios, embryo, yolk sac and gestational sac were segmented, and the location of the umbilical cord at the placenta was marked.

2.2 Model-Based Simulation: Detailed, Arbitrary Content

New content is simulated from surface models using a Monte-Carlo ray tracing method [12,13]. In this method, scatterers are handled using a convolution-based

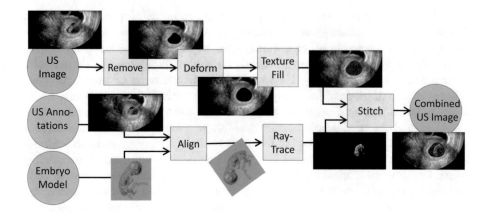

Fig. 1. Framework overview which may include segmenting out the embryo, deforming the gestational sac and surrounding tissue, texture filling of removed parts and stitching with the aligned rendered embryo model.

US simulation, while large-scale structures (modeled surfaces) are handled using ray-tracing, ignoring the wave effects. Scatters were parameterization at a fine and coarse level using normal distributions (μ_s, σ_s), and a density (ρ_s) which gives a probability threshold above which a scatterer will provide an image contribution (i.e. convolution will be performed). Monte-Carlo ray-tracing allowes to simulate tissue interactions, like soft shadows and fuzzy reflections. Furthermore it makes it possible to parameterize surface properties, such as interface roughness (random variation of reflected/refracted ray direction) and interface thickness. Probe and tissue configurations, as well as rendering parameters were set according to the work in [13]. Three hand-crafted embryo models with increasing anatomical complexity and crown-rump lengths, respectively, of 10, 28, and 42 mm were used to represent gestational ages 7, 9.5, and 11 weeks [11], with the largest model consisting of $\approx$1 million triangles, taking <1 s for ray-tracing.

2.3   Tissue Deformations

Incorporating new content can require to remove or create space, e.g. to simulate growth of the fetus. The surrounding tissue should accordingly deform. We simulated a homogeneous increase of the empty (zero intensity) gestational sac by dilating its mask with a spherical structure element of radius r. To get a deformation which has a controllable amount of strain, we used the signed distance map with respect to the new structure. We defined the motion magnitude $m(\mathbf{x})$ from distance map $D(\mathbf{x})$ by

$$m(\mathbf{x}) = \begin{cases} \max(D(\mathbf{x}) + 1.1\,r, 0) & \text{if } D(\mathbf{x}) < 0 \\ \max(-s\,D(\mathbf{x}) + 1.1\,r, 0) & \text{otherwise.} \end{cases}$$

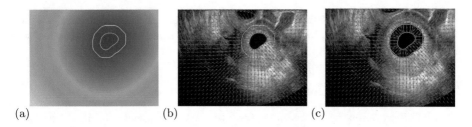

(a)   (b)   (c)

Fig. 2. (a) Distance map w.r.t. yellow contour, (b) moving image with intensities in gestational sac set to zero and motion field overlaid, (c) transformed image showing enlargement of gestational sac to planned region and deformation of surrounding tissue.

where s is the scaling factor. The direction of the displacement field is given by the gradient of $D(\mathbf{x})$, see Fig. 2. We scaled r by 1.1 to ensure that the dilated structure is filled with zero intensities and used $s = 0.1$.

2.4   Texture Filling

Regions consisting of homogeneous tissue, like the gestational sac, might be simulated by texture filling. We employ the method from Efros and Leung [5] for texture filling, as it performed significantly better than other methods for reproducing homogeneous tissue regions in B-mode US images [14]. It is based on filling an image region iteratively starting at its border by matching the intensity of valid voxels in border patches to exemplar patches.

Texture filling is organized via 3 mask images, namely M_f, M_v and M_p. For target image I, voxels to be *filled* are indicated by $M_f > 0$ and *valid* voxels which should not be changed are marked by $M_v > 0$. Exemplar patches of size $7 \times 7 \times 7$ are extracted from regions where $M_p > 0$ for all patch voxels from source image P.

For filling the gestational sac inclusive the embryo, P is the original image and patches are extracted from inside the gestational sac (M_g) excluding the embryo (M_e): $M_p = M_g - M_e$. The target image I is also the original image, which should be filled inside the gestational sac including the embryo, i.e. $M_f = M_g + M_e$, and which has valid voxels inside the US field of view (FOV) excluding M_g and M_e.

Filling starts with non-filled voxels at the border of M_v, i.e. $B = \{\mathbf{x} \mid M_f(\mathbf{x}) > 0, M_v(\mathbf{y}) > 0\}$, where $\mathbf{y}$ is in the 26-connected 3D neighborhood of $\mathbf{x}$. Patches centered at these border voxels B are processed in descending order of their numbers of valid voxels. For each border voxel $\mathbf{x} \in B$, its surrounding patch is compared to all the example patches using sum of squared differences (SSD). Candidate patches for filling the current voxel are those with SSD of all valid voxel values below a given threshold θ. If no matching patch is found, θ is increased by 10%. From these candidates only those with SSD smaller than the minimal SSD_{min} plus a given tolerance ($1.3\,SSD_{min}$) are accepted. Then, one of the accepted patches is randomly chosen and the intensity of its central voxel is assigned to the border voxel $\mathbf{x}$. Finally the masks M_v and M_f are updated by setting $M_v(\mathbf{x}) = 1$ and $M_f(\mathbf{x}) = 0$. The above is iterated until all voxels are filled. As our 3D implementation runs very slow and the mechanically-swept probe anyhow collects volumes slice-wise, we performed texture filling slice-wise in 2D for all slices which include M_f.

2.5 Compounding Contents

Overlapping content of US volumes (real or simulated) was combined by stitching [7]. This preserves speckle patterns and avoids image blurring/degradation of common mean/median approaches by determining a cut interface, such that each voxel comes from a single volume. This interface is found by capturing the transition quality between neighboring voxels by edge potential in a graphical model, which is then optimized via graph-cut [10]. In details, neighboring voxels $\mathbf{x}$ and $\mathbf{y}$ in overlapping volumes V_1 and V_2 have edge potential p based on their image intensity and image gradients [7]:

$$p(\mathbf{x}, \mathbf{y}) = \frac{||V_1(\mathbf{x}) - V_2(\mathbf{x})|| + ||V_1(\mathbf{y}) - V_2(\mathbf{y})||}{||\nabla^e_{V_1}(\mathbf{x})|| + ||\nabla^e_{V_1}(\mathbf{y})|| + ||\nabla^e_{V_2}(\mathbf{x})|| + ||\nabla^e_{V_2}(\mathbf{y})|| + \epsilon} \tag{1}$$

where $\nabla^e_{V_i}$ is the gradient in V_i along the graph edge e and $\epsilon = 10^{-5}$ to avoid division by zero. This encourages cutting when intensities match (numerator small) and at image edges (denumerator large) where seams are likely not visible. A graph G is constructed for only the overlapping voxels, with source s or sink t of the graph being connected to all boundary voxels of the corresponding image. Finally, the minimum cost cut of this graph is found using [3], giving a partition of G such that $\min \sum_{\mathbf{x} \in V_1, \mathbf{y} \in V_2 | e = (\mathbf{x}, \mathbf{y}) \in E} p(\mathbf{x}, \mathbf{y})$.

Even with optimal cuts, there can still be artifacts along stitched interfaces where no suitable seams exists, e.g. due to a quite small overlap and view-dependent artifacts like shadows. We reduced these artifacts by blending the volumes across the seam using a sigmoid function with a small kernel $\sigma = 3$ voxels.

3 Results

There is a wide range of potential applications for the proposed US hybrid simulation framework. We demonstrate its usefulness on four examples.

Case A: Normal Pregnancy, Similar size, Similar location. (Fig. 3) Replacement of a 10 week embryo by a 9 week model with know dimensions. Model placement required removal of real embryo, texture synthesis and stitching. Boundaries are clearly visible for simple fusion, which disappear with stitching.

Case B: Normal Pregnancy, Similar size, Different Location. (Fig. 4) Illustration of placing the 9 week embryo model at a different location for the same patient as in case A. High quality texture synthesis is required to realistically fill the regions where the real embryo was.

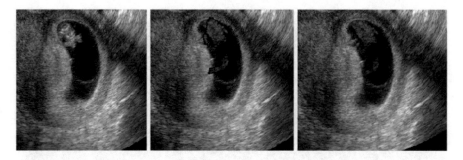

Fig. 3. Simulating an embryo at a similar location. (left) original volume, with rendered embryo inserted by (middle) simple fusion or (right) stitching.

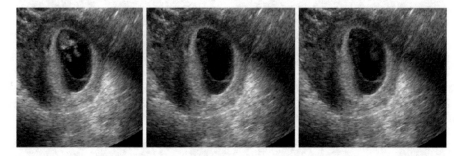

Fig. 4. Simulating an embryo at a different location. (left) original volume, (middle) with original embryo removed and gestational sac filled with texture, and (right) with ray-traced embryo inserted at a different location and stitched with original image.

Case C: Normal Pregnancy, Simulation of Growth. (Fig. 5) A two week development of a 9 week embryo was simulated. This requires all components of the proposed framework including deformation simulation. Challenges include creation of a smooth deformation and realistic speckle patterns within and on the boundary of the gestational sac.

Case D: Ectopic Pregnancy. (Fig. 6) As abnormality we simulated an ectopic pregnancy. Guided by an US specialist in obstetrics and gynecology, we replaced normal tissue close to the ovaries by the model of a 7 week embryo and its gestational sac. Simulation parameters were set empirically for visually best matching of speckle pattern to the surrounding, with resulting image realism confirmed qualitatively by an sonographer in gynecology.

4   Conclusions

We propose a hybrid ultrasound simulation framework, where particular anatomy including rare cases is generated from anatomical models, while normal variability is covered by fusing it with real image data to reduce modeling efforts. Successful combination of these two data sources has been demonstrated for four cases

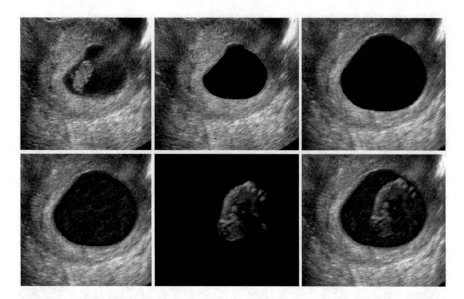

Fig. 5. Simulating of growth (top, left to right) original volume, content of gestational sac removed, expansion of gestational sac, (bottom, left to right) speckle pattern simulation, generated embryo model, content compounding.

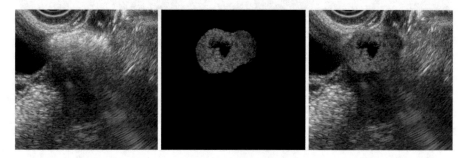

Fig. 6. Simulating ectopic pregnancy, showing (left) original volume, (middle) generated gestational sac with embryo model, and (right) compounded content.

within the context of obstetric examinations. Computations took <10 mins. Volumes fused offline can be used in real-time image-based simulation, e.g. [9].

Acknowledgment. Funding was provided by Innosuisse Swiss Innovation Agency.

References

1. Arkhurst, W., et al.: A virtual reality training system for pediatric sonography. Int. Congress Ser. **1230**, 483–487 (2001)
2. Blum, T., Rieger, A., Navab, N., Friess, H., Martignoni, M.: A review of computer-based simulators for ultrasound training. Simul. Healthcare **8**, 98–108 (2013)

3. Boykov, Y., Kolmogorov, V.: An experimental comparison of min-cut/max-flow algorithms for energy minimization in vision. IEEE Trans. Pattern Anal. Mach. Intell. **26**(9), 1124–1137 (2004)
4. Bürger, B., Bettinghausen, S., Radle, M., Hesser, J.: Real-time GPU-based ultrasound simulation using deformable mesh models. IEEE Trans. Med. Imaging **32**(3), 609–618 (2013)
5. Efros, A., Leung, T.: Texture synthesis by non-parametric sampling. In: IEEE International Conference on Computer Vision (ICCV), pp. 1033–1038 (1999)
6. Ehricke, H.: SONOSim3D: a multimedia system for sonography simulation and education with an extensible case database. Eur. J. Ultrasound **7**(3), 225–300 (1998)
7. Flach, B., Makhinya, M., Goksel, O.: PURE: panoramic ultrasound reconstruction by seamless stitching of volumes. In: Tsaftaris, S.A., Gooya, A., Frangi, A.F., Prince, J.L. (eds.) SASHIMI 2016. LNCS, vol. 9968, pp. 75–84. Springer, Cham (2016). https://doi.org/10.1007/978-3-319-46630-9_8
8. Gao, H., et al.: A fast convolution-based methodology to simulate 2-D/3-D cardiac ultrasound images. IEEE Trans. Ultrason. Ferroelectr. Freq. Control **56**(2), 404–409 (2009)
9. Goksel, O., Salcudean, S.E.: B-mode ultrasound image simulation in deformable 3-D medium. IEEE Trans. Med. Imaging **28**(11), 1657–1669 (2009)
10. Kwatra, V., Schödl, A., Essa, I., Turk, G., Bobick, A.: Graphcut textures: image and video synthesis using graph cuts. ACM Trans. Graph. (ToG). **22**, 277–286 (2003)
11. Loughna, P., Chitty, L., Evans, T., Chudleigh, T.: Fetal size and dating: charts recommended for clinical obstetric practice. Ultrasound **17**(3), 160–166 (2009)
12. Mattausch, O., Goksel, O.: Monte-Carlo ray-tracing for realistic interactive ultrasound simulation. In: Eurographics Workshop on Visual Computing for Biology and Medicine (VCBM), pp. 1–9, Bergen, Norway, September 2016. https://doi.org/10.2312/vcbm.20161285
13. Mattausch, O., Makhinya, M., Goksel, O.: Realistic ultrasound simulation of complex surface models using interactive Monte-Carlo path tracing, vol. 37, pp. 202–213 (2018)
14. Mattausch, O., Ren, E., Bajka, M., Vanhoey, K., Goksel, O.: Comparison of texture synthesis methods for content generation in ultrasound simulation for training. In: SPIE Medical Imaging, p. 1013523 (2017)
15. Maul, H., et al.: Ultrasound simulators: experience with the SonoTrainer and comparative review of other training systems. Ultrasound Obstet. Gynecol. **24**(5), 581–585 (2004)
16. Reichl, T., Passenger, J., Acosta, O., Salvado, O.: Ultrasound goes GPU: real-time simulation using CUDA. In: SPIE Medical Imaging, p. 726116 (2009)
17. Salehi, M., Ahmadi, S.-A., Prevost, R., Navab, N., Wein, W.: Patient-specific 3D ultrasound simulation based on convolutional ray-tracing and appearance optimization. In: Navab, N., Hornegger, J., Wells, W.M., Frangi, A.F. (eds.) MICCAI 2015. LNCS, vol. 9350, pp. 510–518. Springer, Cham (2015). https://doi.org/10.1007/978-3-319-24571-3_61
18. Sclaverano, S., Chevreau, G., Vadcard, L., Mozer, P., Troccaz, J.: BiopSym: a simulator for enhanced learning of ultrasound-guided prostate biopsy. Stud. Health Technol. Inform. **142**, 301–306 (2009)
19. Tahmasebi, A.M., Abolmaesumi, P., Hashtrudi-Zaad, K.: A haptic-based ultrasound training/examination system (HUTES). In: IEEE International Conference on Robotics and Automation (ICRA), pp. 3130–3131 (2007)

Image Segmentation Methods: General Image Segmentation Methods, Measures and Applications

Esophageal Gross Tumor Volume Segmentation Using a 3D Convolutional Neural Network

Sahar Yousefi[1,2]([✉]), Hessam Sokooti[1], Mohamed S. Elmahdy[1],
Femke P. Peters[1], Mohammad T. Manzuri Shalmani[2], Roel T. Zinkstok[1],
and Marius Staring[1,3]

[1] Leiden University Medical Center, Leiden, The Netherlands
s.yousefi.lkeb@lumc.nl
[2] Sharif University of Technology, Tehran, Iran
[3] Delft University of Technology, Delft, The Netherlands

Abstract. Accurate gross tumor volume (GTV) segmentation in esophagus CT images is a critical task in computer aided diagnosis (CAD) systems. However, because of the difficulties raised by the contrast similarity between esophageal GTV and its neighboring tissues in CT scans, this problem has been addressed weakly. In this paper, we present a 3D end-to-end method based on a convolutional neural network (CNN) for this purpose. We leverage design elements from DenseNet in a typical U-shape. The proposed architecture consists of a contractile path and an extending path that includes dense blocks for extracting contextual features and retrieves the lost resolution respectively. Using dense blocks leads to deep supervision, feature re-usability, and parameter reduction while aiding the network to be more accurate. The proposed architecture was trained and tested on a dataset containing 553 scans from 49 distinct patients. The proposed network achieved a Dice value of 0.73 ± 0.20, and a 95% mean surface distance of 3.07 ± 1.86 mm for 85 test scans. The experimental results indicate the effectiveness of the proposed method for clinical diagnosis and treatment systems.

Keywords: Convolutional Neural Network · Gross tumor volume
Esophagus · CT segmentation

1 Introduction

One of the most critical challenges in radiotherapy (RT) treatment planning is a robust strategy for delineation of the gross tumor volume (GTV). Manual segmentation of the GTV is time consuming, subject to error, and involves valuable human resources. Hence, a great deal of effort has been devoted to automating the process for different organs in CT images. Esophageal cancer is the eighth common form of cancer worldwide with 456,000 new cases yearly, and the sixth most fatal form of cancer [1]. RT is one of the treatment options, both in

© Springer Nature Switzerland AG 2018
A. F. Frangi et al. (Eds.): MICCAI 2018, LNCS 11073, pp. 343–351, 2018.
https://doi.org/10.1007/978-3-030-00937-3_40

palliative and curative settings. Delineation of the GTV is not trivial due to short and long term shape changes, and sometimes poor visibility on CT scans used for RT treatment planning. Therefore, physicians use a combination of clinical history, endoscopic findings, and other imaging modalities in conjunction with CT imaging for manual delineation of the esophageal GTV. Obtaining this data is hard, time consuming and expensive. Thus, developing an automatic and reliable esophageal GTV segmentation approach is desirable. However, automatic esophageal GTV segmentation in CT scans has been addressed rarely, and is much harder than segmenting the esophagus due to the difficulties raised by the versatile shape, the poor contrast of the tumor with respect to adjacent tissues, and the existence of foreign bodies in the esophageal lumen.

Lately, convolutional neural networks (CNNs) have attracted a great deal of attention for medical image analysis [2]. However, very few CNN segmentation techniques have been proposed in the context of esophagus segmentation and most of them are highly user interactive. Fechter et al. [3] proposed a fully CNN (FCNN) for segmenting the esophagus in 3D CT images. Because of poor visibility of the transition from the esophagus to the stomach, only the region between the lower tip of the heart and the upper side of the stomach was considered. An active contour model and a random walker were used as post-processing steps. The network achieved an average Dice value of 0.76 ± 0.11 for 20 test scans. A semi-automatic two-stage FCNN for 2D esophagus segmentation was proposed in [4], extracting an ROI in the first stage, and performing the segmentation in the second stage. A Dice value of 0.72 ± 0.07 was reported for 30 test scans. Hao et al. [5] used an FCNN as a pre-processing step for extracting a ROI in 2D CT scans. Then a graph cut method for segmenting the tumor was applied. An average Dice value of 0.75 ± 0.04 was reported for 4 test scans.

In this paper, we propose a 3D end-to-end CNN for esophageal tumor segmentation. The proposed architecture, called 3D-DenseUnet, is related to fully convolutional DenseNet (FC-DenseNet) [6,7], but uses 3D convolutions rather than 2D. In this paper we leverage the idea of dense blocks, arranging them in a typical U-shape. This improves the flow of information and gradients throughout the network and strengthens feature propagation and feature re-usability. Different from [7], two techniques of bottleneck layers and feature compression are used in order to increase the feature maps in a tractable fashion. Also, we adapt the loss function particularly for our dataset. To the best of our knowledge this is the first end-to-end method that addresses automatic 3D tumor segmentation in esophageal CT scans of the whole chest region.

2 Proposed Network Architecture

The proposed DenseUnet, see Fig. 1, is a 3D network composed of a contractile path to extract contextual features and an expanding path to recover the input patch resolution. Each path consists of three main components: dense blocks, down-sampling units, and up-sampling units. Since memory usage in 3D CNNs is a challenging issue, training is performed using 3D patches rather than complete scans. The input patch size is $47 \times 47 \times 47$ voxels, i.e. encompassing the GTV, while the output is probabilistic with size $33 \times 33 \times 33$ voxels, concentric

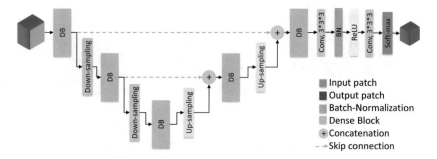

Fig. 1. The architecture of 3D-DenseUnet. The network contains dense blocks, down-sampling units and up-sampling units. The gray dashed arrows between the contractile path and the expansive path demonstrate the skip connections.

with the input. In the contractile path at each level, there is a dense block. The two first contractile levels are followed by down-sampling units which reduce the number of parameters and make the network capture more contextual information. At the third level of the network, a dense block and an up-sampling unit are stacked. Up-sampling layers and skip connections assist the network to retrieve the lost resolution after the down-sampling units. At the final step, the network is followed by one conv($3 \times 3 \times 3$)-BN-ReLU (where BN is batch normalization and ReLU a rectified linear unit), another convolutional layer with linear activation, and a soft-max layer in order to compute a probabilistic output which can be classified as GTV and background.

Figure 2 illustrates the structure of the main components of the proposed network. In each dense block, one conv($1 \times 1 \times 1$)-BN-ReLU and one conv($3 \times 3 \times 3$)-BN-ReLU are stacked. Dense blocks with direct connectivity between all the subsequent layers, improve the information flow between the layers and make the network more accurate [6]. Also, due to its feature reusing capability, dense blocks can perform deep supervision [7]. Unlike FC-Densenet, we employ a feature reduction technique to avoid feature explosion. In each dense block conv($1 \times 1 \times 1$) layers are used as bottleneck layers, which reduce the number of input feature maps and thus improve computational efficiency [6]. Also, in each down-sampling unit there is one conv($1 \times 1 \times 1$)-BN-ReLU which compresses the feature maps with a coefficient θ. A down-sampling unit is followed by one $2 \times 2 \times 2$ max-pooling layer with a stride of $2 \times 2 \times 2$. The up-sampling unit consists of one conv($3 \times 3 \times 3$)-BN-ReLU and one $3 \times 3 \times 3$ transposed convolutional layer with a stride of $2 \times 2 \times 2$. It has been shown that using bottleneck layers and compression aids in preventing overfitting [6].

Optimization is done by the Adam optimizer, with a constant learning rate of 10^{-4}. As the GTV is quite small in comparison with the background, the data is severely imbalanced. To tackle this issue [8], we employ the Dice similarity coefficient as a loss function of the network similar to [9]:

$$\mathrm{DSC}_{\mathrm{GTV}} = \frac{2 \sum_i^N s_i g_i}{\sum_i^N s_i^2 + \sum_i^N g_i^2}, \tag{1}$$

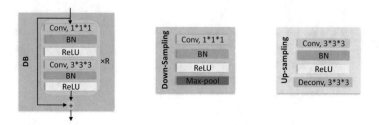

Fig. 2. Main elements of the proposed network, from left to right: dense block, down-sampling unit, and up-sampling unit. Here, deconv stands for transposed convolutional layer. For each dense block, R is the number of dense sub-blocks which output is connected to all subsequent sub-blocks.

where $s_i \in S$ is the binary segmentation of the GTV predicted by the network and $g_i \in G$ is the ground truth segmentation.

3   Materials and Implementation

3.1   Dataset

This study includes two different datasets of chest CT scans. The first dataset was from 21 distinct patients who were treated for esophageal cancer between 2012 and 2014. For each patient, there were five repeat CT scans captured at different time points. For three time points, there was one 3D CT scan, and for two time points there were one 3D CT scan and one 4D CT scan, consisting of 10 breathing phases. The second dataset contains 29 distinct patients who were treated for esophageal cancer in 2016 and 2017, with a single 3D CT scan per patient. In both datasets, for each scan there was a corresponding esophageal GTV segmentation, delineated by a single experienced physician. Each volume contains 58-108 slices of 512×512 pixels and an average voxel size of $0.98 \times 0.98 \times 3$ mm^3 which was resampled to a voxel size of $1 \times 1 \times 3$ mm^3.

3.2   Augmentation and Training Details

We implemented DenseUnet in Google's Tensorflow. The experiments are carried out using a GeForce GTX1080 Ti with 11 GB of GPU memory. For training the network, the dataset was divided into three distinct sets: 30 patients (390 volumes) for training, 6 patients (78 volumes) for validation, and 13 patients (85 volumes) for testing. In order to manage the GPU memory consumption and parallelize the patch selection during the training process, the patches were extracted randomly from the torso region, using a multi-threaded daemon process on the CPU and were fed to the network on the GPU. At the testing time the fully convolutional nature of the network is used, with zero padding to yield equal output size. The batch size is 20 and the number of training iterations

Table 1. Configuration details of the proposed network and DeepUnet$_{122}$. DB refers to dense block, R is the number of the sub-blocks for each DB, f_1 and f_2 denote the number of feature maps for the bottleneck and conv($3 \times 3 \times 3$) layers in each DB, respectively. Each conv($1 \times 1 \times 1$) layer produces $4f_1$ feature maps. m denotes the number of feature maps, and θ is the compression coefficient.

	Patch size	DeepUnet$_{122}$				DenseUnet$_{188}$				DenseUnet$_{122}$			
		R	f_1	f_2	m	R	f_1	f_2	m	R	f_1	f_2	m
Input	$47 \times 47 \times 47$												
DB + Down-sampling	$22 \times 22 \times 22$	3	4	16	8	3	4	4	13	3	16	8	12
DB + Down-sampling	$11 \times 11 \times 11$	4	4	32	16	7	4	4	41	4	32	16	38
DB	$11 \times 11 \times 11$	4	64	64	64	9	4	4	77	4	32	16	102
Up-sampling + DB	$19 \times 19 \times 19$	4	32	32	100	7	4	4	146	4	8	4	105
Up-sampling + DB	$35 \times 35 \times 35$	3	4	64	64	3	2	2	67	3	8	2	44
conv($3 \times 3 \times 3$)-BN-ReLU	$33 \times 33 \times 33$				16				16				22
conv($3 \times 3 \times 3$) + softmax	$33 \times 33 \times 33$				2				2				2
θ		0.5				1				0.5			
# parameters (M)		1.1				0.7				1.2			

is $\sim$10k. During every training iteration, the input patches were augmented by white noise extracted from a Gaussian distribution with zero mean and a random standard deviation between 0 and 5.

Table 1 summarizes the structure of the network. We used two different configurations of the proposed network, where we vary the number of the sub-blocks and also feature maps inside each sub-block.

4   Experiments and Results

Evaluation of the proposed method was done by the Dice Similarity Coefficient (DSC), and mean surface distance (MSD). As in some cases the networks additionally segment areas far away from the GTV, we also report the MSD for the 95% best cases. In addition, precision and recall were reported.

The performance of DenseUnet with two configurations was compared with U-Net [10] and a modified version of U-Net dubbed DeepUnet$_{122}$. The number of layers for the 3D U-Net network was 23 and the number of parameters 1.2M. The DeepUnet$_{122}$ architecture is similar to DenseUnet$_{122}$ but without the loop connections inside the dense blocks. In both U-Net and DeepUnet$_{122}$, the Dice loss function was used instead of cross-entropy [10], to enable a fair comparison. Hence, the 3D U-Net in this paper is similar to V-Net [9].

Figure 3(a–d) depicts the DSC, MSD (mm), recall and precision for all networks on the test set. Figure 3(e) shows the cumulative frequency of the number of the scans for different DSC values. As can be seen, for U-Net, 20 cases have a DSC ≤ 0.5, for DeepUnet$_{122}$ still 15 cases are ≤ 0.5, while this number is 10 and 8 for DenseUnet$_{188}$ and DenseUnet$_{122}$, respectively. A few cases have a low

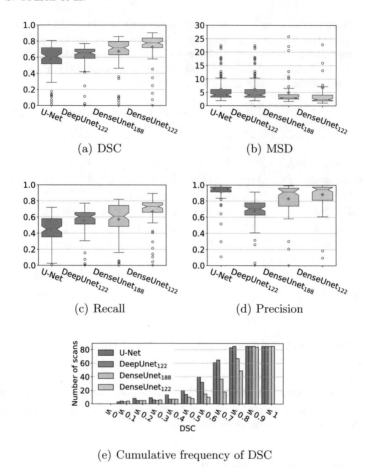

(a) DSC

(b) MSD

(c) Recall

(d) Precision

(e) Cumulative frequency of DSC

Fig. 3. Comparison of the networks. The red marks and red lines show the mean and median, respectively. For (b), a few outliers larger than 30 are not shown.

DSC for all networks. A closer inspection revealed that in some cases there was a feeding tube, surgical clips or air pockets in the esophageal lumen present in the GTV. These cases were rarely seen in the training set. Figure 4 exemplifies the segmentation results for two normal GTVs, a GTV with a large air pocket in the lumen, and a GTV with a feeding tube present.

Table 2 yields a quantitative comparison of the segmentation performance for the networks. As can be seen, DenseUnet$_{188}$ has the best value of MSD but DenseUnet$_{122}$ has the best values in terms of DSC, 95% MSD and median MSD. So, we propose DenseUnet$_{122}$ as the final network.

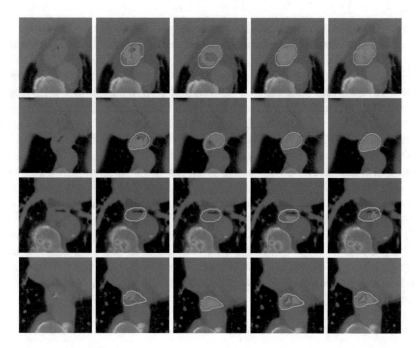

Fig. 4. Example results, from left to right: original images; U-Net; DeepUnet$_{122}$; DenseUnet$_{188}$; DenseUnet$_{122}$. The green contours depict the ground truth and the red overlays the network output. The 3rd and 4th rows show an example of the GTV containing an air cavity in the lumen and a feeding tube, respectively.

Table 2. Comparison of the different networks. The best results are shown in bold. Here, med stands for median. The higher MSD for DenseUnet$_{122}$ is related to some false positives far away from the GTV, which is visible in the MSD.

	U-Net[10]		DeepUnet$_{122}$		DenseUnet$_{188}$		DenseUnet$_{122}$	
	$\mu \pm \sigma$	med	$\mu \pm \sigma$	med	$\mu \pm \sigma$	med	$\mu \pm \sigma$	med
DSC	0.57 ± 0.20	0.61	0.59 ± 017	0.65	0.67 ± 0.19	0.71	$\mathbf{0.73 \pm 0.20}$	**0.78**
MSD (mm)	6.21 ± 5.02	4.06	6.10 ± 5.90	4.00	$\mathbf{4.97 \pm 6.23}$	3.00	6.83 ± 19.21	**2.36**
95% MSD (mm)	5.32 ± 3.63	3.94	5.07 ± 2.98	3.88	3.55 ± 1.93	2.89	$\mathbf{3.07 \pm 1.86}$	**2.31**
Precision	0.91 ± 0.13	0.94	0.68 ± 0.17	0.70	0.83 ± 0.21	0.91	0.88 ± 0.15	0.94
Recall	0.44 ± 0.18	0.45	0.55 ± 0.18	0.60	0.57 ± 0.19	0.61	0.66 ± 0.21	0.73

5   Discussion and Conclusion

We proposed a 3D end-to-end fully convolutional CNN, called DenseUnet, for the segmentation of the esophageal GTV in CT images. DenseUnet leverages the ideas of dense blocks, in conjunction with down-sampling and up-sampling paths. This enables the network to extract contextual features deeply while retrieving image resolution and alleviating the problem of feature map explosion. We applied the proposed network to segment esophageal GTVs in 3D chest CT scans for the first time.

We trained and tested the proposed method on 553 chest CT scans from 49 distinct patients and achieved a DSC value of 0.73 ± 0.20, and a 95% MSD of 3.07 ± 1.86 mm for the test scans, thereby outperforming U-Net. Eight (8/85) scans had a DSC < 0.50, mostly caused by the presence of air cavities and foreign bodies in the GTV, which was rarely seen in the training data.

To further enhance the robustness of the network we consider to increase the training data set (more foreign bodies) and use more elaborate data augmentation. Dilated convolutions may decrease the network size, and consequently make better use of the available training data as well. Combining with ROI-extraction techniques may lower the number of false positives.

In conclusion, the proposed network obtained promising results for the challenging problem of esophageal cancer segmentation on chest CT scans, comparing favorably to U-Net and earlier results found in the literature. The method therefore may assist the clinical workflow, especially when considering an online adaptive RT setting.

Acknowledgements. Denis Shamonin is acknowledged for the torso extraction code.

References

1. Thrift, A.P.: The epidemic of oesophageal carcinoma: where are we now? Cancer Epidemiol. **41**, 88–95 (2016)
2. Litjens, G., et al.: A survey on deep learning in medical image analysis. Med. Image Anal. **42**, 60–88 (2017)
3. Fechter, T., Adebahr, S., Baltas, D., Ayed, I.B., Desrosiers, C., Dolz, J.: A 3D fully convolutional neural network and a random walker to segment the esophagus in CT. arXiv preprint arXiv:1704.06544 (2017)
4. Trullo, R., Petitjean, C., Nie, D., Shen, D., Ruan, S.: Fully automated esophagus segmentation with a hierarchical deep learning approach. In: IEEE ICSIPA, pp. 503–506 (2017)
5. Hao, Z., Liu, J., Liu, J.: Esophagus Tumor segmentation using fully convolutional neural network and graph cut. In: Jia, Y., Du, J., Zhang, W. (eds.) CISC 2017. LNEE, vol. 460, pp. 413–420. Springer, Singapore (2018). https://doi.org/10.1007/978-981-10-6499-9_39
6. Huang, G., Liu, Z., Weinberger, K.Q., van der Maaten, L.: Densely connected convolutional networks. In: IEEE CVPR, pp. 4700–4708 (2017)
7. Jégou, S., Drozdzal, M., Vazquez, D., Romero, A., Bengio, Y.: The one hundred layers tiramisu: fully convolutional densenets for semantic segmentation. In: IEEE CVPR Workshops, pp. 1175–1183 (2017)
8. Sudre, C.H., Li, W., Vercauteren, T., Ourselin, S., Jorge Cardoso, M.: Generalised dice overlap as a deep learning loss function for highly unbalanced segmentations. In: Cardoso, M.J., et al. (eds.) DLMIA/ML-CDS -2017. LNCS, vol. 10553, pp. 240–248. Springer, Cham (2017). https://doi.org/10.1007/978-3-319-67558-9_28

9. Milletari, F., Navab, N., Ahmadi, S.A.: V-Net: fully convolutional neural networks for volumetric medical image segmentation. In: International Conference on 3D Vision, pp. 565–571 (2016)
10. Çiçek, Ö., Abdulkadir, A., Lienkamp, S.S., Brox, T., Ronneberger, O.: 3D U-Net: learning dense volumetric segmentation from sparse annotation. In: Ourselin, S., Joskowicz, L., Sabuncu, M.R., Unal, G., Wells, W. (eds.) MICCAI 2016. LNCS, vol. 9901, pp. 424–432. Springer, Cham (2016). https://doi.org/10.1007/978-3-319-46723-8_49

Deep Learning Based Instance Segmentation in 3D Biomedical Images Using Weak Annotation

Zhuo Zhao[1], Lin Yang[1], Hao Zheng[1], Ian H. Guldner[2], Siyuan Zhang[2], and Danny Z. Chen[1(✉)]

[1] Department of Computer Science and Engineering, University of Notre Dame, Notre Dame, IN 46556, USA
dchen@nd.edu
[2] Department of Biological Sciences, Harper Cancer Research Institute, University of Notre Dame, Notre Dame, IN 46556, USA

Abstract. Instance segmentation in 3D images is a fundamental task in biomedical image analysis. While deep learning models often work well for 2D instance segmentation, 3D instance segmentation still faces critical challenges, such as insufficient training data due to various annotation difficulties in 3D biomedical images. Common 3D annotation methods (e.g., full voxel annotation) incur high workloads and costs for labeling enough instances for training deep learning 3D instance segmentation models. In this paper, we propose a new weak annotation approach for training a fast deep learning 3D instance segmentation model without using full voxel mask annotation. Our approach needs only 3D bounding boxes for all instances and full voxel annotation for a small fraction of the instances, and uses a novel two-stage 3D instance segmentation model utilizing these two kinds of annotation, respectively. We evaluate our approach on several biomedical image datasets, and the experimental results show that (1) with full annotated boxes and a small amount of masks, our approach can achieve similar performance as the best known methods using full annotation, and (2) with similar annotation time, our approach outperforms the best known methods that use full annotation.

1 Introduction

3D instance segmentation seeks to segment all instances of the objects of interest (RoI) in 3D images. This is a fundamental task in computer vision and biomedical image analysis. Recent successes at acquiring 3D biomedical image data [8] put even higher demand on 3D instance segmentation. However, annotation of 3D biomedical images to produce sufficient training data for deep learning models is often highly expensive and time-consuming, because only experts can annotate biomedical images well and no direct annotation technique is yet available

---

Z. Zhao and L. Yang—These authors contributed equally to this work.

© Springer Nature Switzerland AG 2018
A. F. Frangi et al. (Eds.): MICCAI 2018, LNCS 11073, pp. 352–360, 2018.
https://doi.org/10.1007/978-3-030-00937-3_41

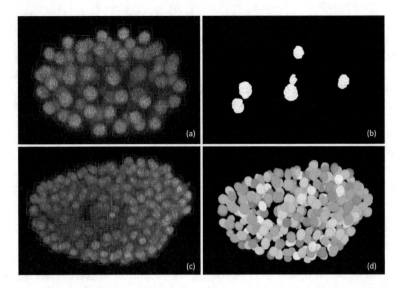

Fig. 1. A training image example and test results for C.elegans developing embryos [8]. (a) Each object instance is labeled by a 3D bounding box; (b) a small fraction of instances are labeled with voxel mask annotation; (c) in stage one, our model uses full box annotation to detect all instances; (d) in stage two, it uses full voxel mask annotation for a small fraction of the instances to segment each detected instance.

for 3D biomedical images. Further, although many 2D weakly supervised methods [4,5,9,11] were developed to reduce annotation efforts, they are not directly applicable to 3D images. A common way to label 3D biomedical images is full annotation (i.e., all voxels of all RoI instances are annotated). This may work for voxel-level 3D segmentation networks [1], but instance segmentation demands much higher workload to annotate a sufficient (large) amount of instances for model training. Hence, using full annotation for 3D instance segmentation is impractical and annotation difficulties are a major obstacle impeding the development of deep learning models for 3D instance segmentation.

Recent 2D instance detection and segmentation methods achieved good performance [2,3,6,7]. However, in addition to the above annotation difficulties for 3D instance segmentation, extending such 2D approaches to 3D directly faces considerable challenges (e.g., GPU memory limit). In [10], 2D pixel segmentation results were stacked as 3D voxel segmentation results, and an algorithm (of high complexity) was then applied to the voxel segmentation results to conduct 3D instance segmentation. Although 2D annotation and the 2D model [10] did not suffer GPU memory issues as much, without taking advantage of 3D context information, the stacked voxel segmentation results were not very accurate, and due to high algorithm complexity [10], processing a dense 3D stack took hours.

To train a fast 3D instance segmentation model without high 3D annotation effort, in this paper, we present an end-to-end deep learning 3D instance segmentation model utilizing weak annotation. Our model needs only 3D bounding boxes for all instances and full voxel annotation for a small amount of instances (Fig. 1(a)–(b)). The model has two stages. In the first stage, the model detects all instances utilizing 3D bounding box annotation; in the second stage, the model segments all detected instances utilizing full voxel annotation for a small amount of instances (Fig. 1(c)–(d)). We adopt the design of VoxRes block [1] to allow information propagating directly in both the forward and backward directions.

We evaluate our 3D instance segmentation approach on several datasets, and the experimental results show that (1) with full annotated boxes and a small amount of masks, our approach can achieve similar performance as the best known methods using full annotation, and (2) with similar annotation time, our approach outperforms the best known methods that use full annotation.

2   Method

Our proposed method consists of two major components: (1) a 3D object detector utilizing 3D bounding box annotation for all instances to predict 3D bounding boxes along with the probabilities of the boxes containing instances; (2) a 3D voxel segmentation model utilizing full voxel annotation for a small amount of instances to segment all instances of all objects of interest (RoI).

2.1   3D Object Detector Using 3D Bounding Box Annotation

We first briefly review 2D region proposal networks (RPN) for object detection, and then present our 3D object detector utilizing 3D bounding box annotation.

Region Proposal Networks (RPN). For object detection tasks, there are often two major steps: generating region proposals and classifying the proposals into different classes. Faster-RCNN [2] proposes an FCN based RPN to generate RoIs from convolutional feature maps directly, and then uses a classifier to classify the generated RoIs into different classes. Different from the previous FCN models for predicting the probability for each pixel, RPN predicts the probabilities for the anchor boxes centering at each feature point (of an instance) and the box regression offset. A multi-task loss for RPN is defined as:

$$L(p_i, t_i) = \frac{1}{N} \sum_i L_{cls}(p_i, p_i^*) + \lambda \frac{1}{N} \sum_i p_i^* L_{reg}(t_i, t_i^*) \qquad (1)$$

where i is the index of an anchor box, p_i is the predicted probability of anchor i, p_i^* is a ground-truth label (0 for negative, 1 for positive), t_i is a 4D vector presenting the shape of the predicted box (two for the box center position and two for the box size), t_i^* presents the ground-truth box associated with a positive anchor, L_{cls} is the log loss over two classes (object and background) for the objectness error, and L_{reg} is the smooth L_1 loss [2] on t_i and t_i^* for box position error. L_{cls} and L_{reg} are normalized by the number of the anchor boxes N.

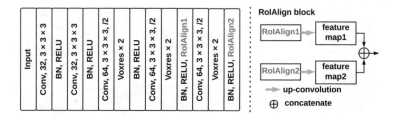

Fig. 2. The backbone and RoIAlign block of the model. RoIAlign is applied to two layers of the backbone. The feature maps after up-convolution are concatenated as the final feature maps.

3D Object Detector Using 3D Bounding Box Annotation. Given the fact that labeling a 3D bounding box for each instance is much cheaper than labeling all voxels of the instance, we propose a 3D object detector utilizing 3D bounding box annotation to detect all the instances in a 3D stack.

Figure 2 shows our FCN based backbone. We adopt the VoxRes block design to allow information propagating in both forward and backward directions directly.

After extracting the feature maps from the backbone, we evaluate a fix number of anchor boxes of different sizes at each location of the feature maps. We first match the anchor boxes to the ground-truth boxes by calculating the maximal Intersection of Union (IoU) between an anchor box and all ground-truth boxes. The anchor boxes having the maximal IoU with some ground-truth boxes are treated as positives, and all the anchor boxes having an IoU over a threshold (0.4 in our experiments) with any ground-truth boxes are also treated as positives. All other boxes are treated as negatives.

A group of convolutional filters is used to predict the shape offset and score of containing an object for all anchor boxes. For a feature layer of size $m \times n \times k$ with p channels, cr filters (c is the number of classes, r is the number of anchor boxes for each feature point) of size $3 \times 3 \times 3 \times p$ are used to predict the instance classes, and $6r$ filters of size $3 \times 3 \times 3 \times p$ are used to predict the box regression offset of all anchor boxes. Hence, the output size for the score of the instance class is $m \times n \times k \times cr$, and the output size for the box regression offset is $m \times n \times k \times 6r$. The regression value $(t_z, t_x, t_y, t_d, t_h, t_w)$ of the predicted 3D box and the value $(t_z^*, t_x^*, t_y^*, t_d^*, t_h^*, t_w^*)$ of the ground-truth box are computed as:

$$
\begin{aligned}
t_z &= (z - z_a)/d_a, t_x = (y - y_a)/h_a, t_y = (x - x_a)/w_a, \\
t_d &= \log(d/d_a), t_h = \log(h/h_a), t_w = \log(w/w_a), \\
t_z^* &= (z^* - z_a)/d_a, t_x^* = (y^* - y_a)/h_a, t_y^* = (x^* - x_a)/w_a, \\
t_d^* &= \log(d^*/d_a), t_h^* = \log(h^*/h_a), t_w^* = \log(w^*/w_a),
\end{aligned}
\tag{2}
$$

where z, x, and y denote the box center coordinates, d, h, and w denote the box size, and z, z_a, and z^* are for the predicted box, anchor box, and ground-truth box, respectively (likewise for x, y, d, w, and h). All anchor boxes are regressed to

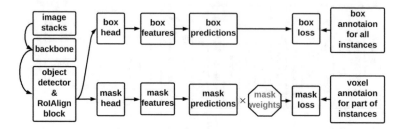

Fig. 3. Illustrating the flow of our method. All boxes contribute to the object detector; only the instances with voxel annotation contribute to the voxel segmentation model.

nearby ground-truth boxes to calculate the predicted boxes. Different from RPN that predicts region proposals (2 classes) and classifies all proposals in another stage, our model predicts the final classes for all objects (c classes). This change works well for biomedical images, while saving memory, because compared to natural scene images, there can be less classes but more instances in one stack (e.g., some types of cells). Thus, changing RPN to an object detector can help focus on locating instances and classifying instances into different classes in one step instead of two steps, which uses less parameters and less GPU memory. We use the same multi-task loss of RPN for our detected boxes, i.e., $L_{box} = L_{cls} + L_{reg}$, but L_{cls} is for all c classes, not only two classes (objects and background). Since all instances have box annotation, the model conducts back-propagation for all boxes (Fig. 3), i.e., all boxes contribute to the object detector.

2.2 3D Voxel Segmentation Using Full Voxel Annotation for a Small Fraction of Instances

Mask-RCNN. Mask-RCNN [3] is used to perform 2D instance segmentation based on RPN. After generating RoIs using RPN, Mask-RCNN uses RoIAlign to align all RoIs to the same size (e.g., 7 × 7). RoIAlign computes the value of each sampling point by bilinear interpolation from the nearby grid points on the feature maps. Using the interpolation value of the nearby grid points instead of using the value of one nearest point can make the predicted mask smoother and more accurate. Then up-convolutional layers are used to calculate the mask for all aligned feature maps.

3D Voxel Segmentation. After detecting the instances for all objects, a 3D voxel segmentation model utilizing full voxel annotation for a small fraction of the instances is used to segment all instances. The corresponding feature maps are cropped from the feature layers of the backbone. To make the detected objects of different sizes share the same segmentation parameters, we extend the RoIAlign design from 2D to a 3D version. All cropped features are aligned to size $s \times s \times s \times p$, where s is the RoIAlign size and p is the channel number of the feature maps. For each sampling point, we first find the 8 nearest neighbor points on the feature maps, and then apply trilinear interpolation to the 8 neighbor points to calculate the value of the sampling point. Then up-convolutional layers are applied to all aligned features for segmenting all the detected instances. To make the model utilize the information from different layers, our 3D RoIAlign is applied to two different layers from the backbone, and the feature maps are concatenated as the final feature maps for 3D RoIAlign (Fig. 2).

Since full annotation methods can be impractical for 3D instance segmentation, our model needs full voxel annotation only for a small fraction of the instances. We add a mask-weight layer before calculating the loss for the voxel masks. Although the model segments all instances (no matter there is corresponding voxel annotation or not), it conducts back-propagation only for those instances having voxel mask annotation (Fig. 3). We add a mask weight layer to set the loss to 0 for these instances without voxel annotation; by this means, only the instances with full voxel annotation contribute to the voxel segmentation model, and all other instances do not affect the voxel segmentation model. The loss for the mask L_{mask} is the average binary cross-entropy loss. The loss for the whole task is $L = L_{box} + L_{mask}$. Experimental results show that, by adding the mask-weight layer, our 3D segmentation model can segment all detected instances utilizing full voxel annotation for only a small fraction of instances.

3   Experiments and Results

We evaluate our 3D instance segmentation model and our weak annotation method on three biomedical image datasets: nuclei of HL60 cells [8], microglia cells (in-house), and C.elegans developing embryos [8]. For nuclei of HL60 cells and C.elegans developing embryos, our objective is different from the original challenge; we only use the data with ground-truth labels as both the training data and test data. We evaluate both the instance detection and instance segmentation performance on the nuclei of HL60 cells and microglia cells. Due to lack of full voxel annotation for the C.elegans embryo dataset, we only evaluate the instance detection performance on this dataset. Based on our experiments, it takes about 15 GB GPU memory during training when a batch contains 4 stacks of size $64 \times 64 \times 128$ each. During testing, a stack of size $64 \times 639 \times 649$ containing 20 instances takes about 10 s on an NVIDIA Tesla P100 GPU.

Nuclei of HL60 Cells and Microglia Cells. Both these two datasets have full voxel annotation for all instances. For these two datasets, the time for an expert to label all the voxels of a cell is about 30 times of that for labeling a 3D bounding box of the cell according to our annotation time statistics. The dataset of HL60 cells has two groups of data: 150 stacks for the 1st group, and 80 stacks for the 2nd group. We use stacks $000, 010, 020, \ldots, 070$ from the 1st group and stacks $000, 010, 020, 030, 040$ from the 2nd group as the training data (13 stacks in total), and use stacks 080–149 from the 1st group and stacks 050–079 from the 2nd group as the test data (100 stacks in total). For microglia cell images,

Table 1. Results on the HL60 cells dataset. AT = approximate annotation time.

Method	AT	Detection F1			Segmentation F1		
		Group 1	Group 2	Mean	Group 1	Group 2	Mean
Our method (20%)	5.5 h	0.9967	**0.9599**	**0.9783**	0.9416	**0.8437**	0.8927
VoxResNet (full)	22.5 h	**0.9988**	0.9543	0.9766	**0.9656**	0.8428	**0.9042**
VoxResNet (4/13)	8.3 h	0.9965	0.9221	0.9593	0.9610	0.7873	0.8742

Table 2. Results on the microglia cells dataset. AT = approximate annotation time.

Method	AT	Detection F1	Segmentation F1
Our method (30%)	54.7 h	**0.9078**	0.8424
VoxResNet (full)	172.9 h	0.9017	**0.8484**
VoxResNet (4/10)	67.5 h	0.8761	0.8307

we use 10 stacks of the 14 total stacks as training data, and the other 4 stacks as test data. For both the datasets, the number c of classes is 2.

To evaluate our 3D voxel segmentation model utilizing full voxel annotation for a small fraction of the instances, for the HL60 cells images, we randomly choose 20% of the cells from each stack as the instances with full voxel masks, and 30% for microglia cells. All the instances have box annotation.

A best-known deep learning method is selected for comparison with our method. VoxResNet [1] is applied to the training data with boundary class to produce voxel segmentation results, and then 3D connected components are computed from the voxel segmentation results as the instance segmentation results. For the comparison method, we evaluate the performance of using full voxel annotation and the performance of using similar annotation time as our method.

For instance detection evaluation, we compute only whether the detected 3D bounding boxes match with some 3D ground-truth bounding boxes. All the detected boxes with IoU larger than 0.4 (note that 0.4 in 3D is more strict than 0.5 in 2D) with some matched ground-truth boxes are taken as true positives. All the other detected boxes are false positives. All ground-truth boxes without matching detected boxes are false negatives. For instance segmentation evaluation, we follow a similar evaluation process as in [10].

Tables 1 and 2 show the results on these two datasets, in which the methods either use a proportion of the full voxel annotation (for our method, all instances have box annotation, and for the comparison method, full annotation is used) or use full annotation in the experiments.

For instance detection, our method using full voxel annotation for only a small part of the instances outperforms the comparison method using full annotation. This is because box annotation contains stronger instance information than voxel annotation, and our model considers the loss for instance detection explicitly (L_{box}). For instance segmentation, due to the resampling operations in RoIAlign, the comparison method using full annotation is better than ours, but ours still outperforms the comparison method with similar annotation time, because locating instances accurately can improve the performance of voxel segmentation. Although our method dose not surpass the comparison method using full annotation, it is still practical due to using much less annotation time.

C.elegans Developing Embryos. For this dataset, we do not have full voxel annotation but only small markers indicating different instances. The dataset is quite dense (e.g., see Fig. 1), and it is difficult (or impractical) to label all voxels of all instances. This dataset has two groups of data; each group contains 190 stacks with markers. To evaluate our detection method, experts labeled 1527 3D bounding boxes for 15 stacks from the first group, and only 67 instances are labeled with full voxel annotation. We use the 190 stacks in the second group for testing. A sample result is given in Fig. 1(c)–(d). We determine the performance of our instance detection by computing the distances between the ground-truth markers and the centers of the detected boxes. The F1 score for this experiment is 0.9495 (using a distance threshold of 5 pixels).

4   Conclusions

In this paper, we presented a new end-to-end 3D instance segmentation approach, and to reduce annotation effort on 3D biomedical images, we proposed a weak annotation method for training our 3D instance segmentation model. Experimental results show that (1) with full annotated boxes and a small amount of masks, our approach can achieve similar performance as the best-known methods using full annotation, and (2) with similar annotation time, our approach outperforms the best-known methods that use full annotation.

Acknowledgment. This research was supported in part by NSF grant CCF-1640081 and the Nanoelectronics Research Corporation (NERC), a wholly-owned subsidiary of the Semiconductor Research Corporation (SRC), through Extremely Energy Efficient Collective Electronics (EXCEL), an SRC-NRI Nanoelectronics Research Initiative under Research Task ID 2698.005, NSF grants CCF-1617735 and CNS-1629914, and NIH grant R01 R01CA194697.

References

1. Chen, H., Dou, Q., Yu, L., Heng, P.A.: VoxResNet: deep voxelwise residual networks for volumetric brain segmentation. arXiv preprint arXiv:1608.05895 (2016)
2. Girshick, R.: Fast R-CNN. arXiv preprint arXiv:1504.08083 (2015)
3. He, K., Gkioxari, G., Dollár, P., Girshick, R.: Mask R-CNN. In: ICCV, pp. 2980–2988 (2017)
4. Hu, R., Dollár, P., He, K., Darrell, T., Girshick, R.: Learning to segment every thing. arXiv preprint arXiv:1711.10370 (2017)
5. Khoreva, A., Benenson, R., Hosang, J., Hein, M., Schiele, B.: Simple does it: weakly supervised instance and semantic segmentation. In: CVPR (2017)

6. Liu, W., et al.: SSD: single shot MultiBox detector. In: Leibe, B., Matas, J., Sebe, N., Welling, M. (eds.) ECCV 2016. LNCS, vol. 9905, pp. 21–37. Springer, Cham (2016). https://doi.org/10.1007/978-3-319-46448-0_2

7. Ren, S., He, K., Girshick, R., Sun, J.: Faster R-CNN: towards real-time object detection with region proposal networks. In: NIPS, pp. 91–99 (2015)

8. Ulman, V., et al.: An objective comparison of cell-tracking algorithms. Nat. Methods **14**, 1141 (2017)

9. Yang, L., Zhang, Y., Chen, J., Zhang, S., Chen, D.Z.: Suggestive annotation: a deep active learning framework for biomedical image segmentation. In: Descoteaux, M., Maier-Hein, L., Franz, A., Jannin, P., Collins, D.L., Duchesne, S. (eds.) MICCAI 2017. LNCS, vol. 10435, pp. 399–407. Springer, Cham (2017). https://doi.org/10.1007/978-3-319-66179-7_46

10. Yang, L., Zhang, Y., Guldner, I.H., Zhang, S., Chen, D.Z.: 3D segmentation of glial cells using fully convolutional networks and k-terminal cut. In: Ourselin, S., Joskowicz, L., Sabuncu, M.R., Unal, G., Wells, W. (eds.) MICCAI 2016. LNCS, vol. 9901, pp. 658–666. Springer, Cham (2016). https://doi.org/10.1007/978-3-319-46723-8_76

11. Zhang, Y., Yang, L., Chen, J., Fredericksen, M., Hughes, D.P., Chen, D.Z.: Deep adversarial networks for biomedical image segmentation utilizing unannotated images. In: Descoteaux, M., Maier-Hein, L., Franz, A., Jannin, P., Collins, D.L., Duchesne, S. (eds.) MICCAI 2017. LNCS, vol. 10435, pp. 408–416. Springer, Cham (2017). https://doi.org/10.1007/978-3-319-66179-7_47

Learn the New, Keep the Old: Extending Pretrained Models with New Anatomy and Images

Firat Ozdemir[1]([⊠])(ID), Philipp Fuernstahl[2], and Orcun Goksel[1](ID)

[1] Computer-assisted Applications in Medicine, ETH Zurich, Zurich, Switzerland
ozdemirf@vision.ee.ethz.ch
[2] CARD Group, University Hospital Balgrist, University of Zurich,
Zurich, Switzerland

Abstract. Deep learning has been widely accepted as a promising solution for medical image segmentation, given a sufficiently large representative dataset of images with corresponding annotations. With ever increasing amounts of annotated medical datasets, it is infeasible to train a learning method always with all data from scratch. This is also doomed to hit computational limits, e.g., memory or runtime feasible for training. Incremental learning can be a potential solution, where new information (images or anatomy) is introduced iteratively. Nevertheless, for the preservation of the collective information, it is essential to keep some "important" (i.e., representative) images and annotations from the past, while adding new information. In this paper, we introduce a framework for applying incremental learning for segmentation and propose novel methods for selecting representative data therein. We comparatively evaluate our methods in different scenarios using MR images and validate the increased learning capacity with using our methods.

Keywords: Segmentation · Class-incremental learning

1 Introduction

With the growing interest in automatic and semi-automatic analysis of patients, available data size for research is continuously increasing. Even for a single anatomical structure, soon it may become infeasible to retrain a network when a newly available data is introduced. On the other hand, one can expect to see variations in image properties across iterations of new data due to various factors, e.g. mechanical differences across imaging device brands, physiological differences across imaged subjects. Furthermore, although various datasets from similar modality are often available, they belong to different studies, hence they have different field-of-view (FOV), image acquisition parameters, and/or annotated anatomy. For instance, some MR modalities (i.e., ultra short TE) are often used to analyze bones and tendons thanks to its high contrast. However, a study

© Springer Nature Switzerland AG 2018
A. F. Frangi et al. (Eds.): MICCAI 2018, LNCS 11073, pp. 361–369, 2018.
https://doi.org/10.1007/978-3-030-00937-3_42

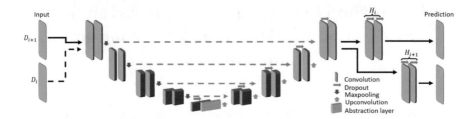

Fig. 1. Schematic of the proposed convolutional network at incremental step $i + 1$. Additional layers ("Head") at step $i+1$ are shown with H_{i+1}. Second layer at coarsest level is called *abstraction layer*. D_i denotes the *exemplar data* in Sect. 2.2.

on diagnosis or healing quantification of Achilles tendon often do not allocate resources for proximal bone tissue annotation. Similarly, for an osteotomy planning, often only bones are annotated to generate surgical guides. Aggregation of annotation knowledge across different anatomy, modality & dataset are not well investigated; however, it is of growing interest in the machine learning community [1,2] as in the form of an "evolving" classifier. To the best of our knowledge, increasing label problem has neither been tackled for segmentation nor in medical community.

For class-incremental learning problem, initial works include finetuning [3]; however, it is well known [4] that this results with "catastrophic forgetting." Later on, learning without forgetting (LwF) [2] has been proposed, which utilizes distillation loss [1] such that when new classes are being added to a network, final activation response of the previous classes are also used for backpropagation. With iCaRL [5], authors extend on LwF by proposing a strategy for selecting an *exemplar* dataset, which keeps a "representative" subset of the earlier training data for the existing classes, and put an upper bound on required memory requirements. In [6], authors suggest a novel way to pick representative samples to train on, for the purpose of maximizing performance for binary segmentation task of gland cells at a next training iteration.

In this work, our novelties are in line with blocks that are necessary to expand class-incremental learning for segmentation task; *extending distillation loss to segmentation* without an assumption on mutual exclusivity of classes. We propose alternative methods for picking representative samples to sustain segmentation accuracy of prior classes. To the best of our knowledge, this is the first work extending distillation loss for class-incremental segmentation.

2   Incremental Head Networks

2.1   Conservation of Prior Knowledge with Distillation

In medical image analysis, a lot of anatomies show similarity in their statistical priors (i.e., bones). Similarly to the idea of finetuning a pretrained VGG [7] network for different digital image classification task, one can train a model with a dataset of anatomy A_x and then finetune it for a new dataset of anatomy A_y, as to utilize knowledge obtained from dataset of A_x when learning A_y. Based on the application, maintaining segmentation capability of anatomy A_x can be equally important (e.g. functional modeling), albeit the two annotated dataset being collected from different patients/studies. It is possible to use distillation loss [1,5] in order to retain the segmentation accuracy of A_x, while exploiting learned prior statistical knowledge to better learn more limited resources of A_y.

Inspired by the idea (LwF [2]) from classification, we propose a segmentation framework for class-incremental learning. At an initial training phase, we train a U-Net [8] like network (cf. Fig. 1 without H_{i+1}) with a first dataset D_{init} using desired classification loss L_c. In order to disambiguate between initial and incremental training, we will refer to the old and new steps as i and $i+1$, respectively. Prior to incremental training, all available dataset $D_a = D_{i+1} \cup D_i$ is passed through the pretrained network in order to produce prediction probabilities for the old classes, including their respective background. For old classes c_i, these predictions p^{c_i} are then used for retaining the network's segmentation accuracy. For incremental training, a new network is then constructed with an additional head H_{i+1} as shown in Fig. 1. The parameters for the network (cf. Fig. 1) except for H_{i+1} are loaded from the previously trained model. During incremental training, for given mini-batch B we optimize the following loss:

$$L_{\text{total}} = \begin{cases} \alpha L_c + (1-\alpha)L_d, & \text{if } B \in D_{i+1} \\ L_d, & \text{otherwise} \end{cases} \tag{1}$$

where $\alpha \in [0,1]$ is a weighting scalar, and L_d is the distillation loss defined as:

$$L_d = \sum_{c_i^{(j)} \in c_i} p_i^{c_i^{(j)}} \log(y^{c_i^{(j)}}) \tag{2}$$

where $p^{c_i^{(j)}}$ and $y^{c_i^{(j)}}$ are the predicted probabilities for class $j \in c_i$ for the initially trained network and the old class heads H_i in the new network.

While it would be ideal to retain all prior training dataset when introducing a new label, this is not a scalable solution due to computational challenges discussed before. An extreme case is to remove all prior data from incremental learning; i.e., $D_i = \{\}$ [2]. The method proposed above is called in the following as LwfSeg. When incrementally learning with datasets of similar properties, LwfSeg may prove sufficient to preserve old class segmentation capacity. Unfortunately, there can be significant amount of variation in image data across different iterations of training, e.g. different MR field inhomogeneity due to different patient profiles, differences across used machine brands. This can lead to a false guidance of the network with an effort to retain old class knowledge.

2.2 Selecting Representative Samples

One can select a subset of the training data to be kept for future incremental learning processes. For classification tasks, a potential approach to choosing representative samples is to observe the feature space right before the final network layer (i.e., embedding space) [5,9], where each input sample is represented with a class-discriminating vector.

Although an intuitive extension for segmentation is to use the embedding space, this is not directly applicable. Finding "most representative" pixels per class in the embedding space is not very helpful. Even if one aggregates a representativeness metric over all pixels at the embedding space as to get a scalar value per input image, it is not clear how to account for the ratio of the foreground pixels accordingly. Therefore, we propose the following two alternatives.

Maximum Set Coverage over Most Certain Sample Abstractions: Using dropout layers, one can compute a trained models confidence for a given input image I through Monte Carlo estimates [10] by getting inference t_{MC} times. A typical way to get a scalar uncertainty value from an image is to aggregate the uncertainty over all pixels. In [6], in a microscopy segmentation context, authors select samples based on maximum uncertainty for maximizing performance gain in a next round of training. An ideal exemplar set should contain slices with high confidence (i.e., least uncertainty) for class-incremental task, in order to prevent "catastrophic forgetting." For typical medical images where foreground labels are underrepresented, or completely missing in a slice when this anatomy is not intersecting, high confidence samples are likely to fall on images with only background. As a remedy, one can choose k_c most *certain* slices for each class among images where corresponding class label exists, creating a "most" *certain* set S_c^j for every class j.

As an effort to further reduce the kept training data, we aim to select a *representative* subset of S_c^j. Similarly to [6], we use spatially averaged activations at the *abstraction-layer* (c.f. Fig. 1) of our network to represent a given image as a vector I_{abs}^R. In an iterative fashion, we then create a *representative* set $S_r^j \subseteq S_c^j$ with k_r elements for each class j in order to maximize set coverage [11] over the full training set S_a, using cosine similarity between each I_{abs}^R. We call this method Abstraction exemplar-based incremental Segmentation (AeiSeg). Although one can use a faster method to pick samples for the set S_r^j, the iterative set coverage approach ensures maximum set coverage even if in future some of the later picked exemplar samples need to be removed; i.e., storage constraints.

Maximum Set Coverage over Content Distance: Albeit being a fast proposition, similarity across spatially averaged activations [6] at *abstraction-layer* have questionable image representation capability, as no objective function directly optimizes for *image representation*. Instead, we use the activations of a pre-trained VGG network at multiple layer levels to describe "content" of an input image, which is inspired by [12]. A VGG network trained on ImageNet [13] has convolutional filters tuned for object recognition and localization task. Hence, its layer responses aim to distinctively represent objects present in a given image invariant to their spatial location. Based on this, a distance metric defined over the activations of such a network can give an accurate relative quantification of any two images from a dataset. Let $R^{l,f}(I_i) \in \mathcal{R}^{w_l, h_l}$ be the activation response of a VGG16 network at layer l, filter f, width w_l and height h_l at the corresponding layer for a given image I_i. We compute the *content distance*

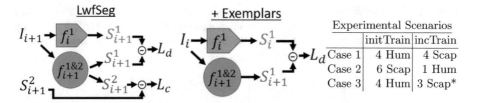

Fig. 2. Learning an incremental network $f_{i+1}^{1\&2}$ for classes 1&2 with new images I_{i+1} and annotations of new structures S_{i+1}^2, given a pre-trained and frozen network f_i^1. Left: representation of LwfSeg. Middle: additional loss in AeiSeg and CoRiSeg for augmenting the new network (left) with exemplar images I_i. Right: experimental scenarios depicting initial (init) and incremental (inc) datasets for humerus (Hum) and scapula (Scap). Case 3 incTrain (*) was conducted on a different MR sequence (water-saturated Dixon).

$$d_{\text{cont}} = \sum_{l \in L, f \in F_l} (R^{l,f}(I_i) - R^{l,f}(I_j))^2 \tag{3}$$

as the mean squared distance between activation responses of two images I_i and I_j, where L and F_l are the sets of all convolutional layers and their respective filters of the trained VGG network. We call this method Content Representativeness-based incremental Segmentation (CoRiSeg).

3   Experiments and Results

Our experimental dataset consists of 9 Dixon sequences of left shoulder collected with 1.5 T at resolution of 0.91 mm × 0.91 mm × 3 mm, corresponding to 192 × 192 × 64 voxel resolution. Humerus and scapula bones were annotated by an expert. Our goal is to combine knowledge from different data for a network that can segment both anatomical structures. We evaluated our proposed method for the three scenarios shown in the table in Fig. 2. One volume each was fixed randomly for validation and testing each of all scenarios. The first scenario (Case 1) tests a typical setting where different anatomies were of interest and thus annotated in separate studies. The second scenario (Case 2) aims to observe advantages of incremental training with minimal effort, i.e., incrementally annotated data, giving insight on an extreme case where a single volume annotation is provided. The last scenario (Case 3) studies the feasibility of combining learned segmentation information from different anatomy and images of different contrast. The methods were implemented with Tensorflow [14] and ran on an Nvidia Titan X GPU. Proposed network is implemented in 2D, hence 64 image samples per volume given in Fig. 2. For a fair comparison, we fixed all parameters across different models to $k_c = 50$, $k_r = 30$, $\alpha = 0.5$, $t_{\text{MC}} = 29$, batch size of 8 images, and trained all models for 1000 epochs. Used network (cf. Fig. 1) has a first convolutional layer with 64 filters and the amount of filters double at every coarsening level. Each convolutional layer is proceeded with

Table 1. Dice coefficient [%] and average symmetric surface distance (SurfDist) [mm] of networks trained only for humerus (HumSeg) and scapula (ScapSeg), finetuning, and our proposed incremental learning methods (cf. table in Fig. 2). Best scores of incremental methods are shown in bold.

	Method	Case 1 Dice hum scap	Case 1 SurfDist hum scap	Case 2 Dice scap hum	Case 2 SurfDist scap hum	Case 3 Dice hum scap	Case 3 SurfDist hum scap
Upper-bound	HumSeg	96.7 -	0.36 -	82.9	- 5.38	96.7 -	0.36 -
Upper-bound	ScapSeg	- 88.1	- 0.67	88.5 -	0.66 -	- 84.6	- 0.93
Baseline	finetuned	0.1 86.2	41.22 1.08	13.4 79.8	16.41 7.54	0.0 **83.8**	65.93 **1.21**
Proposed	LwfSeg	95.9 **87.5**	**0.88** **1.51**	73.2 87.3	6.08 **7.12**	66.0 79.1	13.32 2.86
Proposed	AeiSeg	96.1 82.9	1.31 2.27	74.8 63.5	7.09 36.52	94.2 76.7	2.68 3.20
Proposed	CoRiSeg	**96.3** 82.8	0.89 2.30	**78.7** **90.2**	**5.38** 13.51	**94.8** 78.7	**1.56** 2.03

a batch normalization and ReLU activation. For CoRiSeg, we use a VGG16 network [7] pre-trained on ImageNet [13]. While a VGG trained on a medical image set would be expected to provide more accurate d_{cont} score, training set of ImageNet is not matchable by any annotated medical database. We used Dice similarity coefficient and average symmetric surface distance for evaluating segmentation performance across tested methods (cf. Table 1). We compared our proposed methods: LwfSeg with its extensions with exemplar sets AeiSeg and CoRiSeg. Upper bound cases are presented with networks trained on only a given anatomy/dataset, i.e., without any incremental learning and hence without the need to preserve "old" (extra) information. We also show results from finetuning for comparison, although catastrophic forgetting is a known problem. In Fig. 3, we showcase qualitative results from different scenarios (cf. table in Fig. 2).

4   Discussions

As seen, with finetuning, the shared network body gets re-tuned to adapt to the new incremental data, almost completely forgetting the initial classes. Proposed segmentation extension of learning without forgetting (LwfSeg) performs relatively well in all cases. For every scenario, both proposed methods using exemplar sets either outperform or achieve performance as close to LwfSeg for the old class. CoRiSeg achieves the highest Dice score for the old data, suggesting that for selecting exemplars the maximum set coverage over content distance is more effective than averaging at abstraction-layer (AeiSeg). In addition, in Case 2, where the incremental dataset is severely handicapped, both LwfSeg and CoRiSeg surprisingly outperform HumSeg. While it is expected for a network trained on 1 volume (64 images) to perform poorly, incremental networks are seen to achieve higher segmentation performance, suggesting that shared-body layers potentially learned to extract *bone-generic knowledge*. Should this be shown for a wider range of bone structures, it would be critically relevant for orthopedic applications in the future. When the incremental

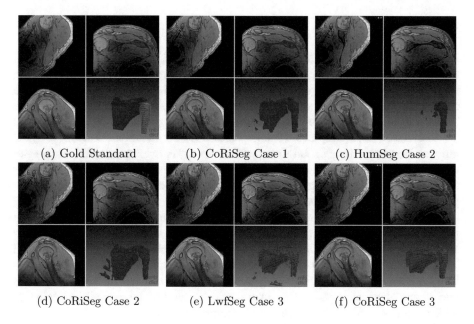

(a) Gold Standard   (b) CoRiSeg Case 1   (c) HumSeg Case 2

(d) CoRiSeg Case 2   (e) LwfSeg Case 3   (f) CoRiSeg Case 3

Fig. 3. Segmentation of the test volume with different methods.

dataset is introduced from a different imaging sequence in Case 3, one can see the great advantage of keeping exemplar samples; i.e., 28.8% increase in Dice score of CoRiSeg compared to LwfSeg. While the performance difference is less obvious for the new class, the change in old class scores suggests distillation loss to have provided false "guidance" on the new dataset with LwfSeg, i.e. trying to retain old class segmentation performance without any exemplar samples. Since finetuning does not need to remember the appearance of humerus (bone) in the other image modality, it outperforms with scapula in Case 3. We expected VGG trained for object classification (on ImageNet) to select better exemplar images for our task. Indeed, compared to CoRiSeg, using the UNet trained by us for d_{cont} yielded 1.6%, 0.7%, and 0.07% worse Dice, respectively, for each Case.

Note the high average symmetric surface distance in some of the proposed incremental methods, i.e., AeiSeg and CoRiSeg in Case 2; LwfSeg in Case 3. These are due to small blobs of false positives far from the target anatomy (cf. Fig. 3). These blobs could possibly be removed with a trivial post processing step (e.g. morphological operations, largest connected region, conditional random fields, user input), which is beyond the objective of this paper. Additional randomized hold-out test sets for Case 3 showed little variation ($\approx$2% Dice) in results, while the proposed AeiSeg and CoRiSeg were still over 27% Dice better than LwfSeg in retaining old class info. We will conduct extensive evaluations in future.

5   Conclusions

In this work, we have proposed a solution for applying class-incremental learning to *segmentation* using a distillation objective function (LwfSeg). However, with increasing size of labels and variability in medical images, we have shown that LwfSeg may become suboptimal without an exemplar dataset. To address this, we have proposed two novel methods to select *representative* images based on abstraction layer response (AeiSeg) and content distance (CoRiSeg); which imposes no restrictions on the incremental data size or #classes. We have evaluated the proposed frameworks on three different scenarios that often exist in medical image analysis community and shown that the proposed methods achieve performance similar to the upper-bound conditions. LwfSeg showed promising efficiency in retaining old class segmentation performance, which was improved further with proposed extensions with exemplar selections. To the best of our knowledge, this work is the first to show class-incremental learning in medical image segmentation (LwfSeg), and its extensions with intelligent exemplar selection (AeiSeg & CoRiSeg), CoRiSeg being our favorite with its intuitive design and higher performance. In the future, we will extend incremental training to additional anatomical structures and imaging modalities.

Acknowledgements. Funded by the Swiss National Science Foundation (SNSF) and a Highly-Specialized Medicine grant of the Canton of Zurich.

References

1. Hinton, G., Vinyals, O., Dean, J.: Distilling the knowledge in a neural network. In: NIPS Deep Learning and Representation Learning Workshop (2015). arXiv:1503.02531
2. Li, Z., Hoiem, D.: Learning without forgetting. IEEE Trans. Pattern Anal. Mach. Intell., 1 (2017). https://doi.org/10.1109/TPAMI.2017.2773081
3. Girshick, R., Donahue, J., Darrell, T., Malik, J.: Rich feature hierarchies for accurate object detection and semantic segmentation. In: Proceedings of the IEEE Conference on Computer Vision and Pattern Recognition (CVPR) (2014)
4. McCloskey, M., Cohen, N.J.: Catastrophic interference in connectionist networks: the sequential learning problem. Psychol. Learn. Motiv. **24**, 109–165 (1989). https://doi.org/10.1016/S0079-7421(08)60536-8
5. Rebuffi, S., Kolesnikov, A., Sperl, G., Lampert, C.H.: iCaRL: incremental classifier and representation learning. In: 2017 IEEE Conference on Computer Vision and Pattern Recognition (CVPR), pp. 5533–5542 (2017). https://doi.org/10.1109/CVPR.2017.587
6. Yang, L., Zhang, Y., Chen, J., Zhang, S., Chen, D.Z.: Suggestive annotation: a deep active learning framework for biomedical image segmentation. In: Descoteaux, M., Maier-Hein, L., Franz, A., Jannin, P., Collins, D.L., Duchesne, S. (eds.) MICCAI 2017. LNCS, vol. 10435, pp. 399–407. Springer, Cham (2017). https://doi.org/10.1007/978-3-319-66179-7_46
7. Simonyan, K., Zisserman, A.: Very deep convolutional networks for large-scale image recognition. arXiv e-prints arXiv:1409.1556v6 (2014)

8. Ronneberger, O., Fischer, P., Brox, T.: U-net: convolutional networks for biomedical image segmentation. In: Navab, N., Hornegger, J., Wells, W.M., Frangi, A.F. (eds.) MICCAI 2015. LNCS, vol. 9351, pp. 234–241. Springer, Cham (2015). https://doi.org/10.1007/978-3-319-24574-4_28

9. Haeusser, P., Mordvintsev, A., Cremers, D.: Learning by association - a versatile semi-supervised training method for neural networks. In: 2017 IEEE Conference on Computer Vision and Pattern Recognition (CVPR), pp. 626-635 (2017). https://doi.org/10.1109/CVPR.2017.74

10. Gal, Y., Ghahramani, Z.: Dropout as a Bayesian approximation: representing model uncertainty in deep learning. In: International Conference on Machine Learning (ICML), pp. 1050–1059 (2016)

11. Hochbaum, D.S.: Approximating covering and packing problems: set cover, vertex cover, independent set, and related problems. In: Approximation Algorithms for NP-Hard Problems, pp. 94–143. PWS Publishing Co., Boston (1997). http://dl.acm.org/citation.cfm?id=241938.241941

12. Gatys, L.A., Ecker, A.S., Bethge, M.: Image style transfer using convolutional neural networks. In: 2016 IEEE CVPR, pp. 2414–2423 (2016). https://doi.org/10.1109/CVPR.2016.265

13. Russakovsky, O., Deng, J., Su, H., Krause, J., et al.: ImageNet large scale visual recognition challenge. Int. J. Comput. Vis. **115**(3), 211–252 (2015). https://doi.org/10.1007/s11263-015-0816-y

14. Abadi, M., Agarwal, A., Barham, P., Brevdo, E., et al.: TensorFlow: large-scale machine learning on heterogeneous systems (2015)

ASDNet: Attention Based Semi-supervised Deep Networks for Medical Image Segmentation

Dong Nie[1,2], Yaozong Gao[3], Li Wang[2], and Dinggang Shen[2(✉)]

[1] Department of Computer Science, University of North Carolina at Chapel Hill,
Chapel Hill, USA
[2] Department of Radiology and BRIC, University of North Carolina at Chapel Hill,
Chapel Hill, USA
dgshen@med.unc.edu
[3] Shanghai United Imaging Intelligence Co., Ltd., Shanghai, China

Abstract. Segmentation is a key step for various medical image analysis tasks. Recently, deep neural networks could provide promising solutions for automatic image segmentation. The network training usually involves a large scale of training data with corresponding ground truth label maps. However, it is very challenging to obtain the ground-truth label maps due to the requirement of expertise knowledge and also intensive labor work. To address such challenges, we propose a novel semi-supervised deep learning framework, called "Attention based Semi-supervised Deep Networks" (ASDNet), to fulfill the segmentation tasks in an end-to-end fashion. Specifically, we propose a fully convolutional confidence network to adversarially train the segmentation network. Based on the confidence map from the confidence network, we then propose a region-attention based semi-supervised learning strategy to include the unlabeled data for training. Besides, sample attention mechanism is also explored to improve the network training. Experimental results on real clinical datasets show that our ASDNet can achieve state-of-the-art segmentation accuracy. Further analysis also indicates that our proposed network components contribute most to the improvement of performance.

1 Introduction

Recent development of deep learning has largely boosted the state-of-the-art segmentation methods [8,11]. Among them, fully convolutional networks (FCN) [8], a variant of convolutional neural networks (CNN), is a recent popular choice for semantic image segmentation in both computer vision and medical image fields [8,11,13]. FCN trains neural networks in an end-to-end fashion by directly

D. Shen—This work was supported by the National Institutes of Health grant 1R01 CA140413.

A. F. Frangi et al. (Eds.): MICCAI 2018, LNCS 11073, pp. 370–378, 2018.
https://doi.org/10.1007/978-3-030-00937-3_43

optimizing intermediate feature layers for segmentation, which makes it outperform the traditional methods that often regard the feature learning and segmentation as two separate tasks. UNet [11], an evolutionary variant of FCN, has achieved excellent performance by effectively combining high-level and low-level features in the network architecture. Generally, while being effective, the training of FCN (or UNet) requires a large amount of labeled data as there are millions of parameters in the network to be optimized. However, it is difficult to acquire a large training set with manually labeled ground-truth maps due to the following three factors: (a) manual annotation requires expertise knowledge; (b) it is time-consuming and tedious to annotate pixel-wise (voxel-wise) label maps; (c) it suffers from large intra- and inter-observer variability.

Several works have been done to address the aforementioned challenges [1, 2, 6]. To relieve the demand for large-scale labeled data, Bai et al. [1] proposed a semi-supervised deep learning framework for cardiac MR image segmentation, in which the segmented label maps from unlabeled data are incrementally included into the training set to refine the network. Baur et al. [2] introduced auxiliary manifold embedding in the latent space to FCN for semi-supervised learning in the MS lesion segmentation. In both cases, the unlabeled data information are fully involved in the model learning. However, certain regions of the unlabeled data may not be suitable for the learning due to their low-quality (automatically-) segmented label maps. To overcome such issues, we propose an attention based semi-supervised learning framework for medical image segmentation. Our framework is composed of two networks: (1) segmentation network and (2) confidence network. Specifically, we propose a fully convolutional adversarial learning scheme (i.e., using confidence network) to better train the segmentation network. The confidence map generated by the confidence network can provide us the trustworthy regions in the segmented label map from the segmentation network. Based on the confidence map, we further propose a region based semi-supervised loss to adaptively use part of unlabeled data for training the network. Since we can adopt unlabeled data to further train the segmentation network, the need of a large-scale training set can be alleviated accordingly. Our proposed algorithm has been applied to the task of pelvic organ segmentation, which is critical for guiding both biopsy and cancer radiation therapy. Experimental results indicate that our proposed algorithm can improve the segmentation accuracy, compared to other state-of-the-art methods. In addition, our proposed training strategies are also proved to be effective.

2 Method

As mentioned above, the proposed ASDNet consists of two subnetworks, i.e., (1) segmentation network (denoted as S) and (2) confidence network (denoted as D). The architecture of our proposed framework is presented in Fig. 1.

To ease the description of the proposed algorithm, we first give the notations used throughout the paper. Given a labeled input image $\mathbf{X} \in R^{H \times W \times T}$ with corresponding ground-truth label map $\mathbf{Y} \in Z^{H \times W \times T}$, we encode it to one-hot format $\mathbf{P} \in R^{H \times W \times T \times C}$, where C is the number of semantic categories in the dataset. The segmentation network outputs the class probability map $\widehat{\mathbf{P}} \in R^{H \times W \times T \times C}$. Similarly, we regard an unlabeled image as $\mathbf{U} \in R^{H \times W \times T}$. Therefore, the whole input image dataset can be defined by $\mathbf{O} = \{\mathbf{X}, \mathbf{U}\}$.

2.1 Segmentation Network with Sample Attention

In ASDNet as shown in Fig. 1, the segmentation network can be any end-to-end segmentation network, such as FCN [8], UNet [11], VNet [9], and DSRe-sUNet [13]. In this paper, we adopt a simplified VNet [9] (internal pool-conv-deconv layers are removed, and thus is denoted as SVNet) as the segmentation network to balance the performance and memory cost.

Multi-class Dice Loss: The class imbalance problem is usually serious in medical image segmentation tasks. To overcome it, we propose using a generalized multi-class Dice loss [12] as the segmentation loss, as defined below in Eq. 1:

$$
L_{Dice}\left(\mathbf{X}, \mathbf{P}; \theta_{\mathbf{s}}\right) = 1 - 2 \frac{\sum\limits_{c=1}^{C} \pi_c \sum\limits_{h=1}^{H} \sum\limits_{w=1}^{W} \sum\limits_{t=1}^{T} P_{h,w,t,c} \widehat{P}_{h,w,t,c}}{\sum\limits_{c=1}^{C} \pi_c \sum\limits_{h=1}^{H} \sum\limits_{w=1}^{W} \sum\limits_{t=1}^{T} P_{h,w,t,c} + \widehat{P}_{h,w,t,c}}, \tag{1}
$$

where π_c is the class balancing weight of category c, $\theta_{\mathbf{S}}$ is the parameters of segmentation network, and we set $\pi_c = 1/\left(\sum\limits_{h=1}^{H} \sum\limits_{w=1}^{W} \sum\limits_{t=1}^{T} P_{h,w,t,c}\right)^2$. $\widehat{\mathbf{P}}$ is the predicted probability maps from the segmentation network: $\widehat{\mathbf{P}} = S\left(\mathbf{X}, \theta_{\mathbf{s}}\right)$.

Multi-class Dice Loss with Sample Attention: Besides the class imbalance problem, the network optimization also suffers from the issue of dominance by easy samples: the large number of easy samples will dominate network training, thus the difficult samples cannot be well considered. To address this issue,

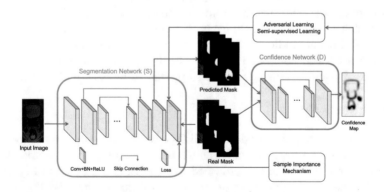

Fig. 1. Illustration of the architecture of our proposed ASDNet, which consists of a segmentation network and a confidence network.

inspired by the focal loss [6] proposed to handle similar issue in detection networks, we propose a sample attention based mechanism to consider the importance of each sample during the training. The multi-class Dice loss with sample attention is thus defined below by Eq. 2:

$$
L_{AttDice}\left(\mathbf{X}, \mathbf{P}; \theta_{\mathbf{s}}\right) = (1 - dsc)^{\beta} \left(1 - 2 \frac{\sum_{c=1}^{C} \pi_c \sum_{h=1}^{H} \sum_{w=1}^{W} \sum_{t=1}^{T} P_{h,w,t,c} \widehat{P}_{h,w,t,c}}{\sum_{c=1}^{C} \pi_c \sum_{h=1}^{H} \sum_{w=1}^{W} \sum_{t=1}^{T} P_{h,w,t,c} + \widehat{P}_{h,w,t,c}} \right),
$$

$$(2)$$

where dsc is the average Dice similarity coefficient of the sample over different categories, e.g., different organ labels. Note that we re-compute the dsc in each iteration, but we don't back-propagate gradient through it when training the networks. β is the sample attention parameter with a range of $[0, 5]$. Following [6], we set β to 2 in this paper.

2.2 Confidence Network for Fully Convolutional Adversarial Learning

Adversarial learning is derived from the recent popular Generative Adversarial Network (GAN) [3]. It has achieved a great success in image generation and segmentation [3,5,10]. Hence, we also incorporate adversarial learning in our architecture to further improve the segmentation network. Instead of using CNN-based discriminator, we propose to use FCN-based discriminator to generate local confidence at local region.

Adversarial Loss of the Confidence Network: The training objective of the confidence network is the summation of binary cross-entropy loss over the image domain, as shown in Eq. 3. Here, we use S and D to denote the segmentation and confidence networks, respectively.

$$
L_D(\mathbf{X}, \mathbf{P}; \theta_{\mathbf{d}}) = L_{BCE}(D(\mathbf{P}, \theta_{\mathbf{d}}), \mathbf{1}) + L_{BCE}(D(S(\mathbf{X}), \theta_{\mathbf{d}}), \mathbf{0}), \tag{3}
$$

where

$$
L_{BCE}\left(\widehat{\mathbf{Q}}, \mathbf{Q}\right) = -\sum_{h=1}^{H} \sum_{w=1}^{W} \sum_{t=1}^{T} Q_{h,w,t} \log\left(\widehat{Q}_{h,w,t}\right) + (1 - Q_{h,w,t}) \log\left(1 - \widehat{Q}_{h,w,t}\right)
$$

$$(4)$$

where $\mathbf{X}$ and $\mathbf{P}$ represent the input data and its corresponding manual label map (one-hot encoding format), respectively. $\theta_{\mathbf{d}}$ is network parameters for the confidence network.

Adversarial Loss of the Segmentation Network: For segmentation network, besides the multi-class Dice loss with sample attention as defined in Eq. 2, there is another loss from D working as "variational" loss. It enforces higher-order consistency between ground-truth segmentation and automatic segmentation. In particular, the adversarial loss ("ADV") to improve S and fool D can be defined by Eq. 5.

$$L_{ADV}\left(\mathbf{O}, \theta_{\mathbf{s}}\right) = L_{BCE}\left(D\left(S\left(\mathbf{O}; \theta_{\mathbf{s}}\right)\right), \mathbf{1}\right) \tag{5}$$

2.3   Region-Attention Based Semi-supervised Learning

Since our discriminator (i.e., confidence network) could provide local confidence information over the image domain, we use such information in the semi-supervised setting to include unlabeled data for improving segmentation accuracy, and the similar strategy has been explored in [5].

Specifically, given an unlabeled image $\mathbf{U}$, the segmentation network will first produce the probability map $\widehat{\mathbf{P}} = S\left(\mathbf{U}\right)$, which will be then used by the trained confidence network to generate a confidence map $\mathbf{M} = D(\widehat{\mathbf{P}})$, indicating where the confident regions of the prediction results are close enough to the ground truth label distribution. The confident regions can be easily obtained by setting a threshold (i.e., γ) to the confidence map. In this way, we can use these confident regions as masks to select parts of unlabeled data and their segmentation results to enrich the set of supervised training data. Thus, our proposed semi-supervised loss can be defined by Eq. 6.

$$L_{semi}\left(\mathbf{U}, \theta_{\mathbf{s}}\right) = 1 - 2\frac{\sum\limits_{c=1}^{C}\pi_c\sum\limits_{h=1}^{H}\sum\limits_{w=1}^{W}\sum\limits_{t=1}^{T}[\mathbf{M}>\gamma]_{h,w,t}\overline{P}_{h,w,t,c}\widehat{P}_{h,w,t,c}}{\sum\limits_{c=1}^{C}\pi_c\sum\limits_{h=1}^{H}\sum\limits_{w=1}^{W}\sum\limits_{t=1}^{T}[\mathbf{M}>\gamma]_{h,w,t}\left(\overline{P}_{h,w,t,c}+\widehat{P}_{h,w,t,c}\right)} \tag{6}$$

where $\overline{\mathbf{P}}$ is the one-hot encoding of $\widehat{\mathbf{Y}}$, and $\widehat{\mathbf{Y}} = \arg\max(\widehat{\mathbf{P}})$. [] is the indicator function. Similar to dsc in Eq. 2, $\overline{\mathbf{P}}$ and the value of indicator function are recomputed in each iteration.

Total Loss for Segmentation Network: By summing the above losses, the total loss to train the segmentation network can be defined by Eq. 7.

$$L_S = L_{AttDice} + \lambda_1 L_{ADV} + \lambda_2 L_{semi}, \tag{7}$$

where λ_1 and λ_2 are the scaling factors to balance the losses. They are selected at 0.03 and 0.3 after trails, respectively.

2.4   Implementation Details

Pytorch[1] is adopted to implement our proposed ASDNet shown in Fig. 1. We adopt Adam algorithm to optimize the network. The input size of the segmentation network is $64 \times 64 \times 16$. The network weights are initialized by the Xavier algorithm, and weight decay is set to be 1e–4. For the network biases, we initialize them to 0. The learning rates for the segmentation and confidence network are initialized to 1e–3 and 1e–4, followed by decreasing the learning rate 10 times every 3 epochs. Four Titan X GPUs are utilized to train the networks.

---

[1] https://github.com/pytorch/pytorch.

3   Experiments and Results

Our pelvic dataset consists of 50 prostate cancer patients from a cancer hospital, each with one T2-weighted MR image and corresponding manually-annotated label map by medical experts. In particular, the prostate, bladder and rectum in all these MRI scans have been manually segmented, which serve as the ground truth for evaluating our segmentation method. Besides, we have also acquired 20 MR images from additional 20 patients, without manually-annotated label maps. All these images were acquired with 3T MRI scanners. The image size is mostly $256 \times 256 \times (120-176)$, and the voxel size is $1 \times 1 \times 1$ mm^3.

Five-fold cross validation is used to evaluate our method. Specifically, in each fold of cross validation, we randomly chose 35 subjects as training set, 5 subjects as validation set, and the remaining 10 subjects as testing set. We use sliding windows to go through the whole MRI for prediction for a testing subject. Unless explicitly mentioned, all the reported performance by default is evaluated on the testing set. As for evaluation metrics, we utilize Dice Similarity Coefficient (DSC) and Average Surface Distance (ASD) to measure the agreement between the manually and automatically segmented label maps.

3.1   Comparison with State-of-the-art Methods

To demonstrate the advantage of our proposed method, we also compare our method with other five widely-used methods on the same dataset as shown in Table 1: (1) multi-atlas label fusion (MALF), (2) SSAE [4], (3) UNet [11], (4) VNet [9], and (5) DSResUNet [13]. Also, we present the performance of our proposed ASDNet.

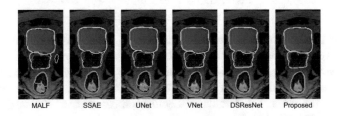

MALF   SSAE   UNet   VNet   DSResNet   Proposed

Fig. 2. Pelvic organ segmentation results of a typical subject by different methods. Orange, silver and pink contours indicate the manual ground-truth segmentation, and yellow, red and cyan contours indicate automatic segmentation.

Table 1 quantitatively compares our method with the five state-of-the-art segmentation methods. We can see that our method achieves better accuracy than the five state-of-the-art methods in terms of both DSC and ASD. The VNet works well in segmenting bladder and prostate, but it cannot work very well for rectum (which is often more challenging to segment due to the long and narrow shape). Compared to UNet, DSResUNet improves the accuracy by a large

Table 1. DSC and ASD on the pelvic dataset by different methods.

Method	DSC			ASD		
	Bladder	Prostate	Rectum	Bladder	Prostate	Rectum
MALF	.867(.068)	.793(.087)	.764(.119)	1.641(.360)	2.791(.930)	3.210(2.112)
SSAE	.918(.031)	.871(.042)	.863(.044)	1.089(.231)	1.660(.490)	1.701(.412)
UNet	.896(.028)	.822(.059)	.810(.053)	1.214(.216)	1.917(.645)	2.186(0.850)
VNet	.926(.018)	.864(.036)	.832(.041)	1.023(.186)	1.725(.457)	1.969(.449)
DSResUNet	.944(.009)	.882(.020)	.869(.032)	.914(.168)	1.586(.358)	1.586(.405)
Proposed	**.970(.006)**	**.911(.016)**	**.906(.026)**	**.858(.144)**	**1.316(.288)**	**1.401(.356)**

margin, indicating that residual learning and deep supervision bring performance gain, and thus it might be a good future direction for us to further improve our proposed method. We also visualize some typical segmentation results in Fig. 2, which further show the superiority of our proposed method.

3.2   Impact of Each Proposed Component

As our proposed method consists of several designed components, we conduct empirical studies below to analyze them.

Impact of Sample Attention: As mentioned in Sect. 2.1, we propose a sample attention mechanism to assign different importance for different samples so that the network can concentrate on hard-to-segment examples and thus avoid dominance by easy-to-segment samples. The effectiveness of sample attention mechanism (i.e., AttSVNet) is further confirmed by the improved performance, e.g., 0.82%, 1.60% and 1.81% DSC performance improvements (as shown in Table 2) for bladder, prostate and rectum, respectively.

Impact of Fully Convolutional Adversarial Learning: We conduct more experiments for comparing with the following three networks: (1) only segmentation network; (2) segmentation network with a CNN-based discriminator [3]; (3) segmentation network with a FCN-based discriminator (i.e., confidence network). Performance in the middle of Table 2 indicates that adversarial learning contributes a little bit to improving the results as it provides a regularization to prevent overfitting. Compared with CNN-based adversarial learning, our proposed FCN-based adversarial learning further improves the performances by 0.90% in average. This demonstrates that fully convolutional adversarial learning works better than the typical adversarial learning with a CNN-based discriminator, which means the FCN-based adversarial learning can better learn structural information from the distribution of ground-truth label map.

Impact of Semi-supervised Loss: We apply the semi-supervised learning strategy with our proposed ASDNet on 50 labeled MRI and 20 extra unlabeled MRI. The comparison methods are semiFCN [1] and semiEmbedFCN [2]. We use the AttSVNet as the basic architecture of these two methods for fair

Table 2. Comparison of the performance of methods with different strategies on the pelvic dataset in terms of DSC.

Method	Bladder	Prostate	Rectum
VNet	.926(.018)	.864(.036)	.832(.041)
SVNet	.920(.015)	.862(.037)	.844(.037)
AttSVNet	.931(.010)	.878(.028)	.862(.034)
AttSVNet+CNN	.938(.010)	.884(.026)	.874(.031)
AttSVNet+FCN	.944(.008)	.893(.022)	.887(.025)
semiFCN	.959(.006)	.895(.024)	.885(.030)
semiEmbedFCN	.964(.007)	.902(.022)	.891(.028)
AttSVNet+Semi	.937(.012)	.878(.036)	.865(.041)
Proposed	**.970(.006)**	**.911(.016)**	**.906(.026)**

comparison. The evaluation of the comparison experiments are all based on the labeled dataset, and the unlabeled data involves only in the learning phase. The experimental results in Table 2 show that our proposed semi-supervised strategy works better than the semiFCN and the semiEmbedFCN. Moreover, it is worth noting that the adversarial learning on the labeled data is important to our proposed semi-supervised scheme. If the segmentation network does not seek to fool the discriminator (i.e., AttSVNet+Semi), the confidence maps generated by the confidence network would not be meaningful.

3.3 Validation on Another Dataset

To show the generalization ability of our proposed algorithm, we conduct additional experiments on the PROMISE12-challenge dataset [7]. This dataset contains 50 subjects, each with a pair of MRI and its manual label map (where only prostate was annotated). Five-fold cross validation is performed to evaluate the performance of all comparison methods. Our proposed algorithm again achieves very good performance in segmenting prostate (i.e., 0.900 in terms of DSC), and it is also very competitive compared to the state-of-the-art methods applied to this dataset in the literature [9,13]. These experimental results indicate a good generalization capability of our proposed ASDNet.

4   Conclusions

In this paper, we have presented a novel attention-based semi-supervised deep network (ASDNet) to segment medical images. Specifically, the semi-supervised learning strategy is implemented by fully convolutional adversarial learning, and also region-attention based semi-supervised loss is adopted to effectively address the insufficient data problem for training the complex networks. By integrating these components into the framework, our proposed ASDNet has achieved significant improvement in terms of both accuracy and robustness.

References

1. Bai, W., et al.: Semi-supervised learning for network-based cardiac MR image segmentation. In: Descoteaux, M., et al. (eds.) MICCAI 2017. LNCS, vol. 10434, pp. 253–260. Springer, Cham (2017). https://doi.org/10.1007/978-3-319-66185-8_29
2. Baur, C., Albarqouni, S., Navab, N.: Semi-supervised deep learning for fully convolutional networks. In: Descoteaux, M. (ed.) MICCAI 2017. LNCS, vol. 10435, pp. 311–319. Springer, Cham (2017). https://doi.org/10.1007/978-3-319-66179-7_36
3. Goodfellow, I., et al.: Generative adversarial nets. In: NIPS (2014)
4. Guo, Y., et al.: Deformable MR prostate segmentation via deep feature learning and sparse patch matching. IEEE TMI **35**, 1077–1089 (2016)
5. Hung, W.-C., et al.: Adversarial learning for semi-supervised semantic segmentation. arXiv preprint arXiv:1802.07934 (2018)
6. Lin, T.-Y., et al.: Focal loss for dense object detection. arXiv preprint arXiv:1708.02002 (2017)
7. Litjens, G.: Evaluation of prostate segmentation algorithms for MRI: the PROMISE12 challenge. MedIA **18**(2), 359–373 (2014)
8. Long, J., et al.: Fully convolutional networks for semantic segmentation. In: CVPR, pp. 3431–3440 (2015)
9. Milletari, F., et al.: V-net: fully convolutional neural networks for volumetric medical image segmentation. In: 3DV, pp. 565–571. IEEE (2016)
10. Nie, D., et al.: Medical image synthesis with context-aware generative adversarial networks. In: Descoteaux, M., et al. (eds.) MICCAI 2017. LNCS, vol. 10435, pp. 417–425. Springer, Cham (2017). https://doi.org/10.1007/978-3-319-66179-7_48
11. Ronneberger, O., Fischer, P., Brox, T.: U-Net: convolutional networks for biomedical image segmentation. In: Navab, N., Hornegger, J., Wells, W.M., Frangi, A.F. (eds.) MICCAI 2015. LNCS, vol. 9351, pp. 234–241. Springer, Cham (2015). https://doi.org/10.1007/978-3-319-24574-4_28
12. Sudre, C.H., et al.: Generalised dice overlap as a deep learning loss function for highly unbalanced segmentations. DLMIA/ML-CDS -2017. LNCS, vol. 10553, pp. 240–248. Springer, Cham (2017). https://doi.org/10.1007/978-3-319-67558-9_28
13. Yu, L., et al.: Volumetric ConvNets with mixed residual connections for automated prostate segmentation from 3D MR images. In: AAAI (2017)

MS-Net: Mixed-Supervision Fully-Convolutional Networks for Full-Resolution Segmentation

Meet P. Shah[1], S. N. Merchant[1], and Suyash P. Awate[2(✉)]

[1] Electrical Engineering Department, Indian Institute of Technology (IIT) Bombay,
Mumbai, India
[2] Computer Science and Engineering Department,
Indian Institute of Technology (IIT) Bombay, Mumbai, India

Abstract. For image segmentation, typical fully convolutional networks (FCNs) need strong supervision through a large sample of high-quality dense segmentations, entailing high costs in expert-raters' time and effort. We propose *MS-Net*, a new FCN to significantly reduce supervision cost, and improve performance, by coupling strong supervision with *weak supervision* through low-cost input in the form of *bounding boxes* and *landmarks*. Our MS-Net enables *instance-level segmentation* at *high spatial resolution*, with feature extraction using *dilated convolutions*. We propose a new loss function using *bootstrapped Dice* overlap for precise segmentation. Results on large datasets show that MS-Net segments more accurately at reduced supervision costs, compared to the state of the art.

Keywords: Instance-level image segmentation
Fully convolutional networks · Weak supervision · Full resolution
Dice loss · Bootstrapped loss

1 Introduction and Related Work

Fully convolutional networks (FCNs) are important for segmentation through their ability to learn multiscale per-pixel features. Unlike FCNs for natural-image analysis, FCNs for medical image segmentation cannot always rely on transfer learning of parameters from networks (pre-)trained for natural-image analysis (VGG-16, ResNet). Thus, for medical image segmentation, training FCNs typically needs strong supervision through a *large number of high-quality dense segmentations*, with per-pixel labels, produced by radiologists or pathologists. However, generating high-quality segmentations is laborious and expensive. We propose a novel FCN, namely, *MS-Net*, to significantly reduce the cost (time and

Suyash P. Awate—Supported by: Nvidia GPU Grant Program, IIT Bombay Seed Grant 14IRCCSG010, Wadhwani Research Centre for Bioengineering (WRCB) IIT Bombay, Department of Biotechnology (DBT) Govt. of India BT/INF/22/SP23026/2017, iNDx Technology.

© Springer Nature Switzerland AG 2018
A. F. Frangi et al. (Eds.): MICCAI 2018, LNCS 11073, pp. 379–387, 2018.
https://doi.org/10.1007/978-3-030-00937-3_44

effort) of expert supervision, and significantly improve performance, by effectively enabling both high-quality/ strong and lower-quality/ *weak* supervision using training data comprising (i) low-cost coarse-level annotations for a majority of images and (ii) high-quality per-pixel labels for a minority of images.

Early convolutional neural networks (CNNs) for microscopy image segmentation [2] learn features from image patches to label the center-pixel in each patch. Later CNNs [1] use an autoencoder design to extract features from entire brain volumes for lesion segmentation. U-Net [11] localizes objects better by extending the symmetric-autoencoder design to combine high-resolution features from the encoding path with upsampled outputs in the decoding path. Also, U-Net training gives larger weights to misclassification at pre-computed pixel locations heuristically estimated to be close to object boundaries. Similarly, DCAN [4] explicitly adds an additional branch in its FCN to predict the pixel locations close to true object contours. V-Net [9] eliminates U-Net's heuristic weighting scheme through a loss function based on the Dice similarity coefficient (DSC) to handle a severe imbalance between the number of foreground and background voxels. These segmentation methods lead to reduced precision near object boundaries because of limited context (patches) [2], tiling [11], or subsampling [9]. All these methods rely *solely* on strong supervision via high-quality, but high-cost, dense segmentations. In contrast, our MS-Net also leverages *weak supervision* through low-cost input in the form of *bounding boxes* and *landmarks*. We improve V-Net's scheme of using DSC by continuously refocusing the learning on a subset of pixels with predicted class probabilities farthest from their true labels.

Instance segmentation methods like Mask R-CNN [5] simultaneously detect (via bounding boxes) and segment (via per-pixel labels) object instances. Mask R-CNN and other architectures [1,2,9,11] cannot preserve full spatial resolution in their feature maps, and are imprecise in localizing object boundaries. For segmenting street scenes, FRRN [10] combines multiscale context and pixel-level localization using two processing streams: one at full spatial resolution to precisely localize object boundaries and another for sequential feature-extraction and pooling to produce an embedding for accurate recognition. We improve over FRRN by leveraging (i) low-cost weak supervision through bounding-boxes and landmarks, (ii) a bootstrapped Dice (BADICE) based loss, and (iii) dilated convolutions to efficiently use larger spatial context for feature extraction.

We propose a novel FCN architecture for instance-level image segmentation at full resolution. We reduce the cost of expert supervision, and improve performance, by effectively coupling (i) strong supervision through dense segmentations with (ii) *weak supervision* through low-cost input via *bounding boxes* and *landmarks*. We propose the BADICE loss function using *bootstrapped DSC*, with feature extraction using *dilated convolutions*, geared for segmentation. Results on large openly available medical datasets show that our MS-Net segments more accurately with reduced supervision cost, compared to the state of the art.

2   Methods

We describe our MS-Net FCN incorporating (i) *mixed supervision* via dense segmentations, bounding boxes, and landmarks, and (ii) the BADICE loss function.

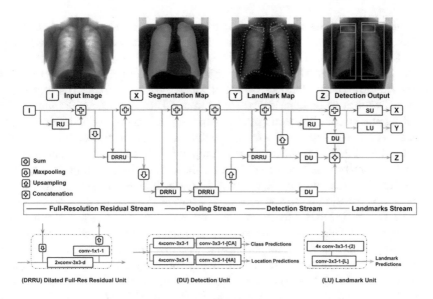

Fig. 1. Our MS-Net: Mixed-Supervision FCN for Full-Resolution Segmentation (abstract structure). We enable *mixed supervision* through a combination of:(i) high-quality *strong supervision* in the form of dense segmentation (per-pixel label) images, and (ii) low-cost *weak supervision* in the form of bounding boxes and landmarks. $N \times$ conv-KxK-D-(S)-[P] denotes: N sequential convolutional layers with kernels of spatial extent (K, K), dilation factor D, spatial stride S, and P output feature maps.

Architecture. Our MS-Net architecture (abstract structure in Fig. 1) has two types of components: (i) a *base network* for full-resolution feature extraction related to the FRRN [10] architecture and (ii) 3 task-specific subnetwork extensions: *segmentation unit* (SU), *landmark unit* (LU), and *detection unit* (DU).

The base network comprises two streams: (i) the *full-resolution residual stream* to determine precise object boundaries and (ii) the *pooling stream* to produce multiscale, robust, and discriminative features. The pooling stream comprises two main components: (i) the *residual unit* (RU) used in residual networks [6] and (ii) the *dilated full-resolution residual unit* (DRRU). The DRRU (Fig. 1) takes in two incoming streams and has an associated dilation factor. Features from each stream are first concatenated and then passed through two 3×3 dilated-convolutional layers, each followed by batch normalization and rectified linear unit (ReLU) activation. The resulting feature map, besides being passed on to the next DRRU, also serves as residual feedback to the full-resolution residual stream afterundergoing channel adjustment using a 1×1 convolutional layer and subsequent bilinear upsampling. We modify FRRN's B model (Table 1 in [10]) replacing their 9 groups of full-resolution residual units with an equal number of DRRUs with dilation factors of $[1, 1, 2, 2, 4, 2, 2, 1]$. The dilated convolutions lend our MS-Net features a larger spatial context to prevent segmentation errors like (i) holes within object regions, where local statistics are closer to the background, and (ii) poor segmentations near image boundaries.

Subnetwork extensions use the features extracted by the base network. The **SU** takes the extracted features into a 1×1 convolutional layer followed by a channel-wise softmax to output a full-resolution dense segmentation map.

The **LU** helps locate landmarks at object boundaries (in this paper) or within objects (in principle). Because LU's output is closely related SU's output, we design LU's input to be identical to SU's input. LU outputs L mask images, each indicating the spatial location (probabilistically) of one of the L landmarks. To do so, the extracted features are fed through four 3×3 convolutional layers with a spatial stride of 2. The resulting feature map is fed through a 1×1 convolutional layer with L output channels to obtain the landmark feature maps at $(1/16)$-th of the full image resolution. The pixel with the highest activation in the l-th feature map corresponds to the spatial location of the l-th landmark of interest.

Each **DU** uses DRRU features from different levels in the upsampling path of the pooling stream, to produce object locations, via bounding boxes, and their class predictions for C target classes. Each ground-truth box is represented by (i) a one-hot C-length vector indicating the true class and (ii) a 4-length vector parametrizing the true bounding-box coordinates. A DU uses a single-stage object-detection paradigm, similar to that used in [7]. For each level, at each pixel, the DU outputs $A := 9$ candidate bounding boxes, termed *anchor boxes* [7], as follows. The DU's class-prediction (respectively, location-prediction) subnetwork outputs a C-class probability vector (respectively, 4-length vector) for each of the A anchors. So, the DU passes a DRRU's T-channel output through four 3×3 convolutional layers, each with 256 filters, and a 3×3 convolutional layer with CA (respectively, $4A$) filters. To define the DU loss, we consider a subset of anchor boxes that are close to some ground-truth bounding box, with a Jaccard similarity coefficient (JSC) (same as intersection-over-union) >0.5. MS-Net training seeks to make this subset of anchor boxes close to their closest ground-truth bounding boxes. DUs share parameters when their inputs have the number of channels. We pool the class predictions and location predictions from DUs at all levels to get output Z (Fig. 1). During testing, Z indicates a final set of bounding boxes after thresholding the class probabilities.

Loss Functions for SU, LU, DU. Correct segmentations for some image regions are easy to get, e.g., regions far from object and image boundaries or regions without image artifacts. To get high-quality segmentations, training should *focus* more on the remaining pixels that are hard to segment. U-net [11] and DCAN [4] restrict focus to a subset of hard-to-segment pixels only

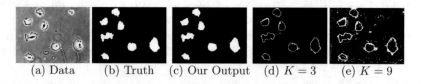

(a) Data   (b) Truth   (c) Our Output   (d) $K = 3$ (e) $K = 9$

Fig. 2. Our BADICE Loss. (a) Input. (b) Ground truth and (c) our segmentation. (d) Top 3% and (e) 9% pixels with class probabilities farthest from the truth.

at object boundaries, thereby failing to capture other hard-to-segment regions, e.g., near image boundaries and image artifacts. In contrast, we use bootstrapped loss, as in [12], by automatically identifying hard-to-segment pixels as the top K percentile with predicted class probabilities farthest from the ground truth; K is a free parameter; typically $K \in [3,9]$. For the **SU**, our BADICE loss is the mean, over C classes, negative DSC over the top-K pixel subset, where we use the differentiable-DSC between N-pixel probability maps P and Q as $2\sum_{n=1}^{N} P_n Q_n / (\sum_{n=1}^{N} P_n^2 + \sum_{n=1}^{N} Q_n^2)$. Indeed, the pixels selected by BADICE (Fig. 2) are near object boundaries as well as other hard-to-segment areas. We find that BADICE leads to faster convergence because the loss-function gradients focus on errors at hard-to-segment pixels and are more informative.

For the **LU**, the loss function, for the l-th landmark, is the cross-entropy between (i) the binary ground-truth mask (having a single non-zero pixel corresponding to the l-th landmark location) and (ii) a 2D probability map generated by a softmax over all pixels in the l-th channel of the LU output. The **DU** loss is the mean, over valid anchors, of the sum of (i) a cross-entropy based focal loss [7] on class predictions and (ii) a regularized-L_1 loss for bounding box coordinates.

Training. We minimize the sum of SU, LU, and DU losses using stochastic gradient descent, using checkpoint-based memory optimizations to process memory-intensive dilated convolutions at full-resolution. We use data augmentation through (i) random image resizing by factors $\in [0.85, 1.25]$ for all datasets and (ii) horizontal and vertical flipping, rotations within $[-25, 25]$ degrees, and elastic deformations for histopathology and microscopy data.

3   Results and Discussion

We evaluate 5 methods (free parameters tuned by cross-validation): (i) MS-Net with strong supervision only, via dense segmentation maps; (ii) MS-Net with strong supervision and weak supervision via bounding boxes only; (iii) MS-Net with strong supervision and weak supervision via bounding boxes and landmarks; (iv) U-Net [11]; (v) DCAN [4]. We evaluate all methods at different levels of strong supervision during training, where a fraction of the images have strong-supervision data and the rest have only weak-supervision data. We evaluate on 5 openly available medical datasets. We measure performance by the mean JSC (mJSC), over all classes, between the estimated and true label maps.

Radiographs: Chest. This dataset (Fig. 3(a)–(b)) has 247 high-resolution (2048^2) chest radiographs (db.jsrt.or.jp/eng.php), with expert segmentations and 166 landmark annotations for 5 anatomical structures (2 lungs, 2 clavicles, heart) [3]. We use the 50-50 training-testing split prescribed by [3]. Qualitatively (Fig. 3(c)–(e)), MS-Net trained with mixed supervision (Fig. 3(c)), i.e., strong supervision via dense label maps and weak supervision via bounding boxes and landmarks, gives segmentations that are much more precise near object boundaries compared to U-net (Fig. 3(d)) and DCAN (Fig. 3(e)) both trained using strong supervision only. Quantitatively (Fig. 4), at all levels of

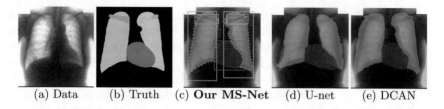

(a) Data   (b) Truth   (c) **Our MS-Net**   (d) U-net   (e) DCAN

Fig. 3. Radiographs: Chest. (a) Data. **(b)** True segmentation. **(c)–(e)** Outputs for networks trained using all strong-supervision and weak-supervision data available.

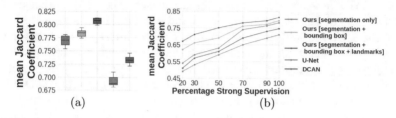

Fig. 4. Radiographs: Chest. (a) mJSC using all training data (strong + weak supervision). Box plots give variability over stochasticity in the optimization. **(b)** mJSC using different levels of strong supervision (remaining data with weak supervision).

strong supervision, (i) all 3 versions of MS-Net outperform U-net and DCAN, and (ii) MS-Net trained with mixed supervision outperforms MS-Net trained without weak supervision using landmarks or bounding boxes.

Histopathology: Gland. This dataset (Fig. 5(a)–(b)) has 85 training slides (37 benign, 48 malignant) and 80 testing slides (37 benign, 43 malignant) of intestinal glands in human colorectal cancer tissues (warwick.ac.uk/fac/sci/dcs/research/tia/glascontest) with dense segmentations. To create weak-supervision, we generate bounding boxes, but cannot easily generate landmarks. For this dataset, we use DSC and Hausdorff distance (HD) for evaluation, because other methods did this in glascontest. Qualitatively, compared to U-net and DCAN, our MS-Net produces segmentations with fewer false positives (Fig. 5(c)–(e); top left) and better labelling near gaps between spatially adjacent glands (Fig. 5(c)–(e); mid right). Quantitatively, at all strong-supervision levels, (i) MS-Net outperforms U-net and DCAN, and (ii) MS-Net trained with mixed supervision outperforms MS-Net without any weak supervision (Fig. 6).

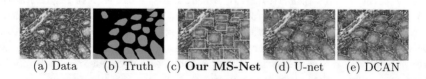

(a) Data   (b) Truth   (c) **Our MS-Net**   (d) U-net   (e) DCAN

Fig. 5. Histopathology: Gland. (a) Data. **(b)** True segmentation. **(c)–(e)** Outputs for networks trained using all strong-supervision and weak-supervision data available.

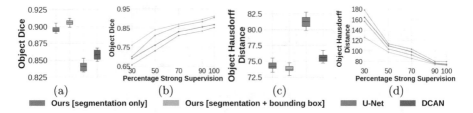

Fig. 6. Histopathology: Gland. (a), (c) mJSC and HD using all training data (strong + weak supervision). Box plots give variability over stochasticity in the optimization. **(b), (d)** mJSC and HD using different levels of strong supervision.

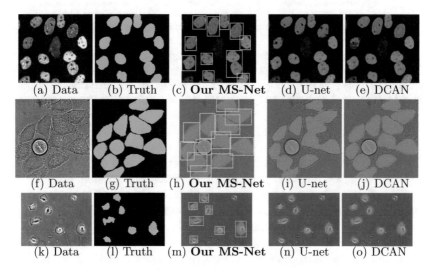

Fig. 7. Microscopy: Cells. (a), (f), (k) Data. **(b), (g), (l)** True segmentation. **(c)–(e), (h)–(j), (m)–(o)** Outputs for nets trained using all strong+weak-supervision data.

Microscopy: Cells. The next three datasets [8] (Fig. 7) have cell images acquired using 3 microscopy techniques: (i) fluorescent counterstaining: 43 images, (ii) phase contrast: 35 images, and (iii) differential interference contrast: 20 images. To evaluate weak-supervision, we generate bounding boxes, but cannot easily generate landmarks. We use a random 60-40% training-testing split. Similar to previous datasets, at all strong-supervision levels, our MS-Net outperforms U-net and DCAN qualitatively (Fig. 7) and quantitatively (Fig. 8). U-net and DCAN produces labels maps with holes within cell regions that appear to be similar to the background (Fig. 7(d)-(e)), while our MS-Net (Fig. 7(c)) avoids such errors via BADICE loss and larger-context features through dilated convolutions for multiscale regularity. MS-Net also clearly achieves better boundary localization (Fig. 7(h)), unlike U-net and DCAN that fail to preserve gaps between objects (loss of precision) (Fig. 7(i)–(j)).

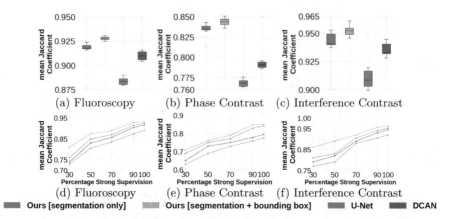

Fig. 8. Microscopy: Cells. mJSC using all training data (strong + weak supervision) for: **(a)** fluoroscopy, **(b)** phase-contrast, and **(c)** differential interference contrast datasets. Box plots give variability over stochasticity in the optimization and train-test splits. **(d)–(f)** mJSC with different levels of strong supervision for the same 3 datasets.

Conclusion. For full-resolution segmentation, we propose *MS-Net* that significantly improves segmentation accuracy and precision, and significantly reduces supervision cost, by effectively coupling (i) strong supervision with (ii) *weak supervision* through low-cost rater input in the form of *bounding boxes* and *landmarks*. We propose (i) BADICE loss using *bootstrapped DSC* to automatically focus learning on hard-to-segment regions and (ii) *dilated convolutions* for larger-context features. Results on 5 large medical open datasets clearly show MS-Net's better performance, even at reduced supervision costs, over the state of the art.

References

1. Brosch, T., Yoo, Y., Tang, L.Y.W., Li, D.K.B., Traboulsee, A., Tam, R.: Deep convolutional encoder networks for multiple sclerosis lesion segmentation. In: Navab, N., Hornegger, J., Wells, W.M., Frangi, A.F. (eds.) MICCAI 2015. LNCS, vol. 9351, pp. 3–11. Springer, Cham (2015). https://doi.org/10.1007/978-3-319-24574-4_1

2. Ciresan, D., Giusti, A., Schmidhuber, J.: Deep neural networks segment neuronal membranes in electron microscopy images. In: Advances in Neural Information Processing System, pp. 2843–2851 (2012)

3. Ginneken, B., Stegmann, M., Loog, M.: Segmentation of anatomical structures in chest radiographs using supervised methods: a comparative study on a public database. Med. Image Anal. **10**(1), 19–40 (2006)

4. Hao, C., Xiaojuan, Q., Lequan, Y., Pheng-Ann, H.: DCAN: deep contour-aware networks for accurate gland segmentation. In: IEEE Computer Vision Pattern Recognition, pp. 2487–2496 (2016)

5. He, K., Gkioxari, G., Dollár, P., Girshick, R.: Mask R-CNN. In: International Conference on Computer Vision, pp. 2980–2988 (2017)

6. He, K., Zhang, X., Ren, S., Sun, J.: Deep residual learning for image recognition. In: IEEE Computer Vision Pattern Recognition, pp. 770–778 (2016)

7. Lin, T., Goyal, P., Girshick, R., He, K., Dollár, P.: Focal loss for dense object detection. In: Intelligence Conference on Computer Vision (2017)

8. Martin, M., et al.: A benchmark for comparison of cell tracking algorithms. Bioinformatics **30**(11), 1609–1617 (2014)

9. Milletari, F., Navab, N., Ahmadi, S.: V-net: Fully convolutional neural networks for volumetric medical image segmentation. In: International Conference on 3D Vision, pp. 565–571 (2016)

10. Pohlen, P., Hermans, A., Mathias, M., Leibe, B.: Full-resolution residual networks for semantic segmentation in street scenes. In: IEEE Computer Vision Pattern Recognition, pp. 3309–3318 (2017)

11. Ronneberger, O., Fischer, P., Brox, T.: U-net: convolutional networks for biomedical image segmentation. In: Navab, N., Hornegger, J., Wells, W.M., Frangi, A.F. (eds.) MICCAI 2015. LNCS, vol. 9351, pp. 234–241. Springer, Cham (2015). https://doi.org/10.1007/978-3-319-24574-4_28

12. Wu, Z., Shen, C., Hengel, A.: Bridging category-level and instance-level semantic image segmentation (2016). arXiv preprint arXiv:1605.06885

How to Exploit Weaknesses in Biomedical Challenge Design and Organization

Annika Reinke[1]([✉]), Matthias Eisenmann[1], Sinan Onogur[1], Marko Stankovic[1], Patrick Scholz[1], Peter M. Full[1], Hrvoje Bogunovic[2], Bennett A. Landman[3], Oskar Maier[4], Bjoern Menze[5], Gregory C. Sharp[6], Korsuk Sirinukunwattana[7], Stefanie Speidel[8], Fons van der Sommen[9], Guoyan Zheng[10], Henning Müller[11], Michal Kozubek[12], Tal Arbel[13], Andrew P. Bradley[14], Pierre Jannin[15], Annette Kopp-Schneider[16], and Lena Maier-Hein[1]([✉])

[1] Division Computer Assisted Medical Interventions (CAMI), German Cancer Research Center (DKFZ), Heidelberg, Germany
{a.reinke,l.maier-hein}@dkfz.de
[2] Christian Doppler Laboratory for Ophthalmic Image Analysis, Department of Ophthalmology, Medical University Vienna, Vienna, Austria
[3] Electrical Engineering, Vanderbilt University, Nashville, TN, USA
[4] Institute Medical Informatics, University of Lübeck, Lübeck, Germany
[5] Institute Advanced Studies, Department of Informatics, Technical University of Munich, Munich, Germany
[6] Department Radiation Oncology, Massachusetts General Hospital, Boston, MA, USA
[7] Institute Biomedical Engineering, University of Oxford, Oxford, UK
[8] Division Translational Surgical Oncology (TCO), National Center for Tumor Diseases Dresden, Dresden, Germany
[9] Department Electrical Engineering, Eindhoven University of Technology, Eindhoven, The Netherlands
[10] Institute Surgical Technology and Biomechanics, University of Bern, Bern, Switzerland
[11] Information System Institute, HES-SO, Sierre, Switzerland
[12] Centre for Biomedical Image Analysis, Masaryk University, Brno, Czech Republic
[13] Department of Electrical and Computer Engineering, McGill University, Montreal, QC, Canada
[14] Science and Engineering Faculty, Queensland University of Technology, Brisbane, QLD, Australia
[15] Laboratoire du Traitement du Signal et de l'Image, INSERM, University of Rennes 1, Rennes, France
[16] Division Biostatistics, German Cancer Research Center (DKFZ), Heidelberg, Germany

Abstract. Since the first MICCAI grand challenge organized in 2007 in Brisbane, challenges have become an integral part of MICCAI conferences. In the meantime, challenge datasets have become widely recognized as international benchmarking datasets and thus have a great influ-

A. Reinke, M. Eisenmann, A. Kopp-Schneider and L. Maier-Hein—Shared first/ senior authors.

A. F. Frangi et al. (Eds.): MICCAI 2018, LNCS 11073, pp. 388–395, 2018.
https://doi.org/10.1007/978-3-030-00937-3_45

ence on the research community and individual careers. In this paper, we show several ways in which weaknesses related to current challenge design and organization can potentially be exploited. Our experimental analysis, based on MICCAI segmentation challenges organized in 2015, demonstrates that both challenge organizers and participants can potentially undertake measures to substantially tune rankings. To overcome these problems we present best practice recommendations for improving challenge design and organization.

1   Introduction

In many research fields, organizing challenges for international benchmarking has become increasingly common. Since the first MICCAI grand challenge was organized in 2007 [4], the impact of challenges on both the research field as well as on individual careers has been steadily growing. For example, the acceptance of a journal article today often depends on the performance of a new algorithm being assessed against the state-of-the-art work on publicly available challenge datasets. Yet, while the publication of papers in scientific journals and prestigious conferences, such as MICCAI, undergoes strict quality control, the design and organization of challenges do not. Given the discrepancy between challenge impact and quality control, the contributions of this paper can be summarized as follows:

1. Based on analysis of past MICCAI challenges, we show that current practice is heavily based on trust in challenge organizers and participants.
2. We experimentally show how "security holes" related to current challenge design and organization can be used to potentially manipulate rankings.
3. To overcome these problems, we propose best practice recommendations to remove opportunities for cheating.

2   Methods

Analysis of Common Practice: To review common practice in MICCAI challenge design, we systematically captured the publicly available information from publications and websites. Based on the data acquired, we generated descriptive statistics on the ranking scheme and several further aspects related to the challenge organization, with a particular focus on segmentation challenges.

Experiments on Rank Manipulation: While our analysis demonstrates the great impact of challenges on the field of biomedical image analysis it also revealed several weaknesses related to challenge design and organization that can potentially be exploited by challenge organizers and participants to manipulate rankings (see Table 2). To experimentally investigate the potential effect of these weaknesses, we designed experiments based on the most common challenge design choices. As detailed in Sect. 3, our comprehensive analysis revealed *segmentation* as the most common algorithm category, *single-metric ranking* with *mean* and *metric-based aggregation* as the most frequently used ranking scheme and the *Dice similarity coefficient (DSC)* as the most commonly used segmentation metric. We thus consider single-metric ranking based on the DSC (aggregate with mean, then rank) as the default ranking scheme for segmentation challenges in this paper. For our analysis, the organizers of the MICCAI 2015 segmentation challenges provided the following datasets for all tasks (n_{tasks} = 50 in total) of their challenges[1] that met our inclusion criteria[2]: For each participating algorithm (n_{algo} = 445 in total) and each test case, the metric values for those metrics $\in$ {DSC, HD, HD95} (HD: *Hausdorff distance (HD)*; HD95: 95% variant) that had been part of the original challenge ranking were provided. Note in this context that the DSC and the HD/HD95 were the most frequently used segmentation metrics in 2015. Based on this data, the following three scenarios were analyzed:

Scenario 1: Increasing One's Rank by Selective Test Case Submission
According to our analysis, only 33% of all MICCAI tasks provide information on missing data handling *and* punish missing submitted values in some way when determining a challenge ranking (see Sect. 3). However, out of the 445 algorithms who participated in the 2015 segmentations tasks we investigated, 17% of participating teams did not submit results for all test cases. For these algorithms, the mean/maximum amount of missing values was 16%/73%. In theory, challenge participants could exploit the practice of missing data handling by only submitting the results on the easiest cases. To investigate this problem in more depth, we used the MICCAI 2015 segmentation challenges with default ranking scheme to perform the following analysis: For each algorithm and each task of each challenge that met our inclusion criteria (see footnote 2), we artificially removed those test set results (i.e. set the result to N/A) whose DSC was below a threshold of $t_{DSC} = 0.5$. We assume that these cases could have been relatively easily identified by visual inspection even without having access to the reference annotations. We then compared the new ranking position of the algorithm with the position in the original (default) ranking.

Scenario 2a: Decreasing a Competitor's Rank by Changing the Ranking Scheme
According to our analysis of common practice, the ranking scheme is not published in 20% of all challenges. Consulting challenge organizers further revealed that roughly 40% of the organizers did not publish the (complete) ranking scheme before the challenge took place. While there may be good reasons to do so (e.g. organizers want to prevent algorithms from overfitting to a certain assessment method), this practice may – in theory – be exploited by challenge organizers to their own benefit. In this scenario, we explored the hypothetical case where the challenge organizers do not want the winning team, according to the default ranking method, to become the challenge winner (e.g. because the winning team is their main competitor). Based on the MICCAI 2015 segmentation challenges,

---

[1] A challenge may comprise several different tasks for which dedicated rankings/leaderboards are provided (if any).

[2] Number of participating algorithms >2 and number of test cases >1.

we performed the following experiment for all tasks that met our inclusion criteria (see footnote 2) and had used both the DSC and the HD/HD95 (leading to $n = 45$ tasks and $n_{algo} = 424$ for Scenario 2a and 2b): We simulated 12 different rankings based on the most commonly applied metrics (DSC, HD, HD95), rank aggregation methods (rank then aggregate vs aggregate then rank) and aggregation operators (mean vs median). We then used Kendall's tau correlation coefficient [6] to compare the 11 simulated rankings with the original (default) ranking. Furthermore, we computed the maximal change in the ranking over all rank variations for the winners of the default ranking and the non-winning algorithms.

Scenario 2b: Decreasing a Competitor's Rank by Changing the Aggregation Method
As a variant of Scenario 2a, we assume that the organizers published the metric(s) they want to use before the challenge, but not the way they want to aggregate metric values. For the three metrics DSC, HD and HD95, we thus varied only the rank aggregation method and the aggregation operator while keeping the metric fixed. The analysis was then performed in analogy to that of scenario 2a.

3   Results

Between 2007 and 2016, a total of 75 grand challenges with a total of 275 tasks have been hosted by MICCAI. 60% of these challenges published their results in journals or conference proceedings. The median number of citations (in May 2018) was 46 (max: 626). Most challenges (48; 64%) and tasks (222; 81%) dealt with segmentation as algorithm category. The computation of the ranking in segmentation competitions was highly heterogeneous. Overall, 34 different metrics were proposed for segmentation challenges (see Table 1), 38% of which were only applied by a single task. The DSC (75%) was the most commonly used metric, and metric values were typically aggregated with the mean (59%) rather than with the median (3%) (39%: N/A). When a final ranking was provided (49%), it was based on one of the following schemes:

Metric-based aggregation (76%): Initially, a *rank for each metric* and algorithm is computed by aggregating metric values over all test cases. If multiple metrics are used (56% of all tasks), the final rank is then determined by aggregating metric ranks.
Case-based aggregation (2%): Initially, a *rank for each test case* and algorithm is computed for one or multiple metrics. The final rank is determined by aggregating test case ranks.
Other (2%): Highly individualized ranking scheme (e.g. [2])
No information provided (20%)

As detailed in Table 2, our analysis further revealed several weaknesses of current challenge design and organization that could potentially be exploited for rank manipulation. Consequences of this practice have been investigated in our experiments on rank manipulation:

Scenario 1: Our re-evaluation of all MICCAI 2015 segmentation challenges revealed that 25% of all 396 non-winning algorithms would have been ranked first if they had systematically not submitted the worst results. In 8% of the 50 tasks investigated, every single participating algorithm (including the one ranked last) could have been ranked first if they had selectively submitted results. Note that a threshold of $t_{DSC} = 0.5$ corresponds to a median of 25% test cases set to N/A. Even when leaving out only the 5% worst results, still 11% of all non-winning algorithms would have been ranked first.

Scenario 2a: As illustrated in Fig. 1, the ranking depends crucially on the metric(s), the rank aggregation method and the aggregation operator. In 93% of the tasks, it was possible to change the winner by changing one or multiple of these parameters. On average, the winner according to the default ranking was only ranked first in 28% of the ranking variations. In two cases, the first place dropped to rank 11. 16% of all (originally non-winning) 379 algorithms became the winner in at least one ranking scheme.

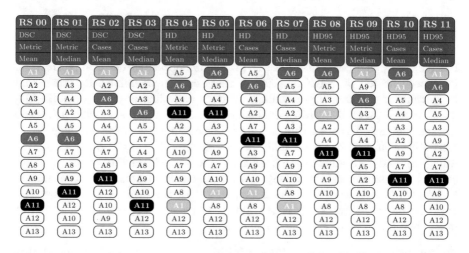

Fig. 1. Effect of different ranking schemes (RS) applied to one example MICCAI 2015 segmentation task. Design choices are indicated in the gray header: *RS xy* defines the different ranking schemes. The following three rows indicate the used *metric* ∈ {DSC, HD, HD95}, the *aggregation method* based on {Metric, Cases} and the *aggregation operator* ∈ {Mean, Median}. *RS 00* (single-metric ranking with DSC; aggregate with mean, then rank) is considered as the default ranking scheme. For each RS, the resulting ranking is shown for algorithms A1 to A13. To illustrate the effect of different RS on single algorithms, A1, A6 and A11 are highlighted.

Scenario 2b: When assuming a fixed metric (DSC/HD/HD95) and only changing the rank aggregation method and/or the aggregation operator (three ranking variations), the winner remains stable in 67% (DSC), 24% (HD) and 31% (HD95) of the experiments. In these cases 7% (DSC), 13% (HD) and 7% (HD95) of all (originally non-winning) 379 algorithms became the winner in at least one ranking scheme. To overcome the problems related to potential cheating, we compiled several best practice recommendations, as detailed in Table 2.

Table 1. Metrics used by MICCAI segmentation tasks between 2007 and 2016.

Metric	Count	%	Metric	Count	%
Dice similarity coefficient (DSC)	206	75	Specificity	15	5
Average surface distance	121	44	Euclidean distance	14	5
Hausdorff distance (HD)	94	34	Volume	12	4
Adjusted rand index	82	30	F1-Score	11	4
Interclass correlation	80	29	Accuracy	11	4
Average symmetric surface distance	52	19	Jaccard index	10	4
Recall	29	11	Absolute surface distance	6	2
Precision	23	8	Time	6	2
95% Hausdorff distance (HD95)	18	7	Area under curve	6	2
Kappa	15	5	Metrics used in <2% of tasks	61	22

4   Discussion

To our knowledge, we are the first to investigate common practice and weaknesses related to MICCAI challenge design and organization. According to our experiments, a number of different ranking design choices (metrics, aggregation method, missing data handling) have a substantial influence on the ranking. Further, the instability of the rankings combined with common practice of reporting/challenge organization can – in theory – be exploited by both challenge participants and organizers to manipulate rankings. Our analysis also revealed that challenge design and organization of MICCAI challenges are highly heterogeneous and lot of relevant information is commonly not reported. While initial valuable steps towards more quality control related to MICCAI challenges have subsequently been taken, these initiatives have so far been focusing on the selection of challenge proposals, while no quality control process has been put in place to monitor the implementation of the proposed design. A weakness of our experimental analysis could be seen in the fact that we simulated the removed test case results by applying a threshold to the DSC values based on the known reference annotations rather than performing a visual inspection. Yet, we strongly believe that the poorly performing cases with a DSC below 0.5 would have also been identified visually. Our approach, in turn, ensured an objective, scalable and reproducible process. Note that an investigation with the HD/HD95 as metric in an analogous manner would not have been reasonable as a threshold would strongly depend on the task/images. Secondly, it is worth

Table 2. Weaknesses of current challenge design and organization that can potentially be exploited by challenge organizers and participants along with best practice recommendations to address existing issues.

Source of problem → Consequence	Best practice recommendation
Ranking schemes are often not published before the challenge → Challenge organizers may tune rankings (cf. Sect. 3)	Challenge organizers should ... ... consider not generating a final ranking at all ... publish the whole challenge design before the challenge ... make changes in the ranking scheme transparent ... publish their evaluation software
Challenge participants often have access to test data → They may do manual corrections of the algorithm output and/or use the knowledge of the test data to tune their algorithms	Challenge organizers should... ... consider releasing more test cases than are used for validation (and keeping the real ones for which annotations are available confidential). ... consider not releasing test data at all and requiring submission of algorithms [1] or ... arrange on-site competitions and ... ask participants to release their source code
Challenge organizers have access to test data annotations → They may manipulate their results	Challenge organizers and members of the organizers' institute(s) ... ... should not be eligible for awards ... should not participate in their own challenge or otherwise ... should make their participation transparent in the leaderboard Provision of (non-competing) baseline algorithms by the organizers, on the other hand, is encouraged
Missing data may be ignored when aggregating metric values → Challenge participants may selectively submit test cases to get a better rank (cf. Sect. 3)	Missing cases should not be allowed or be punished, e.g. by ... assigning the last rank to those cases in case-based aggregation (see e.g. [7]) ... setting the result to the worst metric value (e.g. 0 for the DSC) in metric-based aggregation, if possible (see e.g. [8])
Sometimes arbitrary number of resubmissions possible → Participants can tune their algorithms based on the performance on the test set	Feedback after a submission should not reveal information on individual cases Only the final submission should be based on the full test set [3]

mentioning that instead of applying the different variations of ranking schemes as used in the challenges we focused on the most commonly used ranking scheme in order to perform a statistical analysis that enables a valid comparison across challenges. Given that all rankings of the challenges investigated are based on the DSC as metric, we consider this procedure as valid. Finally, it could be argued that our work is of limited practical value as challenge organizers and participants are fair in general. While this may hold true for the majority, we expect every "security hole" to be exploited sooner or later [5]. Furthermore, our study not only investigates the effect of challenge weaknesses in the context of cheating but also demonstrates the instabilities of rankings for the first time.

In conclusion, we believe that the insights of this study along with the best practice recommendations provided should be carefully considered in future MICCAI challenges. A key message from this paper is to make the challenge design, organization and results as transparent as possible.

Acknowledgments. We thank all of the organizers of the 2015 segmentation challenges who are not co-authoring this paper. We further thank A. Laha, D. Mindroc-Filimon, B. Pekdemir and J. Yoganathan (DKFZ, Germany) for helping with the comprehensive challenge capturing. Finally, we acknowledge support from the European Union through the ERC starting grant COMBIOSCOPY under the New Horizon Framework Programme under grant agreement ERC-2015-StG-37960.

References

1. Boettiger, C.: An introduction to docker for reproducible research. ACM SIGOPS Oper. Syst. Rev. **49**(1), 71–79 (2015). https://doi.org/10.1145/2723872.2723882
2. Carass, A., et al.: Longitudinal multiple sclerosis lesion segmentation: resource and challenge. NeuroImage **148**, 77–102 (2017). https://doi.org/10.1016/j.neuroimage.2016.12.064
3. Dwork, C., Feldman, V., Hardt, M., Pitassi, T., Reingold, O., Roth, A.: The reusable holdout: preserving validity in adaptive data analysis. Science **349**(6248), 636–638 (2015). https://doi.org/10.1126/science.aaa9375
4. van Ginneken, B., Heimann, T., Styner, M.: 3D Segmentation in the Clinic: A Grand Challenge, pp. 7–15 (2007)
5. Ioannidis, J.P.: Why most published research findings are false. PLoS Med. **2**(8), e124 (2005). https://doi.org/10.1371/journal.pmed.0020124
6. Kendall, M.G.: A new measure of rank correlation. Biometrika **30**(1/2), 81–93 (1938)
7. Maier, O., et al.: ISLES 2015 - a public evaluation benchmark for ischemic stroke lesion segmentation from multispectral MRI. Med. Image Anal. **35**, 250–269 (2017). https://doi.org/10.1016/j.media.2016.07.009
8. Maška, M., et al.: A benchmark for comparison of cell tracking algorithms. Bioinformatics **30**(11), 1609–1617 (2014). https://doi.org/10.1093/bioinformatics/btu080

Accurate Weakly-Supervised Deep Lesion Segmentation Using Large-Scale Clinical Annotations: Slice-Propagated 3D Mask Generation from 2D RECIST

Jinzheng Cai[1,2(✉)], Youbao Tang[1], Le Lu[1], Adam P. Harrison[1], Ke Yan[1], Jing Xiao[3], Lin Yang[2], and Ronald M. Summers[1]

[1] National Institutes of Health Clinical Center, Bethesda, MD 20892, USA
{youbao.tang,le.lu,adam.harrison,ke.yan,rms}@nih.gov
[2] University of Florida, Gainesville, FL 32611, USA
jimmycai@ufl.edu, lin.yang@bme.ufl.edu
[3] Ping An Insurance (Group) Company of China, Ltd.,
Shenzhen 510852, People's Republic of China
xiaojing661@pingan.com.cn

Abstract. Volumetric lesion segmentation from computed tomography (CT) images is a powerful means to precisely assess multiple time-point lesion/tumor changes. However, because manual 3D segmentation is prohibitively time consuming, current practices rely on an imprecise surrogate called response evaluation criteria in solid tumors (RECIST). Despite their coarseness, RECIST markers are commonly found in current hospital picture and archiving systems (PACS), meaning they can provide a potentially powerful, yet extraordinarily challenging, source of weak supervision for full 3D segmentation. Toward this end, we introduce a convolutional neural network (CNN) based weakly supervised slice-propagated segmentation (WSSS) method to (1) generate the initial lesion segmentation on the axial RECIST-slice; (2) learn the data distribution on RECIST-slices; (3) extrapolate to segment the whole lesion slice by slice to finally obtain a volumetric segmentation. To validate the proposed method, we first test its performance on a fully annotated lymph node dataset, where WSSS performs comparably to its fully supervised counterparts. We then test on a comprehensive lesion dataset with 32,735 RECIST marks, where we report a mean Dice score of 92% on RECIST-marked slices and 76% on the entire 3D volumes.

1 Introduction

Given the prevailing clinical adoption of the response evaluation criteria in solid tumors (RECIST) [4] for cancer patient monitoring, many modern hospitals' picture archiving and communication systems (PACS) store tremendous amounts

---

J. Cai and Y. Tang—Equal contribution.

A. F. Frangi et al. (Eds.): MICCAI 2018, LNCS 11073, pp. 396–404, 2018.
https://doi.org/10.1007/978-3-030-00937-3_46

of lesion diameter measurements linked to computed tomography (CT) images. In this paper, we tackle the challenging problem of leveraging existing RECIST diameters to produce fully volumetric lesion segmentations in 3D. From any input CT image with the RECIST diameters, we first segment the lesion on the RECIST-marked image (RECIST-slice) in a weakly supervised manner, followed by generalizing the process into other successive slices to obtain the lesion's full volume segmentation.

Inspired by related work [3,6,8,10] of weakly supervised segmentation in computer vision, we design our lesion segmentation in an iteratively slice-wise propagated fashion. More specifically, with the bookmarked long and short diameters on the RECIST-slice, we initialize the segmentation using unsupervised learning methods, e.g., GrabCut [13]. Afterward, we iteratively refine the segmentation using a supervised convolutional neural network (CNN), which can accurately segment the lesion on RECIST-slices. Importantly, the resulting CNN model, trained from all RECIST-slices, can capture the appearance of lesions in CT slices. Thus, the model is capable of detecting lesion regions from images other than the RECIST-slices. With more slices segmented, more image data can be extracted and used to further fine-tune the model. As such, the proposed weakly supervised segmentation model is a slice-wise label-map propagation process, from the RECIST-slice to the whole lesion volume. Therefore, we leverage a large amount of retrospective (yet clinically annotated) imaging data to automatically achieve the final 3D lesion volume measurement and segmentation.

To compare the proposed weakly supervised slice-propagated segmentation (WSSS) against a fully-supervised upper performance limit, we first validate on a publicly-available lymph node (LN) dataset [12], consisting of 984 LNs with full pixel-wise annotations. After demonstrating comparable performance to fully-supervised approaches, we then evaluate WSSS on the DeepLesion dataset [16], achieving mean DICE scores of 92% and 76% on the RECIST-slices and lesion volumes, respectively.

2   Method

In the DeepLesion dataset [16], each CT volume contains an axial slice marked with RECIST diameters that represent the longest lesion axis and its perpendicular counterpart. RECIST diameters can act as a means of weakly supervised training data. Thus, we leverage weakly supervised principles to learn a CNN model using CT slices with no extra pixel-wise manual annotations. Formally, we denote elements in DeepLesion as $\{(V^i, R^i)\}$ for $i \in \{1, \ldots, N\}$, where N is the number of lesions, V^i is the CT volume of interest, and R^i is the corresponding RECIST diameter. To create the 2D training data for the segmentation model, the RECIST-slice and label pairs, X^i and Y^i, respectively, must be generated, and $X^i = V^i_r$ is simply the RECIST-slice, i.e., the axial slice at index r that contains R. For notational clarity, we drop the superscript i for the remainder of this discussion.

2.1 Initial RECIST-Slice Segmentation

We adopt GrabCut [13] to produce the initial lesion segmentation on RECIST-slices. GrabCut is initialized with image foreground and background seeds, Y^s, and produces a segmentation using iterative energy minimization. The resulting mask is calculated to minimize an objective energy function conditioned on the input CT image and seeds:

$$Y = \arg\min_{\tilde{Y}} E_{gc}(\tilde{Y}, Y^s, X), \qquad (1)$$

where we follow the original definition of the energy function E_{gc} in [13].

Given the fact that the quality of GrabCut's initialization will largely affect the final result, we propose to use the spatial prior information, provided by R, to compute high quality initial seeds, $Y^s = S(R)$, where $S(R)$ produces four categories: regions of background (BG), foreground (FG), *probable* background (PBG), and *probable* foreground (PFG). More specifically, if the lesion bounding box tightly around the RECIST axes is $[w, h]$, a $[2w, 2h]$ region of interest (ROI) is cropped from the RECIST-slice. The outer 50% of the ROI is assigned to BG whereas 10% of the image region, obtained from a dilation around R is assigned to FG. The remaining 40% is divided between PFG and PBG based on the distances to FG and BG. Figure 1 visually depicts the training mask generation process (see the "RECIST to Mask" part). We use FG and BG as GrabCut seed regions, leaving the rest as regions where the initial mask is estimated.

2.2 RECIST-Slice Segmentation

We represent our CNN model as a mapping function $\hat{Y} = f(X; \theta)$, where θ represents the model parameters. Our goal is to minimize the differences between $\hat{Y}$ and the imperfect GrabCut mask Y, which contains 3 groups, namely the RECIST pixel indices $\mathcal{R}$, the estimated lesion (foreground) pixel indices $\mathcal{F}$, and the estimated background pixel indices set $\mathcal{B}$. Formally, the indices sets are defined to satisfy the constraints as $Y = Y_{\mathcal{R}} \cup Y_{\mathcal{F}} \cup Y_{\mathcal{B}}$, and $\mathcal{R} \cap \mathcal{F} = \mathcal{R} \cap \mathcal{B} = \mathcal{F} \cap \mathcal{B} = \emptyset$. Thus, we define CNN's training objective containing 3 loss parts as,

$$L = L_{\mathcal{R}} + \alpha L_{\mathcal{F}} + \beta L_{\mathcal{B}}, \qquad (2)$$

$$= \frac{1}{|\mathcal{R}|} \sum_{i \in \mathcal{R}} -\log \hat{y}_i + \alpha \frac{1}{|\mathcal{F}|} \sum_{i \in \mathcal{F}} -\log \hat{y}_i + \beta \frac{1}{|\mathcal{B}|} \sum_{i \in \mathcal{B}} -\log (1 - \hat{y}_i), \qquad (3)$$

where $\hat{y}_i$ is the ith pixel in $\hat{Y}$, $|\cdot|$ represents the set cardinality and α, β are positive weights to balance the losses. Empirically, we set α, and β to small values at the start of model training when $\mathcal{F}, \mathcal{B}$ regions are estimated with low confidence. Afterwards, we set α, and β to larger values, *e.g.*, 1, when training converges.

2.3 Weakly Supervised Slice-Propagated Segmentation

To obtain volumetric measurements, we follow a similar strategy as with the RECIST-slices, except in this slice-propagated case, we must infer R for off-RECIST-slices and also incorporate inference results $\hat{Y}$ from the CNN model. These two priors are used together for slice-propagated CNN training.

RECIST Propagation: A simple way to generate off-RECIST-slice diameters $\hat{R}$ is to take advantage of the fact that RECIST-slice R lies on the maximal cross-sectional area of the lesion. The rate of reduction of off-RECIST-slice endpoints is then calculated by their relative offset distance to the RECIST-slice. Propagated RECIST endpoints are then projected from the actual RECIST endpoints by the Pythagorean theorem using physical Euclidean distance. The "3D RECIST Propagation" part in Fig. 1 depicts the propagation across CT slices. Given the actual RECIST on the rth slice, $\hat{R}_{r-1}$ and $\hat{R}_{r-2}$ are the estimated RECISTs on the first and second off-RECIST-slices, respectively.

Off-RECIST-Slice Segmentation: For slice r, offset from the RECIST-slice, we update the seed generation function from Sect. 2.1 to now take both the inference from the RECIST-slice trained CNN, $\hat{Y}$, and the estimated RECIST, $\hat{R}$: $Y^s = S(\hat{Y}, \hat{R}, R)$. More specifically, $\hat{Y}$ is first binarized by adjusting the threshold so that it covers at least 50% of R's pixels. Regions in $\hat{Y}$ that associate with high foreground probability values, $i.e.$, >0.8, and overlap with $\hat{R}$ will be set as FG together with $\hat{R}$. Similarly, regions with high background probabilities and that have no overlap with $\hat{R}$ will be assigned as BG. The remaining pixels are left as uncertain using the same distance criteria as in the 2D mask generation case and fed into GrabCut for lesion segmentation. In the limited cases where the CNN fails to detect any foreground regions, we fall back to seed generation in Sect. 2.1, except we use $\hat{R}$ as input. The GrabCut mask is then generated using Eq. (1) as before. This procedure is also visually depicted in Fig. 1 (see the "CNN Output to Mask" part).

Slice-Propagated CNN Training: To generate lesion segmentations in all CT slices from 2D RECIST annotations, we train the CNN model in a slice-propagated manner. The CNN first learns lesion appearances based on the RECIST-slices. After the model converges, we then apply this CNN model to slices $[V_{r-1}, V_{r+1}]$ from the entire training set to compute initial predicted probability maps $[\hat{Y}_{r-1}, \hat{Y}_{r+1}]$. Given these probability maps, we create initial lesion segmentations $[Y_{r-1}, Y_{r+1}]$ using GrabCut and the seed generation explained above. These segmentations are employed as training labels for the CNN model on the $[V_{r-1}, V_{r+1}]$ slices, ultimately producing the finally updated segmentations $[\hat{Y}_{r-1}, \hat{Y}_{r+1}]$ once the model converges. As this procedure proceeds iteratively, we can gradually obtain the converged lesion segmentation result across CT slices, and then stack the slice-wise segmentations $[\ldots, \hat{Y}_{r-1}, \hat{Y}_r, \hat{Y}_{r+1}, \ldots]$ to produce a volumetric segmentation. We visually depict this process in Fig. 1 from RECIST-slice to 5 successive slices.

3   Materials and Results

Datasets: The DeepLesion dataset [16] is composed of $32,735$ bookmarked CT lesion instances (with RECIST measurements) from $10,594$ studies of $4,459$

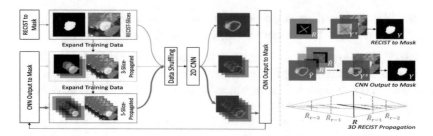

Fig. 1. Overview of the proposed method. **Right:** we use CNN outputs to gradually generate extra training data for lesion segmentation. Arrows colored in red, orange, and blue indicate slice-propagated training at its 1st, 2nd, and 3rd steps, respectively. **Left:** regions colored with red, orange, green, and blue inside the initial segmentation mask Y present FG, PFG, PBG, and BG, respectively.

patients. Lesions have been categorized into 8 subtypes: lung, mediastinum (MD), liver, soft-tissue (ST), abdomen (AB), kidney, pelvis, and bone. For quantitative evaluation, we segmented $1,000$ testing lesion RECIST-slices manually. Out of these 1000, 200 lesions ($\sim$3,500 annotated slices) are fully segmented in 3D as well. Additionally, we also employ the lymph node (LN) dataset [12], which consists of 176 CT scans with complete pixel-wise annotations. Enlarged LN is a lesion subtype and producing accurate segmentation is quite challenging even with fully supervised learning [9]. Importantly, the LN dataset can be used to evaluate our WSSS method against an upper-performance limit, by comparing results with a fully supervised approach [9].

Pre-processing: For the LN dataset, annotation masks are converted into RECIST diameters by measuring its major and minor axes. For robustness, up to 20% random noise is injected into the RECIST diameter lengths to mimic the uncertainty of manual annotation by radiologists. For both datasets, based on the location of RECIST bookmarks, CT ROIs are cropped at two times the extent of the lesion's longest diameters so that sufficient visual context is preserved. The dynamic range of each lesion ROI is then intensity-windowed properly using the CT windowing meta-information in [16]. The LN dataset is separated at the patient level, using a split of 80% and 20% for training and testing, respectively. For the DeepLesion [16] dataset, we randomly select $28,000$ lesions for training.

Evaluation: The mean DICE similarity coefficient (mDICE) and the pixel-wise precision and recall are used to evaluate the quantitative segmentation accuracy.

3.1   Initial RECIST-Slice Segmentation

We denote the proposed GrabCut generation approach in Sect. 2.1 as GrabCut-R. To demonstrate our modifications in GrabCut-R are effective, we have compared it with general initialization methods, *i.e.*, densely connected conditional random fields (DCRF) [7], GrabCut, and GrabCut^i [6]. First, we

Table 1. Performance in generating Y, the initial RECIST-slice segmentation. Mean DICE scores are reported with standard deviation for methods that defined in Sect. 3.1.

Method	Lymph Node			DeepLesion (on RECIST-Slice)		
	Recall	Precision	mDICE	Recall	Precision	mDICE
RECIST-D	0.35±0.09	**0.99±0.05**	0.51±0.09	0.39±0.13	**0.92±0.14**	0.53±0.14
DCRF	0.29±0.20	0.98±0.05	0.41±0.21	0.72±0.26	0.90±0.15	0.77±0.20
GrabCut	0.10±0.25	0.32±0.37	0.11±0.26	0.62±0.46	0.68±0.44	0.62±0.46
GrabCut^i	0.53±0.24	0.92±0.10	0.63±0.17	0.94±0.11	0.81±0.16	0.86±0.11
GrabCut-R	**0.83±0.11**	0.86±0.11	**0.83±0.06**	**0.94±0.10**	0.89±0.10	**0.91±0.08**

define a bounding box (bbox) which is tightly covering the extent of RECIST marks. To initialize GrabCut, we set areas inside and outside the bbox as BG and PFG, respectively. To initialize GrabCut^i, we set the central 20% bbox region as FG, regions outside the bbox as BG, and the rest as PFG, which is similar to the setting of bbox^i in [6]. We then test DCRF [7] using the same bbox^i as the unary potentials and intensities to compute pairwise potentials. Since the DCRF is moderately sensitive to parameter variations, we record the best configuration we found and have it reported in Table 1. Finally, we measure results as we directly use the RECIST diameters, but dilated to 20% of bbox area, to generate the initial segmentation. We denote this approach RECIST-D, which produces the best precision, but at the cost of very low recall. From Table 1, we observe that GrabCut-R significantly outperforms all its counterparts on both of the Lymph Node and the DeepLesion datasets, demonstrating the validity of our mask initialization process.

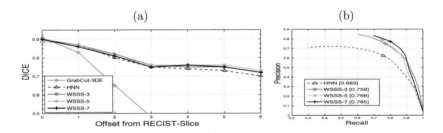

Fig. 2. WSSS on DeepLesion. (a) depicts mean Dice scores on *2D slices* as a function of offsets with respect to the RECIST-slice. (b) depicts *volumetric* precision-recall curves.

3.2   CNN Based RECIST-Slice Segmentation

We use holistically nested networks (HNNs) [15] as our baseline CNN model, which has been adapted successfully for lymph node [9], pancreas [2], and lung segmentation [5]. In all experiments, deep learning is implemented in Tensorflow [1] and Tensorpack [14]. The initial learning rate is 5×10^{-5}, dropping to

1×10^{-5} when the model training-validation plot plateaus. Given the results of Y, *i.e.*, >90% mDICE, we simply set the balance weights in Eq. (2) as $\alpha = \beta = 1$.

Following Sect. 3.1, we select three ways to generate training masks on the RECIST-slice: the RECIST-D, GrabCut-R and the fully annotated ground truth (GT). As Table 2 demonstrates, on the LN dataset [12], HNNs trained using masks Y generated from RECIST-D, GrabCut-R, and GT achieve 61%, 70%, and 71% mDICE scores, respectively. This observation demonstrates the robustness and effectiveness of using GrabCut-R labels, which only performs slightly worse than using the GT. On the DeepLesion [16] testset of $1,000$ annotated RECIST-slices, HNN trained on GrabCut-R outperforms the deep model learned from RECIST-D by a margin of 25% in mean DICE (90.6% versus 64.4%). GrabCut post-processing, denoted with the suffix "-GC", further improves the results from 90.6% to 91.5%.

We demonstrate our weakly supervised approach, trained on a large quantity of "imperfectly-labeled" object masks, can outperform fully-supervised models trained on fewer data. To do this, we separated the $1,000$ annotated testing images into five folds and report the mean DICE scores using fully-supervised HNN [15] and UNet [11] models on this smaller dataset. Impressively, the 90.6% DICE score of the weakly supervised approach considerably outperforms the fully supervised HNN and UNet mDICE of 83.7% and 72.8%, respectively. Coupled with an approach like ours, this demonstrates the potential in exploiting large-scale, but "imperfectly-labeled", datasets.

Table 2. Results of using different training masks, where GT refers to the manual segmentations. All results report mDICE $\pm$ std. GT results for the DeepLesion dataset are trained on the subset of $1,000$ annotated slices. See Sect. 3.2 for method details.

Method	Lymph node		DeepLesion (on RECIST-slice)	
	CNN	CNN-GC	CNN	CNN-GC
UNet + GT	**0.729±0.08**	0.838±0.07	0.728±0.18	0.838±0.16
HNN + GT	0.710±0.18	**0.845±0.06**	0.837±0.16	0.909±0.10
HNN + RECIST-D	0.614±0.17	0.844±0.06	0.644±0.14	0.801±0.12
HNN + GrabCut-R	0.702±0.17	0.844±0.06	**0.906±0.09**	**0.915±0.10**

Table 3. Mean DICE scores for lesion volumes. "HNN" is the HNN [15] trained on GrabCut-R from RECIST slices and "WSSS-7" is the proposed approach trained on 7 successive CT slices. See Sect. 3.3 for method details.

Method	Bone	AB	MD	Liver	Lung	Kidney	ST	Pelvis	Mean
GrabCut-3DE	0.654	0.628	0.693	0.697	0.667	0.747	0.726	0.580	0.675
HNN	0.666	0.766	0.745	0.768	0.742	0.777	**0.791**	**0.736**	0.756
WSSS-7	**0.685**	0.766	**0.776**	**0.773**	0.757	**0.800**	0.780	0.728	0.762
WSSS-7-GC	0.683	**0.774**	0.771	0.765	**0.773**	**0.800**	0.787	0.722	**0.764**

3.3 Weakly Supervised Slice-Propagated Segmentation

In Fig. 2a, we show the segmentation results on 2D CT slices arranged in the order of offsets with respect to the RECIST-slice. GrabCut with 3D RECIST estimation (GrabCut-3DE), which is generated from RECIST propagation, produces good segmentations (~91%) on the RECIST-slice but degrades to 55% mDICE when the offset rises to 4. This is mainly because 3D RECIST approximation often is not a robust estimation across slices. In contrast, the HNN trained with only RECIST slices, *i.e.*, the model from Sect. 3.2, generalizes well with large slice offsets, achieving mean DICE scores of >70% even when the offset distance ranges to 6. However, performance is further improved at higher slice offsets when using the proposed slice-propagated approach with 3 axial slices, *i.e.*, WSSS-3, and even further when using slice-propagated learning with 5 and 7 axial slices, *i.e.*, WSSS-5, and WSSS-7, respectively. This propagation procedure is stopped at 7 slices as we observed the performance had converged. The current results demonstrate the value of using the proposed WSSS approach to generalize beyond 2D RECIST-slices into full 3D segmentation. We observe that improvements in mean DSC are not readily apparent, given the normalizing effect of that metric. However, when we measure F1-scores aggregated over the entire dataset (Fig. 2b, WSSS-7 improves over HNN from 0.683 to 0.785 (i.e., a lot of more voxels have been correctly segmented).

Finally, we reported the categorized 3D segmentation results. As demonstrated in Table 3, WSSS-7 propagates the learned lesion segmentation from the RECIST-slice to the off-RECIST-slices improving the 3D segmentation results from baseline 0.68 Dice score to 0.76. From the segmentation results of WSSS-7, we observe that the Dice score varies from 0.68 to 0.80 on different lesion categories, where the kidney is the easiest one and bone is the most challenging one. This suggests future investigation of category-specific lesion segmentation may yield further improvements.

4 Conclusion

We present a simple yet effective weakly supervised segmentation approach that converts massive amounts of RECIST-based lesion diameter measurements (retrospectively stored in hospitals' digital repositories) into full 3D lesion volume segmentation and measurements. Importantly, our approach does not require pre-existing RECIST measurement on processing new cases. The lesion segmentation results are validated quantitatively, *i.e.*, 91.5% mean DICE score on RECIST-slices and 76.4% for lesion volumes. We demonstrate that our slice-propagated learning improves performance over state-of-the-art CNNs. Moreover, we demonstrate how leveraging the weakly supervised, but large-scale data, allows us to outperform fully-supervised approaches that can only be trained on subsets where full masks are available. Our work is potentially of high importance for automated and large-scale tumor volume measurement and management in the domain of precision quantitative radiology imaging.

Acknowledgement. This research was supported by the Intramural Research Program of the National Institutes of Health Clinical Center and by the Ping An Insurance Company through a Cooperative Research and Development Agreement. We thank Nvidia for GPU card donation.

References

1. Abadi, M., Agarwal, A., Barham, P., et al.: TensorFlow: large-scale machine learning on heterogeneous systems (2015). https://www.tensorflow.org/
2. Cai, J., Lu, L., Xie, Y., Xing, F., Yang, L.: Improving deep pancreas segmentation in CT and MRI images via recurrent neural contextual learning and direct loss function. In: MICCAI (2017)
3. Dai, J., He, K., Sun, J.: Boxsup: exploiting bounding boxes to supervise convolutional networks for semantic segmentation. In: IEEE ICCV, pp. 1635–1643 (2015)
4. Eisenhauer, E., Therasse, P.: New response evaluation criteria in solid tumours: revised RECIST guideline (version 1.1). Eur. J. Cancer **45**, 228–247 (2009)
5. Harrison, A.P., Xu, Z., George, K., Lu, L., Summers, R.M., Mollura, D.J.: Progressive and multi-path holistically nested neural networks for pathological lung segmentation from CT images. In: MICCAI, pp. 621–629 (2017)
6. Khoreva, A., Benenson, R., Hosang, J., Hein, M., Schiele, B.: Simple does it: weakly supervised instance and semantic segmentation. In: IEEE CVPR (2017)
7. Krähenbühl, P., Koltun, V.: Efficient inference in fully connected CRFs with gaussian edge potentials. In: NIPS, pp. 1–9 (2012)
8. Lin, D., Dai, J., Jia, J., He, K., Sun, J.: Scribblesup: scribble-supervised convolutional networks for semantic segmentation. In: IEEE CVPR, pp. 3159–3167 (2016)
9. Nogues, I., Lu, L., Wang, X., Roth, H., Bertasius, G., Lay, N., et al.: Automatic lymph node cluster segmentation using holistically-nested neural networks and structured optimization in ct images. In: MICCAI, pp. 388–397 (2016)
10. Papandreou, G., Chen, L.C., Murphy, K.P., Yuille, A.L.: Weakly-and semi-supervised learning of a deep convolutional network for semantic image segmentation. In: IEEE ICCV, pp. 1742–1750 (2015)
11. Ronneberger, O., Fischer, P., Brox, T.: U-net: convolutional networks for biomedical image segmentation. In: MICCAI, pp. 234–241 (2015)
12. Roth, H., Lu, L., Seff, A., Cherry, K., Hoffman, J., Liu, J., et al.: A new 2.5D representation for lymph node detection using random sets of deep convolutional neural network observations. In: MICCAI, pp. 520–527 (2014)
13. Rother, C., Kolmogorov, V., Blake, A.: Grabcut: interactive foreground extraction using iterated graph cuts. ACM TOG **23**(3), 309–314 (2004)
14. Wu, Y., et al.: Tensorpack (2016). https://github.com/tensorpack/
15. Xie, S., Tu, Z.: Holistically-nested edge detection. In: ICCV, pp. 1395–1403 (2015)
16. Yan, K., Wang, X., Lu, L., Zhang, L., Harrison, A., et al.: Deep lesion graphs in the wild: relationship learning and organization of significant radiology image findings in a diverse large-scale lesion database. In: CVPR (2018)

Semi-automatic RECIST Labeling on CT Scans with Cascaded Convolutional Neural Networks

Youbao Tang[1](✉), Adam P. Harrison[3], Mohammadhadi Bagheri[2], Jing Xiao[4], and Ronald M. Summers[1]

[1] Imaging Biomarkers and Computer-Aided Diagnosis Laboratory, National Institutes of Health Clinical Center, Bethesda, MD 20892, USA
youbao.tang@nih.gov
[2] Clinical Image Processing Service, National Institutes of Health Clinical Center, Bethesda, MD 20892, USA
[3] NVIDIA, Santa Clara, CA 95051, USA
[4] Ping An Insurance Company of China, Shenzhen 510852, China

Abstract. Response evaluation criteria in solid tumors (RECIST) is the standard measurement for tumor extent to evaluate treatment responses in cancer patients. As such, RECIST annotations must be accurate. However, RECIST annotations manually labeled by radiologists require professional knowledge and are time-consuming, subjective, and prone to inconsistency among different observers. To alleviate these problems, we propose a cascaded convolutional neural network based method to semi-automatically label RECIST annotations and drastically reduce annotation time. The proposed method consists of two stages: lesion region normalization and RECIST estimation. We employ the spatial transformer network (STN) for lesion region normalization, where a localization network is designed to predict the lesion region and the transformation parameters with a multi-task learning strategy. For RECIST estimation, we adapt the stacked hourglass network (SHN), introducing a relationship constraint loss to improve the estimation precision. STN and SHN can both be learned in an end-to-end fashion. We train our system on the DeepLesion dataset, obtaining a consensus model trained on RECIST annotations performed by multiple radiologists over a multi-year period. Importantly, when judged against the inter-reader variability of two additional radiologist raters, our system performs more stably and with less variability, suggesting that RECIST annotations can be reliably obtained with reduced labor and time.

1 Introduction

Response evaluation criteria in solid tumors (RECIST) [1] measures lesion or tumor growth rates across different time points after treatment. Today, the majority of clinical trials evaluating cancer treatments use RECIST as an objective response measurement [2]. Therefore, the quality of RECIST annotations

This is a U.S. government work and not under copyright protection in the U.S.; foreign copyright protection may apply 2018
A. F. Frangi et al. (Eds.): MICCAI 2018, LNCS 11073, pp. 405–413, 2018.
https://doi.org/10.1007/978-3-030-00937-3_47

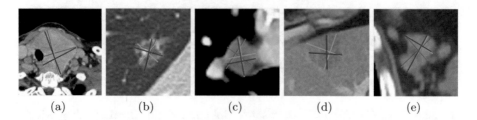

$$(a) \qquad\qquad (b) \qquad\qquad (c) \qquad\qquad (d) \qquad\qquad (e)$$

Fig. 1. Five examples of RECIST annotations labeled by three radiologists. For each image, the RECIST annotations from different observers are indicated by diameters with different colors. Better viewed in color.

will directly affect the assessment result and therapeutic plan. To perform RECIST annotations, a radiologist first selects an axial image slice where the lesion has the longest spatial extent. Then he or she measures the diameters of the in-plane longest axis and the orthogonal short axis. These two axes constitute the RECIST annotation. Figure 1 depicts five examples of RECIST annotations labeled by three different radiologists with different colors.

Using RECIST annotation face two main challenges. (1) Measuring tumor diameters requires a great deal of professional knowledge and is time-consuming. Consequently, it is difficult and expensive to manually annotate large-scale datasets, e.g., those used in large clinical trials or retrospective analyses. (2) RECIST marks are often subjective and prone to inconsistency among different observers [3]. For instance, from Fig. 1, we can see that there is large variation between RECIST annotations from different radiologists. However, consistency is critical in assessing actual lesion growth rates, which directly impacts patient treatment options [3]. To overcome these problems, we propose a RECIST estimation method that uses a cascaded convolutional neural network (CNN) approach. Given region of interest (ROI) cropped using a bounding box roughly drawn by a radiologist, the proposed method directly outputs RECIST annotations. As a result, the proposed RECIST estimation method is semi-automatic, drastically reducing annotation time while keeping the "human in the loop". To the best of our knowledge, this paper is the first to propose such an approach. In addition, our method can be readily made fully automatic as it can be trivially connected with any effective lesion localization framework.

From Fig. 1, the endpoints of RECIST annotations can well represent their locations and sizes. Thus, the proposed method estimates four keypoints, i.e., the endpoints, instead of two diameters. Recently, many approaches [4–7] have been proposed to estimate the keypoints of the human body, e.g., knee, ankle, and elbow, which is similar to our task. Inspired by the success and simplicity of stacked hourglass networks (SHN) [4] for human pose estimation, this work employs SHN for RECIST estimation. Because the long and short diameters are orthogonal, a new relationship constraint loss is introduced to improve the accuracy of RECIST estimation. Regardless of class, the lesion regions may have large variability in sizes, locations and orientations in different images. To make our method robust to these variations, the lesion region first needs to be normalized

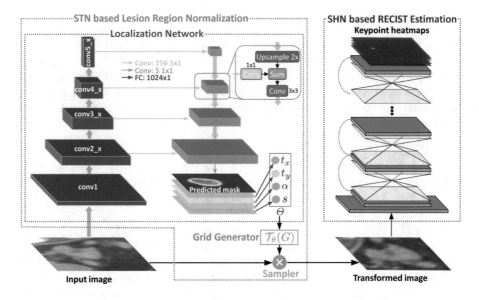

Fig. 2. The framework of the proposed method. The predicted mask and keypoint heatmaps are rendered with a color map for visualization purposes.

before feeding into the SHN. In this work, we use the spatial transformer network (STN) [8] for lesion region normalization, where a ResNet-50 [9] based localization network is designed for lesion region and transformation parameter prediction. Experimental results over the DeepLesion dataset [10] compare our method to the multi-rater annotations in that dataset, plus annotations from two additional radiologists. Importantly, our method closely matches the multi-rater RECIST annotations and, when compared against the two additional readers, exhibits less variability than the inter-reader variability.

In summary, this paper makes the following main contributions: (1) We are the first to automatically generate RECIST marks in a roughly labeled lesion region. (2) STN and SHN are effectively integrated for RECIST estimation, and enhanced using multi-task learning and an orthogonal constraint loss, respectively. (3) Our method evaluated on a large-scale lesion dataset achieves lower variability than manual annotations by radiologists.

2   Methodology

Our system assumes the axial slice is already selected. To accurately estimate RECIST annotations, we propose a cascaded CNN based method, which consists of an STN for lesion region normalization and an SHN for RECIST estimation, as shown in Fig. 2. Here, we assume that every input image always contains a lesion region, which is roughly cropped by a radiologist. The proposed method can directly output an estimated RECIST annotation for every input.

2.1 Lesion Region Normalization

The original STN [8] contains three components, i.e., a localization network, a grid generator, and a sampler, as shown in Fig. 2. The STN can implicitly predict transformation parameters of an image and can be used to implement any parameterizable transformation. In this work, we use STN to explicitly predict translation, rotation and scaling transformations of the lesion. Therefore, the transformation matrix $\mathbf{M}$ can be formulated as:

$$
\mathbf{M} = \overbrace{\begin{bmatrix} 1 & 0 & t_x \\ 0 & 1 & t_y \\ 0 & 0 & 1 \end{bmatrix}}^{Translation} \overbrace{\begin{bmatrix} \cos(\alpha) & -\sin(\alpha) & 0 \\ \sin(\alpha) & \cos(\alpha) & 0 \\ 0 & 0 & 1 \end{bmatrix}}^{Rotation} \overbrace{\begin{bmatrix} s & 0 & 0 \\ 0 & s & 0 \\ 0 & 0 & 1 \end{bmatrix}}^{Scaling} = \begin{bmatrix} s\cos(\alpha) & -s\sin(\alpha) & t_x \\ s\sin(\alpha) & s\cos(\alpha) & t_y \\ 0 & 0 & 1 \end{bmatrix}
$$

$$(1)$$

From (1) there are four transformation parameters in $\mathbf{M}$, denoted as $\theta = \{t_x, t_y, \alpha, s\}$. The goal of the localization network is to predict the transformation that will be applied to the input image. In this work, a localization network based on ResNet-50 [9] is designed as shown in Fig. 2. The purple blocks of Fig. 2 are the first five blocks of ResNet-50. Importantly, unlike many applications of STN, the true θ can be obtained easily for transformation parameters prediction (TPP) by settling on a canonical layout for RECIST marks.

As Sect. 3 will outline, the STN also benefits from additional supervisory data, in the form of lesion pseudo-masks. To this end, we generate a lesion pseudo-mask by constructing an ellipse from the RECIST annotations. Ellipses are a rough analogue to a lesion's true shape. We denote this task lesion region prediction (LRP). Finally, to further improve prediction accuracy, we introduce another branch (green in Fig. 2) to build a feature pyramid, similar to previous work [11], using a top-down pathway and skip connections. The top-down feature maps are constructed using a ResNet-50-like structure. Coarse-to-fine feature maps are first upsampled by a factor of 2, and corresponding fine-to-coarse maps are transformed by 256 1×1 convolutional kernels. These are summed, and resulting feature map will be smoothed using 256 3×3 convolutional kernels. This ultimately produces a 5-channel 32×32 feature map, with one channel dedicated to the LRP. The remaining TPP channels are inputted to a fully connected layer outputting four transformation values, as shown in Fig. 2.

According to the predicted θ, a 2×3 matrix Θ can be calculated as

$$
\Theta = \begin{bmatrix} s\cos(\alpha) & -s\sin(\alpha) & t_x \\ s\sin(\alpha) & s\cos(\alpha) & t_y \end{bmatrix}
$$

$$(2)$$

With Θ, the grid generator $\mathcal{T}_\theta(G)$ will produce a parametrized sampling grid (PSG), which is a set of coordinates (x_i^s, y_i^s) of source points where the input image should be sampled to get the coordinates (x_i^t, y_i^t) of target points of the desired transformed image. Thus, the elements in PSG can be formulated as

$$
\begin{bmatrix} x_i^s \\ y_i^s \end{bmatrix} = \begin{bmatrix} s\cos(\alpha) & -s\sin(\alpha) & t_x \\ s\sin(\alpha) & s\cos(\alpha) & t_y \end{bmatrix} \begin{bmatrix} x_i^t \\ y_i^t \\ 1 \end{bmatrix}
$$

$$(3)$$

Armed with the input image and PSG, we use bilinear interpolation as a differentiable sampler to generate the transformed image. We set our canonical space to (1) center the lesion region, (2) make the long diameter horizontal, and 3) remove most of THE background.

2.2   RECIST Estimation

After obtaining the transformed image, we need to estimate the positions of keypoints, i.e., the endpoints of long/short diameters. If the keypoints can be estimated precisely, RECIST annotation will be accurate. To achieve this goal, a network should have a coherent understanding of the whole lesion region and output high-resolution pixel-wise predictions. We use SHN [4] for this task, as they have the capacity to capture the above features and have been successfully used in human pose estimation.

SHN is composed of stacked hourglass networks, where each hourglass network contains a downsampling and upsampling path, implemented by convolutional, max pooling, and upsampling layers. The topology of these two parts is symmetric, which means that for every layer present on the way down there is a corresponding layer going up and they are combined with skip connections. Multiple hourglass networks are stacked to form the final SHN by feeding the output of one as input into the next, as shown in Fig. 2. Intermediate supervision is used in SHN by applying a loss at the heatmaps produced by each hourglass network, with the goal or improving predictions after each hourglass network. The outputs of the last hourglass network are accepted as the final predicted keypoint heatmaps. For SHN training, ground-truth keypoint heatmaps consist of four 2D Gaussian maps (with standard deviation of 1 pixel) centered on the endpoints of RECIST annotations. The final RECIST annotation is obtained according to the maximum of each heatmap. In addition, as the two RECIST axes should always be orthogonal, we also measure the cosine angle between them, which should always be 1. More details on SHN can found in Newell *et al.* [4].

2.3   Model Optimization

We use mean squared error (MSE) loss to optimize our network, where all loss components are normalized into the interval $[0, 1]$. The STN losses are denoted L_{LRP} and L_{TPP}, which measure error in the predicted masks and transformation parameters, respectively. Training first focuses on LRP: $L_{STN} = 10L_{LRP} + L_{TPP}$. After convergence, the loss focuses on the TPP: $L_{STN} = L_{LRP} + 10L_{TPP}$. We first give a larger weight to L_{LRP} to make STN focus more on LRP. After convergence, L_{TPP} is weighted more heavily, so that the optimization is emphasized more on TPP. For SHN training, the losses are denoted L_{HM} and L_{cos}, respectively, which measure error in the predicted heat maps and cosine angle, respectively. Each contribute equally to the total SHN loss.

The STN and SHN networks are first trained separately and then combined for joint training. During joint training, all losses contribute equally. Compared with training jointly and directly from scratch, our strategy has faster convergence and better performance. We use stochastic gradient descent with a momentum of 0.9, an initial learning rate of $5e^{-4}$, which is divided by 10 once the validation loss is stable. After decreasing the learning rate twice, we stop training. To enhance robustness we augment data by random translations, rotations, and scales.

3   Experimental Results and Analyses

The proposed method is evaluated on the DeepLesion (DL) dataset [10], which consists of $32,735$ images bookmarked and measured via RECIST annotations by multiple radiologists over multiple years from $10,594$ studies of $4,459$ patients. 500 images are randomly selected from 200 patients as a test set. For each test image, two extra RECIST annotations are labeled by another two experienced radiologists (R1 and R2). Images from the other $3,759$ and 500 patients are used as training and validation datasets, respectively. To mimic the behavior of a radiologist roughly drawing a bounding box around the entire lesion, input images are generated by randomly cropping a subimage whose region is 2 to 2.5 times as large as the lesion itself with random offsets. All images are resized to 128×128. The performance is measured by the mean and standard deviation

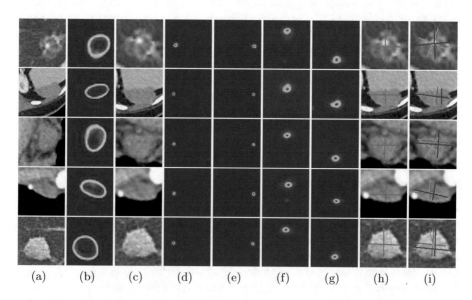

(a)   (b)   (c)   (d)   (e)   (f)   (g)   (h)   (i)

Fig. 3. Given the input test image (a), we can obtain the predicted lesion mask (b), the transformed image (c) from the STN, and the estimated keypoint heatmaps (d)–(g) from the SHN. From (d)–(g), we obtain the estimated RECIST (h), which is close to the annotations (i) labeled by radiologists. Red, green, and blue marks denote DL, R1, and R2 annotations, respectively.

Table 1. The mean and standard deviation of the differences of keypoint locations (Loc.) and diameter lengths (Len.) between radiologist RECIST annotations and also those obtained by different experimental configurations of our method. The unit of all numbers is pixel in the original image resolution.

Reader	DL		R1		R2		Overall	
	Loc.	Len.	Loc.	Len.	Loc.	Len.	Loc.	Len.
Long diameter								
DL	-	-	8.16±10.2	4.11±5.87	9.10±11.6	5.21±7.42	8.63±10.9	4.66±6.71
R1	8.16±10.2	4.11±5.87	-	-	6.63±11.0	3.39±5.62	7.40±10.6	3.75±5.76
R2	9.10±11.6	5.21±7.42	6.63±11.0	3.39±5.62	-	-	7.87±11.3	4.30±6.65
$\overline{SHN}$	10.2±12.3	6.73±9.42	10.4±12.4	6.94±9.83	10.8±12.6	7.13±10.4	10.5±12.5	6.93±9.87
STN+$\overline{SHN}$	7.02±9.43	3.85±6.57	7.14±11.4	3.97±5.85	8.74±11.2	4.25±6.57	7.63±10.4	4.02±6.27
STN+$\overline{SHN}$	5.94±8.13	3.54±5.18	6.23±9.49	3.62±5.31	6.45±10.5	3.90±6.21	6.21±9.32	3.69±5.59
STN+SHN	5.14±7.62	3.11±4.22	5.75±8.08	3.27±4.89	5.86±9.34	3.61±5.72	5.58±8.25	3.33±4.93
Short diameter								
DL	-	-	7.69±9.07	3.41±4.72	8.35±9.44	3.55±5.24	8.02±9.26	3.48±4.99
R1	7.69±9.07	3.41±4.72	-	-	6.13±8.68	2.47±4.27	6.91±8.91	2.94±4.53
R2	8.35±9.44	3.55±5.24	6.13±8.68	2.47±4.27	-	-	7.24±9.13	3.01±4.81
$\overline{SHN}$	9.31±11.8	5.02±7.04	9.59±12.0	5.19±7.35	9.83±12.1	5.37±7.69	9.58±11.8	5.19±7.38
STN+$\overline{SHN}$	6.59±8.46	3.25±5.93	7.63±8.99	3.35±6.41	8.16±9.18	4.18±6.48	7.46±8.93	3.59±6.22
STN+$\overline{SHN}$	5.52±7.74	2.79±4.57	5.71±8.06	2.87±4.62	6.01±8.39	2.96±5.09	5.75±8.01	2.87±4.73
STN+SHN	4.47±6.26	2.68±4.31	4.97±7.02	2.76±4.52	5.41±7.59	2.92±4.98	4.95±6.95	2.79±4.57

of the differences of keypoint locations and diameter lengths between RECIST estimations and radiologist annotations.

Figure 3 shows five visual examples of the results. Figure 3(b) and (c) demonstrate the effectiveness of our STN for lesion region normalization. With the transformed image (Fig. 3(c)), the keypoint heatmaps (Fig. 3(d)–(g)) are obtained using SHN. Figure 3(d) and (e) are the heatmaps of the left and right endpoints of long diameter, respectively, while Fig. 3(f) and (g) are the top and bottom endpoints of the short diameter, respectively. Generally, the endpoints of long diameter can be found more easily than the ones of the short diameter, explaining why the highlighted spots in Fig. 3(d) and (e) are smaller. As Fig. 3(h) demonstrates, the RECIST estimation correspond well with those of the radiologist annotations in Fig. 3(i). Note the high inter-reader variability.

To quantify this inter-reader variability, and how our approach measures against it, we compare the DL, R1, R2 annotations and those of our method against each other, computing the mean and standard deviation of differences between axis locations and lengths. From the first three rows of each portion of Table 1, the inter-reader variability of each set of annotations can be discerned. The visual results in Fig. 3(h) and (i) suggest that our method corresponds well to the radiologists' annotations. To verify this, we compute the mean and standard deviation of the differences between the RECIST marks of our proposed method (STN+SHN) against those of three sets of annotations, as listed in the last row of each part of Table 1. From the results, the estimated RECIST marks obtain the least mean difference and standard deviation in both location and length, suggesting the proposed method produces more stable RECIST annotations than the radiologist readers on the DeepLesion dataset. Note that the estimated RECIST marks are closest to the multi-radiologist annotations from the DL dataset, most likely because these are the annotations used to train our system. As such, this also suggest our method is able to generate a model that aggregates training input from multiple radiologists and learns a common knowledge that is not overfitted to any one rater's tendencies.

To demonstrate the benefits of our enhancements to standard STN and SHN, including the multi-task losses, we conduct the following experimental comparisons: (1) using SHN with only loss L_{HM} ($\overline{\text{SHN}}$), which can be considered as the baseline; (2) using only the L_{TPP} and L_{HM} loss for the STN and SHN, respectively (denoted $\overline{\text{STN}}+\overline{\text{SHN}}$); (3) using both the L_{TPP} and L_{LRP} losses for the STN, but only the L_{HM} loss for the SHN (STN+$\overline{\text{SHN}}$); (4) the proposed method with all L_{TPP}, L_{LRP}, L_{HM}, and L_{cos} losses (STN+SHN). These results are listed in the last four rows of each part in Table 1. From the results, we can see that (1) the proposed method (STN+SHN) achieves the best performance. (2) $\overline{\text{STN}}+\overline{\text{SHN}}$ outperforms $\overline{\text{SHN}}$, meaning that when lesion regions are normalized, the keypoints of RECIST marks can be estimated more precisely. (3) STN+$\overline{\text{SHN}}$ outperforms $\overline{\text{STN}}+\overline{\text{SHN}}$, meaning the localization network with multi-task learning can predict the transformation parameters more precisely than with only a single task TPP. (4) STN+SHN outperforms STN+$\overline{\text{SHN}}$, meaning the accuracy of keypoint heatmaps can be improved by introducing the cosine loss to measure axis orthogonality. All of the above results demonstrate the effectiveness of the proposed method for RECIST estimation and the implemented modifications to improve performance.

4   Conclusions

We propose a semi-automatic RECIST labeling method that uses a cascaded CNN, comprised of enhanced STN and SHN. To improve the accuracy of transformation parameters prediction, the STN is enhanced using multi-task learning and an additional coarse-to-fine pathway. Moreover, an orthogonal constraint loss is introduced for SHN training, improving results further. The experimental results over the DeepLesion dataset demonstrate that the proposed method is highly effective for RECIST estimation, producing annotations with less variability than those of two additional radiologist readers. The semi-automated approach only requires a rough bounding box drawn by a radiologist, drastically reducing annotation time. Moreover, if coupled with a reliable lesion localization framework, our approach can be made fully automatic. As such, the proposed method can potentially provide a highly positive impact to clinical workflows.

Acknowledgments. This research was supported by the Intramural Research Program of the National Institutes of Health Clinical Center and by the Ping An Insurance Company through a Cooperative Research and Development Agreement. We thank Nvidia for GPU card donation.

References

1. Eisenhauer, E.A., Therasse, P., et al.: New response evaluation criteria in solid tumours: revised RECIST guideline. Eur. J. Cancer **45**(2), 228–247 (2009)
2. Kaisary, A.V., Ballaro, A., Pigott, K.: Lecture Notes: Urology. Wiley, Hoboken (2016). 84
3. Yoon, S.H., Kim, K.W., et al.: Observer variability in RECIST-based tumour burden measurements: a meta-analysis. Eur. J. Cancer **53**, 5–15 (2016)
4. Newell, A., Yang, K., Deng, J.: Stacked hourglass networks for human pose estimation. In: European Conference on Computer Vision, pp. 483–499 (2016)
5. Chu, X., Yang, W., et al.: Multi-context attention for human pose estimation. In: IEEE Computer Society Conference on Computer Vision and Pattern Recognition, pp. 5669–5678 (2017)
6. Cao, Z., Simon, T., et al.: Realtime multi-person 2D pose estimation using part affinity fields. In: IEEE Computer Society Conference on Computer Vision and Pattern Recognition, pp. 1302–1310 (2017)
7. Yang, W., Li, S., et al.: Learning feature pyramids for human pose estimation. In: IEEE Computer Society Conference on Computer Vision and Pattern Recognition, pp. 1290–1299 (2017)
8. Jaderberg, M., Simonyan, K., et al.: Spatial transformer networks. In: Advances in Neural Information Processing Systems, pp. 2017–2025 (2015)
9. He, K., Zhang, X., et al.: Deep residual learning for image recognition. In: IEEE Computer Society Conference on Computer Vision and Pattern Recognition, pp. 770–778 (2016)
10. Yan, K., Wang, X., et al.: Deep Lesion Graphs in the Wild: Relationship Learning and Organization of Significant Radiology Image Findings in a Diverse Large-scale Lesion Database. arXiv:1711.10535 (2017)
11. Lin, T.Y. and Dollár, P., et al.: Feature pyramid networks for object detection. In: IEEE Computer Society Conference on Computer Vision and Pattern Recognition, pp. 936–944 (2017)

Image Segmentation Methods: Multi-organ Segmentation

A Multi-scale Pyramid of 3D Fully Convolutional Networks for Abdominal Multi-organ Segmentation

Holger R. Roth[1(✉)], Chen Shen[1], Hirohisa Oda[1], Takaaki Sugino[1],
Masahiro Oda[1], Yuichiro Hayashi[1], Kazunari Misawa[2],
and Kensaku Mori[1,3,4(✉)]

[1] Graduate School of Informatics, Nagoya University, Nagoya, Japan
`rothhr@mori.m.is.nagoya-u.ac.jp, kensaku@is.nagoya-u.ac.jp`
[2] Aichi Cancer Center, Nagoya, Japan
[3] Information Technology Center, Nagoya University, Nagoya, Japan
[4] Research Center for Medical Bigdata, National Institute of Informatics,
Tokyo, Japan

Abstract. Recent advances in deep learning, like 3D fully convolutional networks (FCNs), have improved the state-of-the-art in dense semantic segmentation of medical images. However, most network architectures require severely downsampling or cropping the images to meet the memory limitations of today's GPU cards while still considering enough context in the images for accurate segmentation. In this work, we propose a novel approach that utilizes auto-context to perform semantic segmentation at higher resolutions in a multi-scale pyramid of stacked 3D FCNs. We train and validate our models on a dataset of manually annotated abdominal organs and vessels from 377 clinical CT images used in gastric surgery, and achieve promising results with close to 90% Dice score on average. For additional evaluation, we perform separate testing on datasets from different sources and achieve competitive results, illustrating the robustness of the model and approach.

1 Introduction

Multi-organ segmentation has attracted considerable interest over the years. The recent success of deep learning-based classification and segmentation methods has triggered widespread applications of deep learning-based semantic segmentation in medical imaging [1,2]. Many methods focused on the segmentation of single organs like the prostate [1], liver [3], or pancreas [4,5]. Deep learning-based multi-organ segmentation in abdominal CT has also been approached recently in works like [6,7]. Most of these methods are based on variants of fully convolutional networks (FCNs) [8] that either employ 2D convolutions on orthogonal cross-sections in a slice-by-slice fashion [3–5,9] or 3D convolutions [1,2,7]. A common feature of these segmentation methods is that they are able to extract features useful for image segmentation directly from the training imaging data,

© Springer Nature Switzerland AG 2018
A. F. Frangi et al. (Eds.): MICCAI 2018, LNCS 11073, pp. 417–425, 2018.
https://doi.org/10.1007/978-3-030-00937-3_48

which is crucial for the success of deep learning. This avoids the need for hand-crafting features that are suitable for detection of individual organs.

However, most network architectures require severely downsampling or cropping the images for 3D processing to meet the memory limitations of today's GPU cards [1,7] while still considering enough context in the images for accurate segmentation of organs.

In this work, we propose a multi-scale 3D FCN approach that utilizes a scale-space pyramid with auto-context to perform semantic image segmentation at a higher resolution while also considering large contextual information from lower resolution levels. We train our models on a large dataset of manually annotated abdominal organs and vessels from pre-operative clinical computed tomography (CT) images used in gastric surgery and evaluate them on a completely unseen dataset from a different hospital, achieving a promising performance compared to the state-of-the-art.

Our approach is shown schematically in Fig. 1. We are influenced by classical scale-space pyramid [10] and auto-context ideas [11] for integrating multi-scale and varying context information into our deep learning-based image segmentation method. Instead of having separate FCN pathways for each scale as explored in other work [12,13], we utilize the auto-context principle to fuse and integrate the information from different image scales and different amounts of context. This helps the 3D FCN to integrate the information of different image scales and image contexts at the same time. Our model can be trained end-to-end using modern deep learning frameworks. This is in contrast to previous work which utilized auto-context using a separately trained models for brain segmentation [13].

In summary, our contributions are (1) introduction of a multi-scale pyramid of 3D FCNs; (2) improved segmentation of fine structures at higher resolution; (3) end-to-end training of multi-scale pyramid FCNs showing improved performance and good learning properties. We perform a comprehensive evaluation on a large training and validation dataset, plus unseen testing on data from different hospitals and public sources, showing promising generalizability.

2   Methods

2.1   3D Fully Convolutional Networks

Convolutional neural networks (CNN) have the ability to solve challenging classification tasks in a data-driven manner. Fully convolutional networks (FCNs) are an extension to CNNs that have made it feasible to train models for pixel-wise semantic segmentation in an end-to-end fashion [8]. In FCNs, feature learning is purely driven by the data and segmentation task at hand and the network architecture. Given a training set of images and labels $\mathbf{S} = \{(X_n, L_n),\ n = 1, \ldots, N\}$, where X_n denotes a CT image and L_n a ground truth label image, the model can train to minimize a loss function $\mathcal{L}$ in order to optimize the FCN model $f(I, \Theta)$, where Θ denotes the network parameters, including the convolutional kernel weights for hierarchical feature extraction.

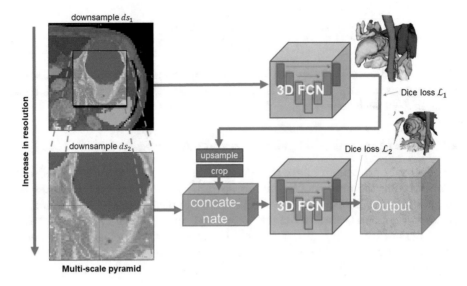

Fig. 1. Multi-scale pyramid of 3D fully convolutional networks (FCNs) for multi-organ segmentation. The lower-resolution-level 3D FCN predictions are upsampled, cropped and concatenated with the inputs of a higher resolution 3D FCN. The Dice loss is used for optimization at each level and training is performed end-to-end.

While efficient implementations of 3D convolutions and growing GPU memory have made it possible to deploy FCN on 3D biomedical imaging data [1,2], image volumes are in practice often cropped and downsampled in order for the network to access enough context to learn an effective semantic segmentation model while still fitting into memory. Our employed network model is inspired by the fully convolutional type 3D U-Net architecture proposed in Çiçek et al. [2].

The 3D U-Net architecture is based on U-Net proposed in [14] and consists of analysis and synthesis paths with four resolution levels each. It utilizes deconvolution [8] (also called transposed convolutions) to remap the lower resolution and more abstract feature maps within the network to the denser space of the input images. This operation allows for efficient dense voxel-to-voxel predictions. Each resolution level in the analysis path contains two $3 \times 3 \times 3$ convolutional layers, each followed by rectified linear units (ReLU) and a $2 \times 2 \times 2$ max pooling with strides of two in each dimension. In the synthesis path, the convolutional layers are replaced by deconvolutions of $2 \times 2 \times 2$ with strides of two in each dimension. These are followed by two $3 \times 3 \times 3$ convolutions, each followed by ReLU activations. Furthermore, 3D U-Net employs shortcut (or skip) connections from layers of equal resolution in the analysis path to provide higher-resolution features to the synthesis path [2]. The last layer contains a $1 \times 1 \times 1$ convolution that reduces the number of output channels to the number of class labels K. This architecture has over 19 million learnable parameters and can be trained to minimize the average Dice loss derived from the binary case in [1]:

$$\mathcal{L}(X, \Theta, L) = -\frac{1}{K} \sum_{k=1}^{K} \left(\frac{2 \sum_i^N p_{i,k} l_{i,k}}{\sum_i^N p_{i,k} + \sum_i^N l_{i,k}} \right). \tag{1}$$

Here, $p_{i,k} \in [0, \ldots, 1]$ represents the continuous values of the *softmax* 3D prediction maps for each class label k of K and $l_{i,k}$ the corresponding ground truth value in L at each voxel i.

2.2 Multi-scale Auto-Context Pyramid Approach

To effectively process an image at higher resolutions, we propose a method that is inspired by the auto-context algorithm [11]. Our method both captures the context information at lower resolution downsampled images and learns more accurate segmentations from higher resolution images in two levels of a scale-space pyramid $\mathbf{F} = \{(f_s(X_s, \Theta_s)), \ s = 1, \ldots, S\}$, with S being the number of levels s in our multi-scale pyramid, and X_s being one of the multi-scale input subvolumes at each level s.

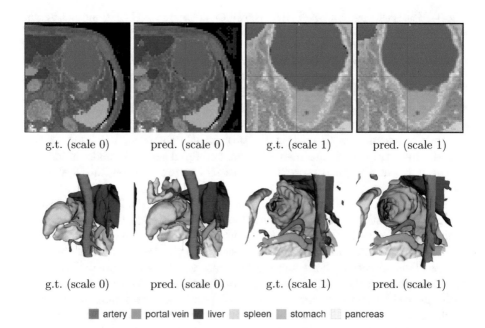

g.t. (scale 0)   pred. (scale 0)   g.t. (scale 1)   pred. (scale 1)

g.t. (scale 0)   pred. (scale 0)   g.t. (scale 1)   pred. (scale 1)

■ artery ■ portal vein ■ liver spleen ■ stomach pancreas

Fig. 2. Axial CT images and 3D surface rendering with ground truth (g.t.) and predictions overlaid. We show the two scales used in our experiments. Each scale's input is of size $64 \times 64 \times 64$ in this setting.

In the first level, the 3D FCN is trained on images of the lowest resolution in order to capture the largest amount of context, downsampled with a factor of $ds_1 = 2S$ and optimized using the Dice loss $\mathcal{L}_1$. This can be thought of as a form of deep supervision [15]. In the next level, we use the predicted segmentation maps as a second input channel to the 3D FCN while learning from the images at a higher resolution, downsampled by a factor of $ds_2 = ds_1/2$, and optimized using Dice loss $\mathcal{L}_2$. For input to this second level of the pyramid, the previous level prediction maps are upsampled by a factor of 2 and cropped in order to spatially align with the higher resolution levels. These predictions can then be fed together with the appropriately cropped image data as a second channel. This approach can be learned end-to-end using modern multi-GPU devices and deep learning frameworks with the total loss being $\mathcal{L}_{\text{total}} = \sum_{s=1}^{L} \mathcal{L}_s (X_s, \Theta_s, L_s)$. This idea is shown schematically in Fig. 1. The resulting segmentation masks for the two-level case are shown in Fig. 2. It can be observed that the second-level auto-context network markedly outperforms the first-level predictions and is able to segment structuress with improved detail, especially at the vessels.

2.3 Implementation and Training

We implement our approach in Keras[1] using the TensorFlow[2] backend. The Dice loss [3] is used for optimization with Adam and automatic differentiation for gradient computations. Batch normalization layers are inserted throughout the network, using a mini-batch size of three, sampled from different CT volumes of the training set. We use randomly extracted subvolumes of fixed size during training, such that at least one foreground voxel is at the center of each subvolume. On-the-fly data augmentation is used via random translations, rotations and elastic deformations similar to [2].

3   Experiments and Results

In our implementation, a constant input and output size of $64 \times 64 \times 64$ randomly cropped subvolumes is used for training in each level. For inference, we employ network reshaping [8] to more efficiently process the testing image with a larger input size while building up the full image in a tiling approach [2]. The resulting segmentation masks for both levels are shown in Fig. 3. It can be observed that the second-level auto-context network markedly outperforms the first-level predictions and is able to segment structures with improved detail. All experiments were performed using a DeepLearning BOX (GDEP Advance) with four NVIDIA Quadro P6000s with 24 GB memory each. Training of 20,000 iterations using this unoptimized implementation took several days, while inference on a full CT scan takes just a few minutes on one GPU card.

Data: Our data set includes 377 contrast-enhanced clinical CT images of the abdomen in the portal-venous phase used for pre-operative planning in gastric surgery. Each CT volume consists of 460–1,177 slices of 512×512 pixels. Voxel dimensions are $[0.59-0.98, 0.59-0.98, 0.5-1.0]$ mm. With $S = 2$, we downsample

---

[1] https://keras.io/.
[2] https://www.tensorflow.org/.

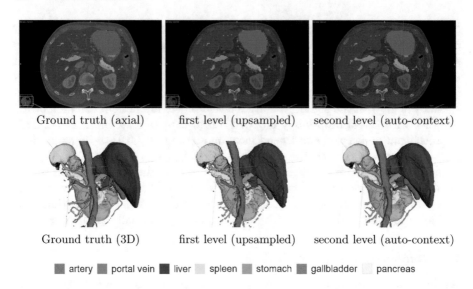

Ground truth (axial)   first level (upsampled)   second level (auto-context)

Ground truth (3D)   first level (upsampled)   second level (auto-context)

■ artery ■ portal vein ■ liver ▨ spleen ■ stomach ■ gallbladder ▨ pancreas

Fig. 3. Axial CT images and 3D surface rendering of predictions from two multi-scale levels in comparison with ground truth annotations. In particular, the vessels are segmented more completely and in greater detail in the second level, which utilizes auto-context information in its prediction.

each volume by a factor of $ds_1 = 4$ in the first level and a factor of $ds_2 = 2$ in the second level. A random 90/10% split of 340/37 patients is used for training and testing the network. We achieve Dice similarity scores for each organ labeled in the testing cases as summarized in Table 1. We list the performance for the first level and second level models when utilizing auto-context trained separately or end-to-end, and compare to using no auto-context in the second level. This shows the impact of using or not using the lower resolution auto-context channel at the higher resolution input while training from the same input resolution from scratch. In our case, each L_n contains $K = 8$ labels consisting of the manual annotations of seven anatomical structures (artery, portal vein, liver, spleen, stomach, gallbladder, pancreas), plus background.

Table 2 compares our results to recent literature and also displays the result using an unseen testing dataset from a different hospital consisting of 129 cases from a distinct research study. Furthermore, we test our model on a public data set of 20 contrast-enhanced CT scans.[3]

---

[3] We utilize the 20 training cases of the VISCERAL data set (http://www.visceral.eu/benchmarks/anatomy3-open) as our test set.

Table 1. Comparison of different levels of our model. End-to-end training gives a statistically significant improvement ($p < 0.001$).

Dice (%)	Artery	Vein	Liver	Spleen	Stomach	Gall.	Pancreas	Avg.
Level 1: initial (low res)								
Avg	75.4	64.0	95.4	94.0	93.7	80.2	79.8	83.2
Std	3.9	5.4	1.0	0.8	7.6	15.5	8.5	06.1
Min	67.4	41.3	91.5	92.6	48.4	27.3	49.7	59.7
Max	82.3	70.9	96.4	95.8	96.5	93.5	90.6	89.4
Level 2: auto-context								
Avg	82.5	76.8	96.7	96.6	95.9	**84.4**	83.4	88.1
Std	4.1	6.4	1.0	0.7	8.0	14.0	8.4	6.1
Min	73.3	46.3	92.9	94.4	48.1	28.0	53.9	62.4
Max	90.0	83.5	97.9	98.0	98.7	96.0	93.4	93.9
End-to-end: auto-context (high-res)								
Avg	**83.0**	**79.4**	**96.9**	**97.2**	**96.2**	83.6	**86.7**	**89.0**
Std	4.4	6.7	1.0	1.0	5.9	17.1	7.4	6.2
Min	73.2	50.2	93.5	94.9	61.4	29.7	60.0	66.1
Max	91.0	87.7	98.3	98.7	98.7	96.4	95.2	95.1
Level 2: no auto-context (high-res)								
Avg	69.9	72.8	86.7	90.9	3.8	73.4	77.0	67.8
Std	6.2	7.0	6.4	5.3	1.3	22.5	10.8	8.5
Min	59.5	47.1	69.9	75.7	0.7	7.8	36.1	42.4
Max	82.1	82.9	95.7	97.0	7.4	95.9	90.9	78.8

*Best average performance is shown in **bold**.

Table 2. We compare our model trained in an end-to-end fashion to recent work on multi-organ segmentation. [9] is using a 2D FCN approach with a majority voting scheme, while [7] employs 3D FCN architectures. Furthermore, we list our performance on an unseen testing dataset from a different hospital and on the public Visceral dataset without any re-training and compare it to the current challenge leaderboard (LB) best performance for each organ. Note that this table is incomprehensive and direct comparison to the literature is always difficult due to the different datasets and evaluation schemes involved.

Dice (%)	Train/Test	Artery	Vein	Liver	Spleen	Stomach	Gall.	Pancreas	Avg.
Ours (end-to-end)	340/37	83.0	79.4	96.9	97.2	96.2	83.6	86.7	89.0
Unseen test	none/129	-	-	95.3	93.6	-	80.8	75.7	86.3
Gibson et al. [7]	72 (8-CV)	-	-	92	-	83	-	66	80.3
Zhou et al. [9][a]	228/12	73.8	22.4	93.7	86.8	62.4	59.6	56.1	65.0
Hu et al. [6]	140 (CV)	-	-	96.0	94.2	-	-	-	95.1
Visceral (LB)	20/10	-	-	95.0	91.1	-	70.6	58.5	78.8
Visceral (ours)[b]	none/20	-	-	94.0	87.2	-	68.2	61.9	77.8

[a]Dice score estimated from Intersection over Union (Jaccard index).
[b]At the time of writing, the testing evaluation servers of the challenge were not available anymore for submitting results.

4   Discussion and Conclusion

The multi-scale auto-context approach presented in this paper provides a simple yet effective method for employing 3D FCNs in medical-imaging settings. No post-processing was applied to any of the network outputs. The improved performance in our approach is effective for all organs tested (apart from the gallbladder, where the differences are not significant). Note that we used different datasets (from different hospitals and scanners) for separate testing. This experiment illustrates our method's generalizability and robustness to differences in image quality and populations. Running the algorithms at a quarter to half of the original resolution improved performance and efficiency in this application. While this method could be extended to using a multi-scale pyramid with the original resolution as the final level, we found that the added computational burden did not add significantly to the segmentation performance. The main improvement comes from utilizing a very coarse image (downsampled by a factor of four) in an effective manner. In this work, we utilized a 3D U-Net-like model for each level of the image pyramid. However, the proposed auto-context approach should in principle also work well for other 3D CNN/FCN architectures and 2D and 3D image modalities.

In conclusion, we showed that an auto-context approach can result in improved semantic segmentation results for 3D FCNs based on the 3D U-Net architecture. While the low-resolution part of the model is able to benefit from a larger context in the input image, the higher resolution auto-context part of the model can segment the image with greater detail, resulting in better overall dense predictions. Training both levels end-to-end resulted in improved performance.

Acknowledgments. This work was supported by MEXT KAKENHI (26108006, 17H00867, 17K20099) and the JPSP International Bilateral Collaboration Grant.

References

1. Milletari, F., Navab, N., Ahmadi, S.A.: V-net: fully convolutional neural networks for volumetric medical image segmentation. In: 3D Vision (3DV), pp. 565–571. IEEE (2016)
2. Çiçek, Ö., Abdulkadir, A., Lienkamp, S.S., Brox, T., Ronneberger, O.: 3D U-Net: learning dense volumetric segmentation from sparse annotation. In: Ourselin, S., Joskowicz, L., Sabuncu, M.R., Unal, G., Wells, W. (eds.) MICCAI 2016 Part II. LNCS, vol. 9901, pp. 424–432. Springer, Cham (2016). https://doi.org/10.1007/978-3-319-46723-8_49
3. Christ, P.F., et al.: Automatic Liver and lesion segmentation in CT using cascaded fully convolutional neural networks and 3D conditional random fields. In: Ourselin, S., Joskowicz, L., Sabuncu, M.R., Unal, G., Wells, W. (eds.) MICCAI 2016 Part II. LNCS, vol. 9901, pp. 415–423. Springer, Cham (2016). https://doi.org/10.1007/978-3-319-46723-8_48

4. Roth, H.R., Lu, L., Farag, A., Sohn, A., Summers, R.M.: Spatial aggregation of holistically-nested networks for automated pancreas segmentation. In: Ourselin, S., Joskowicz, L., Sabuncu, M.R., Unal, G., Wells, W. (eds.) MICCAI 2016 Part II. LNCS, vol. 9901, pp. 451–459. Springer, Cham (2016). https://doi.org/10.1007/978-3-319-46723-8_52

5. Zhou, Y., Xie, L., Shen, W., Wang, Y., Fishman, E.K., Yuille, A.L.: A fixed-point model for pancreas segmentation in abdominal CT scans. In: Descoteaux, M., Maier-Hein, L., Franz, A., Jannin, P., Collins, D.L., Duchesne, S. (eds.) MICCAI 2017 Part I. LNCS, vol. 10433, pp. 693–701. Springer, Cham (2017). https://doi.org/10.1007/978-3-319-66182-7_79

6. Hu, P., Wu, F., Peng, J., Bao, Y., Chen, F., Kong, D.: Automatic abdominal multi-organ segmentation using deep convolutional neural network and time-implicit level sets. Int. J. Comput. Assist. Radiol. Surg. **12**(3), 399–411 (2017)

7. Gibson, E., et al.: Towards image-guided pancreas and biliary endoscopy: automatic multi-organ segmentation on abdominal CT with dense dilated networks. In: Descoteaux, M., Maier-Hein, L., Franz, A., Jannin, P., Collins, D.L., Duchesne, S. (eds.) MICCAI 2017 Part I. LNCS, vol. 10433, pp. 728–736. Springer, Cham (2017). https://doi.org/10.1007/978-3-319-66182-7_83

8. Long, J., Shelhamer, E., Darrell, T.: Fully convolutional networks for semantic segmentation. In: IEEE CVPR, pp. 3431–3440 (2015)

9. Zhou, X., Takayama, R., Wang, S., Hara, T., Fujita, H.: Deep learning of the sectional appearances of 3D CT images for anatomical structure segmentation based on an FCN voting method. Med. Phys. **44**, 5221–5233 (2017)

10. Adelson, E.H., Anderson, C.H., Bergen, J.R., Burt, P.J., Ogden, J.M.: Pyramid methods in image processing. RCA Eng. **29**(6), 33–41 (1984)

11. Tu, Z., Bai, X.: Auto-context and its application to high-level vision tasks and 3D brain image segmentation. IEEE Trans. Pattern Anal. Mach. Intell. **32**(10), 1744–1757 (2010)

12. Chen, L.C., Yang, Y., Wang, J., Xu, W., Yuille, A.L.: Attention to scale: scale-aware semantic image segmentation. In: Proceedings of the IEEE Conference on Computer Vision and Pattern Recognition, pp. 3640–3649 (2016)

13. Salehi, S.S.M., Erdogmus, D., Gholipour, A.: Auto-context convolutional neural network (auto-net) for brain extraction in magnetic resonance imaging. IEEE Trans. Med. Imaging **36**(11), 2319–2330 (2017)

14. Ronneberger, O., Fischer, P., Brox, T.: U-Net: convolutional networks for biomedical image segmentation. In: Navab, N., Hornegger, J., Wells, W.M., Frangi, A.F. (eds.) MICCAI 2015 Part III. LNCS, vol. 9351, pp. 234–241. Springer, Cham (2015). https://doi.org/10.1007/978-3-319-24574-4_28

15. Lee, C.Y., Xie, S., Gallagher, P., Zhang, Z., Tu, Z.: Deeply-supervised nets. In: Artificial Intelligence and Statistics, pp. 562–570 (2015)

3D U-JAPA-Net: Mixture of Convolutional Networks for Abdominal Multi-organ CT Segmentation

Hideki Kakeya[1(✉)], Toshiyuki Okada[1], and Yukio Oshiro[2]

[1] Faculty of Engineering, Information and Systems,
University of Tsukuba, Tsukuba, Japan
kake@iit.tsukuba.ac.jp
[2] Ibaraki Medical Center, Tokyo Medical University, Ami, Japan

Abstract. This paper introduces a new type of deep learning scheme for fully-automated abdominal multi-organ CT segmentation using transfer learning. Convolutional neural network with 3D U-net is a strong tool to achieve volumetric image segmentation. The drawback of 3D U-net is that its judgement is based only on the local volumetric data, which leads to errors in categorization. To overcome this problem we propose 3D U-JAPA-net, which uses not only the raw CT data but also the probabilistic atlas of organs to reflect the information on organ locations. In the first phase of training, a 3D U-net is trained based on the conventional method. In the second phase, expert 3D U-nets for each organ are trained intensely around the locations of the organs, where the initial weights are transferred from the 3D U-net obtained in the first phase. Segmentation in the proposed method consists of three phases. First rough locations of organs are estimated by probabilistic atlas. Second, the trained expert 3D U-nets are applied in the focused locations. Post-process to remove debris is applied in the final phase. We test the performance of the proposed method with 47 CT data and it achieves higher DICE scores than the conventional 2D U-net and 3D U-net. Also, a positive effect of transfer learning is confirmed by comparing the proposed method with that without transfer learning.

Keywords: Convolutional neural networks · Deep learning · Transfer learning
U-net · 3D U-net · Multi-organ segmentation · Mixture of experts

1 Introduction

Multilayer neural networks attracted great attention in the 1980s and in the early 1990s. The most influential work was the invention of error back-propagation learning [1], which is still used in current deep neural networks. During those years several types of network architectures were tried, such as Neocognitron [2] and mixture of experts [3]. After the long ice age of neural networks from the late 1990s to around 2010, the idea of deep convolutional neural networks (CNNs), which inherited some features of Neocognitron, was proposed [4] and realized unprecedented performance in the area of image recognition. Owing to the rapid progress of graphical processor units (GPUs),

© Springer Nature Switzerland AG 2018
A. F. Frangi et al. (Eds.): MICCAI 2018, LNCS 11073, pp. 426–433, 2018.
https://doi.org/10.1007/978-3-030-00937-3_49

fast training of deep convolutional neural networks has been enabled with a low-cost PC, which leads to the current boom of deep learning.

Deep learning using a CNN can be a strong tool in the area of medical imaging also. Since the proposal of U-net [5], which is based on fully convolutional network (FCN) [6], deep CNNs have been applied to various biomedical image segmentation tasks and have outperformed the conventional algorithms. To apply deep CNNs to 3D volume data, 3D U-net has been proposed [7], where 3-dimensional convolutions are applied to attain volumetric segmentation. 3D U-net is easily applied to multi-organ CT segmentation, which is an important pre-process for computer-aided diagnosis and therapy.

The drawback of 3D U-net is that its judgement is based only on the local volumetric data, which often leads to errors in multi-organ segmentation. Some modifications of learning have been tried to overcome this problem. For example, Roth et al. proposed a hierarchical 3D FCN that takes a coarse-to-fine approach, where the network is trained to delineate the organ of interest roughly in the first stage and is trained for detailed segmentation in the second stage [8]. A probabilistic approach can be merged with FCNs [9], but the performance is not improved significantly.

Before the rise of deep learning, several approaches to multiple organ segmentation from 3D medical images had been proposed. These approaches commonly utilize a number of radiological images with manual tracing of organs, called atlases, as training data, and can be classified into multi-atlas label fusion, machine learning, and statistical atlas approaches.

Statistical atlas approaches have been most commonly applied to abdominal organ segmentation. Explicit prior models constructed from atlases, such as the probabilistic atlas (PA) [10, 11] and statistical shape models [12, 13] are used in these approaches.

Okada et al. proposed abdominal multi-organ segmentation method using conditional shape-location and unsupervised intensity priors (S-CSL-UI), assuming that variation of shape and location of abdominal organs were constrained by the organs whose segmentation was stable and relatively accurate [14]. The method using hierarchical modeling interrelation of organs improved the accuracy and stability of segmentation, and it demonstrated effective reduction of the search space. These methods, however, have been outperformed by CNNs.

In this paper, we propose a new 3D U-net learning scheme, which we name 3D U-JAPA-net (Judgement Assisted by PA). The proposed scheme utilizes not only CNNs but also PA information to overcome the drawbacks of the conventional 2D U-net and 3D U-net. Also, the proposed method comprises transfer learning [15] and mixture of experts to make effective use of PA information so that more accurate multi-organ segmentation may be attained.

2   Methods

The goal in this paper is to realize fully-automated segmentation of 8 abdominal organs: liver; spleen; left and right kidneys; pancreas; gallbladder (GB); aorta; and inferior vena cava (IVC). For this purpose, we compare the performances of the following 5 methods: S-CSL-UI; 2D U-net; 3D U-net; Mixture of 3D U-nets; and 3D U-JAPA-net, which we propose in this paper.

A U-net consists of a contracting path and an expansive path. The contracting path follows the typical architecture of a convolutional network. It consists of repeated application of two 3×3 convolutions, each followed by a rectified linear unit (ReLU) and a 2×2 max pooling operation. At each down-sampling step, the number of feature channels is doubled. Every step in the expansive path consists of an up-sampling of the feature map followed by a 2×2 up-convolution that halves the number of feature channels, a concatenation with the feature map from the contracting path, and two 3×3 convolutions, each followed by a ReLU. Cropping is needed due to the loss of border pixels in every convolution. At the final layer, a 1×1 convolution is used to map each 64-component feature vector to the desired number of classes.

3D U-net is a simple expansion of 2D U-net, where both convolution and max pooling operates in 3 dimensions like $3 \times 3 \times 3$ or $2 \times 2 \times 2$. In [7], batch normalization (BN) [16] is introduced before each ReLU. Though 3D U-net can reflect the 3D structure of CT data, size of calculation becomes huge when the input data size is large.

3D U-JAPA-net, which we introduce here, is an expansion of 3D U-net. The learning scheme of 3D U-JAPA-net is shown in Fig. 1.

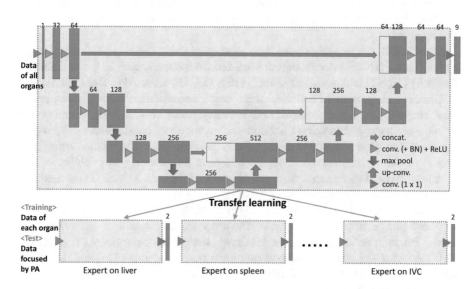

Fig. 1. Learning scheme of 3D U-JAPA-net. Blue boxes represent feature maps and the numbers of feature maps are denoted on top of each box. (Color figure online)

In the first learning phase, a 3D U-net with 9 output layers corresponding each class (8 organs and background) is trained using the whole data inside the bounding boxes of all organs. Also, we prepare PA for each organ based on the training data with the method in [14]. After the first training converges, the weights of this network are transferred to 8 expert 3D U-nets for each organ, each of which has 2 output layers (the organ and the background). Therefore the initial weights of 8 networks are the same except for those connected to the final output layer. In the second learning phase, each expert 3D U-net specialized for each organ accepts volumetric data including the corresponding organ, and the weights are modified by the gradient descent method.

In the test phase, the trained network specialized for each organ accepts data including the voxels whose PA values of that organ are non-zero. If the output "organ" is larger than the output "background" in the final layer, that voxel is labeled as part of that organ.

To see the effect of transfer learning in the above scheme, we also test the system where the first learning phase is removed from 3D U-JAPA-net, which means that each expert network starts from random weights before training.

Since the judgement is given by voxel unit in the U-net based systems, debris emerges in the result. We apply largest component selection as the post-process to remove debris for all the U-net based systems.

3   Experiments and Results

We compared the performances of the following 5 methods: S-CSL-UI; 2D U-net; 3D U-net; Mixture of 3D U-nets for each organ without transfer learning (3D M-U-nets); and 3D U-JAPA-net.

Each method was tested to segment 8 abdominal organs: liver; spleen; left and right kidneys; pancreas; GB; aorta; and IVC. We used 47 CT data from 47 patients with normal organs obtained in the late arterial phase at the same hospital and applied two-fold cross-validations to evaluate the performance of each method. The resolution of each CT slice image was 512×512 pixels. Among 47 CT data, 9 data had 159 slices and the voxel size was $0.625 \times 0.625 \times 1.25$ [mm^3]. The voxel size of other 37 data was $0.781 \times 0.781 \times 0.625$ [mm^3] and the numbers of slices were between 305 and 409. The last one, consisting of 345 slices, had $0.674 \times 0.674 \times 0.625$ [mm^3] voxels.

For 2D U-net, the slice images were first down-sampled to 256×256 pixels. Then the same algorithm in [5] was used, where 3×3 convolutions were applied twice in each layer and the max pooling and up-conversion were applied 4 times. For 3D U-net, the input to the network was a $132 \times 132 \times 116$ voxel tile of the image with 1 channel. After that, the same algorithm in [7] was used, where $3 \times 3 \times 3$ convolutions were applied twice in each layer, while the max pooling and up-conversion were applied 3 times. The output of the final layer becomes $44 \times 44 \times 28$ voxels due to the repeated truncation in every convolution.

We applied dropout of connections in the bottom layer to avoid over-fitting both in 2D U-net and 3D U-net. Data augmentation was not applied in this experiment for simplicity. Also, the training data and the test data are made so that the output voxels may not overlap in order to reduce the calculation time.

As for 3D U-JAPA-net, the above 3D U-net was used both in the first and the second stages of training. When the weights were transferred from the trained network to the expert network for each organ, the connections between the last layer and the second last layer were randomized, for the numbers of output layers were different between the 3D U-net in the first stage of training and the expert 3D U-nets for each organ.

All the U-net components were implemented with TensorFlow framework [17]. The PC we used was composed of Intel Core i7-8700 K CPU, 32 GB main memory, and NVIDIA GeForce GTX 1080 Ti GPU with 11 GB video memory. The detail of training was as follows: training epochs = 30; learning rate = 1.0×10^{-4}; batch size = 3. It took 2.5 h to train 2D-U-net with this PC. As for 3D U-net, it took 16 h to train all organs and it took between 40 and 130 min to train each organ respectively except for the liver, which took 9.5 h to train because of its large size.

Figure 2 shows the DICE scores given by the 5 segmentation methods. The results of paired t-tests between the proposed method and the other methods are indicated in the figure. As the figure shows, the proposed method attains notably better performance than the conventional methods. The performance given by the mixture of experts without transfer learning is poorer, which shows that transfer learning is effective to attain high DICE scores.

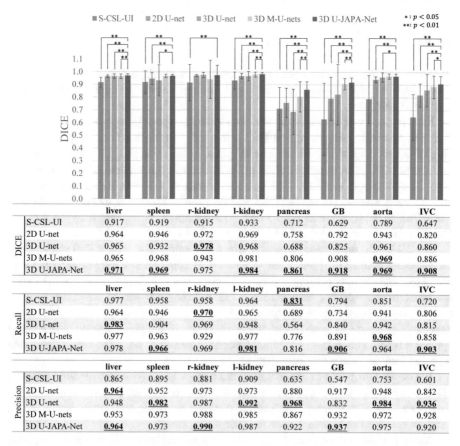

		liver	spleen	r-kidney	l-kidney	pancreas	GB	aorta	IVC
DICE	S-CSL-UI	0.917	0.919	0.915	0.933	0.712	0.629	0.789	0.647
	2D U-net	0.964	0.946	0.972	0.969	0.758	0.792	0.943	0.820
	3D U-net	0.965	0.932	**0.978**	0.968	0.688	0.825	0.961	0.860
	3D M-U-nets	0.965	0.968	0.943	0.981	0.806	0.908	**0.969**	0.886
	3D U-JAPA-Net	**0.971**	**0.969**	0.975	**0.984**	**0.861**	**0.918**	**0.969**	**0.908**

		liver	spleen	r-kidney	l-kidney	pancreas	GB	aorta	IVC
Recall	S-CSL-UI	0.977	0.958	0.958	0.964	**0.831**	0.794	0.851	0.720
	2D U-net	0.964	0.946	**0.970**	0.965	0.689	0.734	0.941	0.806
	3D U-net	**0.983**	0.904	0.969	0.948	0.564	0.840	0.942	0.815
	3D M-U-nets	0.977	0.963	0.929	0.977	0.776	0.891	**0.968**	0.858
	3D U-JAPA-Net	0.978	**0.966**	0.969	**0.981**	0.816	**0.906**	0.964	**0.903**

		liver	spleen	r-kidney	l-kidney	pancreas	GB	aorta	IVC
Precision	S-CSL-UI	0.865	0.895	0.881	0.909	0.635	0.547	0.753	0.601
	2D U-net	**0.964**	0.952	0.973	0.973	0.880	0.917	0.948	0.842
	3D U-net	0.948	**0.982**	0.987	**0.992**	**0.968**	0.832	**0.984**	**0.936**
	3D M-U-nets	0.953	0.973	0.988	0.985	0.867	0.932	0.972	0.928
	3D U-JAPA-Net	**0.964**	0.973	**0.990**	0.987	0.922	**0.937**	0.975	0.920

Fig. 2. Results of eight abdominal organ segmentation by five methods. Bold numbers are the highest DICE/recall/precision rates for each organ.

Figure 3 shows an example of segmentation results, which effectively demonstrate usefulness of the proposed method. 3D U-JAPA-net can recall part of pancreas and GB that other U-net based systems miss. Also, the leakage, which stands out in S-CSL-UI, is not apparent in the other methods including 3D U-JAPA-net.

The effect of increase in training data was tested by comparing 2-fold and 4-fold cross-validations of 3D U-JAPA-net. The result is shown in Table 1. The DICE score is improved significantly in the segmentation of pancreas ($p = 0.012$) by applying 4-fold cross-validation.

The performances of the proposed method and the prior method [8], which is also a modified version of 3D U-net, are compared in Table 2. DICE scores obtained by the proposed method are distinctively higher, which indicates the excellence of the proposed method.

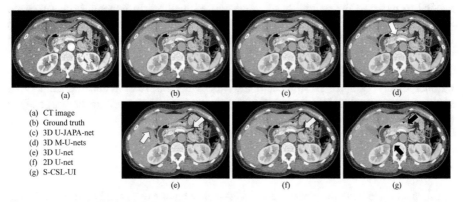

(a) CT image
(b) Ground truth
(c) 3D U-JAPA-net
(d) 3D M-U-nets
(e) 3D U-net
(f) 2D U-net
(g) S-CSL-UI

Fig. 3. An illustrative segmentation results obtained by five methods. White arrows show the failed regions by the conventional priors. Black arrows show the leakages by the conventional priors. (Color figure online)

Table 1. Comparison of 3D U-JAPA-net DICE scores obtained by two-fold and four-fold cross-validations.

	Liver	Spleen	r-kidney	l-kidney	Pancreas	GB	Aorta	IVC
2-fold	0.971	0.969	0.975	0.984	0.861]*	0.918	0.969	0.908
4-fold	0.971	0.969	0.986	0.985	0.882]*	0.915	0.966	0.907

Table 2. Comparison of two modified versions of 3D U-net.

		Roth et al. [8]			3D U-JAPA-net		
		Liver	Spleen	Pancreas	Liver	Spleen	Pancreas
DICE	Mean	0.954	0.928	0.822	0.971	0.969	0.882
	Std	0.020	0.080	0.102	0.014	0.014	0.070
	Median	0.960	0.954	0.845	0.974	0.973	0.901
Subjects		150 (testing)			47 (4-fold cross validation)		

4   Discussion

When 2D U-net and 3D U-net are compared, 2D U-net is good at segmenting larger organs, while 3D U-net is adept at segmenting smaller organs. Since 2D U-net covers larger areas in a single slice, it can grasp wider areas with a single shot, which leads to the above characteristic of performance.

3D U-JAPA-net overcomes the drawback of 3D U-net, which covers a smaller area in each slice, with the help of PA and outperforms both 2D U-net and 3D U-net in segmentation of almost all organs. Improvement by 3D U-JAPA net is especially significant in segmentation of pancreas, GB, and IVC, which have been difficult to segment properly for the conventional methods. The effect of transfer learning is significant in these organs, which shows the validity of the proposed method.

The number of data used here is limited and further study with a larger data size is needed to increase the reliability of the proposed method. In general, however, deep neural networks can attain better performance when the number of training data increases. A higher DICE score may be obtained if we use a larger data set for training with the proposed method.

In this paper PA has been used to see where the value is non-zero or not, for the number of CT samples is small and the values are discrete. When the number of samples is increased and the probabilities become more reliable, arithmetic usage of the probability values can raise DICE scores.

5   Conclusion

In this paper, we have proposed 3D U-JAPA-net, which uses not only the raw CT data but also the probabilistic atlas of organs to reflect the information on organ locations to realize fully-automated abdominal multi-organ CT segmentation. As a result of the 2-fold cross-validation with 47 CT data from 47 patients, the proposed method has marked significantly higher DICE scores than the conventional 2D U-net and 3D U-net in the segmentation of most organs.

The proposed method can be easily implemented for those who can use TensorFlow or similar deep learning tools, for all needed to be done in the proposed method is to make a probabilistic atlas, train a 3D U-net, copy the trained weights to the mixture of 3D U-nets, and train those 3D U-nets. The method described here is worth a trial for those who want to make a reliable fully-automated multi-organ segmentation system with little effort.

Acknowledgements. This research is partially supported by the Grant-in-Aid for Scientific Research, JSPS, Japan, Grant number: 17H00750.

References

1. Rumelhart, D.E., Hinton, G.E., Williams, R.J.: Learning representations by back-propagating errors. Nature **323**(6088), 533–536 (1986)
2. Fukushima, K., Miyake, S., Ito, T.: Neocognitron: a neural network model for a mechanism of visual pattern recognition. IEEE Trans. Syst. Man Cybern. **SMC-13**(3), 826–834 (1983)
3. Jacobs, R.A., Jordan, M.I., Nowlan, S.J., Hinton, G.E.: Adaptive mixtures of local experts. Neural Comput. **3**(1), 79–87 (1991)
4. Krizhevsky, A., Sutskever, I., Hinton, G.E.: ImageNet classification with deep convolutional neural networks. Adv. Neural. Inf. Process. Syst. **1**, 1097–1105 (2012)
5. Ronneberger, O., Fischer, P., Brox, T.: U-Net: convolutional networks for biomedical image segmentation. In: Navab, N., Hornegger, J., Wells, W.M., Frangi, A.F. (eds.) MICCAI 2015. LNCS, vol. 9351, pp. 234–241. Springer, Cham (2015). https://doi.org/10.1007/978-3-319-24574-4_28
6. Long, J., Shelhamer, E., Darrell, T.: Fully convolutional networks for semantic segmentation. arXiv:1411.4038 (2014)
7. Çiçek, Ö., Abdulkadir, A., Lienkamp, S.S., Brox, T., Ronneberger, O.: 3D U-Net: learning dense volumetric segmentation from sparse annotation. In: Ourselin, S., Joskowicz, L., Sabuncu, M., Unal, G., Wells, W. (eds.) MICCAI 2016, LNCS, vol. 9901, pp. 424–432. Springer, Cham (2016). https://doi.org/10.1007/978-3-319-46723-8_49
8. Roth, H., et al.: Hierarchical 3D fully convolutional networks for multi-organ segmentation. arXiv:1704.06382 (2017)
9. Yang, Y., Oda, M., Roth, H., Kitasaka, T., Misawa, K., Mori, K.: Study on utilization of 3D fully convolutional networks with fully connected conditional random field for automated multi-organ segmentation form CT volume. J. JSCAS **19**(4), 268–269 (2017)
10. Park, H., Bland, P.H., Meyer, C.R.: Construction of an abdominal probabilistic atlas and its application in segmentation. IEEE Trans. Med. Imag. **22**(4), 483–492 (2003)
11. Zhou, X., et al.: Constructing a probabilistic model for automated liver region segmentation using non-contrast Xray torso CT images. In: Larsen, R., Nielsen, M., Sporring, J. (eds.) MICCAI 2006, LNCS, vol. 4191, pp. 856–863. Springer, Berlin (2006). https://doi.org/10.1007/11866763_105
12. Heimann, T., Meinzer, H.-P.: Statistical shape models for 3D medical image segmentation: a review. Med. Image Anal. **13**(4), 543–563 (2009)
13. Lamecker, H., Lange, T., Seebaß, M.: Segmentation of the liver using a 3D statistical shape model. Technical report. Zuse Institute, Berlin (2004)
14. Okada, T., Linguraru, M.G., Hori, M., Summers, R.M., Tomiyama, N., Sato, Y.: Abdominal multi-organ segmentation from CT images using conditional shape–location and unsupervised intensity priors. Med. Image Anal. **26**(1), 1–18 (2015)
15. Pratt, L.Y.: Discriminability-based transfer between neural networks. NIPS Conf.: Adv. Neural Inf. Process. Syst. **5**, 204–211 (1993)
16. Ioffe, S., Szegedy, C.: Batch normalization: accelerating deep network training by reducing internal covariate shift. arXiv:1502.03167 (2015)
17. Abadi, M., Agarwal, A., Barham, P., et al.: TensorFlow: large-scale machine learning on heterogeneous systems. arXiv:1603.04467 (2016)

Training Multi-organ Segmentation Networks with Sample Selection by Relaxed Upper Confident Bound

Yan Wang[1(✉)], Yuyin Zhou[1], Peng Tang[2], Wei Shen[1,3], Elliot K. Fishman[4], and Alan L. Yuille[1]

[1] Johns Hopkins University, Baltimore, USA
ywang372@jhu.edu
[2] Huazhong University of Science and Technology, Wuhan, China
[3] Shanghai University, Shanghai, China
[4] Johns Hopkins University School of Medicine, Baltimore, USA

Abstract. Convolutional neural networks (CNNs), especially fully convolutional networks, have been widely applied to automatic medical image segmentation problems, e.g., multi-organ segmentation. Existing CNN-based segmentation methods mainly focus on looking for increasingly powerful network architectures, but pay less attention to data sampling strategies for training networks more effectively. In this paper, we present a simple but effective sample selection method for training multi-organ segmentation networks. Sample selection exhibits an exploitation-exploration strategy, i.e., exploiting hard samples and exploring less frequently visited samples. Based on the fact that very hard samples might have annotation errors, we propose a new sample selection policy, named Relaxed Upper Confident Bound (RUCB). Compared with other sample selection policies, e.g., Upper Confident Bound (UCB), it exploits a range of hard samples rather than being stuck with a small set of very hard ones, which mitigates the influence of annotation errors during training. We apply this new sample selection policy to training a multi-organ segmentation network on a dataset containing 120 abdominal CT scans and show that it boosts segmentation performance significantly.

1 Introduction

The field of medical image segmentation has made significant advances riding on the wave of deep convolutional neural networks (CNNs). Training convolutional deep networks (CNNs), especially fully convolutional networks (FCNs) [6], to automatically segment organs from medical images, such as CT scans, has become the dominant method, due to its outstanding segmentation performance. It also sheds lights to many clinical applications, such as diabetes inspection, organic cancer diagnosis, and surgical planning.

To approach human expert performance, existing CNN-based segmentation methods mainly focus on looking for increasingly powerful network architectures,

© Springer Nature Switzerland AG 2018
A. F. Frangi et al. (Eds.): MICCAI 2018, LNCS 11073, pp. 434–442, 2018.
https://doi.org/10.1007/978-3-030-00937-3_50

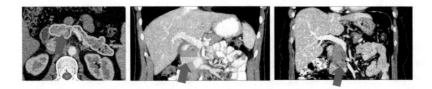

Fig. 1. Examples in a abdominal CT scans dataset which have annotations errors. Left: vein is included in pancreas segmentation; Middle & Right: missing pancreas header.

e.g., from plain networks to residual networks [5,10], from single stage networks to cascaded networks [13,16], from networks with a single output to networks with multiple side outputs [8,13]. However, there is much less study of how to select training samples from a fixed dataset to boost performance.

In the training procedure of current state-of-the-art CNN-based segmentation methods [4,11,12,17], training samples (2D slices for 2D FCNs and 3D sub-volumes for 3D FCNs) are randomly selected to iteratively update network parameters. However, some samples are much harder to segment than others, e.g., those which contain more organs with indistinct boundaries or with small sizes. It is known that using hard sample selection, or called bootstrapping[1], for training deep networks yields faster training, higher accuracy, or both [7,14,15]. Hard sample selection strategies for object detection [14] and classification [7,15] base their selection on the training loss for each sample, but some samples are hard due to annotation errors, as shown in Fig. 1. This problem may not be significant for the tasks in natural images, but for the tasks in medical images, such as multi-organ segmentation, which usually require very high accuracy, and thus the influence of annotation errors is more significant. Our experiments show that the training losses of samples (such as the samples in Fig. 1) with annotation errors are very large, and even larger than real hard samples.

To address this problem, we propose a new hard sample selection policy, named Relaxed Upper Confident Bound (RUCB). Upper Confident Bound (UCB) [2] is a classic policy to deal with *exploitation-exploration* trade-offs [1], e.g., exploiting hard samples and exploring less frequently visited samples for sample selection. UCB was used for object detection in natural images [3], but UCB is easy to be stuck with some samples with very large losses, as the selection procedure goes on. In our RUCB, we relax this policy by selecting hard samples from a larger range, but with higher probability for harder samples, rather than only selecting some very hard samples as the selection procedure goes on. RUCB can escape from being stuck with a small set of very hard samples, which can mitigate the influence of annotation errors. Experimental results on a dataset containing 120 abdominal CT scans show that the proposed Relaxed Upper Confident Bound policy boosts multi-organ segmentation performance significantly.

---

[1] In this paper, we only consider the bootstrapping procedure that selects samples from a fixed dataset.

2   Methodology

Given a 3D CT scan $V = (v_j, j = 1, ..., |V|)$, the goal of multi-organ segmentation is to predict the label of all voxels in the CT scan $\hat{Y} = (\hat{y}_j, j = 1, ..., |V|)$, where $\hat{y}_j \in \{0, 1, ..., |\mathcal{L}|\}$ denotes the predicted label for each voxel v_j, i.e., if v_j is predicted as a background voxel, then $\hat{y}_j = 0$; and if v_j is predicted as an organ in the organ space $\mathcal{L}$, then $\hat{y}_j = 1, ..., |\mathcal{L}|$. In this section, we first review the basics of the Upper Confident Bound policy [2], then elaborate our proposed Relaxed Upper Confident Bound policy on sample selection for multi-organ segmentation.

2.1   Upper Confident Bound (UCB)

The Upper Confident Bound (UCB) [2] policy is widely used to deal with the exploration versus exploitation dilemma, which arises in the multi-armed bandit (MAB) problem [9]. In a K-armed bandit problem, each arm $k = 1, ..., K$ is recorded by an unknown distribution associated with an unknown expectation. In each trial $t = 1, ..., T$, a learner takes an action to choose one of K alternatives $g(t) \in \{1, ..., K\}$ and collects a reward $x_{g(t)}^{(t)}$. The objective of this problem is to maximize the long-run cumulative expected reward $\sum_{t=1}^{T} x_{g(t)}^{(t)}$. But, as the expectations are unknown, the learner can only make a judgement based on the record of the past trails.

At trial t, the UCB selects the alternative k maximizing $\bar{x}_k + \sqrt{\frac{2 \ln n}{n_k}}$, where $\bar{x}_k = \sum_{t=1}^{n} x_k^{(t)}/n_k$ is the average reward obtained from the alternative k based on the previous trails, $x_k^{(t)} = 0$ if x_k is not chosen in the t-th trail. n_k is the number of times alternative k has been selected so far and n is the total number of trail done. The first term is the exploitation term, whose value is higher if the expected reward is larger; and the second term is the exploration term, which grows with the total number of actions that have been taken but shrinks with the number of times this particular action has been tried. At the beginning of the process, the exploration term dominates the selection, but as the selection procedure goes on, the one with the best expected reward will be chosen.

2.2   Relaxed Upper Confident Bound (RUCB) Boostrapping

Fully convolutional networks (FCNs) [6] are the most popular model for multi-organ segmentation. In a typical training procedure of an FCN, a sample (e.g., a 2D slice) is randomly selected in each iteration to calculate the model error and update model parameters. To train this FCN more effectively, a better strategy is to use hard sample selection, rather than random sample selection. As sample selection exhibits an exploitation-exploration trade-off, i.e., exploiting hard samples and exploring less frequently visited samples, we can directly apply UCB to select samples, where the reward of a sample is defined as the network loss function w.r.t. it. However, as the selection procedure goes on, only a small set of samples with the very large reward will be selected for next iteration according to UCB. The selected sample may not be a proper hard sample, but a sample with annotation errors, which inevitably exist in medical image data as well as other image data. Next, we introduce our Relaxed Upper Confident Bound (RUCB) policy to address this issue.

Procedure. We consider that training an FCN for multi-organ segmentation, where the input images are 2D slices from axial directions. Given a training set $S = \{(\mathbf{I}_i, \mathbf{Y}_i)\}_{i=1}^{M}$, where $\mathbf{I}_i$ and $\mathbf{Y}_i$ denote a 2D slice and its corresponding label map, and M is the number of the 2D slices, like the MAB problem, each slice $\mathbf{I}_i$ is set to be associated with the number of times it was selected n_i and the average reward obtained through the training $\bar{J}_i$. After training an initial FCN with randomly sampling slices from the training set, it is boostrapped several times by sampling hard and less frequently visited slices. In the sample selection procedure, rewards are assigned to each training slice once, then the next slice to train FCN is chosen by the proposed RUCB. The reward of this slice is fed into RUCB and the statistics in RUCB are updated. This process is then repeated to select another slice based on the updated statistics, until a max-iteration N is reached. Statistics are reset to 0 before beginning a new boostrapping phase since slices that are chosen in previous rounds may no longer be informative.

Relaxed Upper Confident Bound. We denote the corresponding label map of the input 2D slice $\mathbf{I}_i \subset \mathbb{R}^{H \times W}$ as $\mathbf{Y}_i = \{y_{i,j}\}_{j=1,\dots,H \times W}$. If $\mathbf{I}_i$ is selected to update the FCN in the t-th iteration, the reward obtained for $\mathbf{I}_i$ is computed by

$$\mathcal{J}_i^{(t)}(\mathbf{\Theta}) = -\frac{1}{H \times W} \left[\sum_{j=1}^{H \times W} \sum_{l=0}^{|\mathcal{L}|} \mathbf{1}\left(y_{i,j} = l\right) \log p_{i,j,l}^{(t)} \right], \qquad (1)$$

where $p_{i,j,l}^{(t)}$ is the probability that the label of the j-th pixel in the input slice is l, and $p_{i,j,l}^{(t)}$ is parameterized by the network parameter $\mathbf{\Theta}$. If $\mathbf{I}_i$ is not selected to update the FCN in the t-th iteration, $\mathcal{J}_i^{(t)}(\mathbf{\Theta}) = 0$. After n iterations, the next slice to be selected by UCB is the one maximizing $\bar{J}_i^{(n)} + \sqrt{2 \ln n / n_i}$, where $\bar{J}_i^{(n)} = \sum_{t=1}^{n} \mathcal{J}_i^{(t)}(\mathbf{\Theta})/n_i$.

Preliminary experiments show that reward defined above is usually around $[0, 0.35]$. The exploration term dominates the exploitation term. We thus normalize the reward to make a balance between exploitation and exploration by

$$\tilde{J}_i^{(n)} = \min \left\{ \beta, \frac{\beta}{2} \frac{\bar{J}_i^{(n)}}{\sum_{i=1}^{M} \bar{J}_i^{(n)}/M} \right\}, \qquad (2)$$

where the min operation ensures that the score lies in $[0, \beta]$. Then the UCB score for $\mathbf{I}_i$ is calculated as

$$q_i^{(n)} = \tilde{J}_i^{(n)} + \sqrt{\frac{2 \ln n}{n_i}}. \qquad (3)$$

Algorithm 1. Relaxed Upper Confident Bound

 Input : FCN parameter Θ, input training slices $\{\mathbf{I}_i\}_{i=1,\dots,M}$;
     parameters α and β, max number of iterations T;
 Output: FCN parameter Θ;
1 total number of times slices are selected $n \leftarrow 0$;
2 number of times slice $\mathbf{I}_1, \dots, \mathbf{I}_m$ are selected $n_1, \dots, n_m \leftarrow 0$;
3 running index $i \leftarrow 0$, $\mathcal{J}_1^{(1)}, \dots, \mathcal{J}_M^{(M)} \leftarrow 0$;
4 **repeat**
5   $i \leftarrow i+1$, $n_i \leftarrow n_i + 1$, $n \leftarrow n+1$;
6   Compute $\mathcal{J}_i^{(i)}$ by Eq. 1;
7   $\bar{J}_i^{(M)} = \sum_{t=1}^{M} \mathcal{J}_i^{(i)}/n_i$;
8 **until** $n = M$;
9 $\forall i$, compute $\tilde{J}_i^{(M)}$ by Eq. 2, compute $q_i^{(M)}$ by Eq. 3;
10 $\mu = \sum_{i=1}^{M} q_i^{(M)}/M$, $\sigma = \mathrm{std}(q_i^{(M)})$; iteration $t \leftarrow 0$;
11 **repeat**
12   $t \leftarrow t+1$, $\alpha \sim \mathcal{U}(0,a)$;
13   $K = \sum_{i=1}^{M}(\mathbf{1}(q_i^{(M)} > \mu + \alpha\sigma))$;
14   randomly select a slice $\mathbf{I}_i$ from the set $\{\mathbf{I}_i | q_i^{(n)} \in \mathcal{D}_K(\{q_i^{(n)}\}_{i=1}^{M})\}$;
15   $n_i \leftarrow n_i + 1$, $n \leftarrow n+1$;
16   Compute $\mathcal{J}_i^{(t)}$ by Eq. 1, $\Theta \leftarrow \arg\min_\Theta \mathcal{J}_i^{(t)}(\Theta)$;
17   $\bar{J}_i^{(n)} = \sum_{t=1}^{n} \mathcal{J}_i^{(t)}/n_i$;
18   $\forall i$, compute $\tilde{J}_i$ by Eq. 2, compute $q_i^{(n)}$ by Eq. 3;
19 **until** $t = T$;

As the selection procedure goes on, the exploitation term of Eq. 3 will dominate the selection, i.e., only some very hard samples will be selected. But, these hard samples may have annotation errors. In order to alleviate the influence of annotation errors, we propose to introduce more randomness in UCB scores to relax the largest loss policy. After training an initial FCN with randomly sampling slices from the training set, we assign an initial UCB score $q_i^{(M)} = \tilde{J}_i^{(M)} + \sqrt{2\ln M/1}$ to each slice $\mathbf{I}_i$ in the training set. Assume the UCB scores of all samples follow a normal distribution $\mathcal{N}(\mu, \sigma)$. Hard samples are regarded as slices whose initial UCB scores are larger than μ. Note that initial UCB scores are only decided by the exploitation term. In each iteration of our bootstrapping procedure, we count the number of samples that lie in the range $[\mu + \alpha \cdot \mathrm{std}(q_i^{(M)}), +\infty]$, denoted by K, where α is drawn from a uniform distribution $[0, a]$ ($a = 3$ in our experiment), then a sample is selected randomly from the set $\{\mathbf{I}_i | q_i^{(n)} \in \mathcal{D}_K(\{q_i^{(n)}\}_{i=1}^{M})\}$ to update the FCN, where $\mathcal{D}_K(\cdot)$ denote the K largest values in a set. Here we count the number of hard samples according to a dynamic range, because we do not know the exact range of hard samples. This dynamic region enables our bootstrapping to select hard samples from a larger range with higher probability for harder samples, rather than only selecting some very hard samples. We name our sample selection policy Relaxed Upper Confident Bound (RUCB), as we choose hard samples in a larger range, which introduces more variance to the hard samples. The training procedure for RUCB is summarized in Algorithm 1.

3   Experimental Results

3.1   Experimental Setup

Dataset: We evaluated our algorithm on 120 abdominal CT scans of normal cases under IRB (Institutional Review Board) approved protocol. CT scans are contrast enhanced images in portal venous phase, obtained by Siemens SOMATOM Sensation64 and Definition CT scanners, composed of (319–1051) slices of (512×512) images, and have voxel spatial resolution of ($[0.523 - 0.977] \times [0.523 - 0.977] \times 0.5$) mm^3. Sixteen organs (including aorta, celiac AA, colon, duodenum, gallbladder, interior vena cava, left kidney, right kidney, liver, pancreas, superior mesenteric artery, small bowel, spleen, stomach, and large veins) were segmented by four full-time radiologists, and confirmed by an expert. This dataset is a high quality dataset, but a small portion of error is inevitable, as shown in Fig. 1. Following the standard corss-validation strategy, we randomly partition the dataset into four complementary folds, each of which contains 30 CT scans. All experiments are conducted by four-fold cross-validation, i.e., training the models on three folds and testing them on the remaining one, until four rounds of cross-validation are performed using different partitions.

Evaluation Metric: The performance of multi-organ segmentation is evaluated in terms of Dice-Sørensen similarity coefficient (DSC) over the whole CT scan. We report the average DSC score together with the standard deviation over all testing cases.

Implementation Details: We use FCN-8s model [6] pre-trained on PascalVOC in caffe toolbox. The learning rate is fixed to be 1×10^{-9} and all the networks are trained for $80K$ iterations by SGD. The same parameter setting is used for all sampling strategies. Three boostrapping phases are conducted, at 20,000, 40,000 and 60,000 respectively, i.e., the max number of iterations for each boostrapping phase is $T = 20,000$. We set $\beta = 2$, since $\sqrt{2\ln n/n_i}$ is in the range of [3.0, 5.0] in boostrapping phases.

3.2   Evaluation of RUCB

We evaluate the performance of the proposed sampling algorithm (RUCB) with other competitors. Three sampling strategies considered for comparisons are (1) uniform sampling (Uniform); (2) online hard example mining (OHEM) [14]; and (3) using UCB policy (i.e., select the slice with the largest UCB score during each iteration) in boostrapping.

Table 1 summarizes the results for 16 organs. Experiments show that images with wrong annotations are with large rewards, even larger than real hard samples after training an initial FCN. The proposed RUCB outperforms over all baseline algorithms in terms of average DSC. We see that RUCB achieves much better performance for organs such as *Adrenal gland* (from 29.33% to 36.76%),

Table 1. DSC (%) of sixteen segmented organs (mean ± standard deviation).

Organs	Uniform	OHEM	UCB	RUCB (ours)
Aorta	81.53 ± 4.50	77.49 ± 5.90	81.02 ± 4.50	81.03 ± 4.40
Adrenal gland	29.33 ± 16.26	31.44 ± 16.71	33.75 ± 16.26	36.76 ± 17.28
Celiac AA	34.49 ± 12.92	33.34 ± 13.86	35.89 ± 12.92	38.45 ± 12.53
Colon	77.51 ± 7.89	73.20 ± 8.94	76.40 ± 7.89	77.56 ± 8.65
Duodenum	63.39 ± 12.62	59.68 ± 12.32	63.10 ± 12.62	64.86 ± 12.18
Gallbladder	79.43 ± 23.77	77.82 ± 23.58	79.10 ± 23.77	79.68 ± 23.46
IVC	78.75 ± 6.54	73.73 ± 8.59	77.10 ± 6.54	78.57 ± 6.69
Left kidney	95.35 ± 2.53	94.24 ± 8.95	95.53 ± 2.53	95.57 ± 2.29
Right kidney	94.48 ± 9.49	94.23 ± 9.19	94.39 ± 9.49	95.40 ± 3.62
Liver	96.03 ± 1.70	90.43 ± 4.74	95.68 ± 1.70	96.00 ± 1.28
Pancreas	77.86 ± 9.92	75.32 ± 10.42	78.25 ± 9.92	78.48 ± 9.86
SMA	45.36 ± 14.36	47.18 ± 12.75	44.63 ± 14.36	49.59 ± 13.62
Small bowel	72.35 ± 13.30	67.44 ± 13.22	72.16 ± 13.30	72.88 ± 13.98
Spleen	95.32 ± 2.17	94.56 ± 2.41	95.16 ± 2.17	95.09 ± 2.44
Stomach	90.62 ± 6.51	86.37 ± 8.53	90.70 ± 6.51	90.92 ± 5.62
Veins	64.95 ± 19.96	60.87 ± 19.02	62.70 ± 19.96	65.13 ± 20.15
AVG	73.55 ± 10.28	71.08 ± 11.20	73.47 ± 10.52	74.75 ± 9.88

Celiac AA (34.49% to 38.45%), *Duodenum* (63.39% to 64.86%), *Right kidney* (94.48% to 95.40%), *Pancreas* (77.86% to 78.48%) and *SMA* (45.36% to 49.59%), compared with Uniform. Most of the organs listed above are small organs which are difficult to segment, even for radiologists, and thus they may have more annotation errors.

OHEM performs worse than Uniform, suggesting that directly sampling among slices with largest average rewards during boostrapping phase cannot help to train a better FCN. UCB obtains even slightly worse DSC compared with Uniform, as it only focuses on some hard examples which may have errors.

To better understand UCB and RUCB, some of the hard samples selected more frequently are shown in Fig. 2. Some slices selected by UCB contain obvious errors such as *Colon* annotation for the first one. Slices selected by RUCB are very hard to segment since it contains many organs including very small ones.

Parameter Analysis. α is an important hyper-parameter for our RUCB. We vary it in the following range: $\alpha \in \{0, 1, 2, 3\}$, to see how the performance of some organs changes. The DSCs of *Adrenal gland* and *Celiac AA* are 35.36 ± 17.49 and 38.07 ± 12.75, 32.27 ± 16.25 and 36.97 ± 12.92, 34.42 ± 17.17 and 36.68 ± 13.73, 32.65 ± 17.26 and 37.09 ± 12.15, respectively. Using a fixed α, the performance decreases. We also test the results when K is a constant number, i.e., $K = 5000$. The DSC of *Adrenal gland* and *Celiac AA* are 33.55 ± 17.02 and 36.80 ± 12.91. Compared with UCB, the results further verify that relaxing the UCB score can boost the performance.

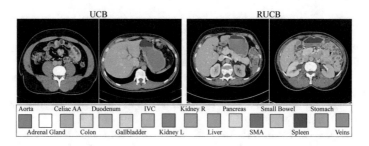

Fig. 2. Visualization of samples selected frequently by left: UCB and right: RUCB. Ground-truth annotations are marked in different colors.

4   Conclusion

We proposed Relaxed Upper Confident Bound policy for sample selection in training multi-organ segmentation networks, in which the exploitation-exploration trade-off is reflected on one hand by the necessity for trying all samples to train a basic classifier, and on the other hand by the demand of assembling hard samples to improve the classifier. It exploits a range of hard samples rather than being stuck with a small set of very hard samples, which mitigates the influence of annotation errors during training. Experimental results showed the effectiveness of the proposed RUCB sample selection policy. Our method can be also used for training 3D patch-based networks, and with other modality medical images.

Acknowledgement. This work was supported by the Lustgarten Foundation for Pancreatic Cancer Research and also supported by NSFC No. 61672336. We thank Prof. Seyoun Park and Dr. Lingxi Xie for instructive discussions.

References

1. Auer, P.: Using confidence bounds for exploitation-exploration trade-offs. J. Mach. Learn. Res. **3**, 397–422 (2002)
2. Auer, P., Cesa-Bianchi, N., Fischer, P.: Finite-time analysis of the multiarmed bandit problem. Mach. Learn. **47**(2), 235–256 (2002)
3. Canévet, O., Fleuret, F.: Large scale hard sample mining with monte carlo tree search. In: Proceedings of the CVPR, pp. 5128–5137 (2016)
4. Çiçek, Ö., Abdulkadir, A., Lienkamp, S.S., Brox, T., Ronneberger, O.: 3D U-Net: learning dense volumetric segmentation from sparse annotation. In: Ourselin, S., Joskowicz, L., Sabuncu, M.R., Unal, G., Wells, W. (eds.) MICCAI 2016. LNCS, vol. 9901, pp. 424–432. Springer, Cham (2016). https://doi.org/10.1007/978-3-319-46723-8_49
5. Fakhry, A., Zeng, T., Ji, S.: Residual deconvolutional networks for brain electron microscopy image segmentation. IEEE Trans. Med. Imaging **36**(2), 447–456 (2017)
6. Long, J., Shelhamer, E., Darrell, T.: Fully convolutional networks for semantic segmentation. In: Computer Vision and Pattern Recognition (2015)

7. Loshchilov, I., Hutter, F.: Online batch selection for faster training of neural networks. CoRR abs/1511.06343 (2015)
8. Merkow, J., Marsden, A., Kriegman, D., Tu, Z.: Dense volume-to-volume vascular boundary detection. In: Ourselin, S., Joskowicz, L., Sabuncu, M.R., Unal, G., Wells, W. (eds.) MICCAI 2016. LNCS, vol. 9902, pp. 371–379. Springer, Cham (2016). https://doi.org/10.1007/978-3-319-46726-9_43
9. Robbins, H.: Some aspects of the sequential design of experiments. Bull. Am. Math. Soc. **58**(5), 527–535 (1952)
10. Ronneberger, O., Fischer, P., Brox, T.: U-Net: Convolutional Networks for Biomedical Image Segmentation. In: Navab, N., Hornegger, J., Wells, W.M., Frangi, A.F. (eds.) MICCAI 2015. LNCS, vol. 9351, pp. 234–241. Springer, Cham (2015). https://doi.org/10.1007/978-3-319-24574-4_28
11. Roth, H., et al.: Hierarchical 3D fully convolutional networks for multi-organ segmentation. CoRR abs/1704.06382 (2017)
12. Roth, H.R., Lu, L., Farag, A., Sohn, A., Summers, R.M.: Spatial aggregation of holistically-nested networks for automated pancreas segmentation. In: Ourselin, S., Joskowicz, L., Sabuncu, M.R., Unal, G., Wells, W. (eds.) MICCAI 2016. LNCS, vol. 9901, pp. 451–459. Springer, Cham (2016). https://doi.org/10.1007/978-3-319-46723-8_52
13. Shen, W., Wang, B., Jiang, Y., Wang, Y., Yuille, A.L.: Multi-stage multi-recursive-input fully convolutional networks for neuronal boundary detection. In: Proceedings of the ICCV, pp. 2410–2419 (2017)
14. Shrivastava, A., Gupta, A., Girshick, R.B.: Training region-based object detectors with online hard example mining. In: CVPR, pp. 761–769 (2016)
15. Simo-Serra, E., Trulls, E., Ferraz, L., Kokkinos, I., Moreno-Noguer, F.: Fracking deep convolutional image descriptors. CoRR abs/1412.6537 (2014)
16. Wang, Y., Zhou, Y., Shen, W., Park, S., Fishman, E.K., Yuille, A.L.: Abdominal multi-organ segmentation with organ-attention networks and statistical fusion. CoRR abs/1804.08414 (2018)
17. Zhou, Y., Xie, L., Shen, W., Wang, Y., Fishman, E.K., Yuille, A.L.: A fixed-point model for pancreas segmentation in abdominal CT scans. In: Descoteaux, M., Maier-Hein, L., Franz, A., Jannin, P., Collins, D.L., Duchesne, S. (eds.) MICCAI 2017. LNCS, vol. 10433, pp. 693–701. Springer, Cham (2017). https://doi.org/10.1007/978-3-319-66182-7_79

Image Segmentation Methods:
Abdominal Segmentation Methods

Bridging the Gap Between 2D and 3D Organ Segmentation with Volumetric Fusion Net

Yingda Xia[1], Lingxi Xie[1(✉)], Fengze Liu[1], Zhuotun Zhu[1],
Elliot K. Fishman[2], and Alan L. Yuille[1]

[1] The Johns Hopkins University, Baltimore, MD 21218, USA
198808xc@gmail.com
[2] The Johns Hopkins University School of Medicine, Baltimore, MD 21287, USA

Abstract. There has been a debate on whether to use 2D or 3D deep neural networks for volumetric organ segmentation. Both 2D and 3D models have their advantages and disadvantages. In this paper, we present an alternative framework, which trains 2D networks on different viewpoints for segmentation, and builds a 3D **Volumetric Fusion Net** (VFN) to fuse the 2D segmentation results. VFN is relatively shallow and contains much fewer parameters than most 3D networks, making our framework more efficient at integrating 3D information for segmentation. We train and test the segmentation and fusion modules individually, and propose a novel strategy, named *cross-cross-augmentation*, to make full use of the limited training data. We evaluate our framework on several challenging abdominal organs, and verify its superiority in segmentation accuracy and stability over existing 2D and 3D approaches.

1 Introduction

With the increasing requirement of fine-scaled medical care, computer-assisted diagnosis (CAD) has attracted more and more attention in the past decade. An important prerequisite of CAD is an intelligent system to process and analyze medical data, such as CT and MRI scans. In the area of medical imaging analysis, organ segmentation is a traditional and fundamental topic [2]. Researchers often designed a specific system for each organ to capture its properties. In comparison to large organs (*e.g.*, the liver, the kidneys, the stomach, *etc.*), small organs such as the pancreas are more difficult to segment, which is partly caused by their highly variable geometric properties [9].

In recent years, with the arrival of the deep learning era [6], powerful models such as convolutional neural networks [7] have been transferred from natural image segmentation to organ segmentation. But there is a difference. Organ segmentation requires dealing with volumetric data, and two types of solutions have been proposed. The first one trains 2D networks from three orthogonal planes and fusing the segmentation results [9,17,18], and the second one suggests training a 3D network directly [4,8,19]. But 3D networks are more computationally

© Springer Nature Switzerland AG 2018
A. F. Frangi et al. (Eds.): MICCAI 2018, LNCS 11073, pp. 445–453, 2018.
https://doi.org/10.1007/978-3-030-00937-3_51

expensive yet less stable when trained from scratch, and it is difficult to find a pre-trained model for medical purposes. In the scenario of limited training data, fine-tuning a pre-trained 2D network [7] is a safer choice [14].

This paper presents an alternative framework, which trains 2D segmentation models and uses a light-weighted 3D network, named **Volumetric Fusion Net** (VFN), in order to fuse 2D segmentation at a late stage. A similar idea is studied before based on either the EM algorithm [1] or pre-defined operations in a 2D scenario [16], but we propose instead to construct generalized linear operations (convolution) and allow them to be learned from training data. Because it is built on top of reasonable 2D segmentation results, VFN is relatively shallow and does not use fully-connected layers (which contribute a large fraction of network parameters) to improve its discriminative ability. In the training process, we first optimize 2D segmentation networks on different viewpoints individually (this strategy was studied in [12,13,18]), and then use the validation set to train VFN. When the amount of training data is limited, we suggest a *cross-cross-augmentation* strategy to enable reusing the data to train both 2D segmentation and 3D fusion networks.

We first apply our system to a public dataset for pancreas segmentation [9]. Based on the state-of-the-art 2D segmentation approaches [17,18], VFN produces a consistent accuracy gain and outperforms other fusion methods, including majority voting and statistical fusion [1]. In comparison to 3D networks such as [19], our framework achieves comparable segmentation accuracy using fewer computational resources, *e.g.*, using 10% parameters and being 3× faster at the testing stage (it only adds 10% computation beyond the 2D baselines). We also generalize our framework to other small organs such as the adrenal glands and the duodenum, and verify its favorable performance.

2   Our Approach

2.1   Framework: Fusing 2D Segmentation into a 3D Volume

We denote an input CT volume by $\mathbf{X}$. This is a $W \times H \times L$ volume, where W, H and L are the numbers of voxels along the *coronal*, *sagittal* and *axial* directions, respectively. The i-th voxel of $\mathbf{X}$, x_i, is the intensity (Hounsfield Unit, HU) at the corresponding position, $i = (1,1,1), \ldots, (W, H, L)$. The ground-truth segmentation of an organ is denoted by $\mathbf{Y}^\star$, which has the same dimensionality as $\mathbf{X}$. If the i-th voxel belongs to the target organ, we set $y_i^\star = 1$, otherwise $y_i^\star = 0$. The goal of organ segmentation is to design a function $\mathbf{g}(\cdot)$, so that $\mathbf{Y} = \mathbf{g}(\mathbf{X})$, with all $y_i \in \{0, 1\}$, is close to $\mathbf{Y}^\star$. We measure the similarity between $\mathbf{Y}$ and $\mathbf{Y}^\star$ by the Dice-Sørensen coefficient (DSC): $\mathrm{DSC}(\mathbf{Y}, \mathbf{Y}^\star) = \frac{2 \times |\mathcal{Y} \cap \mathcal{Y}^\star|}{|\mathcal{Y}| + |\mathcal{Y}^\star|}$, where $\mathcal{Y}^\star = \{i \mid y_i^\star = 1\}$ and $\mathcal{Y} = \{i \mid y_i = 1\}$ are the sets of foreground voxels.

There are, in general, two ways to design $\mathbf{g}(\cdot)$. The first one trains a 3D model to deal with volumetric data directly [4,8], and the second one works by cutting the 3D volume into slices, and using 2D networks for segmentation. Both 2D and 3D approaches have their advantages and disadvantages. We appreciate the ability of 3D networks to take volumetric cues into consideration (radiologists also exploit 3D information to make decisions), but, as shown in Sect. 3.2, 3D networks are sometimes less stable, arguably because we need to train all weights from scratch, while the 2D networks can be initialized with pre-trained models from the computer vision literature [7]. On the other hand, processing volumetric data (*e.g.*, 3D convolution) often requires heavier computation in both training and testing (*e.g.*, requiring 3× testing time, see Table 1).

In mathematical terms, let $\mathbf{X}_l^{\mathrm{A}}$, $l = 1, 2, \ldots, L$ be a 2D slice (of $W \times H$) along the *axial* view, and $\mathbf{Y}_l^{\mathrm{A}} = \mathbf{s}^{\mathrm{A}}(\mathbf{X}_l^{\mathrm{A}})$ be the segmentation score map for $\mathbf{X}_l^{\mathrm{A}}$. $\mathbf{s}^{\mathrm{A}}(\cdot)$ can be a 2D segmentation network such as FCN [7], or a multi-stage system such as a coarse-to-fine framework [18]. Stacking all $\mathbf{Y}_l^{\mathrm{A}}$'s yields a 3D volume $\mathbf{Y}^{\mathrm{A}} = \mathbf{s}^{\mathrm{A}}(\mathbf{X})$. This slicing-and-stacking process can be performed along each axis independently. Due to the large image variation in different views, we train three segmentation models, denoted by $\mathbf{s}^{\mathrm{C}}(\cdot)$, $\mathbf{s}^{\mathrm{S}}(\cdot)$ and $\mathbf{s}^{\mathrm{A}}(\cdot)$, respectively. Finally, a fusion function $\mathbf{f}[\cdot]$ integrates them into the final prediction:

$$\mathbf{Y} = \mathbf{f}\left[\mathbf{X}, \mathbf{Y}^{\mathrm{C}}, \mathbf{Y}^{\mathrm{S}}, \mathbf{Y}^{\mathrm{A}}\right] = \mathbf{f}\left[\mathbf{X}, \mathbf{s}^{\mathrm{C}}(\mathbf{X}), \mathbf{s}^{\mathrm{S}}(\mathbf{X}), \mathbf{s}^{\mathrm{A}}(\mathbf{X})\right]. \tag{1}$$

Note that we allow the image $\mathbf{X}$ to be incorporated. This is related to the idea known as auto-contexts [15] in computer vision. As we shall see in experiments, adding $\mathbf{X}$ improves the quality of fusion considerably. Our goal is to equip $\mathbf{f}[\cdot]$ with partial abilities of 3D networks, *e.g.*, learning simple, local 3D patterns.

2.2   Volumetric Fusion Net

The VFN approach is built upon the 2D segmentation volumes from three orthogonal (*coronal, sagittal* and *axial*) planes. Powered by state-of-the-art deep networks, these results are generally accurate (*e.g.*, an average DSC of over 82% [18] on the NIH pancreas segmentation dataset [9]). But, as shown in Fig. 2, some *local* errors still occur because 2 out of 3 views fail to detect the target. Our assumption is that these errors can be recovered by learning and exploiting the 3D image patterns in its surrounding region.

Regarding other choices, majority voting obviously cannot take image patterns into consideration. The STAPLE algorithm [1], while being effective in multi-atlas registration, does not have a strong ability of fitting image patterns from training data. We shall see in experiments that STAPLE is unable to improve segmentation accuracy over majority voting.

Motivated by the need to learn *local* patterns, we equip VFN with a small input region (64^3) and a shallow structure, so that each neuron has a small receptive field (the largest region seen by an output neuron is 50^3). In comparison, in the 3D network VNet [8], these numbers are 128^3 and 551^3, respectively. This brings twofold benefits. First, we can sample more patches from the training data, and the number of parameters is much less, and so the risk of over-fitting is alleviated. Second, VFN is more computationally efficient than 3D networks, *e.g.*, adding 2D segmentation, it needs only half the testing time of [19].

The architecture of VFN is shown in Fig. 1. It has three down-sampling stages and three up-sampling stages. Each down-sampling stage is composed of two

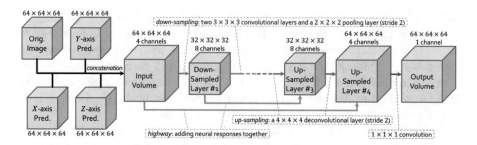

Fig. 1. The network structure of VFN. We only display one down-sampling and one up-sampling stages, but there are 3 of each. Each down-sampling stage shrinks the spatial resolution by 1/2 and doubles the number of channels. We build 3 highway connections (2 are shown). We perform batch normalization and ReLU activation after each convolutional and deconvolutional layer.

$3 \times 3 \times 3$ convolutional layers and a $2 \times 2 \times 2$ max-pooling layer with a stride of 2, and each up-sampling stage is implemented by a single $4 \times 4 \times 4$ deconvolutional layer with a stride of 2. Following other 3D networks [8,19], we also build a few residual connections [5] between hidden layers of the same scale. For our problem, this enables the network to preserve a large fraction of 2D network predictions (which are generally of good quality) and focus on refining them (note that if all weights in convolution are identical, then VFN is approximately equivalent to majority voting). Experiments show that these highway connections lead to faster convergence and higher accuracy. A final convolution of a $1 \times 1 \times 1$ kernel reduces the number of channels to 1.

The input layer of VFN consists of 4 channels, 1 for the original image and 3 for 2D segmentations from different viewpoints. The input values in each channel are normalized into $[0, 1]$. By this we provide equally-weighted information from the original image and 2D multi-view segmentation results, so that VFN can fuse them at an early stage and learn from data automatically. We verify in experiments that image information is important – training a VFN without this input channel shrinks the average accuracy gain by half.

2.3   Training and Testing VFN

We train VFN from scratch, *i.e.*, all weights in convolution are initialized as random white noises. Note that setting all weights as 1 mimics majority voting, and we find that both ways of initialization lead to similar testing performance. All $64 \times 64 \times 64$ volumes are sampled from the region-of-interest (ROI) of each training case, defined as the bounding box covering all foreground voxels padded by 32 pixels in each dimension. We introduce data augmentation by performing random 90°-rotation and flip in 3D space (each cube has 24 variants). We use a Dice loss to avoid background bias (a voxel is more likely to be predicted as background, due to the majority of background voxels in training). We train VFN for 30,000 iterations with a mini-batch size of 16. We start with a learning

Table 1. Comparison of segmentation accuracy (DSC, %) and testing time (in minutes) between our approach and the state-of-the-arts on the NIH dataset [9]. Both [18] and [17] are reimplemented by ourselves, and the default fusion is majority voting.

Approach	Average	Min	1/4-Q	Med	3/4-Q	Max	Time (m)
Roth *et al.* [9]	71.42 ± 10.11	23.99	–	–	–	86.29	6–8
Roth *et al.* [10]	78.01 ± 8.20	34.11	–	–	–	88.65	2–3
Roth *et al.* [11]	81.27 ± 6.27	50.69	–	–	–	88.96	2–3
Cai *et al.* [3]	82.4 ± 6.7	60.0	–	–	–	90.1	N/A
Zhu *et al.* [19]	84.59 ± 4.86	69.62	–	–	–	91.45	4.1
Zhou *et al.* [18]	82.50 ± 6.14	56.33	81.63	84.11	86.28	89.98	0.9
[18] + NLS	82.25 ± 6.57	56.86	81.54	83.96	86.14	89.94	1.1
[18] + VFN	$\mathbf{84.06} \pm 5.63$	62.93	81.98	85.69	87.62	91.28	1.0
Yu *et al.* [17]	84.48 ± 5.03	62.23	82.50	85.66	87.82	91.17	1.3
[17] + NLS	84.47 ± 5.03	62.22	82.42	85.59	87.78	91.17	1.5
[17] + VFN	$\mathbf{84.63} \pm 5.07$	61.58	82.42	85.84	88.37	91.57	1.4

rate of 0.01, and divide it by 10 after 20,000 and 25,000 iterations, respectively. The entire training process requires approximately 6 h in a Titan-X-Pascal GPU. In the testing process, we use a sliding window with a stride of 32 in the ROI region (the minimal 3D box covering all foreground voxels of multi-plane 2D segmentation fused by majority voting). For an average pancreas in the NIH dataset [9], testing VFN takes around 5 s.

An important issue in optimizing VFN is to construct the training data. Note that we cannot reuse the data used for training segmentation networks to train VFN, because this will result in the input channels contain very accurate segmentation, which limits VFN from learning meaningful local patterns and generalizing to the testing scenarios. So, we further split the training set into two subsets, one for training the 2D segmentation networks and the other for training VFN with the testing segmentation results.

However, under most circumstances, the amount of training data is limited. For example, in the NIH pancreas segmentation dataset, each fold in cross-validation has only 60 training cases. Partitioning it into two subsets harms the accuracy of both 2D segmentation and fusion. To avoid this, we suggest a **cross-cross-augmentation** (CCA) strategy, described as follows. Suppose we split data into K folds for cross-validation, and the k_1-th fold is left for testing. For all $k_2 \neq k_1$, we train 2D segmentation models on the folds in $\{1, 2, \ldots, K\} \backslash \{k_1, k_2\}$, and test on the k_2-th fold to generate training data for the VFN. In this way, all data are used for training both the segmentation model and the VFN. The price is that a total of $K(K-1)/2$ extra segmentation models need to be trained, which is more costly than training K models in a standard cross-validation. In practice, this strategy improves the average segmentation accuracy by $\sim 1\%$ in each fold. Note that we perform CCA only on the NIH dataset due to the limited amount of data – in our own dataset, we perform standard training/testing split, requiring <10% extra training time and ignorable extra testing time.

3   Experiments

3.1   The NIH Pancreas Segmentation Dataset

We first evaluate our approach on the NIH pancreas segmentation dataset [9] containing 82 abdominal CT volumes. The width and height of each volume are both 512, and the number of slices along the *axial* axis varies from 181 to 466. We split the dataset into 4 folds of approximately the same size, and apply cross-cross-augmentation (see Sect. 2.3) to improve segmentation accuracy.

Results are summarized in Table 1. We use two recent 2D segmentation approaches as our baseline, and compare VFN with two other fusion approaches, namely majority voting and non-local STAPLE (NLS) [1]. The latter was verified more effective than its former local version. We measure segmentation accuracy using DSC and report the average accuracy over 82 cases. Based on [18], VFN improves majority voting significantly by an average of 1.69%. The improvement over 82 cases is consistent (the student's t-test reports a p-value of 6.9×10^{-7}), although the standard deviation over 82 cases is relatively large – this is mainly caused by the difference in difficulties from case to case. Figure 2 shows an example on which VFN produces a significant accuracy gain. VFN does not improve [17] significantly, arguably because [17] has almost reached the human-level agreement (we invited a radiologist to segment this dataset individually, and she achieves an average accuracy of ∼86%). Note that the other approaches without CCA used both the training and validation folds for training, and so all numbers are comparable in Table 1.

Due to our analysis in Sect. 2.2, NLS does not produce any accuracy gain over either [18] and [17]. NLS is effective in multi-atlas registration, where the

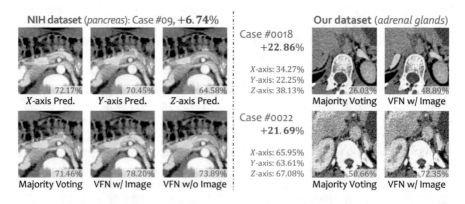

Fig. 2. Two typical examples, each with the original image, segmentation results from three viewpoints, and different fusion results. In each label map, red, green and yellow indicate ground-truth, prediction and overlap, respectively.

labels come from different images and the annotation is relatively accurate [1]. But in our problem, segmentation results from 2D networks can be noisy, thus recovering these errors requires learning local image patterns from training data, which is what VFN does to outperform NLS.

To reveal the importance of image information, we train a VFN without the image channel in the input layer. Based on [18], this version produces approximately half of the improvement (1.69%) by the full model. We show an example in Fig. 2, in which the right part of the pancreas is missing in both *sagittal* and *axial* planes, but the high confidence in the *coronal* plane and the continuity of image intensities suggest its presence in the final segmentation.

3.2 Our Multi-organ Dataset

The radiologists in our team collected a dataset with 300 high-resolution CT scans. These scans were performed on some potential renal donors. Four experts in abdominal anatomy annotated 11 abdominal organs, taking 3−4 h for each scan, and all annotations were verified by an experienced board certified Abdominal Radiologist. Except for the *pancreas*, we choose several challenging targets, including the *adrenal glands*, the *duodenum*, and the *gallbladder* (easy cases such as the *liver* and the *kidneys* are not considered). We use 150 cases for training 2D segmentation models, 100 cases for training VFN, and test on the remaining 50 cases. The data split is random but identical for different organs.

Results are shown in Table 2. Again, our approach consistently improves 2D segmentation, which demonstrates the transferability of our methodology. In *pancreas*, based on [17], we obtain a p-value of 2.7×10^{-5} over 50 testing cases. In *adrenal glands*, although the average accuracy gains are not large, the improvement is significant in some badly segmented cases, *e.g.*, Fig. 2 shows two examples with more than 20% accuracy boosts. Refining bad segmentations makes our segmentation results more reliable. By contrast, the 3D network [19] produces unstable performance ([19] was designed for pancreas segmentation, thus works reasonably well in *pancreas*), which is mainly caused by the limited training data especially for small organs such as *adrenal glands* and *gallbladder*.

Table 2. Comparison of segmentation accuracy (DSC, %) on our multi-organ dataset. The baseline for [18] and [17] is majority voting. The numbers of [17] are different from those in their original paper, because we are using a different dataset.

Approach	Adrenal g.	Duodenum	Gallbladder	Pancreas
Zhu *et al.* [19]	36.74 ± 25.14	68.80 ± 14.38	42.01 ± 29.47	85.25 ± 6.04
Zhou *et al.* [18]	66.09 ± 18.19	71.65 ± 13.15	90.39 ± 5.30	84.52 ± 6.23
[18] + VFN	$\mathbf{69.24} \pm 17.42$	$\mathbf{72.77} \pm 12.80$	$\mathbf{91.40} \pm 5.19$	$\mathbf{86.39} \pm 6.20$
Yu *et al.* [17]	71.40 ± 12.87	77.48 ± 8.70	91.81 ± 4.90	87.22 ± 5.90
[17] + VFN	$\mathbf{72.09} \pm 13.61$	$\mathbf{77.77} \pm 8.46$	$\mathbf{92.15} \pm 5.05$	$\mathbf{88.06} \pm 5.33$

Therefore, we conclude that 2D segmentation followed by 3D fusion is currently a very promising idea to bridge the gap between 2D and 3D segmentation approaches, particularly if there is limited training data.

4   Conclusions

In this paper, we discuss an important topic in medical imaging analysis, namely bridging the gap between 2D and 3D organ segmentation approaches. We propose to train more stable 2D segmentation networks, and then use a light-weighted 3D fusion module to fuse their results. In this way, we enjoy the benefits of exploiting 3D information to improve segmentation, as well as avoiding the risk of over-fitting caused by tuning 3D models (which have $10\times$ more parameters) on a limited amount of training data. We verify the effectiveness of our approach on two datasets, one of which contains several challenging organs.

Based on our work, a promising direction is to train the segmentation and fusion modules in a joint manner, so that the 2D networks can incorporate 3D information in the training process by learning from the back-propagated gradients of VFN. Another issue involves training VFN more efficiently, *e.g.*, using hard example mining. These topics are left for future research.

Acknowledgements. This work was supported by the Lustgarten foundation for pancreatic cancer research. We thank Prof. Seyoun Park, Prof. Wei Shen, Dr. Yan Wang and Yuyin Zhou for instructive discussions.

References

1. Asman, A.J., Landman, B.A.: Non-local statistical label fusion for multi-atlas segmentation. Med. Image Anal. **17**(2), 194–208 (2013)
2. Boykov, Y., Jolly, M.-P.: Interactive organ segmentation using graph cuts. In: Delp, S.L., DiGoia, A.M., Jaramaz, B. (eds.) MICCAI 2000. LNCS, vol. 1935, pp. 276–286. Springer, Heidelberg (2000). https://doi.org/10.1007/978-3-540-40899-4_28
3. Cai, J., Lu, L., Xie, Y., Xing, F., Yang, L.: Pancreas segmentation in MRI using graph-based decision fusion on convolutional neural networks. In: Descoteaux, M., Maier-Hein, L., Franz, A., Jannin, P., Collins, D.L., Duchesne, S. (eds.) MICCAI 2017. LNCS, vol. 10435, pp. 674–682. Springer, Cham (2017). https://doi.org/10.1007/978-3-319-66179-7_77
4. Çiçek, Ö., Abdulkadir, A., Lienkamp, S.S., Brox, T., Ronneberger, O.: 3D U-net: learning dense volumetric segmentation from sparse annotation. In: Ourselin, S., Joskowicz, L., Sabuncu, M.R., Unal, G., Wells, W. (eds.) MICCAI 2016. LNCS, vol. 9901, pp. 424–432. Springer, Cham (2016). https://doi.org/10.1007/978-3-319-46723-8_49
5. He, K., Zhang, X., Ren, S., Sun, J.: Deep residual learning for image recognition. In: CVPR (2016)
6. Krizhevsky, A., Sutskever, I., Hinton, G.E.: Imagenet classification with deep convolutional neural networks. In: NIPS (2012)
7. Long, J., Shelhamer, E., Darrell, T.: Fully convolutional networks for semantic segmentation. In: CVPR (2015)

8. Milletari, F., Navab, N., Ahmadi, S.A.: V-net: fully convolutional neural networks for volumetric medical image segmentation. In: 3DV (2016)
9. Roth, H.R., et al.: Deeporgan: multi-level deep convolutional networks for automated pancreas segmentation. In: MICCAI (2015)
10. Roth, H.R., Lu, L., Farag, A., Sohn, A., Summers, R.M.: Spatial aggregation of holistically-nested networks for automated pancreas segmentation. In: Ourselin, S., Joskowicz, L., Sabuncu, M.R., Unal, G., Wells, W. (eds.) MICCAI 2016. LNCS, vol. 9901, pp. 451–459. Springer, Cham (2016). https://doi.org/10.1007/978-3-319-46723-8_52
11. Roth, H.R., et al.: Spatial aggregation of holistically-nested convolutional neural networks for automated pancreas localization and segmentation. arXiv:1702.00045 (2017)
12. Setio, A.A.A., et al.: Pulmonary nodule detection in CT images: false positive reduction using multi-view convolutional networks. IEEE Trans. Med. Imaging **35**(5), 1160–1169 (2016)
13. Su, H., Maji, S., Kalogerakis, E., Learned-Miller, E.: Multi-view convolutional neural networks for 3D shape recognition. In: Proceedings of the IEEE International Conference on Computer Vision, pp. 945–953 (2015)
14. Tajbakhsh, N., et al.: Convolutional neural networks for medical image analysis: full training or fine tuning? IEEE TMI **35**(5), 1299–1312 (2016)
15. Tu, Z., Bai, X.: Auto-context and its application to high-level vision tasks and 3D brain image segmentation. IEEE TPAMI **32**(10), 1744–1757 (2010)
16. Yang, H., Sun, J., Li, H., Wang, L., Xu, Z.: Deep fusion net for multi-atlas segmentation: application to cardiac MR images. In: Ourselin, S., Joskowicz, L., Sabuncu, M.R., Unal, G., Wells, W. (eds.) MICCAI 2016. LNCS, vol. 9901, pp. 521–528. Springer, Cham (2016). https://doi.org/10.1007/978-3-319-46723-8_60
17. Yu, Q., Xie, L., Wang, Y., Zhou, Y., Fishman, E.K., Yuille, A.L.: Recurrent saliency transformation network: incorporating multi-stage visual cues for small organ segmentation. arXiv:1709.04518 (2017)
18. Zhou, Y., Xie, L., Shen, W., Wang, Y., Fishman, E.K., Yuille, A.L.: A fixed-point model for pancreas segmentation in abdominal CT scans. In: Descoteaux, M., Maier-Hein, L., Franz, A., Jannin, P., Collins, D.L., Duchesne, S. (eds.) MICCAI 2017. LNCS, vol. 10433, pp. 693–701. Springer, Cham (2017). https://doi.org/10.1007/978-3-319-66182-7_79
19. Zhu, Z., Xia, Y., Shen, W., Fishman, E.K., Yuille, A.L.: A 3D coarse-to-fine framework for automatic pancreas segmentation. arXiv:1712.00201 (2017)

Segmentation of Renal Structures
for Image-Guided Surgery

Junning Li[(⊠)], Pechin Lo, Ahmed Taha, Hang Wu, and Tao Zhao

Intuitive Surgical, 1020 Kifer Road, Sunnyvale, CA 94086, USA
{Junning.Li,Pechin.Lo,Ahmed.Taha,Hang.Wu,
Tao.Zhao}@intusurg.com

Abstract. Anatomic models of kidneys may help surgeons make plans or guide surgical procedures, in which segmentation is a prerequisite. We develop a convolutional neural network to segment multiple renal structures from arterial-phase CT images, including parenchyma, arteries, veins, collecting systems, and abnormal structures. To the best of our knowledge, this is the first work dedicated to jointly segment these five renal structures. We introduce two novel techniques. First, we generalize the sequential residual architecture to residual graphs. With this generalization, we convert a popular multi-scale architecture (U-Net) to a residual U-Net. Second, we solve the unbalanced data problem which commonly exists in medical image segmentation by weighting pixels with multi-scale entropy. Our multi-scale entropy map combines information theory and scale analysis to capture spatial complexity of a multi-class label map. The two techniques significantly improve segmentation accuracy. Trained on 400 CT scans and tested on another 100, our algorithm achieves median Dice indices 0.96, 0.86, 0.8, 0.62, and 0.29 respectively for renal parenchyma, arteries, veins, collecting systems and abnormal structures.

1 Introduction

Kidney cancer has 63,990 estimated new cases and causes 14,400 deaths in 2017 in United States alone [1]. Laparoscopic partial nephrectomy has become increasingly popular due to the preservation of kidneys' healthy part and the reduced invasiveness. Minimally invasive surgeries by the da Vinci[TM] surgical systems have increased significantly over the past 20 years, with approximately 877,000 procedures in 2017.

The da Vinci[TM] system not only offers surgeons with dexterity and precision, but is also a great platform to enable image-guided surgery. The system has a stereo endoscope and a stereo viewer that make augmented reality possible. The endoscope is stably held by a robotic arm which provides a stable view, and its position is tracked in real-time through the robotic kinematics. The TilePro[TM] feature through which external videos can be piped in enables augmented reality without further integration.

Visualizing segmented renal structures (such as parenchyma, arteries, veins, ureters, and tumors) in 3D has many clear advantages over native CT images. Preoperatively, it can help surgeons assess the 3D relationship of different structures and create the best plan. Intra-operatively, the model can provide real-time guidance. More specifically, there are three benefits: (1) It enables selective arterial clamping to

A. F. Frangi et al. (Eds.): MICCAI 2018, LNCS 11073, pp. 454–462, 2018.
https://doi.org/10.1007/978-3-030-00937-3_52

improve the health of the preserved part of the kidney, compared to total clamping in complex procedures that need more time. (2) It enables the awareness of critical structures (major blood vessels and collecting systems) close to a tumor and helps reduce surgical complication. (3) Overlaying tumors not visible from outside of the kidney can help surgeons to localize tumors quickly in the absence of tactile feedback.

Image-guided laparoscopic partial nephrectomy has been studied in many previous works [2, 3]. The reported works are focused on registration and augmented reality. Efficient and low cost segmentation of the renal structures is a prerequisite for any image guidance. Manual segmentation by using interactive tools is time consuming, prohibiting the adoption of such use. In this work, we try to automate the segmentation of renal structures.

To assist surgical planning and guidance, we segment the following five structures: kidney parenchyma, renal arteries (including aorta), renal veins (including IVC), collecting systems (including renal calyces, renal pelvis and ureters), and abnormal structures (including tumors and cysts). We use the arterial-phase CT images as the input due to its wide availability in different renal scan protocols. Kidney parenchyma and arteries has higher contrast while other structures are not enhanced thus difficult to disambiguate from the background.

Previous works on kidney segmentation employed random forests [4, 5], multi-atlases [6], and deep learning [7, 8]. Some [4–7] focused on segmentation of the kidney body, while others [8] focused on blood vessels and collecting systems. Deep convolutional neural networks have revolutionized a lot of image analysis tasks including medical image segmentation. A fully convolutional network [9–11] whose the output network is a probabilistic map of the same size as the input is an end-to-end approach that solves feature learning and classification jointly.

We develop a single convolutional neural network to segment all the aforementioned structures. Our network structure is inspired by the popular U-Net [9] and the ResNet [12]. Our work presents a number of contributions:

- To the best of our knowledge, this is the first work dedicated to jointly segment kidney body and its internal structures.
- We generalize the sequential residual architecture [12] to direct acyclic graphs. With this generalization, we convert a popular multi-scale architecture U-Net [9] to a residual U-Net.
- We propose an elegant approach to encode the importance of pixels to solve the problems of unbalanced data, both inter-class data and intra-class, which are common in medical image segmentation.
- We show notable improvement made by the two new techniques on a dataset of 500 CT images.

2   Residual U-Net

2.1   Residual Graphs

The residual architecture [12] has significantly improved deep neural networks' performance in image recognition. The original residual network (ResNet) is a sequential accumulation of many (possibly nonlinear) functions, as shown in Fig. 1(a). It directly propagates the optimization gradient from the end to the beginning, so leads to a better training process.

However, not all models are sequential, for example, the popular U-Net [9], as shown in Fig. 1(d). In the model, the output of filter f_{pre} takes two paths. One goes down, forwarding information from fine scales to coarse scales. The other merges at filter f_{post} with context information extracted from coarse scales. Such a structure is not sequential, but a directed acyclic graph with branching and merging.

We propose the following residual architecture for directed acyclic graphs, fully compatible with original sequential one. Let $G = \{V, \vec{E}\}$ be a directed acyclic graph where V is its vertices and $\vec{E}$ is its directed edges. Given a vertex $a \in V$, let $acs(a)$, excluding a itself, denote the vertices in V which can reach a via directed paths in $\vec{E}$. The residual graph derived from G is composed by functions on vertices. The function f_a on a vertex a takes the summation of $acs(a)$ as its input, that is:

$$\text{input } of\ f_a = \sum_{b \in acs(a)} f_b.$$

For instance, Fig. 1(c) shows the residual graph derived from the graph in Fig. 1 (b). In Fig. 1(c), the input of f_4 is the summation of f_1 and f_2; the input of f_5 is the summation of f_2 and f_3; the input of f_6 is the summation of $f_1, f_2, ..., f_5$.

2.2   Multi-scale Residual Network

We combine the residual graph with the U-Net into a Res. U-Net, as shown in Fig. 1 (e). Data flow from fine scales to coarse scales through two channels: the green which

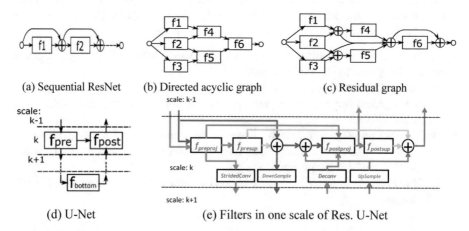

(a) Sequential ResNet   (b) Directed acyclic graph   (c) Residual graph

(d) U-Net   (e) Filters in one scale of Res. U-Net

Fig. 1. (a) An example of sequential residual network. (b) An example of directed acyclic graph. (c) The residual graph derived from (b). (d) The U-Net architecture. Downward arrows represent down-sampling or strided convolutions. Upward arrows represent up-sampling or deconvolution. (e) The Res. U-Net architecture. It consists of two threads. The first thread is scale-specific features: the green channels. It follows a similar architecture to the U-Net. The second thread is the residual architecture, including the red, the orange and the blue channels.

is scale-specific features and the red which is the accumulation of supervision features. The green and the red channels, concatenated together, are projected to a high-dimensional feature space through $f_{preproj}$, and then compressed by f_{presup}. The output of f_{presup} is added to the red channel to keep the accumulation updated. The green channel after $f_{preproj}$ and the red channel after f_{presup}, are forwarded to a coarser scale $k + 1$, respectively through strided convolution and down-sampling. Data flow from coarse scales to fine scales through two channels, the green, and the blue, respectively through de-convolution and up-sampling. The blue is the accumulation of supervision features from the coarsest scale to the current scale. The blue channel is added to the red channel to keep the accumulation updated. The accumulated features, concatenated with green channels, are projected to a high-dimensional feature space through $f_{postproj}$, and then compressed by $f_{postsup}$. The outputs of f_{presup} and $f_{postsup}$ are added to the blue channel to keep it as the accumulation. When the blue channel travels to the first scale, it is the accumulation of all scales.

The Res. U-Net consists of two threads. The first thread is scale-specific features: the green channels. It follows a similar architecture to the U-Net. It branches at $f_{preproj}$ and then merges at $f_{postproj}$. The second thread is the residual architecture, including the red, the orange and the blue channels. We consider the pair of $f_{preproj}$ and f_{presup} and the pair of $f_{postproj}$ and $f_{postsup}$ as processing units in the residual architecture. f_{presup} or $f_{postsup}$ produces the output of a processing unit. $f_{preproj}$ or $f_{postproj}$ produces intermediate features. The input to a processing unit always includes summation of f_{presup} or $f_{postsup}$ from its ancestor processing units.

Parameters of the Res. U-Net used in our experiment are in Table 1.

Table 1. Profile of the Res. U-Net used in the experiment, in the format of W × H × D: C where W, H and D are respectively the width, height and depth of convolution kernels and C is the number of output channels. Strided convolutions and deconvolutions stride by 2.

k	$f_{preproj}$: Relu (Conv)	f_{presup}: Conv	StridedConv: Relu (Conv)	Deconv: Relu (Conv)	$f_{postproj}$: Relu (Conv)	$f_{postsup}$: Conv
1	$1 \times 1 \times 1$: 8	$1 \times 1 \times 1$: 5	$3 \times 3 \times 3$: 16	$3 \times 3 \times 3$: 8	$3 \times 3 \times 3$: 8	$1 \times 1 \times 1$: 5
2	$1 \times 1 \times 1$: 16	$1 \times 1 \times 1$: 5	$3 \times 3 \times 3$: 32	$3 \times 3 \times 3$: 16	$3 \times 3 \times 3$: 16	$1 \times 1 \times 1$: 5
3	$1 \times 1 \times 1$: 32	$1 \times 1 \times 1$: 5	$3 \times 3 \times 3$: 64	$3 \times 3 \times 3$: 32	$3 \times 3 \times 3$: 32	$1 \times 1 \times 1$: 5
4	$1 \times 1 \times 1$: 64	$1 \times 1 \times 1$: 5	$3 \times 3 \times 3$: 128	$3 \times 3 \times 3$: 64	$3 \times 3 \times 3$: 64	$1 \times 1 \times 1$: 5
5	$1 \times 1 \times 1$: 128	$1 \times 1 \times 1$: 5	$3 \times 3 \times 3$: 256	$3 \times 3 \times 3$: 128	$3 \times 3 \times 3$: 128	$1 \times 1 \times 1$: 5

3 Multi-scale Categorical Entropy

Uniform weighting in model training may yield unsatisfactory segmentation. For example, it will make a model tend to label pixels into a class overwhelmingly greater in size than others [13]. Besides inter-class unbalance, it is also problematic for intra-class pixels. For example, it will undesirably make thin vessels less important than thick ones simply because the later take a lesser number of pixels. By intuition, we would like to have a pixel-wise weight map with the following properties: (1) edges are important because they define the boundary; (2) complicated structures, though

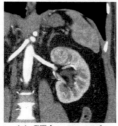 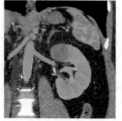 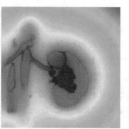

| (a) CT image patch | (b) Manual segmentation | (c) Multi-scale entropy map |

Fig. 2. An example of multi-scale entropy map. (a) A patch of a CT image. (b) Manual segmentation, with green for parenchyma, red for arteries, blue for veins, yellow for collecting systems and purple for masses. (c) The entropy map derived with smoothing kernel sizes 1, 2, 4, 8, 16, 32, 64, 128, and 256. It emphasizes edges, complicated structures, and areas near the foreground.

possibly small, are important, for example, branching thin vessels; (3) the further away a point is from the foreground, the less important it is.

We propose using multi-scale entropy to weight pixels. Given a multi-channel probabilistic map y and a series of scale levels $\sigma_0 < \ldots < \sigma_n$, the multi-scale entropy s is defined as:

$$y_\delta = \kappa_\sigma * y, \text{ for } \sigma \in \{\sigma_0, \ldots, \sigma_n\}, \tag{1}$$

$$\text{RelativeEntropy}_{\sigma_i|\sigma_{i+1}}(p) = \sum_c y_{\sigma_i}(p)[c]\ln\frac{y_{\sigma_i}(p)[c]}{y_{\sigma_{i+1}}(p)[c]}, \tag{2}$$

$$s_{\sigma_i|\sigma_{i+1}} = \kappa_{|\sigma_{i+1}-\sigma_i|} * \text{RelativeEntropy}_{\sigma_i|\sigma_{i+1}}, \tag{3}$$

$$s = \sum_i s_{\sigma_i|\sigma_{i+1}}, \tag{4}$$

where κ_σ is a Gaussian kernel of width δ, and $y_{\sigma_i}(p)[c]$ is c-th channel's probability at a point p in y_{σ_i}. Equation (1) generates a series of smoothed probabilistic maps y_δ s from the original map y. Equation (2) calculates the relative entropy between two smoothed probabilistic maps y_{σ_i} and $y_{\sigma_{i+1}}$. It captures how complex the label map is at a scale. Equation (3) smooths the relative entropy map to the resolution of σ_{i+1}. Equation (4) sums up relative entropy at different scales. $\sigma_0, \ldots, \sigma_n$ usually increase exponentially. Figure 2 shows an entropy map derived with $\sigma = 1, 2, 4, 8, 16, 32, 64, 128$, and 256. It emphasizes edges, complicated structures, and areas near the foreground.

4   Experiments

4.1   Data

The dataset consists of 500 subjects' arterial-phase renal CT images. The average spacing   is   0.757 mm × 0.757 mm × 0.906 mm,   with   standard   deviation

0.075 mm × 0.075 mm × 0.327 mm. The dataset is randomly divided into two disjoint subsets, one of 400 subjects for training and the other of 100 subjects for testing.

The renal parenchyma, arteries, veins, collecting system, and abnormal structures are manually labelled. Abnormal structures (including tumors, cysts, etc.) are jointly labelled into one class "mass". In total there are five foreground classes.

4.2 Methods and Evaluation

The following methods are compared: (1) the U-Net trained with uniform weighting on pixels; (2) the Res. U-Net trained with uniform weighting on pixels; (3) the Res. U-Net trained with multi-scale entropy weighting on pixels. All methods use multi-class cross entropy as their loss function to handle multiple anatomical structures. For method (3), multi-scale entropy map derived from manual segmentation is used to weight pixel's contribution to the loss function. Each method is iteratively trained with 5000 batches consisting of $b = 12$ patches. 3D patches of size $67 \times 67 \times 67$ are randomly and evenly sampled from each class (including the background), and randomly rotated. The learning rate is initially $0.00025 * \sqrt{b - 1}$, and exponentially decays to $0.00001 * \sqrt{b - 1}$ at the last batch. The Adam optimizer [14] is employed to minimize the loss function. It takes about 24 h to train a model with a Quadro P6000 GPU.

The following indices are used to evaluate the methods.

- AUC: the area under the receiver operating characteristic curve. For each foreground class, a binary mask is be derived by thresholding its probabilistic map. Precision and sensitivity, defined as follows, are calculated by comparing the binary mask with the manual segmentation:

$$\text{Precision} = \frac{\text{TruePositive}}{\text{TotalPositive}}, \text{Sensitivity} = \frac{\text{TruePositive}}{\text{GrandTruth}}.$$

This procedure is applied to every image, and then the precision or the sensitivity is averaged over all images. To eliminate the arbitrariness of the threshold value, different thresholds are used, from 0.05 to 0.95 with a step size of 0.05. The averaged precision and sensitivity pairs at different threshold values form a curve. The larger the area under the curve (AUC), the better a model is. The AUC is calculated separately for each class.

- Median Dice indices. Given the multi-class probabilistic maps of an image, a mutually exclusive multi-class segmentation can be derived by labelling each pixel with the class holding the highest probability. The Dice index, defined as follows, are calculated for each class:

$$\text{Dice} = \frac{\text{TruePositive}}{(\text{TotalPositive} + \text{GrandTruth})/2}.$$

This procedure is applied to every image and the median is summarized.

4.3   Results

Table 2 shows the accuracy of the three methods, evaluated on the testing dataset. All the methods achieve excellent accuracy (AUC $\geq$ 0.97, and Dice $\geq$ 0.94) for parenchyma, and high accuracy (AUC from 0.84 to 0.91, and Dice from 0.81 to 0.86) for arteries. They show relatively large variance for veins and collecting system. For veins, the AUC ranges from 0.58 to 0.82 and the Dice ranges from 0.62 to 0.80. For collecting systems, the AUC ranges from 0.52 to 0.66 and the Dice ranges from 0.54 to 0.62. None of the models performs well with masses, with AUC from 0.05 to 0.22 and Dice from 0.06 to 0.29.

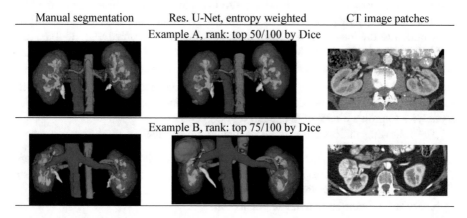

Fig. 3. Visual examples of results by the Res. U-Net weighted by multi-scale entropy. The color code is green for parenchyma, red for arteries, blue for veins, yellow for collecting systems and purple for masses.

Table 2. Segmentation performance.

	U-Net, uniform	Res. U-Net, uniform	Res. U-Net, entropy
Parenchyma	AUC = 0.97, Dice = 0.94	AUC = 0.98, Dice = 0.95	AUC = 0.98, Dice = 0.96
Artery	AUC = 0.84, Dice = 0.81	AUC = 0.90, Dice = 0.85	AUC = 0.91, Dice = 0.86
Vein	AUC = 0.58, Dice = 0.62	AUC = 0.77, Dice = 0.75	AUC = 0.82, Dice = 0.80
Col. Sys.	AUC = 0.53, Dice = 0.54	AUC = 0.61, Dice = 0.58	AUC = 0.66, Dice = 0.62
Mass	AUC = 0.05, Dice = 0.06	AUC = 0.13, Dice = 0.22	AUC = 0.22, Dice = 0.29

For all the classes, the Res. U-Net with entropy weighting performs the best; the Res. U-Net with uniform weighting performs the second; and the U-Net with uniform weighting performs the last. The Res. U-Net improves the accuracy for veins from AUC = 0.58 and Dice = 0.62 to AUC = 0.77 and Dice = 0.75, by more than 0.12. The entropy weighting further improves the accuracy to AUC = 0.82 and Dice = 0.80, by 0.05. The Res. U-Net improves the accuracy for collecting systems from AUC = 0.53 and Dice = 0.54 to AUC = 0.61 and Dice = 0.58, by about 0.04. The entropy weighting further improves the accuracy to AUC = 0.66 and Dice = 0.62, by another 0.04. The same trend can also be found for masses.

Most previous works [4–7] focused on the kidney body, with the best reported Dice index equal to 0.96 [4]. Our method achieves the same level of accuracy. We also evaluated the deeply supervised U-Net in [8] for blood vessels and collecting systems. Its AUCs are 0.78 for arteries, 0.45 for veins, and 0.32 for collecting systems. Please note that the evaluation conducted in [8] only involved connected components overlapping the ground truth and that the evaluation in this paper does not involves such post-processing depending on the ground truth. Figure 3 shows visual examples of results by the Res. U-Net weighted by multi-scale entropy. Their Dice indices respectively rank the top 50th and 75th among 100 images, where better Dice indices imply smaller rank numbers. It in average takes 17.7 s to segment a 3D volume.

5 Conclusions

The residual neural network significantly improves performance by propagating optimization forces directly to different layers. We generalize it from its original sequential structure to directed acyclic graphs. The proposed Res. U-Net, derived from the popular U-Net with a branching and merging structure, conducts multi-scale processing with the residual architecture. It significantly improves segmentation of renal veins and collecting systems.

In addition to inter-class balance, intra-class pixels should also be weighted according to their importance. Our multi-scale entropy captures the spatial complexity of a multi-class label map. It jointly considers distance, edges and shapes. The Res. U-Net trained with multi-scale entropy considerably improves accuracy for renal veins and collecting systems.

References

1. Cancer Stat Facts: Kidney and Renal Pelvis Cancer. https://seer.cancer.gov/statfacts/html/kidrp.html
2. Hughes-Hallett, A., et al.: Augmented reality partial nephrectomy: examining the current status and future perspectives. Urology **83**, 266–273 (2014)
3. Su, L., Vagvolgyi, B., Agarwal, R., Reiley, C., Taylor, R., Hager, G.: Augmented reality during robot-assisted laparoscopic partial nephrectomy: toward real-time 3D-CT to stereoscopic video registration. Urology **73**, 896–900 (2009)

4. Cuingnet, R., Prevost, R., Lesage, D., Cohen, L.D., Mory, B., Ardon, R.: Automatic detection and segmentation of kidneys in 3D CT images using random forests. In: Ayache, N., Delingette, H., Golland, P., Mori, K. (eds.) MICCAI 2012. LNCS, vol. 7512, pp. 66–74. Springer, Heidelberg (2012). https://doi.org/10.1007/978-3-642-33454-2_9

5. Khalifa, F., Soliman, A., Dwyer, A., Gimelfarb, G., ElBaz, A.: A random forest-based framework for 3D kidney segmentation from dynamic contrast-enhanced CT images. In IEEE International Conference on Image Processing (2016)

6. Yang, G., et al.: Automatic kidney segmentation in CT images based on multi-atlas image registration. In: Annual International Conference of the IEEE on Engineering in Medicine and Biology Society (2014)

7. Sharma, K., et al.: Automatic segmentation of kidneys using deep learning for total kidney volume quantification in autosomal dominant polycystic kidney disease. Sci. Rep. **7**, 2049 (2017)

8. Taha, A., Lo, P., Li, J., Zhao, T.: Kid-Net: convolution networks for kidney vessels segmentation from CT-volumes. In: Medical Image Computing and Computer-Assisted Intervention (2018)

9. Ronneberger, O., Fischer, P., Brox, T.: U-Net: convolutional networks for biomedical image segmentation. In: Navab, N., Hornegger, J., Wells, W.M., Frangi, A.F. (eds.) MICCAI 2015. LNCS, vol. 9351, pp. 234–241. Springer, Cham (2015). https://doi.org/10.1007/978-3-319-24574-4_28

10. Merkow, J., Marsden, A., Kriegman, D., Tu, Z.: Dense volume-to-volume vascular boundary detection. In: Ourselin, S., Joskowicz, L., Sabuncu, M.R., Unal, G., Wells, W. (eds.) MICCAI 2016. LNCS, vol. 9902, pp. 371–379. Springer, Cham (2016). https://doi.org/10.1007/978-3-319-46726-9_43

11. Milletari, F., Navab, N., Ahmadi, S.-A.: V-Net: fully convolutional neural networks for volumetric medical image segmentation. In: International Conference on 3D Vision (2016)

12. He, K., Zhang, X., Ren, S., Sun, J.: Deep residual learning for image recognition. In: IEEE Conference on Computer Vision and Pattern Recognition (2016)

13. Huang, C., Li, Y., Loy, C.C., Tang, X.: Learning deep representation for imbalanced classification. In: IEEE Conference on Computer Vision and Pattern Recognition (2016)

14. Kingma, D., Ba, J.: Adam: a method for stochastic optimization. In: International Conference for Learning Representations

Kid-Net: Convolution Networks for Kidney Vessels Segmentation from CT-Volumes

Ahmed Taha[1(✉)], Pechin Lo[2], Junning Li[2], and Tao Zhao[2]

[1] University of Maryland, College Park, USA
ahmdtaha@cs.umd.edu
[2] Intuitive Surgical, Inc., Sunnyvale, USA
{pechin.lo,junning.li,tao.zhao}@intusurg.com

Abstract. Semantic image segmentation plays an important role in modeling patient-specific anatomy. We propose a convolution neural network, called Kid-Net, along with a training schema to segment kidney vessels: artery, vein and collecting system. Such segmentation is vital during the surgical planning phase in which medical decisions are made before surgical incision. Our main contribution is developing a training schema that handles unbalanced data, reduces false positives and enables high-resolution segmentation with a limited memory budget. These objectives are attained using dynamic weighting, random sampling and $3D$ patch segmentation.

Manual medical image annotation is both time-consuming and expensive. Kid-Net reduces kidney vessels segmentation time from matter of hours to minutes. It is trained end-to-end using $3D$ patches from volumetric CT-images. A complete segmentation for a $512 \times 512 \times 512$ CT-volume is obtained within a few minutes (1–2 mins) by stitching the output $3D$ patches together. Feature down-sampling and up-sampling are utilized to achieve higher classification and localization accuracies. Quantitative and qualitative evaluation results on a challenging testing dataset show Kid-Net competence.

Keywords: CT-volumes · Segmentation · Kidney · Biomedical
Convolution · Neural networks

1 Introduction and Related Work

After its success in classification [9] and action recognition [5], convolution neural networks (CNN) began achieving promising results in challenging semantic segmentation tasks [1,12,14]. One key pillar is its ability to learn features from raw input data – without relying on hand-crafted features. A second recent pillar is the ability to precisely localize these features when combining convolution features at different scales. Such localization approach eliminate the need for traditional hand-crafted post processing like Dense-CRF [2,8]. Thus, end-to-end CNN training for challenging segmentation problems becomes feasible. This sheds light on semantic segmentation applications in medical field.

© Springer Nature Switzerland AG 2018
A. F. Frangi et al. (Eds.): MICCAI 2018, LNCS 11073, pp. 463–471, 2018.
https://doi.org/10.1007/978-3-030-00937-3_53

Semantic segmentation for human anatomy using volumetric scans like MRI and CT-volumes is an important medical application. It is a fundamental step to perform or plan surgical procedures. Recent work uses automatic segmentation to do computer assisted diagnosis [13,15], interventions [17] and segmentation from sparse annotations [4]. Recently, U-shaped networks [14] managed to train fully $2D$ convolution network for semantic segmentation in an end-to-end fashion. These architectures have two contradicting phases that carry out complementary tasks. The down-sampling phase detects features, while the up-sampling phase accurately localizes the detected features. Such combination is proven essential in recent literature [4,11,12] to acquire precise segmentation.

Inspired by U-shaped networks, we propose Kid-Net to segment $3D$ patches from volumetric CT-images. We agree with [12] that $3D$ convolutions are better than slice-wise approaches when processing volumetric scans. We build on [12] architecture by processing volumetric patches to enable high resolution segmentation and thus bypass GPU memory constraints. Despite the promising results, such vanilla model suffers due to unbalanced data. This leads to our main contribution which is balancing both intra-foreground and background-foreground classes within independent patches. This achieves the best results as presented in the experiments section. Accordingly, manual preprocessing like cropping or down-sampling workarounds are no longer needed for high resolution CT-volume segmentation.

In this work, we aim to segment kidney vessels: artery, vein and collecting system (ureter). This task is challenging for a number of reasons. First, the CT-volume is huge to fit in memory. To avoid processing the whole CT-volume, we process $3D$ patches individually. Second, foreground and background classes are unbalanced and most patches are foreground-free. Another major challenge is obtaining the groundtruth for training. Medical staff annotate our data; their prior knowledge leads to incomplete groundtruth. Vessels far from kidney are considered less relevant and thus ignored. Figure 1 shows a CT-slice with the three foreground classes. It highlights the problem difficulty even for a well-informed technician.

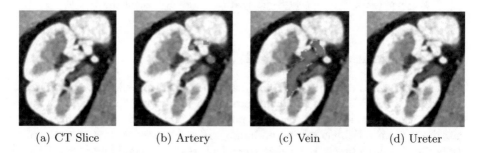

(a) CT Slice   (b) Artery   (c) Vein   (d) Ureter

Fig. 1. CT slice contains three foreground classes: artery (red), vein (blue) and collecting system (orange). Best seen in color and zoom

2   Method

Inspired by U-Net structure [14], Kid-Net is divided into two main phases: down-sampling and up-sampling. Figure 2 shows these phases and how Kid-Net up-sampling phase is different from U-Net. In U-Net, down-sampled features are repeatedly up-sampled and concatenated with the corresponding feature till a single segmentation result, with the original image resolution, is obtained. Kid-Net is similar to U-Net but adds residual links extension in which each down-sampled feature is independently up-sampled 2^n times till the original resolution is restored. Thus unlike U-Net, Kid-Net generates multiple segmentation results that are averaged to obtain a final segmentation result. These residual links follow Junning et. al [10] Residual-U-Net design. Sequential non-linear functions accumulation improves deep neural networks performance in image recognition. In our paper, residual links are added in up-sampling phase only for simplicity

Kid-Net segments kidney vessels from CT-volumes. The foreground classes are artery, vein and collecting system (ureter) vessels. To avoid the large memory requirement of CT-volumes, Kid-Net is trained using $3D$ CT-volume patches from $R^{96 \times 96 \times 96}$. Without any architecture modification, wider context through bigger patches, within GPU memory constraints, are feasible. Kid-Net outputs a soft-max probability maps for artery, vein, collecting system and background. Instead of training for individual foreground classes independently, our network is trained to detect the three foreground classes. Such approach has two advantages; first, a single network decision per voxel fills in for a heuristic-based approach to merge multiple networks decisions. Second, this approach aligns with [6] recommendation that learning tasks with less data benefit largely from joint training with other tasks.

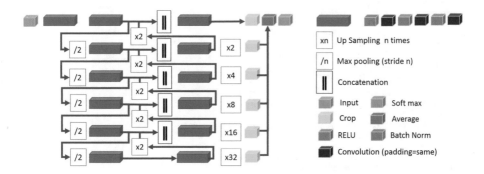

Fig. 2. KID-Net architecture. The two contradicting phases are colored in blue. The down-sampling and up-sampling phases detect and localize features respectively. The segmentation result, at different scale levels, are averaged to compute the final segmentation. Best seen in color and zoom

While training Kid-Net with $3D$ patches bypasses GPU memory constraints, a new challenge surfaces–unbalanced data. Patches majority are foreground-free.

Even when a foreground class exists, it occupies a small percentage. In this paper, we leverage recent work [4,11], that addresses tiny structures precise localization, to tackle unbalanced data. As follows, a two-fold approach is proposed to hinder bias against the tiny structured foreground classes.

The first fold assigns dynamic weights to individual voxels based on their classes and patches significance. A major challenge in medical image processing is detecting small structures. Vessels in direct contact with kidney are tiny and their resolution is limited by acquisition. Tiny vessels are challenging to annotate, more valuable to acquire. Thus, patches containing smaller vessels are more significant, have higher weight. Patch weight is inversely proportional to the vessel volume inside it. Foreground classes are also assigned higher weights to hinder the network background bias. The key idea is to measure the average foreground classes volumes per patch dynamically during training. Then, assign higher weights to classes with smaller average volumes and vice versa.

A policy that a vessel volume × weight must equal $1/n$ is imposed where n is the number of classes including the background class. Thus, all classes contribute equally from a network perspective. To account for data augmentation, vessels volumes are measured during training. Enforcing equal contribution (volume × weight) from all classes is our objective. To do so, we use the moving average procedure outlined in Algorithm 1.

Algorithm 1. Our proposed moving average procedure assigns voxels dynamic weights (VW_c) based on their classes and patch weight. Patch Weight (PW) is inversely proportional to its foreground volume. Class weight (CW) is inversely proportional to its average volume per patch. Initially $V_c = \frac{1}{n}$ for every class c. Our settings $\alpha = 0.001$, $n = 4$.

Require: α : Convergence Rate
Require: P : Current 3D patch with axis x, y, z
Require: n : Number of classes (background included)
Require: V_c : Class (c) moving average volume
Require: PW : Current patch weight
Require: CW_c : Class (c) weight
   for all c in classes **do**
      // Measure class (c) volume in patch P
      $V_c(P) = \left(\sum_x \sum_y \sum_z P(x,y,z) == c \right) / size(P)$
      // Update class (c) moving average volume
      $V_c = V_c \times (1 - \alpha) + V_c(P) \times \alpha$
      // Update class weight based on its moving average volume
      $CW_c = 1 / (n \times V_c)$
   end for
   // Set patch weight based on foreground volume
   if P contains background only **then**
      $PW = 1$
   else
      // Foreground volume $\sum_{c=1}^{n-1} V_c(P) < 1$
      $PW = 1 - log(\sum_{c=1}^{n-1} V_c(P))$
   end if
   $VW_c = PW * CW_c$ (Voxel weight is function of PW and CW_c)

Due to background relative huge volume, it's assigned tiny class weight. So the network produces a lot of false positives – it is cheap to mis-classify a background voxel. To tackle this undesired phenomena, we propose our second complementary fold – Random Sampling. Random Background voxels are sampled and assigned high weights. Such method is most effective in limiting false positives because high loss is incurred for these voxels if mis-classified. Figure 3 shows our sampling schema. Two bands are constructed around kidney vessels using morphological kernel, a binary circular dilation of radii two and four. Misclassifications within the first band (<2 voxels away from the vessel) are considered marginal errors. In a given patch, the sampled background voxels are equivalent to the foreground vessel volume, where 20% and 80% come from the red band and the volume beyond this band respectively. If a patch is foreground-free, 1% voxels are randomly sampled.

While using advanced U-shaped architectures can lead to marginal improvements, dynamic weighting and random sampling are indispensable. Both weighting and sampling are done during training phase while patches are fed into the network.

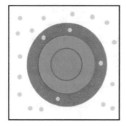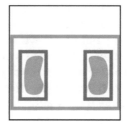

Fig. 3. (Left) Background sampling approach. Foreground vessel, in green, surrounded by two bands, blue and red, at distance 2 and 4 voxels. Equivalent foreground volume, 20% and 80%, is randomly sampled from the red band and the volume beyond this band respectively. (Right) Experiments evaluation regions. The first region is the whole region of interest defined per subject ground truth outlined in blue. The second region is the kidney bounding box outlined in green.

3   Experiments

In our experiments, we use volumetric CT-scans from 236 subjects. The average spacing is $0.757 \times 0.757 \times 0.906$ mm, with standard deviation $0.075 \times 0.075 \times 0.327$ mm. Kid-Net is trained using $3D$ patches from 99 cases, while 30 and 107 cases are used for validation and testing respectively. Training patches are presliced to reduce I/O bottleneck. They are uniformly sliced from CT-scans random points at background, collecting system, artery and vein centerlines. Training with foreground-free patches is mandatory. When eliminated, performance degrades because the network learns that every patch has a foreground object, and segments accordingly, which is false.

Two training schema, with and without random sampling, are evaluated. In both schema dynamic weighting following Algorithm 1 is applied. Training without both dynamic weighting and random sampling leads to a degenerate segmentation – background class-bias. Kid-Net is trained using Keras API [3], Adam optimizer [7], and a categorical cross entropy loss function. Segmentation results are evaluated using dice-coefficient – F1 score [16].

Both artery and vein have tree-structure; they are thick near aorta and vena cava, while fine at terminals near renal artery and renal vein. These fine vessels are most difficult to annotate, i.e. most valuable to acquire. Dice-coefficient is biased against fine details in such tree-structure. To overcome such limitation, we evaluate the two regions depicted in Fig. 3. The first region is based on the ground truth region of interest. This evaluates the whole tree-structure including the thick branches– aorta and vena cava. The second region is the kidney bounding box. It targets fine vessels in direct contact with the kidney.

The ground truth region of interest (ROI) is subject dependent. During evaluation, we clip our output in z-axis, based on the per subject ground truth ROI. It is worth-noting that the ground truth annotation is incomplete for two reasons. First, vessels in direct connect with kidney are challenging to annotate due to their tiny size, thus the ground truth is a discretized vessel islands – 12 islands on average. Second, vessels far from kidney have little value, for kidney surgery, to annotate and so are typically missing. To avoid penalizing valid segmentations, we evaluate predictions overlapping with known ground-truth vessel islands. This evaluation approach reduces the chances of falsely penalizing unannotated detections. It also aligns with the premise that neural networks assist, but not replace, human especially in medical applications.

Table 1. Quantitative evaluation for different training schema in two evaluation regions. Dynamic Weighting (DW) plus Random Sampling (RS) achieves the highest accuracies. Artery F1 score is the highest.

	Whole ROI		Kidney bounding box	
	DW	DW+RS	DW	DW+RS
Artery	0.86	**0.88**	0.72	**0.72**
Vein	**0.59**	0.57	0.60	**0.67**
Ureter	0.32	**0.62**	0.41	**0.63**

Table 1 summarizes the quantitative results and highlights our network ability to segment both coarse and fine vessels around the kidney. Artery segmentation is the most accurate because all scans are done during arterial phase. This suggests that better vein and ureter segmentations are feasible if venous and waste-out scans are available. The thick aorta boosts artery segmentation F1 score in the whole ROI. In the kidney bounding box, tiny artery vessels become more challenging, and F1 score relatively decreases. The same argument explains vein vessels F1 score. Since arterial scans are used, concealed vena cava penalizes F1 score severely in the whole ROI region. This observation manifests in Fig. 4,

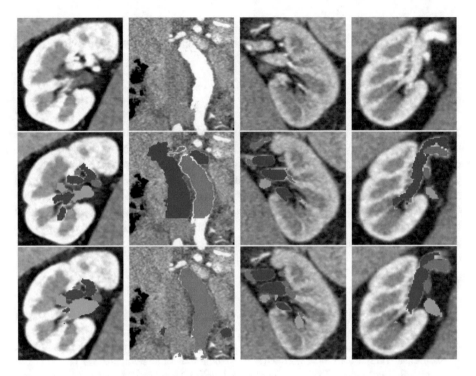

Fig. 4. Qualitative evaluation results. Rows contain raw CT slice, ground truth annotation, and Kid-Net segmentation respectively. Artery, vein, and ureter are highlighted in red, blue, and orange. Best seen in color and zoom

second column. While aorta is easy to segment and boosts F1 score, vena cava is more challenging and thus F1 score degrades.

Among the three kidney vessels, the collecting system is the most challenging. Due to their tiny size, it is difficult to manually annotate or automatically segment. Ureter vessels ground truth annotations are available only within the kidney proximity–far ureter are less relevant. This explains why ureter F1 score is similar in both evaluation regions. Ureter class is assigned the highest weight due to its relative small size. This leads to a lot of false ureter positives. While random sampling has limited effect on artery and vein F1 score, its merits manifest in ureter segmentation. It boosts segmentation accuracy by 30% and 22% in the whole ROI and kidney bounding box respectively. Thus, It is concluded that both dynamic weights and random sampling are essential to achieve accurate tiny vessels segmentation.

Figure 4 shows qualitative results and highlights vessels around the kidney. All CT-slices are rendered using soft tissue window–level = 40, width = 400. Vein and collecting system segmentation are the most challenging. The second column shows a shortcoming case due to a concealed vein. Fine vessels near kidney are the most difficult to annotate. Manually annotating such vessels can be cumbersome and time consuming. Thats why Kid-Net is valuable; its training schema enables fine anatomy segmentation in high resolution CT-volumes, and voids GPU memory constraints.

4   Conclusion

We propose Kid-Net, a convolution neural network for kidney vessels segmentation. Kid-Net achieves great performance segmenting different vessels by processing $3D$ patches. Fitting a whole CT-volume in memory, to train a neural network, is no longer required. We propose a two-fold solution to balance foreground and background distributions in a training dataset. Dynamically weighting voxels resolves unbalanced data. Assigning higher weights to randomly sampled background voxels effectively reduces false positives. The proposed concepts are applicable to other fine segmentation tasks.

References

1. Bertasius, G., Shi, J., Torresani, L.: Semantic segmentation with boundary neural fields. In: CVPR (2016)
2. Chen, L.C., Papandreou, G., Kokkinos, I., Murphy, K., Yuille, A.L.: DeepLab: semantic image segmentation with deep convolutional nets, atrous convolution, and fully connected CRFs. arXiv preprint arXiv:1606.00915 (2016)
3. Chollet, F., et al.: Keras (2015). https://github.com/fchollet/keras
4. Çiçek, Ö., Abdulkadir, A., Lienkamp, S.S., Brox, T., Ronneberger, O.: 3D U-Net: learning dense volumetric segmentation from sparse annotation. In: MICCAI (2016)
5. Ji, S., Xu, W., Yang, M., Yu, K.: 3D convolutional neural networks for human action recognition. IEEE Trans. Pattern Anal. Mach. Intell. 3(5), 221–231 (2013)
6. Kaiser, L., Gomez, A.N., Shazeer, N., Vaswani, A., Parmar, N., Jones, L., Uszkoreit, J.: One model to learn them all. arXiv preprint arXiv:1706.05137 (2017)
7. Kingma, D., Ba, J.: Adam: A method for stochastic optimization. arXiv preprint arXiv:1412.6980 (2014)
8. Krähenbühl, P., Koltun, V.: Efficient inference in fully connected CRFs with Gaussian edge potentials. In: NIPS (2011)
9. Krizhevsky, A., Sutskever, I., Hinton, G.E.: ImageNet classification with deep convolutional neural networks. In: NIPS (2012)
10. Li, J., Lo, P., Taha, A., Wu, H., Zhao, T.: Segmentation of renal structures for image-guided surgery. In: MICCAI (2018)
11. Merkow, J., Marsden, A., Kriegman, D., Tu, Z.: Dense volume-to-volume vascular boundary detection. In: IJCARS (2016)
12. Milletari, F., Navab, N., Ahmadi, S.A.: V-Net: fully convolutional neural networks for volumetric medical image segmentation. In: 3D Vision (3DV) (2016)
13. Porter, C.R., Crawford, E.D.: Combining artificial neural networks and transrectal ultrasound in the diagnosis of prostate cancer. Oncology 17, 1395–1418 (2003)
14. Ronneberger, O., Fischer, P., Brox, T.: U-Net: Convolutional networks for biomedical image segmentation. arXiv preprint arXiv:1505.04597 (2015)

15. Shin, H.C., et al.: Deep convolutional neural networks for computer-aided detection: CNN architectures, dataset characteristics and transfer learning. IEEE TMI **35**, 1285 (2016)
16. Sørensen, T.: A method of establishing groups of equal amplitude in plant sociology based on similarity of species and its application to analyses of the vegetation on Danish commons. Biol. Skr. **5**, 1–34 (1948)
17. Zettinig, O., et al.: Multimodal image-guided prostate fusion biopsy based on automatic deformable registration. IJCARS **10**, 1997–2007 (2015)

Local and Non-local Deep Feature Fusion for Malignancy Characterization of Hepatocellular Carcinoma

Tianyou Dou[1], Lijuan Zhang[2], Hairong Zheng[2], and Wu Zhou[1(✉)]

[1] School of Medical Information Engineering,
Guangzhou University of Chinese Medicine, Guangzhou, China
zhouwu@gzucm.edu.cn
[2] Shenzhen Institutes of Advanced Technology, Chinese Academy of Sciences,
Shenzhen, China

Abstract. Deep feature derived from convolutional neural network (CNN) has demonstrated superior ability to characterize the biological aggressiveness of tumors, which is typically based on convolutional operations repeatedly processed within a local neighborhood. Due to the heterogeneity of lesions, such local deep feature may be insufficient to represent the aggressiveness of neoplasm. Inspired by the non-local neural networks in computer vision, the non-local deep feature may be remarkably complementary for lesion characterization. In this work, we propose a local and non-local deep feature fusion model based on common and individual feature analysis by extracting common and individual components of local and non-local deep features to characterize the biological aggressiveness of lesions. Specifically, we first design a non-local subnetwork for non-local deep feature extraction of neoplasm, and subsequently combine local and non-local deep features with a specific designed fusion subnetwork based on common and individual feature analysis. Experimental results of malignancy characterization of clinical hepatocellular carcinoma (HCC) with Contrast-enhanced MR images demonstrate several intriguing features of the proposed local and non-local deep feature fusion model as follows: (1) Non-local deep feature outperforms local deep feature for lesion characterization; (2) The fusion of local and non-local deep feature yields further improved performance of lesion characterization; (3) The fusion method of common and individual feature analysis outperforms the method of simple concatenation and the method of deep correlation model.

1 Introduction

Hepatocellular carcinoma (HCC) is the most common primary hepatic malignancy, ranking second in the world for the cause of death from tumors [1]. Malignancy of HCC is an important prognostic factor that affects recurrence and survival after liver transplantation or surgical resection in clinical practice [2]. MR imaging has played a significant role in the diagnosis of HCC, in which

© Springer Nature Switzerland AG 2018
A. F. Frangi et al. (Eds.): MICCAI 2018, LNCS 11073, pp. 472–479, 2018.
https://doi.org/10.1007/978-3-030-00937-3_54

there are a variety of studies that address the malignancy characterization of HCC by identifying imaging features [3,4]. However, such morphological features are generally dependent on empirical manual design, which are often insufficient to characterize the heterogeneity of the tumor.

Deep features relied on data-driven learning from samples demonstrate superior ability to characterize tumors [5]. Recently, deep feature in the arterial phase of Contrast-enhanced MR has been verified to outperform texture features for malignancy characterization of HCC [6]. Such local deep feature is typically based on convolutional operations repeatedly processed within a local neighborhood. More recently, a non-local neural network has been illustrated for the task of video classification in computer vision, which is based on a non-local operation that allows distant pixels to make contribution to the response at a position as a weighted mean of features from all the distant pixels [7]. We hypothesize that such non-local deep feature may be remarkably applicable and complementary to local deep feature for malignancy characterization of HCC.

More importantly, it is essential to take full advantage of the local and non-local deep features by optimal fusion for lesion characterization. One simple way for fusing information is concatenating deep features [8] or integrating multi-modal results based on weighted summation [9]. Recently, deep correlational model has been proposed to extract maximum correlated representation of deep features from multimodal by canonic correlation analysis for lesion characterization [10]. However, only shared or correlated component of deep features between modals are extracted, neglecting the influence of separation of deep features across modals for characterization. As a matter of fact, a common part to be shared and a modal-specific part from features of the color and depth information have been recovered to represent the implicit relationship between different modalities for RGB-D object recognition [11,12]. We hypothesize that both the correlated component and separated component between local and non-local deep features of neoplasm may play significant roles in malignancy characterization of HCC.

In this work, we propose a local and non-local deep feature fusion model to characterize the malignancy of HCC. The proposed model first extracts local and non-local deep feature of neoplasm separately, and subsequently recovers common and individual components of local and non-local deep features based on common and individual feature analysis. Specifically, the learned common and individual features can reflect the implicit relationship of local and non-local deep features, which further improve the performance of malignancy characterization of HCC.

2   Method

2.1   Local Deep Feature Extraction

The local deep feature extraction consists of multiple repetitions of convolutional layer with activation function. Given the input feature of image x in CNN, the local deep feature y is obtained by $y = \sigma(Wx + b)$, where W is a convolutional filter based on a convolutional operation that sums up the weighted input in a local neighborhood, b is the bias term, σ is the rectified linear unit (ReLU) active function.

2.2 Non-local Deep Feature Extraction

The non-local deep feature extraction is based on the conventional non-local mean operation defined in deep neural network as follows [7]

$$y_i = \frac{1}{C(x)} \sum_{\forall j} f(x_i, x_j) g(x_j) \tag{1}$$

where i is the index of a position to be computed and j is the index of all possible positions. x is the input image and y is the output non-local feature of the same size as x. A similarity function f computes a scalar that manifests approximation between i and j. The function g computes a representation of the input image at the position j. The response is normalized by a factor $C(x)$.

In this work, the g is considered in the form of a linear embedding as $g(x_j) = W_g x_j$, where W_g is a weight matrix to be learned. Furthermore, the similarity function f is considered by the embedded Gaussian as $f(x_i, x_j) = e^{\theta(x_i)^T \phi(x_j)}$, where $\theta(x_i) = W_\theta x_i$, and $\phi(x_j) = W_\phi x_j$ are two embeddings.

We set $C(x) = \sum_{\forall j} f(x_i, x_j)$, and for a given i, $\frac{1}{C(x)} f(x_i, x_j)$ becomes the softmax computation along the dimension j. Therefore, the output non-local deep feature y becomes

$$y = softmax(x^T W_\theta^T W_\phi x) W_g x \tag{2}$$

where W_g, W_θ and W_ϕ are three weight matrices to be learned. Inspired by the work of [7] in video classification, an implementation of the non-local deep feature map y of neoplasm is described in Fig. 1. Different from the work of [7] in video classification, we conduct the non-local operation directly for the non-local deep feature extraction of neoplasm without considering the residual connection.

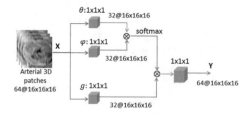

Fig. 1. An implementation of the 3D non-local deep feature map. $\otimes$ denotes matrix multiplication, and "$1 \times 1 \times 1$" denotes $1 \times 1 \times 1$ convolutions. Note that the softmax operation is performed on each row, and we set the number of channels in x to 64.

2.3   Correlation and Individual Feature Analysis

Given two local and non-local deep feature sets $\{Y_i \in R^{(I_i \times J)}, i = 1, 2\}$, the Correlation and individual feature analysis is to extract common and individual components between the two deep feature sets Y_1 and Y_2 in disciplines. Each feature set Y_i is typically decomposed into three terms as follows [13]:

$$Y_i = J_i + A_i + R_i, \quad i = 1, 2 \tag{3}$$

where $J_i \in R^{(I_i \times J)}$ and $A_i \in R^{(I_i \times J)}$ are low-rank matrices, denoting common component between sets and individual component associated with each set, respectively. $R_i \in R^{(I_i \times J)}$ is a matrix denoting residual noise. In order to facilitate the identification of common and individual components, the rows of J and A_i should be mutually orthogonal. Hence, the common component J_i and individual component A_i can be represented by the original deep feature Y_i as

$$J_i = V_i^T V_i Y_i, \quad A_i = Q_i^T Q_i Y_i \tag{4}$$

where V_i is the mapping matrix that projects the original deep feature Y_i into the common component J_i, and Q_i is the mapping matrix that projects the original deep feature Y_i into the individual component A_i. As J_i and A_i should be unrelated and not contaminated by each other, the mapping matrix V_i and Q_i should be orthogonal to each other as $V_i^T Q_i = 0$.

The purpose of extracting the common and individual components between the two local and non-local deep features $\{Y_i \in R^{(I_i \times J)}, i = 1, 2\}$ is solving the constrained least-squares problem:

$$\begin{aligned} min \quad & ||V_1 Y_1 - V_2 Y_2||_F^2, \\ s.t. \quad & Y_i = V_i^T V_i Y_i + Q_i^T Q_i Y_i, i = 1, 2 \\ & V_i^T Q_i = 0, i = 1, 2 \end{aligned} \tag{5}$$

Where $|| \cdot ||_F$ is the Frobenius norm. In this work, alternating optimization is adopted to minimize the constraint least squares problem for all the variable V_i and Q_i. Based on the Lagrange multiplier criterion, the Lagrange function to minimize the constrained least-squares problem is

$$\begin{aligned} \iota(\phi, \theta) = & ||V_1 Y_1 - V_2 Y_2||_F^2 + \sum_{i=1}^{2} \phi_i ||Y_i - V_i^T V_i Y_i - Q_i^T Q_i Y_i||_F^2 \\ & + \sum_{i=1}^{2} \theta_i ||V_i^T Q_i||_F^2 \end{aligned} \tag{6}$$

Where ϕ_i and θ_i are the positive Lagrange multipliers related to the two linear constraints. In this work, we first learn the mapping matrices V_i to map the local and non-local deep features Y_i into the common feature space J_i separately, and then we use Singular Value Decomposition (SVD) to construct the orthogonal basis Q_i of the matrix V_i. Finally, the common component J_i and individual component A_i are obtained by V_i and Q_i according to Eq. (4).

2.4   Local and Nonlocal Deep Feature Fusion Framework

Figure 2 showed the proposed local and non-local deep feature fusion framework. With respect to the extraction of 3D local deep feature by conventional CNN, the convolutional layer was determined by convolving the extracted 3D patches ($16 \times 16 \times 16$) with a 3D convolution filter ($3 \times 3 \times 3$) to get the convolution feature maps of the original 3D patch, followed by a pooling layer to perform downsampling operation along the 3D dimensions. In addition, the non-local deep feature can be obtained by the non-local operation as demonstrated in the previous Sect. 2.2. Subsequently, the fusion layer performed the correlation and individual feature analysis to recover common and individual components from the local and non-local deep features. The common component J_1 or J_2 and the individual component A_1 and A_2 are concatenated as the output of local and non-local deep feature fusion, followed by the fully-connected layer and the softmax layer to yield the classification results of low-grade or high-grade of HCC.

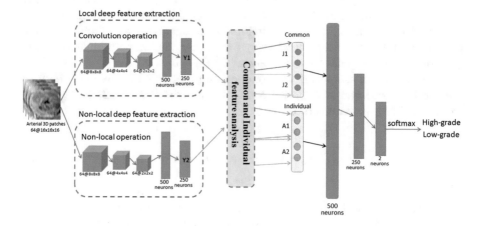

Fig. 2. The proposed local and non-local deep feature fusion framework.

2.5   The Implementation

The proposed framework is implemented by python on the platform of TensorFlow, and the configuration of GPUs used in this work is NVIDIA GeForce GTX1080. The whole network is trained in an end-to-end manner. For the optimization, we use the well-known Adam algorithm [14] for Stochastic Optimization to minimize the objective function. The number of iterations is set to 15000. The initialization of the learning rate is set to 1e-4, and the decay of the learning rate is set to 0.99.

3   Results

The accuracy, sensitivity and specificity are quantitatively computed for malignancy characterization of HCC, and the 4-fold cross-validation with 10 repetitions is adopted to evaluate the performance of the proposed framework.

3.1   Subjects, MR Imaging and Histology Information

Forty-six HCC patients with 46 HCCs are included for this retrospective study from October 2011 to September 2015. Contrast-enhanced MR images with Gd-DTPA agent administration are acquired with a 3.0T MR scanner (Signa Excite HD 3.0T, GE Healthcare, Milwaukee, WI, USA), including pre-contrast, arterial, portal venous, and delayed phase images. The pathological information of HCCs is retrieved from the clinical histology report, including Edmondson grade I (1), II (20), III (24) and IV (1) for these forty-six HCCs. Clinically, Edmondson grade I and II are low-grade, and Edmondson grade III and IV are high-grade, resulting in 21 low-grade and 25 high-grade HCCs for this study. Note that the clinical data has been used in the work of [4,6].

3.2   Performance of Local and Nonlocal Deep Feature

Table 1 showed the characterization performance of local, non-local and the proposed local and non-local fusion of deep features from the arterial phase of Contrast-enhanced MR in 2D and 3D, respectively. First, it can be found that 3D deep feature outperformed 2D deep feature either in local or non-local circumstances for malignancy characterization of HCC, which demonstrated that 3D CNN or 3D Non-local Neural network encoded sufficiently spatial information in volumetric data compared with 2D CNN or 2D Non-local Neural network. Furthermore, non-local deep feature showed better performance than local deep feature for malignancy characterization both in 2D and 3D, indicating that non-local deep feature may embed more image feature from vascularity and cellularity of neoplasm to characterize the aggressiveness of HCC. Finally, the proposed local and non-local deep feature fusion yielded best results both in 2D and 3D when taking advantage of local and non-local deep features.

3.3   Comparison of Deep Feature Fusion Methods

Table 2 showed the performance comparison of local and non-local deep feature fusion by direct concatenation, deep correlation model and the common and individual feature in 2D and 3D, respectively. Compared with the performance of local or non-local deep features in 2D and 3D as tabulated in Table 1, all the fusion methods could obtain improved results as shown in Table 2. Comparatively, the proposed fusion method based on common and individual feature analysis yielded better results than direct concatenation and deep correlation model both in 2D and 3D circumstances. Furthermore, the individual component between local and non-local deep features also yielded promising results

Table 1. Performance comparison of local, non-local and the proposed local and non-local fusion of deep features in 2D and 3D from the arterial phase of Contrast-enhanced MR.(%).

	Accuracy	Sensitivity	Specificity
2D local	84.61 ± 7.25	87.60 ± 11.81	83.00 ± 17.19
2D non-local	86.32 ± 7.93	87.61 ± 12.16	87.24 ± 10.83
2D local and non-local fusion	89.74 ± 8.88	91.51 ± 8.55	88.17 ± 16.12
3D local	87.69 ± 7.05	86.96 ± 9.99	89.53 ± 11.58
3D non-local	90.00 ± 6.01	86.95 ± 9.35	93.42 ± 8.24
3D local and non-local fusion	93.16 ± 4.36	94.14 ± 8.92	91.30 ± 11.26

for malignancy characterization of HCC, especially in 3D. Specifically, the common feature yielded slightly better results than that of the deep correlation model, demonstrating that the common component recovered by the common and individual feature analysis has more advantage than that from the canonical correlation analysis, which is consistent with the previous finding in [13].

Table 2. Performance comparison of local and non-local deep feature fusion in 2D and 3D by direct concatenation, deep correlation model and the common and individual feature analysis(%).

	Accuracy	Sensitivity	Specificity
2D direct concatenation	88.03 ± 8.20	92.44 ± 11.77	86.01 ± 12.37
2D deep correlation model	88.89 ± 9.67	93.94 ± 6.92	85.81 ± 14.07
2D common feature	89.74 ± 6.28	92.35 ± 6.98	89.09 ± 10.16
2D individual feature	88.89 ± 8.20	92.70 ± 6.71	87.39 ± 13.13
2D common and individual feature analysis	90.60 ± 4.83	93.77 ± 7.35	87.50 ± 9.43
3D direct concatenation	91.45 ± 7.64	93.52 ± 9.80	90.22 ± 12.02
3D deep correlation model	90.60 ± 6.04	87.70 ± 9.40	91.45 ± 11.22
3D common feature	91.45 ± 5.67	91.16 ± 8.71	91.91 ± 7.64
3D individual feature	92.31 ± 6.28	91.78 ± 9.84	91.30 ± 12.71
3D common and individual feature analysis	93.16 ± 4.36	94.14 ± 8.92	91.30 ± 11.26

4   Conclusion

The proposed local and non-local deep feature fusion model yields superior performance for malignancy characterization of HCC in comparison of local deep feature, non-local deep feature, and the fusion methods of direct concatenation and deep correlation model, providing a novel strategy for the biological aggressiveness prediction and treatment planning of neoplastic diseases.

Acknowledgment. This research is supported by the grant from National Natural Science Foundation of China (NSFC: 81771920). The authors highly thank Prof. Changhong Liang, Prof. Zaiyi Liu and Dr. Guangyi Wang in the Department of Radiology, Guangdong General Hospital for providing MR images and clinical histology reports of HCCs for this research.

References

1. Park, J.W., Chen, M., Colombo, M., et al.: Global patterns of hepatocellular carcinoma management from diagnosis to death: the BRIDGE study. Liver Int. **35**(9), 2155–2166 (2015)
2. Bruix, J., Sherman, M.: Management of hepatocellular carcinoma. Hepatology **42**, 1208–1236 (2005)
3. Nishie, A., Tajima, T., Asayama, Y., et al.: Diagnostic performance of apparent diffusion coefficient for predicting histological grade of hepatocellular carcinoma. Eur. J. Radiol. **80**(2), e29–e33 (2011)
4. Zhou, W., Zhang, L., Wang, K., et al.: Malignancy characterization of hepatocellular carcinomas based on texture analysis of contrast-enhanced MR images. J. Magn. Reson. Imaging **45**(5), 1476–1484 (2017)
5. Litjens, G., Kooi, T., Bejnordi, B.E., et al.: A survey on deep learning in medical image analysis. Med. Image Anal. **42**(9), 60–88 (2017)
6. Wang, Q., Zhang, L., Xie, Y., Zheng, H., Zhou, W.: Malignancy characterization of hepatocellular carcinoma using hybrid texture and deep feature. In: Proceedings of the 24th IEEE International Conference Image Processing, pp. 4162–4166 (2017)
7. Wang, X., Girshick, R., Gupta A., He K.: Non-local neural networks. arXiv:1711.07971 (2017)
8. Setio, A.A.A., Ciompi, F., Litjens, G., et al.: Pulmonary nodule detection in CT images: false positive reduction using multi-view convolutional networks. IEEE Trans. Med. Imaging **35**(5), 1160–1169 (2016)
9. Ciompi, F., de Hoop, B., Van Riel, S.J., et al.: Automatic classification of pulmonary peri-fissural nodules in computed tomography using an ensemble of 2D views and a convolutional neural network out-of-the box. Med. Image Anal. **26**, 195–202 (2015)
10. Yao, J., Zhu, X., Zhu, F., Huang, J.: Deep correlational learning for survival prediction from multi-modality data. MICCAI 2017. LNCS, vol. 10434, pp. 406–414. Springer, Cham (2017). https://doi.org/10.1007/978-3-319-66185-8_46
11. Wang, A, Cai, J, Lu, J, Cham, T.: MMSS: multi-modal sharable and specific feature learning for RGB-D object recognition. In: IEEE International Conference on Computer Vision, pp. 1125–1133 (2015)
12. Wang, Z., Lin, R., Lu, J., Feng, J., Zhou, J.: Correlated and individual multi-modal deep learning for RGB-D object recognition. arXiv:1604.01655v2 [cs.CV] (2016)
13. Panagakis, Y., Nicolaou, M.A., Zafeiriou, S., Pantic, M.: Robust correlated and individual component analysis. IEEE Trans. Pattern Anal. Mach. Intel. **38**(8), 1665–1678 (2016)
14. Kingma, D.P., Ba, J.L.: Adam: a method for stochastic optimization. arXiv:1412.6980 [cs.LG] (2014)

A Novel Bayesian Model Incorporating Deep Neural Network and Statistical Shape Model for Pancreas Segmentation

Jingting Ma[1(✉)], Feng Lin[1], Stefan Wesarg[3], and Marius Erdt[1,2]

[1] School of Computer Science and Engineering, Nanyang Technological University,
Singapore, Singapore
{jma012,asflin,merdt}@ntu.edu.sg
[2] Fraunhofer Singapore, Nanyang Technological University, Singapore, Singapore
[3] Visual Healthcare Technologies, Fraunhofer IGD, Darmstadt, Germany
stefan.wesarg@igd.fraunhofer.de

Abstract. Deep neural networks have achieved significant success in medical image segmentation in recent years. However, poor contrast to surrounding tissues and high flexibility of anatomical structure of the interest object are still challenges. On the other hand, statistical shape model based approaches have demonstrated promising performance on exploiting complex shape variabilities but they are sensitive to localization and initialization. This motivates us to leverage the rich shape priors learned from statistical shape models to improve the segmentation of deep neural networks. In this work, we propose a novel Bayesian model incorporating the segmentation results from both deep neural network and statistical shape model for segmentation. In evaluation, experiments are performed on 82 CT datasets of the challenging public NIH pancreas dataset. We report 85.32 % of the mean DSC that outperforms the state-of-the-art and approximately 12 % improvement from the predicted segment of deep neural network.

Keywords: Bayesian model · Deep neural networks
Statistical shape model · Pancreas segmentation

1 Introduction

With the rapid development of Convolutional Neural Networks (CNNs) in semantic segmentation, deep neural networks like U-Net [1], SegNet [2] have become a popular trend in medical image segmentation and achieved remarkable success in segmentation of many organs, e.g. liver, lung and spleen. However, segmentation of challenging organs such as pancreas still remains difficulties due to the relatively small region in the whole volume, highly complex anatomical structure and significantly ambiguous boundary. On the other hand, usually the amount of labeled medical image data is limited which inhibits the segmentation from achieving considerable accuracy. To tackle these challenges, we aim to

© Springer Nature Switzerland AG 2018
A. F. Frangi et al. (Eds.): MICCAI 2018, LNCS 11073, pp. 480–487, 2018.
https://doi.org/10.1007/978-3-030-00937-3_55

propose a robust segmentation approach for pancreas, which is one of the most challenging organs.

Numerous works focus on pancreas segmentation in literature, and the majority of them adopt deep neural networks with various refinement methods. In [3,4], a coarse-to-fine framework is designed where the coarse network is trained to obtain the rough segment and remove the background regions, afterwards the shrunken region is passed to the fine network for precise segmentation. In [5], a Recurrent Neural Network (RNN) combining with CNN layers is employed to exploit spatial relations among successive slices. On the other hand, traditional machine learning approaches are demonstrated to be useful in segmentation framework for locally fine-tuning, e.g., random forests are utilized in feature extraction and classification following the deep neural networks in [6,7] and Gaussian Mixture Model is employed to refine the U-Net in [8].

Considering of the ambiguities on boundary, it is well worth to leverage the 3D shape variabilities to distinguish the non-visible boundary, this motivates us to employ statistical shape models in segmentation framework. Through back projection onto the shape model, the corruptness on input shape is supposed to be corrected. Owing to the high variability of pancreas shape, we adopt the robust kernel statistical shape model presented in [9] as it has compelling advantages in handling corrupted and highly deformable training data than conventional PCA models. However, the model based approaches are sensitive to initialization, thus a deep neural network plays an important role in providing a rough segmentation for shape model initialization. With this motivation, we integrate the segmentation from deep neural network and statistical shape model within a Bayesian model for pancreas segmentation. A novel optimization principle joint with image feature and shape prior is proposed to guide segmentation. Our approach is demonstrated to be promising and efficient in terms of evaluation.

2   Method

In this section, we elaborate our segmentation approach starting with the deep neural network architecture, followed by the Bayesian model. Let us assume we have a set of 3D CT volumes $I = \{I_1, \ldots, I_N\}$ and corresponding ground truth mask $Y = \{Y_1, \ldots Y_N\}$ for training. We extract shapes $S = \{S_1, \ldots, S_N\}$ from the ground truth mask to train the robust kernel statistical shape model [9], defined as $RKSSM(S|\Phi; V; K)$, where Φ represents the implicit feature space, V decides the eigenvectors in kernel space, K is the robust kernel matrix with elements $K_{ij} = \kappa(S_i, S_j) = \Phi(S_i)^T \Phi(S_j)$ and κ is the kernel trick function.

2.1   Dense-UNet Segmentation Network

DenseNet [10] has advantages in narrowing the network width, reusing features and significantly alleviating the problem of gradient vanishing. Therefore, we adopt the DenseNet in U-Net architecture by simply replacing the stacked

Conv − Relu and a following max pooling operation at each downsampling step with a 3-layer dense block with the growth rate of 4, meanwhile, keeping the upsampling path and concatenation unchanged. We use the Dice coefficient loss with a smooth value according to the most of related works that $\mathcal{L}(Z,Y) = 1 - \frac{2\times\sum_i z_i y_i + 0.1}{\sum_i(z_i^2 + \sum_i y_i^2) + 0.1}$, where Z represents the predicted mask. Our Dense-UNet is trained with 2D slices extracted from 3D training images from Axial view, Sagittal view and Coronal view respectively, resulting in three predicted segment Z^A, Z^S and Z^C. Due to the *ReLu* activation in the output layer, the intensity range in predicted segment is in $[0, 255]$. To make use of the predicted segments in further Bayesian model, we generate probability maps $\Pi = \{\Pi_1, \ldots, \Pi_N\}$ by merging the three predicted segments and feeding into a sigmoid logistic function:

$$\Pi_i = \frac{1}{1 + \exp(-\frac{S_i^A + S_i^Z + S_i^C}{255})}, \tag{1}$$

where Π_i indicates the probability map of the ith image. Using the sigmoid function to compute probability map is because (1) this is a binary segmentation task with 2 classes in total, and (2) considering the uncertain accuracy of Dense U-Net, we make the probability for each pixel in range $[0.5, 1]$ that "1" indicates the pixel has a considerable probability of being *ROI* (Region of Interest) and "0.5" indicates the pixel is unsure to be *ROI* or *NOI* (Non of Interest). Apparently, the intersection region of Z^A, Z^S and Z^C is assigned higher probabilities, and uncertain or corrupted areas receive lower probabilities.

2.2 Bayesian Model

Let the shape model $RKSSM$ fed into Π for initialization (cf. Fig. 1(b)), we have an initial shape of segmentation $C = \{x_1, \ldots, x_{n_P}\}$, where landmark x_i represents the ith pixel in the test image. Given the test image I, probability map Π and the shape model $RKSSM$, assume the optimal shape C can be derived using Bayes' rule as follows:

$$p(C|I, \Pi) \propto p(I, \Pi|C)\, p(C), \tag{2}$$

term $p(I, \Pi|C)$ is maximum likelihood estimation of C based on image and probability map and term $p(C)$ is considered as the prior distribution of the shape model. Shape C is guided towards the most probable mode by maximizing the posteriori in Eq. 2, which is equivalent to simply minimizing its negative logarithm leading to the energy function:

$$E(C) = -\log(p(I, \Pi|C)) - \log(p(C)), \tag{3}$$

the first term related to the intensity feature is solved via a Gaussian Mixture Model and the second term related to the shape prior is solved with the shape model. The optimal solution is reached by adapting the gradient descent to the energy. The overall procedure of segmentation algorithm is summarized in Algorithm 1.

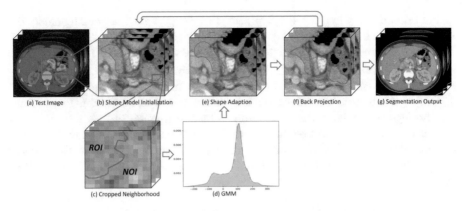

(a) Test Image   (b) Shape Model Initialization   (e) Shape Adaption   (f) Back Projection   (g) Segmentation Output

ROI

NOI

(c) Cropped Neighborhood   (d) GMM

Fig. 1. This figure illustrates the pipeline of segmentation approach: given the test image with probability map (a), the shape model is initialized to fit the detected region (b); considering the neighborhood region around each landmark (c), a Gaussian Mixture Model is trained (d) to guide shape adaption (e); afterwards, project the shape onto statistical shape model (f); we obtain the segmentation output (g) when the convergence is reached.

Gaussian Mixture Model Joint with Probability Map. To find the maximum likelihood of $p(I, \Pi | C)$, we train a Gaussian Mixture Model (GMM) based on the image intensity as the pixels are statistically independent from each other. In contrast to conventional mixture models, the probability map Π is adopted as prior weights of different components in the model. Let $X = \{x_1, \ldots, x_{n_K}\}$ be a D-dimension image with n_K pixels, the probability density function of GMM is defined as:

$$\mathcal{P}(X|\Pi, \Theta) = \prod_{i=1}^{n_K} \{\pi_i \Psi(x_i|\Theta_R) + (1 - \pi_i) \Psi(x_i|\Theta_N)\}, \qquad (4)$$

given that $\Psi(X|\Theta_R)$ follows Gaussian distribution where the parameters Θ_R consists of mean value and standard deviation of image intensity, $\Psi(X|\Theta_N)$ is defined in the same way. This GMM contains two independent components $\Psi(X|\Theta_R)$ and $\Psi(X|\Theta_N)$ representing ROI and NOI. As a result, the probability of pixel x_i being each component can be estimated from GMM in Eq. 4, we define $w_R(x_i)$ and $w_N(x_i)$ as the probability of pixel x_i being ROI and NOI:

$$w_R(x_i) = \frac{\pi_i \Psi(x_i|\Theta_R)}{\pi_i \Psi(x_i|\Theta_R) + (1 - \pi_i)\Psi(x_i|\Theta_N)}$$
$$w_N(x_i) = \frac{(1 - \pi_i)\Psi(x_i|\Theta_N)}{\pi_i \Psi(x_i|\Theta_R) + (1 - \pi_i)\Psi(x_i|\Theta_N)}. \qquad (5)$$

To release the non-related pixels' influence on GMM, only the neighborhood around each landmark is considered in training (cf. Fig. 1(c)). Let $\Omega(x_i)$ donate the cubic neighborhood around the center x_i with radius r, thus each neighborhood contains $(2r + 1)^3$ pixels. Let $\Omega^+(x_i)$ be the region inside the shape within $\Omega(x_i)$ and $\Omega^-(x_i) = \Omega(x_i) - \Omega^+(x_i)$ be the outside region (cf. Fig. 1(c)). Therefore, the parameters Θ_R, Θ_N are trained within $\int_{x_i \in C} \Omega^+(x_i)dx$ and $\int_{x_i \in C} \Omega^-(x_i)dx$ respectively. Similarly, we obtain the mean probability μ_{wR} and μ_{wN} of being ROI and NOI by only considering the pixels in region $\int_{i=1}^{n_P} \Omega(x_i)dx$. In this way, more precise probabilities can be obtained by shrinking the region of neighborhood, leading to finer segmentation.

Theoretically, it would be ideal that the pixels inside shape C have the highest probability of being ROI and the pixels outside shape C have the highest probability of being NOI. Inspired by the popular Mumford-Shah function [11], we form the energy function term:

$$-\log(p(I, \Pi|C)) = \int_{i=1}^{n_P} \int_{j \in \Omega(x_i)} \left(w_R(x_j) - \mu_{wR}\right)^2 + \left(w_N(x_j) - \mu_{wN}\right)^2 \\ + \left(w_R(x_j) - \mu_{wR}\right)\left(w_N(x_j) - \mu_{wN}\right)dx, \tag{6}$$

at this stage, the landmarks are fitting to superior positions automatically in terms of the probability rules in Eq. 5. Since the pixels are statistically independent without global constraint, assume the landmark x_i will move along the outward curvature normal with direction $\overrightarrow{\jmath}(x_i)$ to reach the optimal, we compute $\frac{\partial(p(I,\Pi|C))}{\partial(C)} = 0$ to obtain the movement direction $\overrightarrow{\jmath}^*(x_i)$ for each landmark that:

$$\overrightarrow{\jmath}^*(x_i) = \frac{(w_R(x_i) - \mu_{wR})^2 - (w_N(x_i) - \mu_{wN})^2}{(w_R(x_i) - \mu_{wR})(w_N(x_i) - \mu_{wN})}, \tag{7}$$

note that for pixels $x_j \in \Omega^+(x_i)$, $\overrightarrow{\jmath}^*(x_j) < 0$, otherwise for pixels $x_j \in \Omega^-(x_i)$, $\overrightarrow{\jmath}^*(x_j) > 0$. Namely, $\overrightarrow{\jmath}^*(x_i) > 0$ indicates x_i moves along the normal to exterior and $\overrightarrow{\jmath}^*(x_i) < 0$ indicates x_i moves along the inverse direction of outward normal to interior.

Shape Prior. Statistical shape models are demonstrated to have a strong ability in global shape constraint. In this work, we employ the RKPCA method in [9] to train such a robust kernel model $RKSSM(S|\Phi; V; K)$. Differently, we use the model statistics to correct the erroneous modes and estimate the uncertain pieces (cf. Fig. 1(e) to (f)), which means we only focus on the back projection process. Subject to the nonlinearity of kernel space, it is sensitive to initialization of clusters. Furthermore, the shape to be projected onto the model at this stage already contains certain pieces that are supposed to be preserved. Consequently, we improve the back projection of kernel model by assigning a supervised initialization to project onto the optimal cluster. Namely, finding the jth shape in training datasets S_j satisfying $\kappa(C, S_j) = \max(\kappa(C, S_i) : i = 1, \ldots, N)$. Employing the shape model in Bayesian model, we consider the prior as:

$$-\log(p(C)) = \left\|\mathbb{P}_n\Phi(C) - \Phi(\hat{C})\right\|^2 + \lambda\left\|S_j - \hat{C}\right\|^2, \tag{8}$$

the first term is the objective function employed in [9] and we add an additional term with a balance λ. $\mathbb{P}_n\Phi(x)$ denotes the projection of $\Phi(x)$ onto the principal subspace of Φ. Afterwards, the shape projection is solved by taking gradient $\frac{\partial(-\log(p(C)))}{\partial(\hat{C})} = 0$ and the reconstructed shape vector is derived by:

$$\hat{C} = \frac{\sum_{i=1}^{N} \gamma_i \kappa(C, S_i) S_i - \lambda S_j}{\sum_{i=1}^{N} \gamma_i \kappa(C, S_i) - \lambda}, \quad \gamma_i = \sum_{k=1}^{N} V_i^j K_j V_i^k. \tag{9}$$

Algorithm 1. Algorithm of Segmentation with Bayesian Model

Input: a set of test images $I = \{I_1, \ldots, I_{n_S}\}$, the probability maps $\Pi = \{\Pi_1, \ldots, \Pi_{n_S}\}$, shape model $RKSSM$, radius $r = 2$
1. Feed shape model to the initial shape C extract from probability map
2. **while** neighborhood radius $r \geq 0$ **do**
3. Train $\mathcal{P}(X|\Pi, \Theta)$ with current shape C in Eq. 4
4.   **while** not converged **do**
5.   Train GMM in Eq. 6
6.   Shape Adaption in terms of Eq. 7 and obtain the new shape C^*
7.   **if** $\|C^* - C\|_2 \leq \epsilon$ **break**
8.   **end while**
9.   Update C by back projection onto $RKSSM$ in Eq. 9
10.   Shrink the neighborhood for fine tuning $r = r - 1$
11. **end while**
Output: the segment $\hat{Y}$ from the final shape $\hat{C}$

---

3   Evaluation

Datasets and Experiments Experiments are conducted on the public NIH pancreas datasets [12], containing 82 abdominal contrast-enhanced 3D CT volumes with size $512 \times 512 \times D$ ($D \in [181, 146]$) under 4-fold cross validation. We take the measures Dice Similarity Coefficient $DSC = 2(|Y_+ \cap \hat{Y}_+|)/(|Y_+| + |\hat{Y}_+|)$ and Jaccard Index $JI = (|Y_+ \cap \hat{Y}_+|)/(|Y_+| \cup |\hat{Y}_+|)$. For statistical shape modeling, we define the kernel trick $\kappa(x_i, x_j) = \exp(-(x_i - x_j)^2/2\sigma^2)$, where the kernel width $\sigma = 150$. In the shape projection, we set the balance term $\lambda = \frac{1}{2\sigma^2}$. We set $r = 2$ at the beginning in shape adaption with GMM. The convergence condition value for shape adaption is $\epsilon = 0.0001$.

Segmentation Results. We compare the segmentation results with related works using the same datasets in Table 1. In terms of the segmentation results, we report the highest 85.32% average DSC with smallest deviation 4.19, and the DSC for the worse case reaches 71.04%. That is to say, our proposed method is robust to extremely challenging cases. We can also find an improvement of JI. More importantly, we can come to the conclusion that the proposed Bayesian model is efficient and robust in terms of the significant improvement (approximately 12% in DSC) from the neural network segmentation. For an intuitive

Table 1. Pancreas segmentation results comparing with the state-of-the-art. '−' indicates the item is not presented.

Method	Mean DSC	Max DSC	Min DSC	Mean JI
Ours	**85.32 ± 4.19**	**91.47**	**71.04**	**74.61 ± 6.19**
Our DenseUNet	73.39 ± 8.78	86.50	45.60	58.67 ± 10.47
Zhu et al. [4]	84.59 ± 4.86	91.45	69.92	−
Cai et al. [5]	82.40 ± 6.70	90.10	60.00	70.60 ± 9.00
Zhou et al. [3]	82.37 ± 5.68	90.85	62.43	−

view, the segmentation procedure of Bayesian model is shown in Fig. 2, where we compare the segmentation at every stage with the ground truth (in red). The DSC for probability map in Fig. 2(b) is 57.30%, and DSC for the final segmentation in Fig. 2(f) is 82.92%. Obviously, we find that the segmentation leads more precise by shrinking the radius of neighborhood.

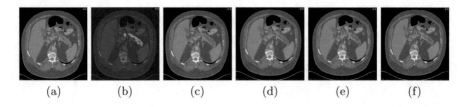

(a)   (b)   (c)   (d)   (e)   (f)

Fig. 2. Figure shows the segmentation procedure of NIH case #4: (a) test image I; (b) probability map Π; (c) initialization for shape model (ground truth mask is in red); (d)–(f) shape adaption with neighborhood radius $r = 2, 1, 0$ respectively.

4 Discussion

Motivated by tackling difficulties in challenging organ segmentation, we integrate deep neural network and statistical shape model within a Bayesian model in this work. A novel optimization principle is proposed to guide segmentation. We conduct experiments on the public NIH pancreas datasets and report the average $DSC = 85.34\%$ that outperforms the state-of-the-art. In future work, we will focus on more challenging segmentation tasks such as the tumor and lesion segmentation.

Acknowledgments. This research is supported by the National Research Foundation, Prime Minister's Office, Singapore under its International Research Centres in Singapore Funding Initiative. This work is partially supported by a grant AcRF RGC 2017-T1-001-053 by Ministry of Education, Singapore.

References

1. Ronneberger, O., Fischer, P., Brox, T.: U-Net: convolutional networks for biomedical image segmentation. In: Navab, N., Hornegger, J., Wells, W.M., Frangi, A.F. (eds.) MICCAI 2015. LNCS, vol. 9351, pp. 234–241. Springer, Cham (2015). https://doi.org/10.1007/978-3-319-24574-4_28

2. Badrinarayanan, V., Kendall, A., Cipolla, R.: SegNet: a deep convolutional encoder-decoder architecture for image segmentation. IEEE Trans. Pattern Anal. Mach. Intell. **39**(12), 2481–2495 (2017)

3. Zhou, Y., Xie, L., Shen, W., Wang, Y., Fishman, E.K., Yuille, A.L.: A fixed-point model for pancreas segmentation in abdominal CT scans. In: Descoteaux, M., Maier-Hein, L., Franz, A., Jannin, P., Collins, D.L., Duchesne, S. (eds.) MICCAI 2017. LNCS, vol. 10433, pp. 693–701. Springer, Cham (2017). https://doi.org/10.1007/978-3-319-66182-7_79

4. Zhu, Z., Xia, Y., Shen, W., Fishman, E.K., Yuille, A.L.:A 3D coarse-to-fine framework for automatic pancreas segmentation. arXiv preprint arXiv:1712.00201 (2017)

5. Cai, J., Lu, L., Xie, Y., Xing, F., Yang, L.: Pancreas segmentation in MRI using graph-based decision fusion on convolutional neural networks. In: Descoteaux, M., Maier-Hein, L., Franz, A., Jannin, P., Collins, D.L., Duchesne, S. (eds.) MICCAI 2017. LNCS, vol. 10435, pp. 674–682. Springer, Cham (2017). https://doi.org/10.1007/978-3-319-66179-7_77

6. Roth, H.R.: Spatial aggregation of holistically-nested convolutional neural networks for automated pancreas localization and segmentation. Med. Image Anal. **45**, 94–107 (2018)

7. Farag, A., Lu, L., Roth, H.R., Liu, J., Turkbey, E., Summers, R.M.: A bottom-up approach for pancreas segmentation using cascaded super-pixels and (deep) image patch labeling. IEEE Trans. Image Process. **26**(1), 386–399 (2017)

8. Guo, Z., et al.: Deep LOGISMOS: deep learning graph-based 3D segmentation of pancreatic tumors on CT scans. arXiv preprint arXiv:1801.08599 (2018)

9. Ma, J., Wang, A., Lin, F., Wesarg, S., Erdt, M.: Nonlinear statistical shape modeling for ankle bone segmentation using a novel kernelized robust PCA. In: Descoteaux, M., Maier-Hein, L., Franz, A., Jannin, P., Collins, D.L., Duchesne, S. (eds.) MICCAI 2017. LNCS, vol. 10433, pp. 136–143. Springer, Cham (2017). https://doi.org/10.1007/978-3-319-66182-7_16

10. Huang, G., Liu, Z., Weinberger, K.Q., van der Maaten, L.: Densely connected convolutional networks. In: Proceedings of the IEEE Conference on Computer Vision and Pattern Recognition, vol. 1, p. 3 (2017)

11. Chan, T.F., Vese, L.A.: Active contours without edges. IEEE Trans. Image Process. **10**(2), 266–277 (2001)

12. Roth, H.R., et al.: DeepOrgan: multi-level deep convolutional networks for automated pancreas segmentation. In: Navab, N., Hornegger, J., Wells, W.M., Frangi, A.F. (eds.) MICCAI 2015. LNCS, vol. 9349, pp. 556–564. Springer, Cham (2015). https://doi.org/10.1007/978-3-319-24553-9_68

Fine-Grained Segmentation Using Hierarchical Dilated Neural Networks

Sihang Zhou[1,2], Dong Nie[2], Ehsan Adeli[3], Yaozong Gao[4], Li Wang[2], Jianping Yin[5], and Dinggang Shen[2(✉)]

[1] College of Computer, National University of Defense Technology, Changsha 410073, Hunan, China
[2] Department of Radiology and BRIC, UNC at Chapel Hill, Chapel Hill, NC, USA
dgshen@med.unc.edu
[3] Stanford University, Stanford, CA 94305, USA
[4] Shanghai United Imaging Intelligence Co., Ltd., Shanghai, China
[5] Dongguan University of Technology, Dongguan 523808, Guangdong, China

Abstract. Image segmentation is a crucial step in many computer-aided medical image analysis tasks, e.g., automated radiation therapy. However, *low tissue-contrast* and large amounts of *artifacts* in medical images, i.e., CT or MR images, corrupt the true boundaries of the target tissues and adversely influence the precision of boundary localization in segmentation. To precisely locate blurry and missing boundaries, human observers often use high-resolution context information from neighboring regions. To extract such information and achieve fine-grained segmentation (high accuracy on the boundary regions and small-scale targets), we propose a novel hierarchical dilated network. In the hierarchy, to maintain precise location information, we adopt dilated residual convolutional blocks as basic building blocks to reduce the dependency of the network on downsampling for receptive field enlargement and semantic information extraction. Then, by concatenating the intermediate feature maps of the serially-connected dilated residual convolutional blocks, the resultant hierarchical dilated module (HD-module) can encourage more smooth information flow and better utilization of both high-level semantic information and low-level textural information. Finally, we integrate several HD-modules in different resolutions in a parallel connection fashion to finely collect information from multiple (more than 12) scales for the network. The integration is defined by a novel late fusion module proposed in this paper. Experimental results on pelvic organ CT image segmentation demonstrate the superior performance of our proposed algorithm to the state-of-the-art deep learning segmentation algorithms, especially in localizing the organ boundaries.

1 Introduction

Image segmentation is an essential component in computer-aided diagnosis and therapy systems, for example, dose planning for imaging-guided radiation

---

D. Shen—This work was supported in part by the National Key R&D Program of China 2018YFB1003203 and NIH grant CA206100.

© Springer Nature Switzerland AG 2018
A. F. Frangi et al. (Eds.): MICCAI 2018, LNCS 11073, pp. 488–496, 2018.
https://doi.org/10.1007/978-3-030-00937-3_56

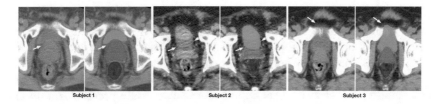

Fig. 1. Illustration of the blurry and vanishing boundaries in pelvic CT images. The green, red and blue masks indicate segmentation ground-truth of bladder, prostate, and rectum, respectively.

therapy (IGRT) and quantitative analysis for disease diagnosis. To obtain reliable segmentation for these applications, not only a robust detection of global object contours is required, a fine localization of tissue boundaries and small-scale structures is also fundamental. Nevertheless, the defection of image quality due to acquisition and process operations of medical images poses challenges to researchers in designing dependable segmentation algorithms.

Take the pelvic CT image as an example. The low soft-tissue-contrast makes the boundaries of target organs vague and hard to detect. This makes the nearby organs visually merged as a whole (see Fig. 1). In addition, different kinds of artifacts, e.g., metal, motion, and wind-mild artifacts, corrupt the real boundaries of organs and, more seriously, split the holistic organs into isolated parts with various sizes and shapes by generating fake boundaries (see Subject 2 in Fig. 1).

Numerous methods have been proposed in the literature to solve the problem of blurry image segmentation. Among the recently proposed algorithms, deep learning methods that are equipped with end-to-end learning mechanisms and representative features have become indispensable components and helped the corresponding algorithms to achieve state-of-the-art performances in many applications. For example, in [9], Oktay *et al.* integrated shape priors into a convolutional network through a novel regularization model to constrain the network of making appropriate estimation in the corrupted areas. In [6], Chen *et al.* introduced a multi-task network structure to simultaneously conduct image segmentation and boundary delineation to achieve better boundary localization performance. A large improvement has been made by the recently proposed algorithms. In the mainstream deep learning-based segmentation methods, to achieve good segmentation accuracy, high-resolution location information (provided by skip connections) is integrated with robust semantic information (extracted by downsampling and convolutions) to allow the network making local estimation with global guidance. However, both these kinds of information cannot help accurately locate the blurry boundaries contaminated by noise and surrounded by fake boundaries, thus posing the corresponding algorithms under potential failure in fine-grained medical image segmentation.

In this paper, to better detect the blurry boundary and tiny semantic structures, we propose a novel hierarchical dilated network. The main idea of our design is to first extract high-resolution context information, which is accurate for localization and abundant in semantics. Then, based on the obtained high-resolution information, we endow our network the ability to infer the precise location of boundaries at blurry areas by collecting tiny but important clues and through observing the surrounding contour tendency in high resolution. To implement this idea, in the designed network, dilation is adopted to replace downsampling for receptive field enlargement to maintain precise location information. Also, by absorbing both the strength of DenseNet (the feature propagation and reuse mechanism) [3] and ResNet (the iterative feature refinement mechanism) [1], we concatenate the intermediate feature maps of several serially-connected dilated residual convolutional blocks and propose our hierarchical dilated module (HD-module). Then, different from the structures of ResNet and DenseNet, which link the dense blocks and residual blocks in a serial manner, we use parallel connections to integrate several deeply supervised HD-modules in different resolutions and construct our proposed hierarchical dilated neural network (HD-Net). After that, a late fusion module is introduced to further merge intermediate results from different HD-modules. In summary, the advantages of the proposed method are three-fold: (1) It can provide a better balance between *what* and *where* by providing high-resolution semantic information, thus helping improve the accuracy on blurry image segmentation; (2) It can endow sufficient context information to tiny structures and achieve better segmentation results on targets with small sizes; (3) It achieves smoother information flow and more elaborate utilization of multi-level (semantic and textural) and multi-scale information. Extensive experiments indicate superior performance of our method to the state-of-the-art deep learning medical image segmentation algorithms.

2   Method

In this section, we introduce our proposed hierarchical dilated neural network (HD-Net) for fine-grained medical image segmentation.

2.1   Hierarchical Dilated Network

Hierarchical Dilated Module (HD-Module). In order to extract high-resolution context information and protect the tiny semantic structure, we select dilated residual blocks as basic building blocks for our network. These blocks can arbitrarily enlarge the receptive field and efficiently extract context information without any compromise on the location precision. Also, the dilation operations eliminate the dependency on downsampling of the networks, thus allowing the tiny but important structures within images to be finely protected for more accurate segmentation. Our proposed hierarchical dilated module is constructed by concatenating the intermediate feature maps of several serially-connected dilated residual convolutional blocks (see Fig. 2). In the designed module, because of the combination of dense connections (concatenation) and residual connections, more smooth information flow is encouraged, and also, more comprehensive multi-level (textural and semantic) and multi-scale information is finely preserved.

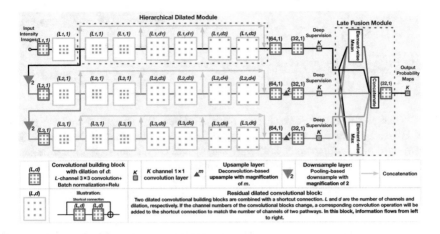

Fig. 2. Proposed hierarchical dilated network (HD-Net).

Hierarchical Dilated Network (HD-Net). To comprehensively exploit the diverse high-resolution semantic information from different scales, we further integrate several HD-modules and propose hierarchical dilated network (HD-Net). As we can see at the bottom of Fig. 2, convolution and downsampling operations tightly integrate three HD-modules from different resolutions into the network. Then, after upsampling and deep supervision operations [6], the intermediate probability maps of the three modules are further combined to generate the final output. The numbers of channels L_1, L_2, and L_3 of the three modules are 32, 48 and 72, respectively. The dilation factors are set as $d_1 = 3, d_2 = 5$ for high-resolution, $d_3 = 2, d_4 = 4$ for medium-resolution, and $d_5 = 2, d_6 = 2$ for low-resolution module. In this setting, when generating the output probability maps, multi-scale information from 12 receptive fields with sizes ranging from 7 to 206 is directly visible to the final convolutional layers, making the segmentation result precise and robust.

Late Fusion Module. Element-wise max or average [6] operations are two common fusion strategies in deep learning research. However, these methods treat all the results equally. Therefore, to better fuse the intermediate deeply supervised results from different sub-networks, we propose a late fusion module that weighs the outputs according to their quality and how they convey complementary information compared to other outputs. Specifically, we first generate the element-wise max and average of original outputs as intermediate results, and then automatically merge all the results through convolution. In this way, the enhanced intermediate results are automatically fused with more appropriate weights, to form an end-to-end model.

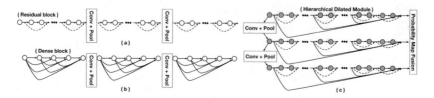

Fig. 3. Sketches of network structures of (a) ResNet, (b) DenseNet and (c) the proposed HD-Net. In the figure, unbroken arcs indicate concatenation, dotted arcs indicate element-wise plus, and straight lines indicate ordinal connections. Solid and hollow circles indicate convolution with and without dilation.

2.2 Comparison with ResNet and DenseNet

As discussed earlier, the proposed HD-Net borrows the advantages of both residual neural networks and dense networks. In this sub-section, we briefly compare the differences between these networks (See Fig. 3 for intuitive comparison).

Intra-block Connections. Residual blocks are constructed in a parallel manner by linking several convolutional layers with identity mapping, while dense blocks are constructed in a serial-parallel manner by densely linking all the preceding layers with the later layers. However, as pointed out by the latest research, although both networks perform great in many applications, the effective paths in residual networks are proved to be relatively shallow [2], which means the information interaction between lower layers and higher layers is not smooth enough. Also, compared to DenseNet, Chen *et al.* [8] argued that too frequent connections from the preceding layers may cause redundancy within the network. To solve the problem of information redundancy of DenseNet, in our network the dilated residual convolutions are selected as basic building blocks. In this building block, dilation can help speed up the process of iterative representation refinement within residual blocks [4], thus making the features extracted by two consecutive dilated residual convolution blocks be more diverse. Moreover, to solve the problem of lacking long-term connections within ResNet, we introduce dense connections into the serially connected dilated residual blocks and encourage a smoother information flow throughout the network.

Inter-block Connections. As far as inter-block connections are concerned, both ResNet and DenseNet use serial connection manners. As can be imagined, this kind of connection may suffer from a risk of blocking the low-layer textural information to be visible to the final segmentation result. Consequently, in our designed network, we adopt a parallel connection between HD-modules to achieve more direct utilization of multi-level information.

The Usage of Downsampling. ResNet and DenseNet mainly use downsampling operations to enlarge receptive field and to extract semantic information.

But in our proposed network, dilation becomes the main source of receptive field enlargement. Downsampling is mainly utilized for improving the information diversity and robustness of the proposed network. This setting also makes the design of parallel connections between modules to be more reasonable.

In summary, thanks to the dilation operations and the hierarchical structure, the high-resolution semantic information in different scales is fully exploited. Hence, HD-Net tends to provide a more detailed segmentation result, making it potentially more suitable for fine-grained medical image segmentation.

3   Experiments

Dataset and Implementation Details. To test the effectiveness of the proposed HD-Net, we adopt a pelvic CT image dataset with 339 scans for evaluation. The contours of the three main pelvic organs, i.e., prostate, bladder, and rectum have been delineated by experienced physicians and serve as ground-truth for segmentation. The dataset is randomly divided into training, validation and testing sets with 180, 59 and 100 samples, respectively. The patch size for all the compared networks is $144 \times 208 \times 5$. The implementations of all the compared algorithms are based on Caffe platform. To make a fair comparison, we use Xavier method to initialize parameters, and employ the Adam optimization method with fixed hyper-parameters for all the compared methods. Among the parameters, the learning rate (lr) is set to 0.001, and the decay rate hyper-parameters β_1 and β_2 are set to 0.9 and 0.999, respectively. The batch size of all compared methods is 10. The models are trained for at least 200,000 iterations until we observe a plateau or over-fitting tendency according to validation losses.

Evaluating the Effectiveness of Dilation and Hierarchical Structure in HD-Net. To conduct such an evaluation, we construct three networks for comparison. The first one is the HD-Net introduced in Sect. 2. The second one is an HD-Net without dilation (denoted by H-Net). The third one is constructed by the HD-module but without the hierarchical structure, i.e., with only one pathway (referred to as D-Net). The corresponding Dice similarity coefficient (DSC) and average surface distance (ASD) of these methods are listed in Table 1. Through the results, we can find that the introduction of dilation can contribute an improvement of approximately 1.3% on Dice ratio and 0.16 mm on ASD, while the introduction of hierarchical structure can contribute an improvement of approximately 2.3% on Dice ratio and 0.34 mm on ASD. It verifies the effectiveness of dilation and hierarchical structure in HD-Net.

Evaluating the Effectiveness of Late Fusion Module. From the reported DSC and ASD in Table 2, we can see that, with the help of the late fusion module, the network performance improves compared with the networks using average fusion (Avg-Fuse), max fusion (Max-Fuse), and simple convolution (Conv-Fuse).

Table 1. Evaluation of dilation and hierarchical structure in HD-Net.

Networks	Prostate	Bladder	Rectum	Prostate	Bladder	Rectum
	DSC (%)			ASD (mm)		
H-Net	86.1 ± 4.9	91.6 ± 8.7	85.5 ± 5.5	1.57 ± 0.78	1.58 ± 2.34	1.39 ± 0.50
D-Net	85.3 ± 4.7	91.5 ± 7.6	84.1 ± 5.4	1.62 ± 0.53	1.75 ± 2.53	1.70 ± 0.69
HD-Net	$\mathbf{87.7 \pm 3.7}$	$\mathbf{93.4 \pm 5.5}$	$\mathbf{86.5 \pm 5.2}$	$\mathbf{1.39 \pm 0.36}$	$\mathbf{1.34 \pm 1.75}$	$\mathbf{1.32 \pm 0.50}$

Table 2. Evaluation of the effectiveness of the proposed late fusion module.

Networks	Prostate	Bladder	Rectum	Prostate	Bladder	Rectum
	DSC (%)			ASD (mm)		
Avg-Fuse	87.0 ± 3.9	93.0 ± 6.2	85.7 ± 5.3	1.50 ± 0.44	1.43 ± 2.04	1.42 ± 0.48
Max-Fuse	87.2 ± 3.9	93.2 ± 5.4	86.1 ± 5.3	1.43 ± 0.37	$\mathbf{1.21 \pm 0.92}$	1.47 ± 0.67
Conv-Fuse	87.3 ± 3.9	93.1 ± 5.4	85.9 ± 5.5	1.45 ± 0.42	1.47 ± 2.41	1.48 ± 0.72
Proposed	$\mathbf{87.7 \pm 3.7}$	$\mathbf{93.4 \pm 5.5}$	$\mathbf{86.5 \pm 5.2}$	$\mathbf{1.39 \pm 0.36}$	1.34 ± 1.75	$\mathbf{1.32 \pm 0.50}$

Comparison with the State-of-the-Art Methods. Table 3 compares our proposed HD-Net with several state-of-the-art deep learning algorithms. Among these methods, U-Net [5] achieved the best performance on ISBI 2012 EM challenge dataset; DCAN [6] has won the 1st prize in 2015 MICCAI Grand Segmentation Challenge 2 and 2015 MICCAI Nuclei Segmentation Challenge; DenseSeg [7] has won the first prize in the 2017 MICCAI grand challenge on 6-month infant brain MRI segmentation.

Table 3 shows the segmentation results of U-Net [5], DCAN [6], DenseSeg [7], as well as our proposed network. As can be seen, all the results from the compared algorithms are reasonably well on predicting the global contour of the target organs; however, our proposed algorithm still outperforms the state-of-the-art methods by approximately 1% in Dice ratio and nearly **10%** in average surface distance for prostate and rectum. By visualizing the segmentation results of a representative sample in Fig. 4, we can see that the improvement mainly comes from the better boundary localization.

Table 3. Comparison with the state-of-the-art deep learning algorithms.

Networks	Prostate	Bladder	Rectum	Prostate	Bladder	Rectum
	DSC (%)			ASD (mm)		
U-Net [5]	86.0 ± 5.2	91.7 ± 5.9	85.5 ± 5.1	1.53 ± 0.49	1.77 ± 1.85	1.47 ± 0.53
DCAN [6]	86.8 ± 4.3	92.7 ± 7.1	84.8 ± 5.8	1.55 ± 0.55	1.72 ± 2.59	1.85 ± 1.13
DenseSeg [7]	86.5 ± 3.8	92.5 ± 7.0	85.2 ± 5.5	1.58 ± 0.53	1.37 ± 1.30	1.53 ± 0.76
Proposed	$\mathbf{87.7 \pm 3.7}$	$\mathbf{93.4 \pm 5.5}$	$\mathbf{86.5 \pm 5.2}$	$\mathbf{1.39 \pm 0.36}$	$\mathbf{1.34 \pm 1.75}$	$\mathbf{1.32 \pm 0.50}$

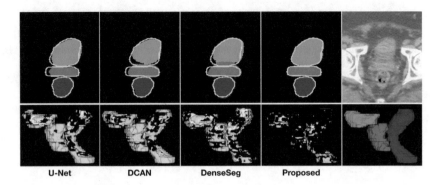

Fig. 4. Illustration of segmentation results. The first row visualizes the axial segmentation results and the corresponding intensity image (yellow curves denote the ground-truth contours). The second row is the 3D difference between the estimated and the ground-truth segmentation results. In these sub-figures, yellow and white portions denote the false positive and false negative predictions, respectively. The last sub-figure shows the 3D ground-truth contours.

4   Conclusion

In this paper, to address the adverse effect of blurry boundaries and also conduct fine-grained segmentation for medical images, we proposed to extract multiple high-resolution semantic information. To this end, we first replace downsampling with dilation for receptive field enlargement for accurate location prediction. Then, by absorbing both the advantages of residual blocks and dense blocks, we propose a new module with better mid-term and long-term information flow and less redundancy, i.e., hierarchical dilated module. Finally, by further integrating several HD-module with different resolutions using our newly defined late fusion module in parallel, we propose our hierarchical dilated network. Experimental results, based on a CT pelvic dataset, demonstrate the superior segmentation performance of our method, especially on localizing the blurry boundaries.

References

1. He, K., Zhang, X., Ren, S., et al.: Deep residual learning for image recognition. In: CVPR, pp. 770–778 (2016)
2. Veit, A., Wilber, M.J., Belongie, S.: Residual networks behave like ensembles of relatively shallow networks. In: NIPS, pp. 550–558 (2016)
3. Huang, G., Liu, Z., Weinberger, K.Q., et al.: Densely connected convolutional networks. In: CVPR, vol. 1, no. 2, p. 3 (2017)
4. Greff, K., Srivastava, R.K., Schmidhuber, J. Highway and residual networks learn unrolled iterative estimation. arXiv preprint arXiv:1612.07771 (2016)
5. Ronneberger, O., Fischer, P., Brox, T.: U-Net: convolutional networks for biomedical image segmentation. In: Navab, N., Hornegger, J., Wells, W.M., Frangi, A.F. (eds.) MICCAI 2015. LNCS, vol. 9351, pp. 234–241. Springer, Cham (2015). https://doi.org/10.1007/978-3-319-24574-4_28

6. Chen, H., Qi, X., Yu, L., et al.: DCAN: deep contour-aware networks for object instance segmentation from histology images. Med Image Anal. **36**, 135–146 (2017)
7. Bui, T.D., Shin, J., Moon, T.: 3D densely convolution networks for volumetric segmentation. arXiv preprint arXiv:1709.03199 (2017)
8. Chen, Y., Li, J., Xiao, H., et al.: Dual path networks. In: NIPS, pp. 4470–4478 (2017)
9. Oktay, O., et al.: Anatomically constrained neural networks (ACNN): application to cardiac image enhancement and segmentation. In: TMI (2017)

Generalizing Deep Models for Ultrasound Image Segmentation

Xin Yang[1], Haoran Dou[2,3], Ran Li[2,3], Xu Wang[2,3], Cheng Bian[2,3],
Shengli Li[4], Dong Ni[2,3(✉)], and Pheng-Ann Heng[1]

[1] Department of Computer Science and Engineering,
The Chinese University of Hong Kong, Shatin, Hong Kong
[2] National-Regional Key Technology Engineering Laboratory for Medical
Ultrasound, School of Biomedical Engineering, Health Science Center,
Shenzhen University, Shenzhen, China
nidong@szu.edu.cn
[3] Medical UltraSound Image Computing (MUSIC) Lab, Shenzhen Maternal
and Child Healthcare Hospital of Nanfang Medical University, Shenzhen, China
[4] Department of Ultrasound, Shenzhen Maternal and Child Healthcare Hospital
of Nanfang Medical University, Shenzhen, China

Abstract. Deep models are subject to performance drop when encountering appearance discrepancy, even on congeneric corpus in which objects share the similar structure but only differ slightly in appearance. This performance drop can be observed in automated ultrasound image segmentation. In this paper, we try to address this general problem with a novel online adversarial appearance conversion solution. Our contribution is three-fold. First, different from previous methods which utilize corpus-level training to model a fixed source-target appearance conversion in advance, we only need to model the source corpus and then we can efficiently convert each single testing image in the target corpus on-the-fly. Second, we propose a self-play training strategy to effectively pre-train all the adversarial modules in our framework to capture the appearance and structure distributions of source corpus. Third, we propose to explore a composite appearance and structure constraints distilled from the source corpus to stabilize the online adversarial appearance conversion, thus the pre-trained models can iteratively remove appearance discrepancy in the testing image in a weakly-supervised fashion. We demonstrate our method on segmenting congeneric prenatal ultrasound images. Based on the appearance conversion, we can generalize deep models at-hand well and achieve significant improvement in segmentation without re-training on massive, expensive new annotations.

1 Introduction

With massive annotated training data, deep networks have brought profound change to the medical image analysis field. However, retraining on newly annotated corpus is often compulsory before generalizing deep models to new imaging conditions [1]. Retraining is even required for congeneric corpora in which

© Springer Nature Switzerland AG 2018
A. F. Frangi et al. (Eds.): MICCAI 2018, LNCS 11073, pp. 497–505, 2018.
https://doi.org/10.1007/978-3-030-00937-3_57

objects share similar structures but only differ slightly in appearances. As shown in Fig. 1(a), there are two congeneric copora S and T, representing a similar anatomical structure, i.e. fetal head, with recognizable appearance difference, like intensity, speckle pattern and structure details. However, a deep model trained on S performs poor in segmenting images from T (Fig. 1).

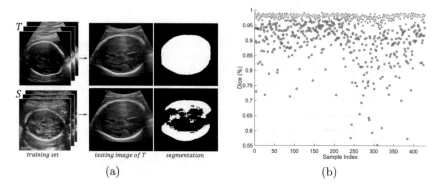

Fig. 1. Segmentation performance drop. (a) the model trained on T segments testing image in T well (red dots in (b)), while the model trained on S gets poor result in segmenting image in T (green dots in (b)). Better view in color version.

In practice, retraining is actually infeasible, because the data collection and expert annotation are expensive and sometimes unavailable. The situation becomes even worse when images are acquired at different sites, experts, protocols and even time points. Ultrasound is a typical imaging modality which suffers from these varying factors. Building a corpus for specific cases and retraining models for these diverse cases turn to be intractable. Unifying the image appearance across different imaging conditions to relive the burden of retraining is emerging as an attractive choice.

Recently, we witnessed many works on medical image appearance conversion. From a corpus level, Lei et al. proposed the convolutional network based low-dose to standard-dose PET translation [11]. With the surge of generative adversarial networks (GANs) [4] for medical image analysis [7], Wolterink et al. utilized GAN to reduce noise in CT images [10]. GAN also enables the realistic synthesis of ultrasound images from tissue labels [9]. Segmentation based shape consistency in cycled GAN was proposed in [5,13] to constrain the translation between CT and MR. Corpus-level conversion models can match the appearance distributions of different corpora from a global perspective. However, these models tend to be degraded on images which have never been modeled during training. From a single image level, style transfer [3] is another flexible and appealing scheme for appearance conversion between any two images. Whereas, it is subjective in choosing the texture level to represent the style of referring ultrasound image and preserve the structure of testing image. Leveraging the well-trained model in source corpus and avoiding the building of heavy target corpus, i.e. just using a single testing image, to realize structure-preserved appearance conversion is still a nontrivial task.

In this paper, we try to address this problem with a novel solution. Our contribution is three-fold. First, different from previous methods which model a corpus-level source-target appearance conversion in advance, our method works in an extreme case. The case is also the real routine clinic scenario where we are blinded to the complete target corpus and only a single testing image from target corpus is available. Our framework only needs to model the source corpus and then it can efficiently convert each testing image in target corpus on-the-fly. Second, under the absence of complete target corpus, we propose a self-play training strategy to effectively pre-train all adversarial modules in our framework to capture both the appearance and structure distributions of source corpus. Third, we propose to explore the mixed appearance and structure constraints distilled from the source corpus to guide and stabilize the online adversarial appearance conversion, thus the pre-trained models can iteratively remove appearance discrepancy in the testing image in a weakly-supervised fashion. We demonstrate the proposed method on segmenting congeneric prenatal ultrasound images. Extensive experiments prove that our method is fast and can generalize the deep models at-hand well, plus achieving significant improvement in segmentation without the re-training on massive, expensive new annotations.

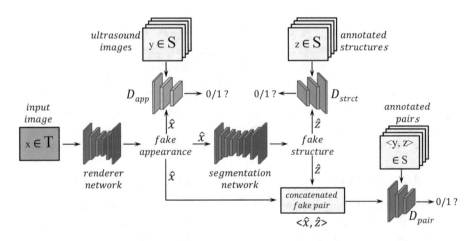

Fig. 2. Schematic view of our proposed framework.

2   Methodology

Figure 2 is the schematic view of our proposed adversarial framework for appearance conversion. System input is a single testing image from the blinded target corpus T. Renderer network renders the testing image and generates fake substitute with the appearance that can not be distinguished by appearance discriminator (D_{app}) from the appearance distribution of source corpus S.

Segmentation network then generates the fake structure on the fake appearance. Fake structure is also expected to fool the structure discriminator (D_{strct}) w.r.t the annotated structures in S. Structure here means shape. To enforce the appearance and structure coherence, the pair of fake appearance and structure is further checked by a pair discriminator (D_{pair}). During the adversarial training, the appearance of testing image and its segmentation will be iteratively fitted to the distributions of S. System outputs the final fake structure as segmentation.

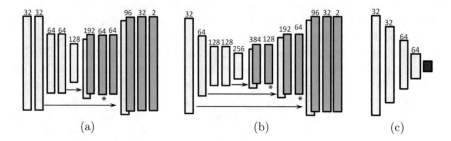

Fig. 3. Architecture of the sub-networks in our framework. Star denotes the site to inject the auxiliary supervision. Arrow denotes skip connection for concatenation.

2.1   Architecture of Sub-networks

We adapt the renderer and segmentor network from U-net [8] featured with skip connections. Renderer (Fig. 3(a)) is designed to efficiently modify the image appearance, thus its architecture is light weighted with less convolutional and pooling layers compared with the segmentor (Fig. 3(b)). Auxiliary supervisions [2] are coupled with renderer and segmentor. Discriminators D_{app}, D_{strct} and D_{pair} share the same architecture design for fake/real classification (Fig. 3(c)), except that D_{pair} gets 2-channel input for the pairs. Definition of objective functions to tune parameters in these 5 sub-networks are elaborated below.

2.2   Objective Functions for Online Adversarial Rendering

Our system is firstly fully trained on the source corpus S to capture both appearance and structure distributions. Then the system iteratively renders a single testing image in corpus T with online updating. In this section, we introduce the diverse objectives we use during the full training and online updating.

Renderer Loss. With a renderer, our goal is to modulate the intensity represented appearance of ultrasound image x into $\hat{x}$ to fit the appearance in S. Severely destroying the content information in x is not expected. Therefore, there is an important $L1$ distance based objective for renderer to satisfy the content-preserved conversion (Eq. 1). α_i is the weight for auxiliary losses.

$$\mathcal{L}_{rend} = \sum_i \alpha_i \parallel x - \hat{x} \parallel_1, i = 0, 1. \tag{1}$$

Appearance Adversarial Loss. Renderer needs to preserve the content in x, but at the same time, it still needs to enable the fake $\hat{x}$ fool the appearance discriminator D_{app} which is trying to determine whether the input is from corpus S or T. Therefore, the adversarial loss for D_{app} is shown as Eq. 2.

$$\mathcal{L}_{D_{app}} = \mathbb{E}_{y \sim S}[\log D_{app}(y)] + 1 - \log(D_{app}(\hat{x})). \tag{2}$$

Segmentor Loss. Segmentor extracts fake structure $\hat{z}$ from $\hat{x}$. Built on limited receptive field, convolutional networks may lose power in boundary deficient areas, like acoustic shadow, in ultrasound images. Therefore, based on classic cross-entropy loss, we adapt the hybrid loss $\mathcal{L}_{seg}$ as proposed in [12] to get Dice coefficient based shape-wise supervision in order to combat boundary deficiency.

Structure Adversarial Loss. Renderer is trying to keep content of x while cheat the D_{app} by minimizing both Eqs. 1 and 2. However, the renderer may stick to x or, on the contrary, collapse on a average mode in S. Structure discriminator D_{strct} here is beneficial to alleviate the problem, since it requires that the structure $\hat{z}$ extracted from $\hat{x}$ must further fit the structure distribution of $z \in S$. The adversarial loss for D_{strct} is shown as Eq. 3.

$$\mathcal{L}_{D_{strct}} = \mathbb{E}_{z \sim S}[\log D_{strct}(z)] + 1 - \log(D_{strct}(\hat{z})). \tag{3}$$

Pair Adversarial Loss. Inspired by the conditional GAN [6], as illustrated in Fig. 2, we further inject a discriminator D_{pair} to determine whether the $\hat{x}$ and $\hat{z}$ in the $<\hat{x}, \hat{z}>$ pair can match each other. Pair adversarial loss for D_{pair} is shown in Eq. 4.

$$\mathcal{L}_{D_{pair}} = \mathbb{E}_{<x,z> \sim S}[\log D_{pair}(<x,z>)] + 1 - \log(D_{pair}(<\hat{x}, \hat{z}>)). \tag{4}$$

Our full objective function is therefore defined as:

$$\mathcal{L}_{full} = \mathcal{L}_{rend} + \mathcal{L}_{D_{app}} + \mathcal{L}_{seg} + \mathcal{L}_{D_{strct}} + \mathcal{L}_{D_{pair}}. \tag{5}$$

2.3 Optimization and Online Rendering

Self-play Full Training. With the images and labels in S, we can only train the segmentor for image-to-label mapping in a supervised way. How to train other adversarial networks without fake samples and further convey the distilled appearance and structure constraints of S to online testing phase? In this section, we propose a self-play scheme to train all sub-networks in a simple way.

Although all samples in S are supposed to share an appearance distribution, the intra-class variation still exists (Fig. 4). Our self-play training scheme roots in this observation. Before training, we can assume that every randomly selected sample from S has the same chance to be located far from the appearance distribution center of S. Thus, in each training epoch, we randomly take a sample from S as a fake sample and the rest as real samples to train our sub-networks. The result of this self-play training is that renderer can learn to convert all samples in S into a more concentrated corpus S' so that the objective $\mathcal{L}_{full}$ can be minimized. Also, segmentor can learn to extract structures from the resulted S'. D_{app}, D_{strct} and D_{pair} also capture the appearance and structure knowledge of S' for classification in online rendering stage. As shown in Fig. 4, with the self-play full training, ultrasound samples in S' present more coherent appearance and enhanced details than that in S. S' will replace S and be used as real samples to tune adversarial modules in the online testing phase.

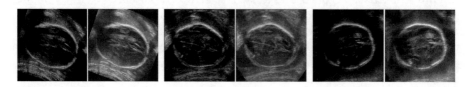

Fig. 4. Illustration of the self-play training based appearance unification on S. In each group, original image in S (left), intensity unified image in S' (right).

Online Rendering for a Single Image. In testing phase, we apply the pre-trained renderer to modify the appearance of testing image to fit S'. D_{app}, D_{strct} and D_{pair} try to distinguish the fake appearance, structure and pair from any randomly selected images or pairs in S' to ensure that the renderer generates reliable conversion. Testing phase is iterative and driven by the minimization of the objective $\mathcal{L}_{full}$ discarding the $\mathcal{L}_{seg}$. The optimization is fast and converges in few iterations. As depicted, our online appearance conversion is image-level, since we can only get a single image from the blinded target corpus. All the adversarial procedures are thus facing a 1-to-many conversion problem, which may cause harmful fluctuations during rendering. However, three designs of our framework alleviate the risk: (i) the composite constraints imposed by D_{app}, D_{strct} and D_{pair} from complementary perspectives, (ii) the loss $\mathcal{L}_{rend}$ restricts the appearance change within a limited range, (iii) S' provides exemplar samples with low intra-class appearance variation (Fig. 4), which is beneficial to smooth the gradient flow in rendering. Detailed ablation study is shown in Sect. 3.

3   Experimental Results

Materials and Implementation Details. We verify our solution on the task of prenatal ultrasound image segmentation. Ultrasound images of fetal head are collected from different ultrasound machines and compose two congeneric datasets. 1372 images acquired using a Siemens Acuson Sequoia 512 ultrasound scanner serve as corpus S with the gestational age from 24 w to 40 w. 1327 images acquired using a Sonoscope C1-6 ultrasound scanner serve as corpus T with the gestational age from 30 w to 34 w. In both S and T, we randomly take 900 images for training, the rest for testing. S and T are collected by different experts and present distinctive image appearance. Experienced experts provide boundary annotations for S and T as ground truth. To avoid unrelated factors to image appearance, like scale and translation, we cropped all images to center around the fetal head region and resize them to the size as 320×320. Segmentation model trained on S drops severely on T, as Fig. 1 and Table 1 show.

We implement the whole framework in *Tensorflow*, using a standard PC with an NVIDIA TITAN Xp GPU. *Code is online available*[1]. In full training, we update the weights of all sub-networks with an Adam optimizer (batch size $= 2$, initial learning rate is 0.001, momentum term is 0.5, total iteration $= 6000$). During the online rendering, we update the weights of all sub-networks with smaller initial learning rate 0.0001. Renderer and segmentor are updated twice as often as the discriminators. We only need less than 25 iterations (about 10 s for each iteration) before achieving a satisfying and stable online rendering.

Table 1. Quantitative evaluation of our proposed framework

Method	Metrics						
	Dice [%]	Conf [%]	Adb [pixel]	Hdb [pixel]	Jaccard [%]	Precision [%]	Recall [%]
Orig-T2T	97.848	95.575	3.7775	25.419	95.799	96.606	99.148
Orig-S2T	88.979	73.493	21.084	73.993	80.801	94.486	84.737
S2T-sp	92.736	84.075	13.917	62.782	86.688	94.971	91.267
S2T-p	93.296	85.127	12.757	58.352	87.619	95.115	**93.262**
S2T	**93.379**	**85.130**	**11.160**	**53.674**	**87.886**	**95.218**	92.633

Quantitative and Qualitative Analysis. We adopt 7 metrics to evaluate the proposed framework on segmenting ultrasound images from T, including Dice coefficient (DSC), Conformity (Conf), Hausdorff Distance of Boundaries (Hdb), Average Distance of Boundaries (Adb), Precision and Recall. We firstly trained two segmentors on the training set of corpus T (Orig-T2T) and corpus S (Orig-S2T) respectively with same settings, and then test them on T. From Table 1, we can see that, compared with Orig-T2T, the deep model Orig-S2T is severely degraded (about 10% in Dice) when testing images from T. As we upgrade the Orig-S2T with the proposed online rendering (denoted as S2T), we achieve a significant improvement (4% in DSC) in the segmentation. This proves the efficacy of our renderer in converting the congeneric ultrasound images to the appearance which can be well-handled by the segmentor.

Ablation study is conducted to verify the effectiveness of D_{strct} and D_{pair}. We remove the D_{pair} in S2T to form the S2T-p, and further remove the D_{strct} in S2T-p to form the S2T-sp. As we can observe in Table 1, without the constraints imposed by D_{strct} and D_{pair}, S2T-sp becomes weak in appearance conversion. Compared to S2T-sp, S2T-p is better in appearance conversion, thus D_{strct} takes more important role than D_{pair} in regularizing the conversion. With Fig. 5(a), we show the intermediate results of the online rendering. As the renderer modulates the appearance of input ultrasound image, the segmentation result is also

---

[1] https://github.com/xy0806/congeneric_renderer.

gradually improved. Figure 5(b) illustrates the Dice improvement curve along with iteration for all the 427 testing images in T. Almost all the rendering come to convergence around 5 iterations (about 50 s in total). The highest averaged Dice improvement (5.378%) is achieved at iteration 23.

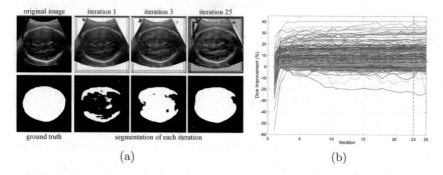

(a)   (b)

Fig. 5. (a) Intermediate rendering and segmentation result. (b) Dice improvement over iteration 0 for all the 427 testing images in T. Green star is average at each iteration.

4   Conclusions

We present a novel online adversarial appearance rendering framework to fit the input image appearance to the well-modeled distribution of source corpus, and therefore relieve the burden of retraining for deep networks when encountering congeneric images with unseen appearance. Our framework is flexible and renders the testing image on-the-fly, which is more suitable for routine clinic applications. The proposed self-play based full training scheme and the composite adversarial modules prove to be beneficial in realizing the weakly-supervised appearance conversion. Our framework is novel, fast and can be considered as an alternative in more tough tasks, like cross-modality translation.

Acknowledgments. The work in this paper was supported by the grant from National Natural Science Foundation of China under Grant 81270707, and the grants from the Research Grants Council of the Hong Kong Special Administrative Region (Project Nos. GRF 14202514 and GRF 14203115).

References

1. Chen, H., Ni, D., et al.: Standard plane localization in fetal ultrasound via domain transferred deep neural networks. IEEE JBHI **19**(5), 1627–1636 (2015)
2. Dou, Q., Yu, L., et al.: 3D deeply supervised network for automated segmentation of volumetric medical images. Med. Image Anal. **41**, 40–54 (2017)
3. Gatys, L.A., Ecker, A.S., Bethge, M.: Image style transfer using convolutional neural networks. In: CVPR, pp. 2414–2423. IEEE (2016)
4. Goodfellow, I., et al.: Generative adversarial nets. In: NIPS, pp. 2672–2680 (2014)

5. Huo, Y., Xu, Z., et al.: Adversarial synthesis learning enables segmentation without target modality ground truth. arXiv preprint arXiv:1712.07695 (2017)
6. Isola, P., Zhu, J.Y., Zhou, T., Efros, A.A.: Image-to-image translation with conditional adversarial networks. arXiv preprint (2017)
7. Nie, D., et al.: Medical image synthesis with context-aware generative adversarial networks. In: Descoteaux, M., Maier-Hein, L., Franz, A., Jannin, P., Collins, D.L., Duchesne, S. (eds.) MICCAI 2017. LNCS, vol. 10435, pp. 417–425. Springer, Cham (2017). https://doi.org/10.1007/978-3-319-66179-7_48
8. Ronneberger, O., Fischer, P., Brox, T.: U-Net: convolutional networks for biomedical image segmentation. In: Navab, N., Hornegger, J., Wells, W.M., Frangi, A.F. (eds.) MICCAI 2015. LNCS, vol. 9351, pp. 234–241. Springer, Cham (2015). https://doi.org/10.1007/978-3-319-24574-4_28
9. Tom, F., Sheet, D.: Simulating patho-realistic ultrasound images using deep generative networks with adversarial learning. arXiv preprint arXiv:1712.07881 (2017)
10. Wolterink, J.M., et al.: Generative adversarial networks for noise reduction in low-dose CT. IEEE Trans. Med. Imaging **36**(12), 2536–2545 (2017)
11. Xiang, L., et al.: Deep auto-context convolutional neural networks for standard-dose PET image estimation from low-dose PET/MRI. Neurocomputing **267**, 406–416 (2017)
12. Yang, X., Bian, C., Yu, L., Ni, D., Heng, P.A.: Hybrid loss guided convolutional networks for whole heart parsing. In: Pop, M., et al. (eds.) STACOM 2017. LNCS, vol. 10663, pp. 215–223. Springer, Cham (2018). https://doi.org/10.1007/978-3-319-75541-0_23
13. Zhang, Z., Yang, L., Zheng, Y.: Translating and segmenting multimodal medical volumes with cycle-and shape-consistency generative adversarial network. arXiv preprint arXiv:1802.09655 (2018)

Inter-site Variability in Prostate Segmentation Accuracy Using Deep Learning

Eli Gibson[1($\boxtimes$)], Yipeng Hu[1], Nooshin Ghavami[1], Hashim U. Ahmed[2],
Caroline Moore[1], Mark Emberton[1], Henkjan J. Huisman[3],
and Dean C. Barratt[1]

[1] University College London, London, UK
eli.gibson@ucl.ac.uk
[2] Imperial College, London, UK
[3] Radboud University Medical Center, Nijmegen, The Netherlands

Abstract. Deep-learning-based segmentation tools have yielded higher reported segmentation accuracies for many medical imaging applications. However, inter-site variability in image properties can challenge the translation of these tools to data from 'unseen' sites not included in the training data. This study quantifies the impact of inter-site variability on the accuracy of deep-learning-based segmentations of the prostate from magnetic resonance (MR) images, and evaluates two strategies for mitigating the reduced accuracy for data from unseen sites: training on multi-site data and training with limited additional data from the unseen site. Using 376 T2-weighted prostate MR images from six sites, we compare the segmentation accuracy (Dice score and boundary distance) of three deep-learning-based networks trained on data from a single site and on various configurations of data from multiple sites. We found that the segmentation accuracy of a single-site network was substantially worse on data from unseen sites than on data from the training site. Training on multi-site data yielded marginally improved accuracy and robustness. However, including as few as 8 subjects from the unseen site, e.g. during commissioning of a new clinical system, yielded substantial improvement (regaining 75% of the difference in Dice score).

Keywords: Segmentation · Deep learning · Inter-site variability
Prostate

1 Introduction

Deep-learning-based medical image segmentation methods have yielded higher reported accuracies for many applications including prostate [8], brain tumors [1] and abdominal organs [7]. Applying these methods in practice, however, remains challenging. Few segmentation methods achieve previously reported accuracies on new data sets. This may be due, in part, to *inter-site* variability in image and

© Springer Nature Switzerland AG 2018
A. F. Frangi et al. (Eds.): MICCAI 2018, LNCS 11073, pp. 506–514, 2018.
https://doi.org/10.1007/978-3-030-00937-3_58

reference segmentation properties at different imaging centres due to different patient populations, clinical imaging protocols and image acquisition equipment.

Inter-site variability has remained a challenge in medical image analysis for decades [9,12]. Data sets used to design, train and validate segmentation algorithms are, for logistical and financial reasons, sampled in clusters from one or a small number of imaging centres. The distribution of images and reference segmentations in this clustered sample may not be representative of the distribution of these data across other centres. Consequently, an algorithm developed for one site may not be optimal for other 'unseen' sites not included in the sample, and reported estimates of segmentation accuracy typically overestimate the accuracy achievable at unseen sites.

Data-driven methods, including deep learning, may be particularly susceptible to this problem because they are explicitly optimized on the clustered training data. Additionally, deep-learning-based methods typically avoid explicit normalization methods, such as bias field correction [12], to mitigate known sources of inter-site variability and high-level prior knowledge, such as anatomical constraints, to regularize models. Instead, normalization and regularization are implicitly learned from the clustered training data. The accuracy of deep-learning-based methods may, therefore, depend more heavily on having training data that is representative of the images to which the method will be applied.

One strategy to mitigate this effect is to use images and reference segmentations sampled from multiple sites to better reflect inter-site variability in the training data. A second approach is to 'commission' the systems: in clinical practice, when introducing new imaging technology, hospital staff typically undertake a commissioning process to calibrate and validate the technology, using subjects or data from their centre. In principle, such a process could include re-training or fine-tuning a neural network using a limited sample of data from that site. These strategies have not been evaluated for deep-learning-based segmentation.

In this study, we aimed to quantify the impact of inter-site variability on the accuracy of deep-learning-based segmentations of the prostate from T2-weighted MRI of three deep-learning-based methods, and to evaluate two strategies to mitigate the accuracy loss at a new site: training on multi-site data and training augmented with limited data from the commissioning site. To identify general trends, we conducted these experiments using three different deep-learning based methods. Specifically, this study addresses the following questions:

1. How accurate are prostate segmentations using networks trained on data from a single site when evaluated on data from the same and unseen sites?
2. How accurate are prostate segmentations using networks trained on data from multiple sites when evaluated on data from the same and unseen sites?
3. Can the accuracy of these prostate segmentations be improved by including a small sample of data from the unseen site?

2   Methods

2.1   Imaging

This study used T2-weighted 3D prostate MRI from 6 sites (256 from one site [SITE1] and 24 from 5 other sites [SITE2–SITE6]), drawn from publicly available data sets and clinical trials requiring manual prostate delineation. Reference standard manual segmentations were performed at one of 3 sites: SITE1, SITE2 or SITE5. Images were acquired with anisotropic voxels, with in-plane voxel spacing between 0.5 and 1.0 mm, and out-of-plane slice spacing between 1.8 and 5.4 mm. All images, without intensity normalization, and reference standard segmentations were resampled from their full field of view ($12 \times 12 \times 5.7 \, cm^3$ – $24 \times 24 \times 17.2 \, cm^3$) to $256 \times 256 \times 32$ voxels before automatic segmentation.

2.2   Experimental Design

We evaluated the segmentation accuracies (Dice score and the symmetric boundary distance (BD)) of networks in three experiments with training data sets taken (1) from a single site, (2) with the same sample size from multiple sites, or (3) from multiple sites but with fewer samples from one 'commissioned' site. Segmentation accuracy was evaluated with 'same-site' test data from sites included in training data, 'unseen-site' test data from sites excluded from the training data, and 'commissioned-site' test data from the commissioned site. No subject was included in both training and test data for the same trained network. Three network architectures (Sect. 2.3) were trained and tested for each data partition.

Experiment 1: Single-site Networks. To evaluate the segmentation accuracy of networks trained on data from one site (referred to as *single-site* hereafter), we trained them on 232 subjects from SITE1, and evaluated them on the remaining 24 subjects from SITE1 and all subjects from the other sites.

Experiment 2: Multi-site Networks. To evaluate the segmentation accuracy of networks trained on data from multiple sites, we used two types of data partitions. First, we conducted a patient-level 6-fold cross-validation (referred to as *patient-level* hereafter) where, in each fold, 16 subjects from each site were used for training, and 8 subjects from each site were used for same-site testing. This same-site evaluation has been used in public challenges, such as the PROMISE12 segmentation challenge [8]. Because this may overestimate the accuracy at a site that has not been seen in training, we conducted a second site-level 6-fold cross-validation (referred to as *site-level* hereafter) where, in each fold, 24 subjects from each of 5 sites were used for training, and 24 subjects from the remaining site were used for unseen-site testing.

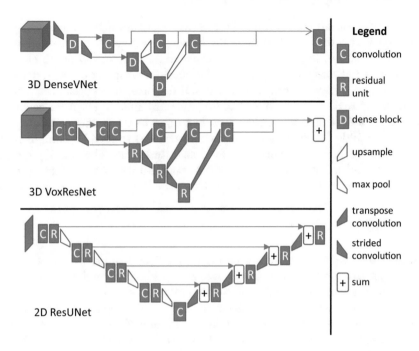

Fig. 1. Architectures of the neural networks.

Experiment 3: Commissioned Networks. To evaluate the utility of commissioning segmentation methods at new imaging centres, we conducted a 6 × 6-fold hierarchical cross-validation where the 6 outer folds correspond to selecting one site as the commissioned site and the 6 inner folds correspond to selecting a subset of subjects from the commissioned site (3 subsets with 8 subjects and 3 subsets with 16). Each network was trained with the 8 or 16 selected subjects from the commissioned site and 24 subjects from each of the other 5 sites (referred to as commission-8 and commission-16, hereafter). In each fold, the remaining subjects from the commissioned site that were excluded from training were used for commissioned-site testing.

2.3 Neural Networks: Architectures and Training

To distinguish general trends from network-specific properties, three different neural network architectures, illustrated in Fig. 1 were used in this study: DenseVNet [4], ResUNet [3], and VoxResNet [2]. Like many recent medical image segmentation networks, these networks are all variants of U-Net architectures [11] comprising a downsampling subnetwork, an upsampling subnetwork and skip connections. ResUNet segments 2D axial slices using a 5-resolution U-Net with residual units [5], max-pooling, and additive skip connections. DenseVNet segments 3D volumes using a 4-resolution V-Net with dense blocks [6] with batch-wise spatial dropout, and convolutional skip connections concatenated prior to a final segmentation convolution. VoxResNet segments 3D volumes using a 4-resolution V-Net with residual units [5], transpose-convolution upsampling, and deep supervision to improve gradient propagation. It is important to note that this study is not designed to compare the absolute accuracy of these networks; accordingly, the network dimensionality and features, hyperparameter choices, and training regimen were not made equivalent, and, apart from setting an appropriate anisotropic input shape, no hyperparameter tuning was done.

For each fold of each experiment, the network was trained by minimizing the Dice loss using the Adam optimizer for 10000 iterations. The training data set was augmented using affine perturbations. Segmentations were post-processed to eliminate spurious segmentations by taking the largest connected component.

3   Results

The described experiments generated more than 2000 segmentations across various data partitioning schemes: single-site networks trained on data from one site, patient-level networks trained on data from all sites, site-level networks trained on data from all sites except the testing site, and commissioned networks trained on 8 or 16 subjects from the commissioned site and all subjects from all other sites. The segmentation accuracies for DenseVNet, VoxResNet and ResUNet are detailed in Table 1, illustrated in Fig. 2 and summarized below.

For single-site networks, the mean accuracy on unseen-site test data was lower than on same-site test data and varied substantially between sites, confirming the same-site evaluation overestimated the unseen-site accuracy due to inter-site variability. The mean Dice score decreased by 0.12 ± 0.15 [0.00–0.47] (mean $\pm$ SD [range]) and the mean boundary distance increased by 2.0 ± 2.6 [0.1–6.9] mm.

For the multi-site training, the mean accuracies generally improved as more training data from the testing site was included, best illustrated in Fig. 2. The patient-level and site-level cross-validations yield two notable observations. First, for the *patient-level* networks, the same-site mean accuracies (Dice: 0.88, 0.84, 0.85; BD: 1.6 mm, 2.0 mm, 1.9 mm) were nearly identical to the same-site testing of the single-site networks (Dice 0.88, 0.85, 0.87; BD: 1.6 mm, 2.0 mm, 1.7 mm), suggesting that it was not inherently more difficult to train the networks on multi-site data than on single-site data. Second, for the *site-level* VoxResNet and ResUNet networks (those with worse generalization), the unseen-site accuracies for multi-site training (Dice: 0.75, 0.75; BD: 4.5 mm, 3.5 mm) were better and less variable than for single-site training (Dice: 0.68, 0,71; BD: 4.9 mm, 4.1 mm), suggesting that training on multi-site data alone yields improvements in generalization. This effect was not observed for DenseVNet, however.

For commissioned networks (with some training data from the testing site), segmentation accuracies on commissioned-site test data regained most of the difference between the *same-site* patient-level and *unseen-site* site-level cross-validations. With only 8 subjects used as commissioning data, segmentation accuracies regained $75 \pm 21\%$ [28–97%] (mean $\pm$ SD [range]) of the Dice score difference (averaged Dice: 0.87, 0.84, 0.83; BD: 1.7 mm, 2.1 mm, 2.3 mm) when the Dice score discrepancy was >0.02. With 16 subjects used as commissioning data, segmentation accuracies regained a 90 ± 12% [66–100%] of the Dice score difference (averaged Dice: 0.87, 0.85, 0.84; BD: 1.7 mm, 1.9 mm, 2.0 mm) when the Dice score discrepancy was >0.02.

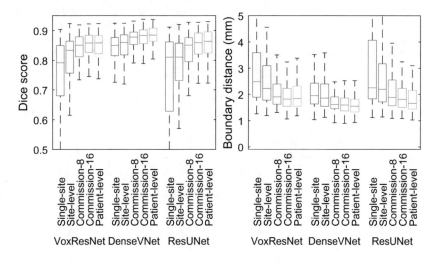

Fig. 2. Box and whisker plots of segmentation accuracies.

4   Discussion

In this work, we demonstrated that multiple deep-learning-based segmentation networks have poor accuracy when applied to data from unseen sites. This challenges the translation of segmentation tools based on these networks to other research sites and to clinical environments.

As illustrated in our study, different medical image analysis methods have different capacities to generalize to new sites. Since this is important for their clinical and research impact, methods' generalization ability should become a metric evaluated by our community. This will require the creation of multi-site datasets, such as PROMISE12 [8] and ADNI [10], to design and evaluate methods. Standardized evaluation protocols, in independent studies and in MICCAI challenges, should include unseen sites in the test set to evaluate generalizability. This will promote the development of methods that generalize better, using established techniques, e.g. dropout as in DenseVNet, or new innovations.

For both single- and multi-site training data set, some sites consistently yielded poorer accuracy when no data from that site was included in training. SITE5 yielded low accuracies in many analyses, likely due to site-specific differences in prostate MRI protocol: for example, the median inter-slice spacing at SITE5 was 4.7 mm compared to 2.8 mm across the other sites. One solution

Table 1. Segmentation accuracies for DenseVNet, VoxResNet and ResUNet.

DenseVNet		SITE1	SITE2	SITE3	SITE4	SITE5	SITE6	Pooled
Training	Testing	Dice coefficient (0–1)						
Single-site	same-site	0.88						
Single-site	unseen-site		0.88	0.84	0.83	0.77	0.85	0.83
Patient-level	same-site	0.87	0.90	0.87	0.88	0.86	0.88	0.88
Site-level	unseen-site	0.87	0.88	0.85	0.74	0.78	0.85	0.83
Commission-8	commissioned-site	0.87	0.89	0.87	0.86	0.86	0.88	0.87
Commission-16	commissioned-site	0.87	0.89	0.88	0.86	0.86	0.88	0.87
		Boundary distance (mm)						
Single-site	same-site	1.6						
Single-site	unseen-site		1.8	2.0	2.2	3.4	2.0	2.3
Patient-level	same-site	1.7	1.5	1.5	1.5	2.0	1.6	1.6
Site-level	unseen-site	1.8	1.7	1.8	4.2	3.2	2.0	2.4
Commission-8	commissioned-site	1.8	1.6	1.6	1.7	2.0	1.7	1.7
Commission-16	commissioned-site	1.8	1.6	1.5	1.7	2.1	1.6	1.7
VoxResNet		SITE1	SITE2	SITE3	SITE4	SITE5	SITE6	Pooled
Training	Testing	Dice coefficient (0–1)						
Single-site	same-site	0.85						
Single-site	unseen-site		0.81	0.83	0.58	0.37	0.80	0.68
Patient-level	same-site	0.84	0.87	0.86	0.84	0.80	0.86	0.84
Site-level	unseen-site	0.83	0.83	0.85	0.66	0.50	0.83	0.75
Commission-8	commissioned-site	0.85	0.86	0.85	0.83	0.79	0.84	0.84
Commission-16	commissioned-site	0.85	0.88	0.86	0.85	0.82	0.85	0.85
		Boundary distance (mm)						
Single-site	same-site	2.0						
Single-site	unseen-site		2.7	2.1	8.1	8.9	2.6	4.9
Patient-level	same-site	2.1	1.9	1.7	1.9	2.7	1.9	2.0
Site-level	unseen-site	2.2	2.2	1.8	5.8	6.6	2.3	3.5
Commission-8	commissioned-site	2.0	1.9	1.8	2.1	2.9	2.0	2.1
Commission-16	commissioned-site	2.0	1.7	1.7	1.8	2.5	1.9	1.9
ResUNet		SITE1	SITE2	SITE3	SITE4	SITE5	SITE6	Pooled
Training	Testing	Dice coefficient (0–1)						
Single-site	same-site	0.87						
Single-site	unseen-site		0.84	0.77	0.48	0.63	0.82	0.71
Patient-level	same-site	0.85	0.88	0.87	0.87	0.81	0.84	0.85
Site-level	unseen-site	0.83	0.84	0.83	0.71	0.51	0.80	0.75
Commission-8	commissioned-site	0.84	0.85	0.86	0.84	0.74	0.82	0.83
Commission-16	commissioned-site	0.84	0.86	0.85	0.86	0.78	0.85	0.84
		Boundary distance (mm)						
Single-site	same-site	1.7						
Single-site	unseen-site		2.0	2.4	8.2	5.9	2.2	4.1
Patient-level	same-site	2.0	1.7	1.6	1.6	2.4	2.1	1.9
Site-level	unseen-site	2.1	2.0	1.9	3.9	8.4	2.5	3.5
Commission-8	commissioned-site	2.1	2.0	1.6	2.0	3.7	2.3	2.3
Commission-16	commissioned-site	2.1	1.8	1.7	1.7	2.8	2.0	2.0

to this problem would be to adjust clinical imaging at this site to be more consistent with other sites; however, such a solution could be very disruptive. Note that this effect almost disappears in the patient-level cross-validation suggesting that these cases are probably not substantially harder to segment, as long as they are represented in the training data to some extent. This suggests that the more practical solution of retraining the segmentation network with some data from each site during the commissioning process may be effective.

The conclusions of this study should be considered in the context of its limitations. Our study focused exclusively on prostate segmentation, where deep-learning-based segmentation methods have become dominant and multi-site data sets are available. Reproducing our findings on other segmentation problems, once appropriate data are available, will be valuable. We observed variability between networks in their generalization to new sites; while we evaluated three different networks, we cannot conclude that all networks will need commissioning with data from each new site. Evaluating each network required training 49 networks, so a more exhaustive evaluation was not feasible for this work.

Our analysis confirmed that the accuracy of deep-learning-based segmentation networks trained and tested on data from one or more sites can overestimate the accuracy at an unseen site. This suggests that segmentation evaluation and especially segmentation challenges should include data from one or more completely unseen sites in the test data to estimate how well methods generalize, and promote better generalization. This also suggests that commissioning segmentation methods at a new site by training networks with a limited number of additional samples from that site could effectively mitigate this problem.

Acknowledgements. This publication presents independent research supported by Cancer Research UK (Multidisciplinary C28070/A19985).

References

1. Bakas, S., Menze, B., Davatzikos, C., Reyes, M., Farahani, K. (eds.): International MICCAI BraTS Challenge (2017)
2. Chen, H., Dou, Q., Yu, L., Qin, J., Heng, P.A.: VoxResNet: deep voxelwise residual networks for brain segmentation from 3D MR images. NeuroImage (2017)
3. Ghavami, N., et al.: Automatic slice segmentation of intraoperative transrectal ultrasound images using convolutional neural networks. In: SPIE Medical Imaging, February 2018
4. Gibson, E., et al.: Automatic multi-organ segmentation on abdominal CT with dense V-networks. IEEE TMI (2018)
5. He, K., Zhang, X., Ren, S., Sun, J.: Identity mappings in deep residual networks. arXiv:1603.05027 (2016)
6. Huang, G., Liu, Z., Weinberger, K.Q., van der Maaten, L.: Densely connected convolutional networks. arXiv:1608.06993 (2016)
7. Landman, B., Xu, Z., Igelsias, J.E., Styner, M., Langerak, T.R., Klein, A.: MICCAI Multi-atlas Labeling Beyond the Cranial Vault - Workshop and Challenge (2015)
8. Litjens, G., et al.: Evaluation of prostate segmentation algorithms for MRI: the PROMISE12 challenge. Med. Image Anal. **18**(2), 359–373 (2014)

9. Mirzaalian, H., et al.: Harmonizing diffusion MRI data across multiple sites and scanners. In: Navab, N., Hornegger, J., Wells, W.M., Frangi, A.F. (eds.) MICCAI 2015. LNCS, vol. 9349, pp. 12–19. Springer, Cham (2015). https://doi.org/10.1007/978-3-319-24553-9_2

10. Mueller, S.G., et al.: The Alzheimer's disease neuroimaging initiative. Neuroimaging Clin. **15**(4), 869–877 (2005)

11. Ronneberger, O., Fischer, P., Brox, T.: U-Net: convolutional networks for biomedical image segmentation. In: Navab, N., Hornegger, J., Wells, W.M., Frangi, A.F. (eds.) MICCAI 2015. LNCS, vol. 9351, pp. 234–241. Springer, Cham (2015). https://doi.org/10.1007/978-3-319-24574-4_28

12. Styner, M.A., Charles, H.C., Park, J., Gerig, G.: Multisite validation of image analysis methods: assessing intra-and intersite variability. In: Medical Imaging 2002: Image Processing, vol. 4684, pp. 278–287. SPIE (2002)

Deep Learning-Based Boundary Detection for Model-Based Segmentation with Application to MR Prostate Segmentation

Tom Brosch$^{(\boxtimes)}$, Jochen Peters, Alexandra Groth, Thomas Stehle, and Jürgen Weese

Philips GmbH Innovative Technologies, Hamburg, Germany
tom.brosch@philips.com

Abstract. Model-based segmentation (MBS) has been successfully used for the fully automatic segmentation of anatomical structures in medical images with well defined gray values due to its ability to incorporate prior knowledge about the organ shape. However, the robust and accurate detection of boundary points required for the MBS is still a challenge for organs with inhomogeneous appearance such as the prostate and magnetic resonance (MR) images, where the image contrast can vary greatly due to the use of different acquisition protocols and scanners at different clinical sites. In this paper, we propose a novel boundary detection approach and apply it to the segmentation of the whole prostate in MR images. We formulate boundary detection as a regression task, where a convolutional neural network is trained to predict the distances between a surface mesh and the corresponding boundary points. We have evaluated our method on the Prostate MR Image Segmentation 2012 challenge data set with the results showing that the new boundary detection approach can detect boundaries more robustly with respect to contrast and appearance variations and more accurately than previously used features. With an average boundary distance of 1.71 mm and a Dice similarity coefficient of 90.5%, our method was able to segment the prostate more accurately on average than a second human observer and placed first out of 40 entries submitted to the challenge at the writing of this paper.

1 Introduction

Model-based segmentation (MBS) [1] has been successfully used for the automatic segmentation of anatomical structures in medical images (e.g., heart [1]) due to its ability to incorporate prior knowledge about the organ shape into the segmentation method. This allows for robust and accurate segmentation, even when the detection of organ boundaries is incomplete. MBS approaches typically use rather simple features for detecting organ boundaries such as strong

© Springer Nature Switzerland AG 2018
A. F. Frangi et al. (Eds.): MICCAI 2018, LNCS 11073, pp. 515–522, 2018.
https://doi.org/10.1007/978-3-030-00937-3_59

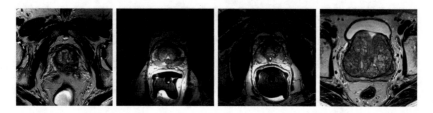

Fig. 1. Example images showing the large variability in image and prostate appearance.

gradients [8] and a set of additional constraints based on intensity value intervals [7] or scale invariant feature transforms [9]. Those features can detect organ boundaries reliably when they operate on well calibrated gray values, as is the case for computed tomography (CT) images. However, defining robust boundary features for the segmentation of organs with heterogeneous texture, such as the prostate, and varying MR protocols and scanners still remains a challenge due to the presence of weak and ambiguous boundaries caused by low signal-to-noise ratio and the inhomogeneity of the prostate, as well as the large variability in image contrast and appearance (see Fig. 1). To increase the robustness of the boundary detection for segmenting the prostate in MR images, Martin et al. [5] have used atlas matching to derive an initial organ probability map and then fine-tuned the segmentation using a deformable model, which was fit to the initial organ probability map and additional image features. Guo et al. [3] have extended this approach by using learned features from sparse stacked autoencoders for multi-atlas matching. Alternatively, Middleton et al. [6] have used a neural network to classify boundary voxels in MR images followed by the adaptation of a deformable model to the boundary voxels for lung segmentation. To speed up the detection of boundary points, Ghesu et al. [2] have used a sparse neural network for classification and restricted the boundary point search to voxels that are close to the mesh and aligned with the triangle normals.

We propose a novel boundary detection approach for fully automatic model-based segmentation of medical images and apply it to the segmentation of the whole prostate in MR images. We formulate boundary detection as a regression task, where a convolutional neural network (CNN) is trained to predict the distances between the mesh and the organ boundary for each mesh triangle, thereby eliminating the need for the time-consuming evaluation of many boundary voxel candidates. Furthermore, we combine the per-triangle boundary detectors into a single network in order to facilitate the calculation of all boundary points in parallel and designed it to be locally adaptive to cope with variations of appearance for different parts of the organ. We have evaluated our method on the Prostate MR Image Segmentation 2012 (PROMISE12) challenge [4] data set with the results showing that the new boundary detection approach can detect boundaries more robustly with respect to contrast and appearance variations and more accurately than previously used features and that the combination of shape-regularized model-based segmentation and deep learning-based boundary detection achieves the highest accuracy on this very challenging task.

2   Method

In this section, we will give a brief introduction to the model-based segmentation framework followed by a description of two network architectures for boundary detection: a global neural network-based boundary detector that uses the same parameters for all triangles, and a triangle-specific boundary detector that uses locally adaptive neural networks to search for the right boundary depending on the triangle index. A comprehensive introduction the model-based segmentation and previously designed boundary detection functions can be found in the papers by Ecabert et al. [1] and Peters et al. [7].

Model-Based Segmentation. The prostate surface is modeled as a triangulated mesh with fixed number of vertices V and triangles T. Given an input image I, the mesh is first initialized based on a rough localization of the prostate using a 3D version of the generalized Hough transformation (GHT) [1], followed by a parametric and a deformable adaptation. Both adaptation steps are governed by the external energy that attracts the mesh surface to detected boundary points. The external energy, E_{ext}, given a current mesh configuration and an image I is defined as

$$E_{\text{ext}} = \sum_{i=1}^{T} \left(\frac{\nabla I(x_i^{\text{boundary}})}{\|\nabla I(x_i^{\text{boundary}})\|} (c_i - x_i^{\text{boundary}}) \right)^2 , \tag{1}$$

where c_i denotes the center of triangle i, x_i^{boundary} denotes the boundary point for triangle i, and $\nabla I(x_i^{\text{boundary}})$ is the image gradient at the boundary point x_i^{boundary}. The boundary point difference $(c_i - x_i^{\text{boundary}})$ is projected onto the image gradient to allow cost-free lateral sliding of the triangles on the organ boundary. For the parametric adaptation, the external energy is minimized subject to the constraint that only affine transformations are applied to the mesh vertices. For the deformable adaptation, the vertices are allowed to float freely, but an internal energy term is added to the energy function, which penalizes deviations from a reference shape model of the prostate.

Neural Network-Based Boundary Detection. For each triangle, the corresponding boundary point is searched for on a line that is aligned with the triangle normal and passes through the triangle center. In previous work (e.g., [7]), candidate points on the search line were evaluated using predefined feature functions and the candidate point with the strongest feature response was selected as a boundary point. In contrast, we directly predict the signed distances d_i, $i \in [1, T]$, of the triangle centers to the organ boundary using neural networks, $f_i^{\text{CNN}} : \mathbb{R}^{D \times H \times W} \mapsto \mathbb{R}$, that process small subvolumes of I with depth D, height H, and width W such that

$$x_i^{\text{boundary}} = c_i + d_i \frac{n_i}{\|n_i\|} \tag{2}$$

with

$$d_i = f_i^{\text{CNN}}\big(S(I; c_i, n_i)\big), \tag{3}$$

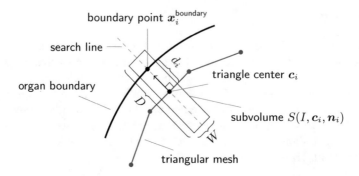

Fig. 2. Illustration of the boundary point search. For simplicity, the boundary point search is illustrated in 2D. The subvolume $S(I, c_i, n_i)$ is extracted from the image I and used by a neural network as input to predict the signed distance d_i of triangle i to its boundary point $x_i^{boundary}$.

where n_i are the normals of triangles i. The subvolumes $S(I, c_i, n_i)$ are sampled on a $D \times H \times W$ grid that is centered at c_i and aligned with n_i (see Fig. 2). The depth of the subvolumes is chosen such that they overlap with the organ boundary for the expected range of boundary distances called the capture range. The physical dimension of the subvolume is influenced by the number of voxels in each dimension of the subvolume and the spacing of the sampling grid. To keep the number of sampling points constant and thereby to allow the same network architecture to be used for different capture ranges, we change the voxel spacing in normal direction to account for different expected maximum distances of a triangle from the organ boundary. The parametric adaptation uses boundary detectors that were trained for an expected capture range of ± 20 mm and a sampling grid spacing of $2 \times 1 \times 1$ mm. We padded the size of the subvolume to account for the reduction of volume size caused by the first few convolutional layers, resulting in a subvolume size of $40 \times 5 \times 5$ voxels or $80 \times 5 \times 5$ mm. After the parametric adaptation, the prostate mesh is already quite well adapted to the organ boundary so we trained a second set of boundary detectors for a capture range of ± 5 mm and a sampling grid spacing of $0.5 \times 1 \times 1$ mm to facilitate the fine adaptation of the surface mesh during the deformable adaptation.

We propose and evaluate two different architectures for the boundary detection networks: a global boundary detector network that uses the same parameters for all triangles, and a locally adaptive network that adds a triangle-specific channel weighting layer to the global network and thereby facilitates the search for different boundary features depending on the triangle index. For both architecture, we combine the per-triangle networks, f_i^{CNN}, into a single network f^{CNN} that predicts all distances in one feedforward pass in order to speed up the prediction of all triangle distances and to allow for the sharing of parameters between the networks f_i^{CNN}:

$$(d_1, d_2, \dots, d_T) = f^{CNN}\big(S(I, c_1, n_1), S(I, c_2, n_2), \dots, S(I, c_T, n_T)\big). \quad (4)$$

Table 1. Network architecture with optional feature selection layer and corresponding dimensions used for predicting boundary point distances for each triangle for a subvolume size of $40 \times 5 \times 5$ voxels.

Layer type	Input dimension	Kernel size	# kernels	Output dimension
Conv + BN + ReLU	$T \times 40 \times 5^2$	$1 \times 7 \times 25$	32	$T \times 34 \times 32$
Conv + BN + ReLU	$T \times 34 \times 32$	$1 \times 7 \times 32$	32	$T \times 28 \times 32$
Conv + BN + ReLU	$T \times 28 \times 32$	$1 \times 7 \times 32$	32	$T \times 22 \times 32$
Conv + BN + ReLU	$T \times 22 \times 32$	$1 \times 22 \times 32$	32	$T \times 1 \times 32$
Conv + BN + ReLU	$T \times 1 \times 32$	$1 \times 1 \times 32$	32	$T \times 1 \times 32$
(Per-triangle weighting)	$T \times 1 \times 32$	—	—	$T \times 1 \times 32$
Conv	$T \times 1 \times 32$	$1 \times 1 \times 32$	1	$T \times 1 \times 1$

To simplify the network architecture, we assume that the width of all subvolumes is equal to their height and additionally reshape all subvolumes from size $D \times W \times W$ to $D \times W^2$. Consequently, the neural network for predicting the boundary distances is a function of the form $f^{\text{CNN}} : \mathbb{R}^{T \times D \times W^2} \mapsto \mathbb{R}^T$. The network input is processed using several blocks of convolutional (Conv), batch normalization (BN), and rectified linear unit (ReLU) layers called CBR blocks as summarized in Table 1, where each $1 \times A \times B$ kernel only operates on the input values and hidden units corresponding to a single triangle. Through the repeated application of valid convolutions, the network input of size $T \times D \times W^2$ is reduced to $T \times 1 \times 1$, where each element of the output vector represents the boundary distance of a particular triangle. Because the kernels are shared between all triangles, the network essentially calculates the same function for each triangle. However, the appearance of the interior and exterior of the organ might vary over the organ boundary and hence a triangle-specific distance function is often required. To allow for the learning of triangle-specific distance estimators, we extend the global network to a locally adaptive network by introducing a new layer that is applied before the last convolutional layer and defined as

$$\boldsymbol{x}_{L-1} = \boldsymbol{F} \odot \boldsymbol{x}_{L-2}, \tag{5}$$

where L is the number of layers of the network, $\boldsymbol{x}_l$ is the output of layer l, $\odot$ denotes element-wise multiplication, and $\boldsymbol{F} \in \mathbb{R}^{T \times 1 \times 32}$ is a trainable parameter matrix with one column per triangle and one row per channel of the output of the last CBR block. The locally adaptive network learns a pool of distance estimators, which are encoded in the convolutional kernels and shared between all triangles, along with triangle-specific weighting vectors encoded in the matrix $\boldsymbol{F}$ that allow the distance estimation to be adapted for different parts of the surface mesh.

Training. Training of the boundary detectors requires a set of subvolumes that are extracted around each triangle and corresponding boundary distances, which can be generated from a set of training images and corresponding reference meshes. To that end, we adapt a method previously used for selecting optimal boundary detectors from a large set of candidates called Simulated Search [7]. At each training iteration, mesh triangles are transformed randomly and independently of each other using three types of basic transformations: (a) random translations along the triangle normal, (b) small translations orthogonal to the triangle normal, and (c) and small random rotations. Then, subvolumes are extracted for each transformed triangle and the distance of the triangle to the reference mesh is calculated. The network parameters are optimized using stochastic gradient descent by minimizing the root mean square error between the predicted and simulated distances. The coarse and fine boundary detectors have been trained with a translation range along the triangle normal of ± 20 mm and ± 5 mm, which matches the capture range of the respective networks.

3 Results

We have evaluated our method on the training and test set from the Prostate MR Image Segmentation 2012 (PROMISE12) challenge[1] [4]. The training set consists of 50 T2-weighted MR images showing a large variability in organ size and shape. The training set contains acquisitions with and without endorectal coils and was acquired from multiple clinical centers using scanners from different vendors, thereby further adding to the variability in appearance and contrasts of the training images. Training of the boundary detection networks took about 6 h on an NVIDIA GeForce 1080 GTX graphics card. Segmentation of the prostate took about 37 s on the GPU and 98 s on the CPU using 8 cores. A comparison of the global and locally adaptive boundary detection networks with previously proposed boundary detection functions [7] was performed on the training set using 5-fold cross-validation. For a direct comparison to state-of-the-art methods, we submitted the segmentation results produced by the locally adaptive method on the test set for evaluation to the challenge.

For the comparison of different boundary detectors, we measured the segmentation accuracy in terms of the average boundary distance (ABD) between the produced and the reference segmentation. We were not able to achieve good segmentation results (ABD = 6.09 mm) using designed boundary detection functions with trained parameters as described in [7], which shows the difficulty of detecting the right boundaries for this data set. Using the global boundary detection network, we were able to achieve satisfying segmentation results with a mean ABD of 2.08 mm. The ABD could be further reduced to 1.48 mm using the locally adaptive network, which produced similar results compared to the global network, except for a few cases where the global network was not able to detect the correct boundary (see Fig. 3(a)) due to the inhomogeneous appearance of the prostate. In those cases, the global network only detected the boundary of the central gland, which produces the correct result for the anterior part of the prostate, but causes errors where the prostate boundary is defined by the peripheral zone. In contrast, locally adaptive networks (see Fig. 3(b)) are able

---

[1] https://promise12.grand-challenge.org/.

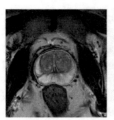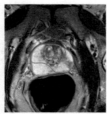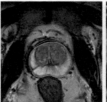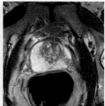

(a) Global boundary detection   (b) Locally adaptive boundary detection

Fig. 3. Comparison of segmentation results (red) and reference meshes (green) using two network architectures. The locally adaptive network correctly detects the prostate hull for the central gland and the peripheral zone, despite the large appearance differences of the two structures.

to switch between the detection of the central gland and the peripheral zone depending on the triangle index, consequently detecting the true boundary in all cases.

A comparison of our method to the best performing methods on the PROMISE12 challenge in terms of the Dice similarity coefficient (DSC), the average boundary distance (ABD), the absolute volume difference (VD), and the 95 percentile Hausdorff distance (HD95) calculated over the whole prostate is summarized in Table 2. The "score" relates a metric to a second observer, where a score of 85 is assigned if a method performs as well as a second observer and a score of 100 corresponds to a perfect agreement with the reference segmentation. At the writing of this paper, our method placed first in the challenge out of 40 entries, although the scores of the top three methods are very close. With

Table 2. Comparison of our method to state-of-the-art methods on the PROMISE12 challenge in terms of the Dice similarity coefficient (DSC), the average boundary distance (ABD), absolute volume difference (VD), and the 95 percentile Hausdorff distance (HD95) calculated over the whole prostate. Our method ranks first in all metrics except for HD95 and performs better on average than a second observer (score > 85).

Rank	Method (Year)	DSC	ABD	VD	HD95	Score
1	**Our method (2018)**	**90.5**	**1.71**	**6.6**	4.94	**87.21**
2	AutoDenseSeg (2018)	90.1	1.83	7.6	5.36	87.19
3	CUMED (2016)	89.4	1.95	7.0	5.54	86.65
4	RUCIMS (2018)	88.8	2.05	8.5	5.59	85.78
5	CREATIS (2017)	89.3	1.93	9.2	5.59	85.74
6	methinks (2017)	87.9	2.06	8.7	5.53	85.41
7	MedicalVision (2017)	89.8	1.79	8.2	5.35	85.33
8	BDSlab (2017)	87.8	2.35	9.1	7.59	85.16
9	IAU (2018)	89.3	1.86	7.7	5.34	84.84
10	UBCRCL (2017)	88.8	1.91	10.6	**4.90**	84.48

a DSC of 90.5%, an average boundary distance of 1.71 mm, and a mean absolute volume difference of 6.6% calculated over the whole prostate, our method achieved the best scores in these three metrics. Our method is second in only one metric, the 95 percentile Hausdorff distance, where our method achieved the second best value (4.94 mm) and is only slightly worse than the fully convolutional neural network approach by UBCRCL, which achieved a distance of 4.90 mm. Overall, our method demonstrated very good segmentation results and performed better on average (score > 85) than a second human observer.

4   Conclusion

We presented a novel deep learning-based method for detecting boundary points for the model-based segmentation of the prostate in MR images. We showed that using neural networks to directly predict the distances to the organ boundary instead of evaluating several boundary candidates using hand-crafted boundary features significantly improves the accuracy and robustness to large contrast variations. The accuracy could be further improved by making the network locally adaptive, which facilitates the learning of boundary detectors that are tuned for specific parts of the boundary. With an average boundary distance of $1.71mm$ and a Dice similarity coefficient of 90.5%, our method was able to segment the prostate more accurately on average than a second human observer and placed first out of 40 submitted entries on this very challenging data set.

References

1. Ecabert, O., et al.: Automatic model-based segmentation of the heart in CT images. IEEE Trans. Med. Imaging **27**(9), 1189–1201 (2008)
2. Ghesu, F.C., et al.: Marginal space deep learning: efficient architecture for volumetric image parsing. IEEE Trans. Med. Imaging **35**(5), 1217–1228 (2016)
3. Guo, Y., Gao, Y., Shen, D.: Deformable MR prostate segmentation via deep feature learning and sparse patch matching. In: Deep Learning for Medical Image Analysis, pp. 197–222. Elsevier (2017)
4. Litjens, G., et al.: Evaluation of prostate segmentation algorithms for MRI: the PROMISE12 challenge. Med. Image Anal. **18**(2), 359–373 (2014)
5. Martin, S., Troccaz, J., Daanen, V.: Automated segmentation of the prostate in 3D MR images using a probabilistic atlas and a spatially constrained deformable model. Med. Phys. **37**(4), 1579–1590 (2010)
6. Middleton, I., Damper, R.I.: Segmentation of magnetic resonance images using a combination of neural networks and active contour models. Med. Eng. Phys. **26**(1), 71–86 (2004)
7. Peters, J., Ecabert, O., Meyer, C., Kneser, R., Weese, J.: Optimizing boundary detection via simulated search with applications to multi-modal heart segmentation. Med. Image Anal. **14**(1), 70–84 (2010)
8. Vincent, G., Guillard, G., Bowes, M.:Fully automatic segmentation of the prostate using active appearance models. In: 2012 MICCAI Grand Challenge: Prostate MR Image Segmentation (2012)
9. Yang, M., Yuan, Y., Li, X., Yan, P.: Medical image segmentation using descriptive image features. In: BMVC, pp. 1–11 (2011)

Deep Attentional Features for Prostate Segmentation in Ultrasound

Yi Wang[1,2], Zijun Deng[3], Xiaowei Hu[4], Lei Zhu[4,5(✉)], Xin Yang[4],
Xuemiao Xu[3], Pheng-Ann Heng[4], and Dong Ni[1,2]

[1] National-Regional Key Technology Engineering Laboratory for Medical
Ultrasound, Guangdong Key Laboratory for Biomedical Measurements and
Ultrasound Imaging, School of Biomedical Engineering, Health Science Center,
Shenzhen University, Shenzhen, China
[2] Medical UltraSound Image Computing (MUSIC) Lab, Shenzhen, China
[3] School of Computer Science and Engineering,
South China University of Technology, Guangzhou, China
[4] Department of Computer Science and Engineering,
The Chinese University of Hong Kong, Hong Kong, China
lzhu@cse.cuhk.edu.hk
[5] Centre for Smart Health, School of Nursing,
The Hong Kong Polytechnic University, Hong Kong, China

Abstract. Automatic prostate segmentation in transrectal ultrasound
(TRUS) is of essential importance for image-guided prostate biopsy
and treatment planning. However, developing such automatic solutions
remains very challenging due to the ambiguous boundary and inhomogeneous intensity distribution of the prostate in TRUS. This paper develops a novel deep neural network equipped with deep attentional feature (DAF) modules for better prostate segmentation in TRUS by fully
exploiting the complementary information encoded in different layers of
the convolutional neural network (CNN). Our DAF utilizes the attention
mechanism to selectively leverage the multi-level features integrated from
different layers to refine the features at each individual layer, suppressing
the non-prostate noise at shallow layers of the CNN and increasing more
prostate details into features at deep layers. We evaluate the efficacy of
the proposed network on challenging prostate TRUS images, and the
experimental results demonstrate that our network outperforms state-
of-the-art methods by a large margin.

1 Introduction

Prostate cancer is the most common noncutaneous cancer and the second leading
cause of cancer-related deaths in men [9]. Transrectal ultrasound (TRUS) is the
routine imaging modality for image-guided biopsy and therapy of prostate cancer. Segmenting prostate from TRUS is of essential importance for the treatment

---

Y. Wang and Z. Deng contributed equally to this work.

© Springer Nature Switzerland AG 2018
A. F. Frangi et al. (Eds.): MICCAI 2018, LNCS 11073, pp. 523–530, 2018.
https://doi.org/10.1007/978-3-030-00937-3_60

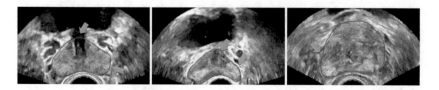

Fig. 1. Example TRUS images. Red contour denotes the prostate boundary. There are large prostate shape variations, and the prostate tissues present inhomogeneous intensity distributions. Orange arrows indicate missing/ambiguous boundaries.

planning [10], and can help surface-based registration between TRUS and preoperative MRI during image-guided interventions [11]. However, accurate prostate segmentation in TRUS remains very challenging due to the missing/ambiguous boundary and inhomogeneous intensity distribution of the prostate in TRUS, as well as the large shape variations of different prostates (see Fig. 1).

The problem of automatic prostate segmentation in TRUS has been extensively exploited in the literature. One main methodological stream utilizes shape statistics for the prostate segmentation. Shen *et al.* [8] presented a statistical shape model for prostate segmentation. Yan *et al.* [14] developed a partial active shape model to address the missing boundary issue in ultrasound shadow area. Another direction is to formulate the prostate segmentation as a foreground classification task. Ghose *et al.* [3] performed supervised soft classification with random forest to identify prostate. In general, all above methods used handcrafted features for segmentations, which are ineffective to capture the high-level semantic knowledge, and thus tend to fail in generating high-quality segmentations when there are ambiguous boundaries in TRUS. Recently, deep neural networks are demonstrated to be a very powerful tool to learn deep features for object segmentation. For TRUS segmentation, Yang *et al.* [15] proposed to learn the shape prior with recurrent neural networks and achieved state-of-the-art segmentation performance.

One of the main advantages of deep neural networks is to generate well-organized features consisting of abundant semantic and fine information. However, directly using these features at individual layers to conduct prostate segmentation cannot guarantee satisfactory results. It is essential to leverage the complementary advantages of features at multiple levels and to learn more discriminative features targeting for accurate and robust segmentation. To this end, we propose to fully exploit the complementary information encoded in multilayer features (MLF) generated by a convolutional neural network (CNN) for better prostate segmentation in TRUS images. Specifically, we develop a novel prostate segmentation network with deep attentional features (DAFs). The DAF is generated at each individual layer by learning the complementary information of the low-level detail and high-level semantics in MLF, thus is more powerful for the better representation of prostate characteristics. Our DAFs at shallow layers can learn highly semantic information encoded in the MLF to suppress its non-prostate regions, while our DAFs at deep layers are able to select the

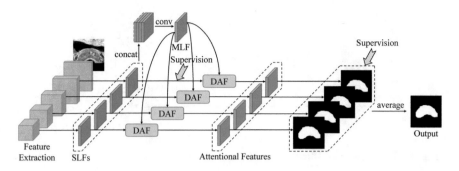

Fig. 2. The schematic illustration of our prostate segmentation network with deep attentional features (DAF). SLF: single-layer features; MLF: multi-layer features.

fine detail features from the MLF to refine prostate boundaries. Experiments on TRUS images demonstrate that our segmentation using deep attentional features outperforms state-of-the-art methods. The code is publicly available at https:// github.com/zijundeng/DAF.

2   Deep Attentional Features for Segmentation

Segmenting prostate from TRUS images is a challenging task especially due to the ambiguous boundary and inhomogeneous intensity distribution of the prostate in TRUS. Directly using low-level or high-level features, or even their combinations to conduct prostate segmentation may often fail to get satisfactory results. Therefore, leveraging various factors such as multi-scale contextual information, region semantics and boundary details to learn more discriminative prostate features is essential for accurate and robust prostate segmentation.

To address above issues, we present a deep neural network with deep attentional features (DAFs). The following subsections present the details of the proposed method and elaborate the novel DAF module.

2.1   Method Overview

Figure 2 illustrates the proposed prostate segmentation network with deep attentional features. Our network takes the TRUS image as the input and outputs the segmentation result in an end-to-end manner. It first produces a set of feature maps with different resolutions by using the CNN. The feature maps at shallow layers have high resolutions but with fruitful detail information while the feature maps at deep layers have low resolutions but with high-level semantic information. The highly semantic features can help to identify the position of prostate and the fine detail is able to indicate the fine boundary of the prostate.

After obtaining the feature maps with different levels of information, we enlarge these feature maps with different resolutions to a quarter of the size of original input image by linear interpolation (the feature maps at the first layer

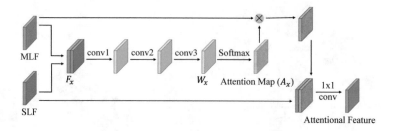

Fig. 3. The schematic illustration of the *deep attentional feature* (*DAF*) module.

are ignored due to the memory limitation). The enlarged feature maps at each individual layer are denoted as "single-layer features (SLF)", and the multiple SLFs are combined together, followed by convolution operations, to generate the "multi-layer features (MLF)". Although the MLF encodes the low-level detail information as well as the high-level semantic information of the prostate, it also inevitably incorporates noise from the shallow layers and losses some subtle parts of the prostate due to the coarse features at deep layers. Hence, the straight-forward segmentation result from the MLF tends to contain lots of non-prostate regions and lose parts of prostate tissues.

In order to refine the features of the prostate ultrasound image, we present a DAF module to generate deep attentional features at each layer in the principle of the attention mechanism. The DAF module leverages the MLF and the SLF as the inputs and produces the refined feature maps; please refer to Sect. 2.2 for the details of our DAF module. Then, we obtain the segmentation maps from the deep attentional features at each layer by using the deeply supervised mechanism [4,13] that imposes the supervision signals to multiple layers. Finally, we get the prostate segmentation result by averaging the segmentation maps at each individual layer.

2.2   Deep Attentional Features

As presented in Sect. 2.1, the feature maps at shallow layers contain the detail information of prostate but also include non-prostate regions, while the feature maps at deep layers are able to capture the highly semantic information to indicate the location of the prostate but may lose the fine details of the prostate's boundaries. To refine the features at each layer, we present a DAF module (see Fig. 3) to generate the deep attentional features by utilizing the attention mechanism to selectively leverage the features at MLF to refine features at the individual layer.

Specifically, given the single-layer feature maps at each layer, we concatenate them with the multi-layer feature maps as F_x, and then produce the unnormalized attention weights W_x (see Fig. 3):

$$W_x = f_a(F_x; \theta),\qquad(1)$$

where θ represents the parameters learned by f_a which contains three convolutional layers. The first two convolutional layers use 3×3 kernels, and the last convolutional layer applies 1×1 kernels.

After that, our DAF module computes the attention map A_x by normalizing W_x across the channel dimension with a Softmax function:

$$a_{i,j}^k = \frac{exp(w_{i,j}^k)}{\sum_k exp(w_{i,j}^k)}, \tag{2}$$

where $w_{i,j}^k$ denotes the value at spatial location (i, j) position and k-th channel on W_x, while $a_{i,j}^k$ denotes the normalized attention weight at spatial location (i, j) and k-th channel on A_x. After obtaining the attention map, we multiply it with the MLF in a element-by-element manner to generate a new refined feature map. The new features are concatenated with the SLF and then we apply a 1×1 convolution operation to produce the final attentional features for the given layer (see Fig. 3).

We apply the DAF module on each layer to refine its feature map. During this process, the attention mechanism is used to generate a set of weights to indicate how much attention should be paid to the MLF for each individual layer. Hence, our DAF enables the features at shallow layers to select the highly semantic features from the MLF in order to suppress the non-prostate regions, while the features at deep layers are able to select the fine detail features from the MLF to refine the prostate boundaries.

3   Experiments

3.1   Materials

Experiments were carried on TRUS images obtained using Mindray DC-8 ultrasound system in the First Affiliate Hospital of Sun Yat-Sen University. Informed consent was obtained from all patients. In total, we collected 530 TRUS images from 17 TRUS volumes which were acquired from 17 patients. The size of each TRUS image is 214×125 with a pixel size of 0.5×0.5 mm. We augmented (i.e., rotated, horizontally flipped) 400 images of 10 patients to 2400 as training dataset, and taken the remaining 130 images from 7 patients as testing dataset. All the TRUS images were manually segmented by an experienced clinician.

3.2   Training and Testing Strategies

Our proposed framework was implemented on PyTorch and used the ResNeXt101 [12] as the feature extraction layers (the orange parts in the left of Fig. 2).

Loss Function. Cross-entropy loss was used for each output of this network. The total loss $\mathcal{L}_t$ was defined as the summation of loss on all predicted score maps:

$$\mathcal{L}_t = \sum_{i=1}^{n} w_i \mathcal{L}_i + \sum_{j=1}^{n} w_j \mathcal{L}_j + w_f \mathcal{L}_f, \tag{3}$$

where w_i and $\mathcal{L}_i$ represent the weight and loss of i-th layer; while w_j and $\mathcal{L}_j$ represent the weight and loss of j-th layer after refining features using our DAF; n is the number of layers of our network; w_f and $\mathcal{L}_f$ are the weight and loss for the output layer. We empirically set all the weights (w_i, w_j and w_f) as 1.

Training Parameters. In order to reduce the risk of overfitting and accelerate the convergence of training, we used the weights trained on ImageNet [2] to initialize the feature extraction layers and other parts were initialized by random noise. The framework was trained on the augmented training set which contained 2400 samples. Stochastic gradient descent (SGD) with the momentum of 0.9 and weight decay of 0.01 was used to train the whole framework. We set the learning rate as 0.005 and it reduced to 0.0001 at 600 iterations. Learning stopped after 1200 iterations. The framework was trained on a single GPU with a mini-batch size of 4, only taking about 20 min.

Inference. In testing, for each input TRUS image, our network produced several output prostate segmentation maps since we added the supervision signals to all layers. We computed the final prediction map (see the last column of Fig. 2) by averaging the segmentation maps at each layer. After getting the final prediction map, we applied the fully connected conditional random field (CRF) [5] to improve the spatial coherence of the prostate segmentation map by considering the relationships of neighborhood pixels.

3.3   Segmentation Performance

We compared results of our method with several advanced methods, including Fully Convolutional Network (FCN) [6], Boundary Completion Recurrent Neural Network (BCRNN) [15], and U-Net [7]. For a fair comparison, we obtain the results of our competitors by using either the segmentation maps provided by corresponding authors, or re-training their models using the public implementations and adjusting training parameters to obtain best segmentation results.

The metrics employed to quantitatively evaluate segmentation included Dice Similarity Coefficient (Dice), Average Distance of Boundaries (ADB, in pixel), Conformity Coefficient (CC), Jaccard Index, Precision, and Recall [1]. A better segmentation shall have smaller ADB, and larger values of all other metrics.

Table 1 lists the metric results of different methods. It can be observed that our method consistently outperforms others on almost all the metrics. Figure 4 visualizes some segmentation results. Apparently, our method obtains the most similar segmented boundaries to the ground truth. Furthermore, as shown in Fig. 4, our method can successfully infer the missing/ambiguous boundaries, and it demonstrates the proposed deep attentional features can efficiently encode complementary information for accurate representation of the prostate tissues.

Table 1. Metric results of different methods (best results are highlighted in bold)

Method	Dice	ADB	CC	Jaccard	Precision	Recall
FCN [6]	0.9188	12.6720	0.8207	0.8513	0.9334	0.9080
BCRNN [15]	0.9239	11.5903	0.8322	0.8602	**0.9446**	0.9051
U-Net [7]	0.9303	7.4750	0.8485	0.8708	0.8985	0.9675
Ours	**0.9527**	**4.5734**	**0.9000**	**0.9101**	0.9369	**0.9698**

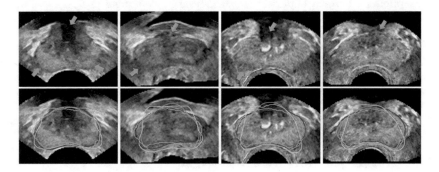

Fig. 4. Visual comparison of prostate segmentation results. Top row: prostate TRUS images with orange arrows indicating missing/ambiguous boundaries; bottom row: corresponding segmentations from our method (blue), U-Net (cyan), BCRNN (green) and FCN (yellow), respectively. Red contours are ground truths. Our method has the most similar segmented boundaries to the ground truth.

4   Conclusion

This paper develops a novel deep neural network for prostate segmentation in ultrasound images by harnessing the deep attentional features. Our key idea is to select the useful complementary information from the multi-level features to refine the features at each individual layer. We achieve this by developing a DAF module, which can automatically learn a set of weights to indicate the importance of the features in MLF for each individual layer by using an attention mechanism. Furthermore, we apply multiple DAF modules in a convolutional neural network to predict the prostate segmentation maps in different layers. Experiments on challenging TRUS prostate images demonstrate that our segmentation using deep attentional features outperforms state-of-the-art methods. In addition, the proposed method is a general solution and has the potential to be used for other medical image segmentation tasks.

Acknowledgments. This work was supported in part by the National Natural Science Foundation of China (61701312; 61571304; 61772206), in part by the Natural Science Foundation of SZU (No. 2018010), in part by the Shenzhen Peacock Plan (KQTD2016053112051497), in part by Hong Kong Research Grants Council (No. 14202514) and Innovation and Technology Commission under TCFS (No. GHP/002/13SZ), and in part by the Guangdong Natural Science Foundation (No. 2017A030311027). Xiaowei Hu is funded by the Hong Kong Ph.D. Fellowship.

References

1. Chang, H.H., Zhuang, A.H., Valentino, D.J., Chu, W.C.: Performance measure characterization for evaluating neuroimage segmentation algorithms. Neuroimage **47**(1), 122–135 (2009)
2. Deng, J., Dong, W., Socher, R., Li, L.J., Li, K., Fei-Fei, L.: ImageNet: a large-scale hierarchical image database. In: CVPR (2009)
3. Ghose, S., et al.: A supervised learning framework of statistical shape and probability priors for automatic prostate segmentation in ultrasound images. Med. Image Anal. **17**(6), 587–600 (2013)
4. Hu, X., Zhu, L., Qin, J., Fu, C.W., Heng, P.A.: Recurrently aggregating deep features for salient object detection. In: AAAI (2018)
5. Krähenbühl, P., Koltun, V.: Efficient inference in fully connected CRFs with Gaussian edge potentials. In: NIPS (2011)
6. Long, J., Shelhamer, E., Darrell, T.: Fully convolutional networks for semantic segmentation. In: CVPR (2015)
7. Ronneberger, O., Fischer, P., Brox, T.: U-Net: convolutional networks for biomedical image segmentation. In: Navab, N., Hornegger, J., Wells, W.M., Frangi, A.F. (eds.) MICCAI 2015. LNCS, vol. 9351, pp. 234–241. Springer, Cham (2015). https://doi.org/10.1007/978-3-319-24574-4_28
8. Shen, D., Zhan, Y., Davatzikos, C.: Segmentation of prostate boundaries from ultrasound images using statistical shape model. IEEE Trans. Med. Imaging **22**(4), 539–551 (2003)
9. Siegel, R.L., Miller, K.D., Jemal, A.: Cancer statistics, 2018. CA: Cancer J. Clin. **68**(1), 7–30 (2018)
10. Wang, Y., et al.: Towards personalized statistical deformable model and hybrid point matching for robust MR-TRUS registration. IEEE Trans. Med. Imaging **35**(2), 589–604 (2016)
11. Wang, Y., Zheng, Q., Heng, P.A.: Online robust projective dictionary learning: shape modeling for MR-TRUS registration. IEEE Trans. Med. Imaging **37**(4), 1067–1078 (2018)
12. Xie, S., Girshick, R., Dollár, P., Tu, Z., He, K.: Aggregated residual transformations for deep neural networks. In: CVPR (2017)
13. Xie, S., Tu, Z.: Holistically-nested edge detection. In: ICCV (2015)
14. Yan, P., Xu, S., Turkbey, B., Kruecker, J.: Discrete deformable model guided by partial active shape model for TRUS image segmentation. IEEE Trans. Biomed. Eng. **57**(5), 1158–1166 (2010)
15. Yang, X., et al.: Fine-grained recurrent neural networks for automatic prostate segmentation in ultrasound images. In: AAAI (2017)

Accurate and Robust Segmentation of the Clinical Target Volume for Prostate Brachytherapy

Davood Karimi[1(✉)], Qi Zeng[1], Prateek Mathur[1], Apeksha Avinash[1],
Sara Mahdavi[2], Ingrid Spadinger[2], Purang Abolmaesumi[1],
and Septimiu Salcudean[1]

[1] Department of Electrical and Computer Engineering,
University of British Columbia, Vancouver, BC, Canada
karimi@ece.ubc.ca
[2] Vancouver Cancer Centre, Vancouver, BC, Canada

Abstract. We propose a method for automatic segmentation of the prostate clinical target volume for brachytherapy in transrectal ultrasound (TRUS) images. Because of the large variability in the strength of image landmarks and characteristics of artifacts in TRUS images, existing methods achieve a poor worst-case performance, especially at the prostate base and apex. We aim at devising a method that produces accurate segmentations on easy and difficult images alike. Our method is based on a novel convolutional neural network (CNN) architecture. We propose two strategies for improving the segmentation accuracy on difficult images. First, we cluster the training images using a sparse subspace clustering method based on features learned with a convolutional autoencoder. Using this clustering, we suggest an adaptive sampling strategy that drives the training process to give more attention to images that are difficult to segment. Secondly, we train multiple CNN models using subsets of the training data. The disagreement within this CNN ensemble is used to estimate the segmentation uncertainty due to a lack of reliable landmarks. We employ a statistical shape model to improve the uncertain segmentations produced by the CNN ensemble. On test images from 225 subjects, our method achieves a Hausdorff distance of 2.7 ± 2.1 mm, Dice score of 93.9 ± 3.5, and it significantly reduces the likelihood of committing large segmentation errors.

1 Introduction

Transrectal ultrasound (TRUS) is routinely used in the diagnosis and treatment of prostate cancer. This study addresses the segmentation of the clinical target volume (CTV) in 2D TRUS images, an essential step for radiation treatment planning [9]. The CTV is delineated on a series of 2D TRUS images from the prostate base to apex. This is a challenging task because image landmarks are often weak or non-existent, especially at the base and apex, and various types of artifacts can be present. Therefore, manual segmentation is tedious and prone to

© Springer Nature Switzerland AG 2018
A. F. Frangi et al. (Eds.): MICCAI 2018, LNCS 11073, pp. 531–539, 2018.
https://doi.org/10.1007/978-3-030-00937-3_61

high inter-observer variability. Several semi- and fully-automatic segmentation algorithms have been proposed based on methods such as level sets, shape and appearance models, and machine learning [7, 10]. However, these methods often require careful initialization and are too slow for real-time segmentation. Moreover, although some of them achieve good average results in terms of, e.g., Dice Similarity Coefficient (DSC), criteria that show worst-case performance such as the Hausdorff Distance (HD) are either not reported or display large variances. This is because some images can be particularly difficult to segment due to weak prostate edges and strong artifacts. This also poses a challenge for deep learning-based methods that have achieved great success in medical image segmentation. Since they have a high representational power and are trained using stochastic gradient descent with uniform sampling of the training data, their training can be dominated by the more typical samples in the training set, leading to poor generalization on less-represented images.

In this paper, we propose a method for segmentation of the CTV in 2D TRUS images that is geared towards achieving good results on most test images while at the same time reducing large segmentation errors. Our contributions are:

1. We propose a novel convolutional neural network (CNN) architecture for segmentation of the CTV in 2D TRUS images.
2. We suggest an adaptive sampling method for CNN training. In brief, our method samples the training images based on how likely they are to contribute to improving the segmentation of difficult images in a validation set.
3. We estimate the segmentation uncertainty based on the disagreement among an ensemble of CNNs and propose a novel method to improve the highly uncertain segmentations with the help of a statistical shape model (SSM).

2   Materials and Methods

2.1   Data

We used the TRUS images of 675 subjects. From each subject, 7 to 14 2D TRUS images of size 415×490 pixels with a pixel size of $0.15 \times 0.15 \, \text{mm}^2$ were acquired. The CTV was delineated in each slice by experienced radiation oncologists. We used the data from 450 subjects for training, including cross-validation, and left the remaining 225 subjects (including a total of 2207 2D images) for test.

2.2   Clustering of the Training Images

We rely on the method of sparse subspace clustering [1] and use a convolutional autoencoder (CAE) for learning low-dimensional image representations as proposed in [4]. As shown in Fig. 1, the encoder part of the CAE learns a low-dimensional representation z^i_{enc} for an input image x^i. Then, a fully-connected layer, which consists of multiplication with a matrix, Γ, without a bias term and nonlinear activation function, transforms this representation into the input to the decoder, z^i_{dec}. The sparse subspace clustering is enforced by requiring:

$$Z_{\text{dec}} \cong Z_{\text{enc}} \varGamma \quad \text{such that:} \quad \text{diag}(\varGamma) = 0 \tag{1}$$

where Z_{enc} is the matrix that has z_{enc}^i for all training images as its columns, and similarly for Z_{dec}, and $\varGamma$ is a sparse matrix with zero diagonal. By enforcing sparsity on $\varGamma$, we require that the representation of the ith image, z_{dec}^i, be approximated as a linear combination of a small number of those of other images in the training set. Note that although the relation between Z_{dec} and Z_{enc} is linear, the clustering method is far from linear because z_{enc}^i is a very rich and highly non-linear representation of the image.

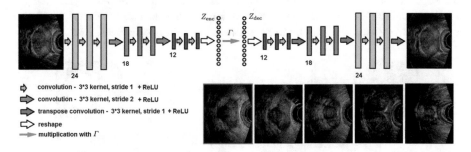

Fig. 1. The CAE architecture used to learn image affinities. On the bottom right, an image (with red borders) is shown along with 4 images with decreasing (left-to-right) similarity to it based on the affinity matrix, $C = |\varGamma| + |\varGamma^{\text{T}}|$, learned by the CAE.

We first train a standard CAE, i.e., with $\varGamma = I$. In this stage, we minimize the standard CAE cost function, i.e., the reconstruction error $\|\hat{X} - X\|_2^2$, where X and $\hat{X}$ denote, respectively, matrices of the input images and the reconstructed images. In the second stage, we introduce $\varGamma$ and train the network by solving:

$$\textbf{minimize} \|\hat{X} - X\|_2^2 + \lambda_1 \|Z_{\text{enc}} - Z_{\text{enc}}\varGamma\|_2^2 + \lambda_2 \|\varGamma\|_1 \quad \textbf{s.t.} \quad \text{diag}(\varGamma) = 0 \tag{2}$$

We empirically chose $\lambda_1 = \lambda_2 = 0.1$. For both training stages, we trained the network for 100 epochs using Adam [5] with a learning rate of 10^{-3}. Once the network is trained, an affinity matrix can be created as $C = |\varGamma| + |\varGamma^{\text{T}}|$, where $C(i,j)$ indicates the similarity between the ith and j^{th} images. Spectral clustering methods can be used to cluster the data based on C, but we will use C directly as explained in Sect. 2.4.

2.3   Proposed CNN Architecture

A simplified representation of our CNN is shown in Fig. 2. Our design is different from widely-used networks such as [8] in that: (1) We apply convolutional filters of varying sizes ($k \in \{3, 5, 7, 9, 11\}$) and strides ($s \in \{1, 2, 3, 4, 5\}$) directly to the input image to extract fine and coarse features. Because small image patches are overwhelmed by speckle and contain little edge information, applying larger filters directly on the image should help the network learn more informative features at different scales, (2) The computed features at each fine scale are forwarded to all coarser layers by applying convolutional kernels of proper sizes and strides. This promotes feature reuse, which reduces the number of network parameters while increasing the richness of the learned representations [3]. Hence, the network extracts features at multiple different resolutions and fields-of-view. These features are then combined via a series of transpose convolutions. (3) In both the contracting and the expanding paths, features go through residual blocks to increase the richness of representations and ease the training. The network outputs a prostate segmentation probability map (in [0,1]). We train the network by maximizing the DSC between this probability map and the ground-truth segmentation. For this, we used Adam with a learning rate of 10^{-4} and performed 200 epochs. The training process is explained in Sect. 2.4.

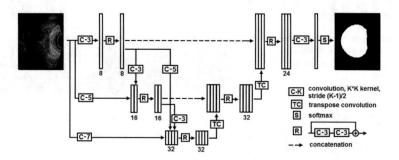

Fig. 2. The proposed CNN architecture. To avoid clutter, the network is shown for a depth of 3. We used a network with a depth of 5; i.e., we also applied C-9 and C-11. Number of feature maps is also shown. All convolutions are followed by ReLU.

2.4 Training a CNN Ensemble with Adaptive Sampling

Due to non-convexity and extreme complexity of their optimization landscape, deep CNNs converge to a local minimum. With small training data, these minima can be heavily influenced by the more prevalent samples in the training set. A powerful approach to reducing the sensitivity to local minima and reducing the generalization error is to learn an ensemble of models [2]. We train $K = 5$ CNN models using 5-fold cross validation. Let us denote the indices of the training and validation images for one of these models with S_{tr} and S_{vl}, respectively. Let e_i denote the "error" committed on the ith validation image by the CNN after the current training epoch. As shown in Fig. 3, for the next epoch we sample the training images according to their similarity to the difficult validation images. Specifically, we compute the probability of sampling the jth training image as:

$$p(j) = q(j)/\Sigma_j q(j) \quad \text{where} \quad q(j) = \Sigma_{i \in S_{\mathrm{vl}}} C(i,j) e(i) \tag{3}$$

We initialize p to a uniform distribution for the first epoch. Importantly, there is a great flexibility in the choice of the error, e. For example, e does not

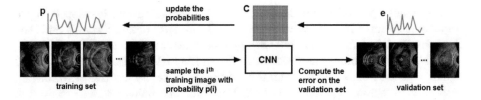

Fig. 3. The proposed training loop with adaptive sampling of the training images.

have to possess requirements such as differentiability. In this work, we chose the Hausdorff Distance (HD) as e. For two curves, X and Y, HD is defined as $\text{HD}(X, Y) = \max\left(\sup_{y \in Y} \inf_{x \in X} \|x - y\|, \sup_{x \in X} \inf_{y \in Y} \|x - y\| \right)$. Although HD is an important measure of segmentation error, it cannot be easily minimized as it is non-differentiable. Our approach provides an indirect way to reduce HD.

2.5 Improving Uncertain Segmentations Using an SSM

Training multiple models enables us to estimate the segmentation (un)certainty by examining the disagreement among the models. For a given image, we compute the average pair-wise DSC between the segmentations produced by the 5 CNNs. If this value is above the empirically-chosen threshold of 0.95, we trust the CNN segmentations because of high agreement among the 5 CNNs trained on different data. In such a case, we will compute the average of the 5 probability maps and threshold it at 0.50 to yield the final segmentation (Fig. 4, top row).

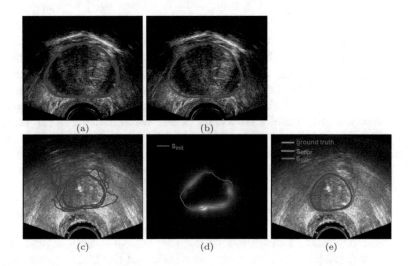

Fig. 4. Top: an "easy" image, (a) the CNNs produce similar results, (b) the final segmentation produced by thresholding the mean probability map. Bottom: a "difficult" image, (c) there is large disagreement between CNNs, (d) the certainty map with s_{init} (red) superimposed, (e) the final segmentation, s_{impr} (blue), obtained using SSM.

If the mean pair-wise DSC among the 5 CNN segmentations is below 0.95, we improve it by introducing prior information in the form of an SSM. We built the SSM from a set of 75 MR images with ground-truth prostate segmentation provided by expert radiologists. From each slice of the MR images, we extracted 100 equally-spaced points on the boundary of the prostate, rigidly (i.e., translation, scale, and rotation) registered them to one reference point set, and computed the SVD of the point sets. We built three separate SSMs for base, mid-gland, and apex. In deciding whether an MRI slice belonged to base, mid-gland, or apex, we assumed that each of these three sections accounted for one third of the prostate length. We use u and V to denote, respectively, the mean shape and the matrix with the n most important shape modes as its columns. We chose $n = 5$ because the top 5 modes explained more than 98% of the shape variance.

If the agreement among the CNN segmentations is below the threshold, we use them to compute: (1) An initial segmentation boundary, s_{init}, by thresholding the average of the 5 probability maps, $\bar{p}$, at 0.5, and (2) a certainty map:

$$Q = \nabla F_{\text{KW}} = \nabla(1 - \bar{p}^2 - (1 - \bar{p})^2) \tag{4}$$

where F_{KW} is based on the Kohavi-Wolpert variance [6]. F_{KW} is 0 where all models agree and increases as the disagreement grows. As shown in Fig. 4(d), Q indicates, roughly, the locations where segmentation boundaries predicted by the 5 models are close, i.e., segmentations are more likely to be correct. Therefore, we estimate an improved segmentation boundary, s_{impr}, as:

$$s_{\text{impr}} = R_{\theta^*}[s^*(Vw^* + u)] + t^*$$
$$\text{where: } \{s^*, t^*, w^*, \theta^*\} = \underset{s,t,w,\theta}{\operatorname{argmin}} \|R_\theta[s(Vw + u)] + t - s_{\text{init}}\|_Q \tag{5}$$

where t, s, and w denote, respectively, translation, scale, and the coefficients of the shape model, R_θ is the rotation matrix with angle θ, and $\|.\|_Q$ denotes the weighted ℓ_2 norm using weights Q computed in Eq. (4). In other words, we fit an SSM to s_{init} while attaching more importance to parts of s_{init} that have higher certainty. Since the objective function in Eq. 5 is non-convex, alternating minimization is used to find a stationary point. We initialize t to the centroid of the initial segmentation, s to 1, and w and θ to zero and perform alternating minimization until the objective function reduces by less than 1% in an iteration. Up to 3 iterations sufficed to converge to a good result (Fig. 4, bottom row).

3   Results and Discussion

We compare our method with the adaptive shape model-based method of [10] and CNN model of [8], which we denote as ADSM and U-NET, respectively. We report three results for our method: (1) Proposed-OneCNN: only one CNN is trained, (2) Proposed-Ensemble: five CNNs are trained as explained in Sect. 2.4 and the final segmentation is obtained by thresholding the average probability map at 0.5, and (3) Proposed-Full: improves uncertain segmentations produced

Table 1. Summary of the comparison of the proposed method with ADSM and U-NET.

		DSC	HD (mm)	95th percentile of HD (mm)
Mid-gland	ADSM	89.9 ± 3.9	3.2 ± 2.0	7.2
	U-NET	92.0 ± 3.6	3.6 ± 2.1	7.3
	Proposed-Full	94.6 ± 3.1	2.5 ± 1.6	4.6
Base	ADSM	86.8 ± 6.6	3.9 ± 2.4	8.0
	U-NET	91.2 ± 4.1	3.8 ± 2.8	8.6
	Proposed-Full	93.6 ± 3.6	2.7 ± 2.0	5.0
Apex	ADSM	84.9 ± 7.4	4.4 ± 3.0	8.4
	U-NET	87.3 ± 5.6	4.6 ± 3.2	9.0
	Proposed-Full	91.2 ± 5.0	3.0 ± 1.9	5.5

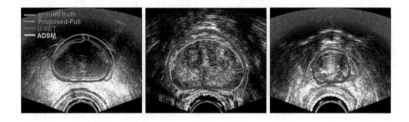

Fig. 5. Example segmentations produced by different methods.

by Proposed-Ensemble as explained in Sect. 2.5. Our comparison criteria are DSC and HD. We also report the 95%-percentile of HD across the test images as a measure of the worst-case performance on the population of test images.

As shown in Table 1, our method outperformed the other methods in terms of DSC and HD. Paired t-tests (at $p = 0.01$) showed that the HD obtained by our method was significantly smaller than the other methods in all three prostate sections. Our method also achieved much smaller values for the 95%-percentile of HD. Figure 5 shows example segmentations produced by different methods.

Table 2 shows the effectiveness of our proposed strategies for improving the segmentations. Proposed-Ensemble and Proposed-Full achieve much better results than Proposed-OneCNN. There is a marked improvement in DSC. The reduction in HD is also substantial. Mean, standard deviation, and the 95%-percentile of HD have been greatly reduced by our proposed strategies. Paired t-tests (at $p = 0.01$) showed that Proposed-Ensemble achieved a significantly lower HD than Proposed-OneCNN and, on images that were processed by SSM fitting, Proposed-Full significantly reduced HD compared with Proposed-Ensemble.

Both the CAE (Fig. 1) and the CNN (Fig. 2) were implemented in Tensor-Flow. On an Nvidia GeForce GTX TITAN X GPU, the training times for the

Table 2. Performance of the proposed method at different stages.

	DSC	HD (mm)	95th percentile of HD (mm)
Proposed-OneCNN	91.8 ± 4.3	3.6 ± 2.6	8.1
Proposed-ensemble	93.5 ± 3.6	3.0 ± 2.1	5.5
Proposed-full	93.9 ± 3.5	2.7 ± 2.1	5.1

CAE and each of the CNNs, respectively, were approximately 24 and 12 h. For a test image, each CNN produces a segmentation in 0.02 s.

4   Conclusion

In the context of prostate CTV segmentation in TRUS, we proposed adaptive sampling of the training data, ensemble learning, and use of prior shape information to improve the segmentation accuracy and robustness and reduce the likelihood of committing large segmentation errors. Our method achieved significantly better results than competing methods in terms of HD, which measures largest segmentation error. Our methods also substantially reduced the maximum errors committed on the population of test images. An important contribution of this work was a method to compute a segmentation certainty map, which we used to improve the segmentation accuracy with the help of an SSM. This certainty map can have many other useful applications, such as in registration of TRUS to pre-operative MRI and for radiation treatment planning. A shortcoming of this work is with regard to our ground-truth segmentations, which have been provided by expert radiation oncologists on TRUS images. These segmentations can be biased at the prostate base and apex. Therefore, a comparison with registered MRI is warranted.

Acknowledgment. This work was supported by Prostate Cancer Canada, the CIHR, the NSERC, and the C.A. Laszlo Chair in Biomedical Engineering held by S. Salcudean.

References

1. Elhamifar, E., Vidal, R.: Sparse subspace clustering: algorithm, theory, and applications. IEEE Trans. Pattern Anal. Mach. Intell. **35**(11), 2765–2781 (2013)
2. Goodfellow, I., Bengio, Y., Courville, A., Bengio, Y.: Deep Learning, vol. 1. MIT Press, Cambridge (2016)
3. Huang, G., Liu, Z., Weinberger, K.Q., van der Maaten, L.: Densely connected convolutional networks. In: Proceedings of the IEEE Conference on Computer Vision and Pattern Recognition, vol. 1, p. 3 (2017)
4. Ji, P., Zhang, T., Li, H., Salzmann, M., Reid, I.: Deep subspace clustering networks. In: Advances in Neural Information Processing Systems, pp. 23–32 (2017)
5. Kingma, D.P., Ba, J.: Adam: a method for stochastic optimization. In: Proceedings of the 3rd International Conference on Learning Representations (ICLR) (2014)

6. Kuncheva, L., Whitaker, C.: Measures of diversity in classifier ensembles and their relationship with the ensemble accuracy. Mach. Learn. **51**(2), 181–207 (2003)
7. Qiu, W., Yuan, J., Ukwatta, E., Fenster, A.: Rotationally resliced 3D prostate trus segmentation using convex optimization with shape priors. Med. phys. **42**(2), 877–891 (2015)
8. Ronneberger, O., Fischer, P., Brox, T.: U-net: convolutional networks for biomedical image segmentation. In: Navab, N., Hornegger, J., Wells, W.M., Frangi, A.F. (eds.) MICCAI 2015. LNCS, vol. 9351, pp. 234–241. Springer, Cham (2015). https://doi.org/10.1007/978-3-319-24574-4_28
9. Sylvester, J.E., Grimm, P.D., Eulau, S.M., Takamiya, R.K., Naidoo, D.: Permanent prostate brachytherapy preplanned technique: the modern seattle method step-by-step and dosimetric outcomes. Brachytherapy **8**(2), 197–206 (2009)
10. Yan, P., Xu, S., Turkbey, B., Kruecker, J.: Adaptively learning local shape statistics for prostate segmentation in ultrasound. IEEE Trans. Biomed. Eng. **58**(3), 633–641 (2011)

Image Segmentation Methods: Cardiac Segmentation Methods

Hashing-Based Atlas Ranking and Selection for Multiple-Atlas Segmentation

Amin Katouzian[1]([✉]), Hongzhi Wang[1], Sailesh Conjeti[2], Hui Tang[1],
Ehsan Dehghan[1], Alexandros Karargyris[1], Anup Pillai[1], Kenneth Clarkson[1],
and Nassir Navab[2]

[1] IBM Almaden Research Center, San Jose, CA, USA
akatouz@us.ibm.com
[2] Computer Aided Medical Procedures, Technische Universität München,
Munich, Germany

Abstract. In this paper, we present a learning based, registration free, atlas ranking technique for selecting outperforming atlases prior to image registration and multi-atlas segmentation (MAS). To this end, we introduce *ensemble hashing*, where each data (image volume) is represented with *ensemble* of hash codes and a learnt distance metric is used to obviate the need for pairwise registration between atlases and target image. We then pose the ranking process as an assignment problem and solve it through two different combinatorial optimization (CO) techniques. We use 43 unregistered cardiac CT Angiography (CTA) scans and perform thorough validations to show the effectiveness and superiority of the presented technique against existing atlas ranking and selection methods.

1 Introduction

In atlas-based segmentation, the goal is to leverage labels in a single fixed (template) atlas for segmenting a target image. The assumption that the spatial appearance of anatomical structures remains almost the same across and within databases is not always held, which results in systematic registration error prior to label propagation. Alternatively, in MAS [2,15], multiple atlases are deployed, encompassing larger span of anatomical variabilities, for compensating large registration errors that may be produced by any single atlas and increasing performance. Thus, the challenge is to optimally select a number of outperforming atlases without compromising segmentation accuracy and computational speed.

For this reason, different atlas selection methods have been proposed based on (1) image similarity between atlases and target image, defined over original space or manifolds [1,11,17], (2) segmentation precision [7], and (3) features representations for supervised learning [12]. Although the aim is to reduce the number of required pairwise registrations between query image and less applicable (dissimilar) atlases, all above mentioned selection techniques themselves rely

© Springer Nature Switzerland AG 2018
A. F. Frangi et al. (Eds.): MICCAI 2018, LNCS 11073, pp. 543–551, 2018.
https://doi.org/10.1007/978-3-030-00937-3_62

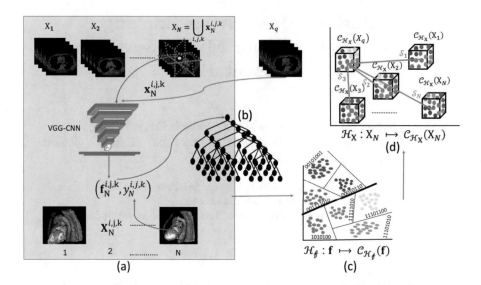

Fig. 1. Overall schematic of proposed method. **Training:** The VGG-convolutional neural network (CNN) [14] is used for feature extraction from 3D atlases (a) and training of mHF H_f (b). The feature space is parsed and hashed $C_{H_f}(f)$ by preserving similarity among each and every organ (c). **Retrieval:** The VGG-CNN features are extracted from query ($\mathbf{X}_q$) and fed to the learnt mHF to generate *ensemble* hash codes $C_{H_X}(\mathbf{X}_q)$. The CO is then used as similarity $\mathcal{S}$ measure for retrieving $\mathcal{N}$ closest matches (d).

on non-rigid registration as a preprocessing step. In fact, at the first glance, registration seems to be inevitable since the selection strategy is often established on the premise of capturing similarity between pairwise images.

This motivated us to investigate potential extension of hashing forests [3] as an alternative solution where similarity can be measured within a registration free regime. The rationale behind the use of hashing forests is further substantiated by [8,10] where the former uses forests for the task of approximate nearest neighbor retrieval and the latter introduced a novel training scheme with guided bagging both applied for segmentation of CT images. Although they can be utilized for the purpose of label propagation as part of MAS, however, their direct generalizations to atlas selection are doubtful due to lack of ranking metric and strategy. In essence, we propose similar idea of preserving similarity in local neighborhoods but what makes our method suitable for atlas ranking is inclusion of hashing in neighborhood approximation, which serves as a basis for defining a definitive metric for ranking through CO techniques [13].

Our work is fundamentally different from [3] from two main perspectives. First, unlike [3], where each data point is represented by a single class sample or hash code (i.e. organ type, Fig. 1(c)) in hashing space, we parse the hashing space with ensemble of codes derived from features representing every organ within the volumetric CT images, Fig. 1(d). Secondly, due to ensemble representations, the retrieval/ranking task becomes a matching or assignment problem in Hamming space that we solve through CO techniques. We use KuhnMunkres (also known as Hungarian) algorithm [9] as well as linear programming (LP) to rank and select the closest atlases to the query. We perform similar validation scheme to [11] and use normalized mutual information (NMI) as similarity measure for atlas selection. Finally, we quantify the overall performance through MAS algorithm proposed by [15].

Our contributions include: **(1)** extending [3] for volumetric data hashing and introducing the concept of *ensemble hashing* for the first time, **(2)** employing hashing for atlas selection and ranking as part of MAS, **(3)** eliminating pairwise registration, which makes atlas selection extremely fast, and **(4)** deploying CO as a solution to atlas ranking problem that will also be shown to be a viable solution for similarity matching in the context of *ensemble hashing*.

2   Methodology

2.1   Volumetric Ensemble Hashing Through mHF

Figure 1 shows the schematic of proposed method and we refer readers to [3] for detailed description about mHF. For a given subset of training atlases $\mathcal{X}_N = \{\mathbf{x}_v : \mathbb{R}^3 \to \mathbb{R}\}_{v=1}^N$ and corresponding labels $\mathcal{Y}_N = \{\mathbf{y}_v : \mathbb{R}^3 \to \mathbb{N}\}_{v=1}^N$ we perform random sampling with minimum rate of $f_{s_{min}}$ to extract features from data represented in three orthogonal planes centered at (i, j, k) spatial coordinate using VGG network $\mathcal{F}_N^{(i,j,k)} = \{\mathbf{f}_v^{(i,j,k)} \in \mathbb{R}^d\}_{v=1}^N$. For simplicity, $\mathcal{X}_N$, $\mathbf{x}_v$, $\mathbf{f}_v^{(i,j,k)}$ are used interchangeably with $\mathcal{X}$, $\mathbf{x}$, $\mathbf{f}$, respectively throughout paper. An n bit hash function h_f is defined that maps $\mathbb{R}^d$ to n-dimensional binary Hamming space $h_f : \mathbb{R}^d \to \{1,0\}^n$ with $\mathcal{C}_{h_f}(\mathbf{f}) = h_f(\mathbf{f})$ codeword. The hashing forest comprises of K independently hashing trees $\mathcal{H}_f = \{h_f^1, \cdots, h_f^K\}$ that encodes each sample point $\mathbf{f}$ from $\mathbb{R}^d$ to nK-dimensional Hamming space $\{1,0\}^{nK}$ such that $\mathcal{H}_f : \mathbf{f} \to \mathcal{C}_{H_f}(\mathbf{f}) = \mathcal{C}_{h_f^1}(\mathbf{f}), \cdots, \mathcal{C}_{h_f^K}(\mathbf{f})$. Given $\mathcal{H}_f$, we encode all organs in training atlases $\mathcal{X} \in \mathbb{R}^{d \times N \times o}$ as $\mathcal{H}_f : \mathcal{F} \to \mathcal{C}_{H_f}(\mathcal{F}) = \mathcal{C}_{h_f^1}(\mathcal{F}), \cdots, \mathcal{C}_{h_f^K}(\mathcal{F}) \in \{1,0\}^{nK \times N \times o}$, where o is the total numbers of organs.

The mHF parses and hashes the latent feature space while preserving similarity among organs, Fig. 1(c). For *ensemble* representation of each volume, we incorporate the coordinates of sampling points (i, j, k) into hashing scheme as follows:

$$\mathcal{H}_\mathcal{X} : \underbrace{\bigcup_{(i,j,k)} \mathbf{f}_N^{(i,j,k)}}_{\mathcal{X}_N} \to \bigcup_{(i,j,k)} C_{\mathcal{H}_f}\left(\mathbf{f}_N^{(i,j,k)}\right) = \underbrace{\bigcup_{(i,j,k)} \left\{ C_{h_f^1}\left(\mathbf{f}_N^{(i,j,k)}\right), \cdots, C_{h_f^K}\left(\mathbf{f}_N^{(i,j,k)}\right) \right\}}_{C_{H_\mathcal{X}}(\mathcal{X}_N)}$$

$$(1)$$

where $C_{H_\mathcal{X}}(\mathcal{X}_N) \in \{1,0\}^{(nk \times N \times n_s)}$ and n_s is the number of sampling points.

2.2   Retrieval Through Combinatorial Optimization (CO)

In classical hashing based retrieval methods, given a query $\mathbf{x}_q$, the inter-sample similarity S could be computed as pairwise Hamming distance D_H between

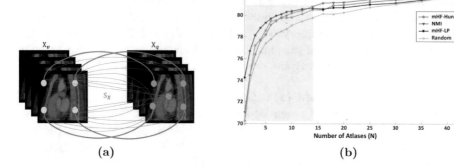

Fig. 2. Distance matching illustration between $\mathcal{X}_v$ and $\mathcal{X}_q$ volumes represented by 4 and 5 sampling points, respectively. The top matches are depicted by thicker edges (a). The MAS performance using different atlas ranking techniques. The average Dice value is reported over all organs when $N = [1{:}9, 10{:}2{:}20, 25, 30, 35, 42]$ (b). The highlighted area covers number of atlases where mHF-LP outperforms or its performance almost becomes equal to NMI ($N = 14$).

the hash codes of query $C_{\mathcal{H}}(\mathbf{x}_q)$ and each sample in training database $C_{\mathcal{H}}(\mathbf{x}_v)$ through logical xor as $S_{\mathbf{x}_{qv}} = D_H(\mathbf{x}_q, \mathbf{x}_v) = C_{\mathcal{H}}(\mathbf{x}_q) \oplus C_{\mathcal{H}}(\mathbf{x}_v) \in \mathbb{N}$. The samples whose hash codes fall within the Hamming ball of radius r centered at $C_{\mathcal{H}}(\mathbf{x}_q)$ *i.e.* $D_H(\mathbf{x}_q, \mathbf{x}_v) \le r$ are considered as nearest neighbors. However, for our problem, the pairwise Hamming distance between hash codes of two volumes is $S_{\mathcal{X}_{qv}} = D_H(\mathcal{X}_q, \mathcal{X}_v) = C_{\mathcal{H}}(\mathcal{X}_q) \oplus C_{\mathcal{H}}(\mathcal{X}_v) \in \mathbb{R}^2$ and finding the nearest neighbors seems intractable.

Both volumes $\mathcal{X}_v$ and $\mathcal{X}_q$ are represented by $n_s^v \times l$ and $n_s^q \times l$ features in latent space, resulting in n_s^v and n_s^q hash codes, where n_s^v and n_s^q are number of sampling points, Fig. 2(a) ($n_s^v = 4$, $n_s^q = 5$). The Similarity $S_{\mathcal{X}}$ can be posed as multipartite Hamming distance matching problem by resolving correspondence between pairwise Hamming tuples of length 2. To this end, we construct set of nodes in each volume, where each node comprises of position of sampling point (i, j, k) and corresponding hash code. The problem now is to find a set of edges that minimizes the matching cost (total weights), which can be tackled by CO methods like assignment problem [4,5] in 2-D Hamming space.

2.3 Similarity Estimation Through Assignment Problem with Dimensionality Reduction

Motivated by [5], we assign costs c_{qv} to pairwise Hamming distances $S_{\mathcal{X}_{qv}}$, which represents the likelihood of matching sampling data in two volumes. The overall cost shall be minimized with respect to c_{qv} as follows:

$$\min \sum_q \sum_v c_{qv} S_{\mathbf{x}_{qv}} \text{ s.t. } \begin{cases} \sum_q c_{qv} = 1 \forall q \\ \sum_v c_{qv} = 1 \forall v \\ c_{qv} \in [0,1] \end{cases} \tag{2}$$

Table 1. The MAS results (Dice: mean $+/-$ Std) for all organs using mHF-Hun, mHF-LP, and NMI atlas selection techniques when $N = [1{:}10,\ 12,\ 14]$ atlases are used.

Organ / Method	ST	A-Ao	D-Ao	R-PA	Ve	R-At	L-At	RV
mHF-Hun	77.91±5.61	77.72±8.92	85.51±7.57	85.44±4.16	88.95±3.75	86.22±5.39	90.69±6.81	86.13±7.80
mHF-LP	**78.95±3.28**	**77.48±1.79**	85.64±1.69	85.29±1.80	**89.64±0.86**	**86.05±1.67**	90.52±1.23	**85.90±1.64**
NMI	77.94±4.08	76.85±2.89	**86.25±1.57**	**85.79±1.73**	88.41±2.24	85.73±2.10	**90.60±1.39**	85.64±2.18

Organ / Method	LV	Myo	L-PA	T-PA	Ao-R	Ao-A	S-VC	I-VC
mHF-Hun	78.94±6.11	84.06±8.27	79.53±10.30	82.23±6.17	65.82±14.38	61.57±9.66	73.82±7.10	60.95±12.06
mHF-LP	78.31±1.67	83.90±1.40	**80.49±2.46**	**82.54±1.64**	**66.14±2.27**	**67.32±2.70**	**75.25±2.76**	61.67±1.57
NMI	**78.53±1.94**	**84.07±1.81**	79.13±2.88	82.49±2.09	63.58±5.39	65.47±7.09	74.58±4.22	**62.30±2.23**

Given n_s^v and n_s^q sampling points, $(n_s^v \times n_s^q)!$ solutions exist, which makes computation of all cost coefficients infeasible as each volume is often represented by 3000 sampling points, on average. To overcome this limitation, we will solve the following LP problem that shares the same optimal solution [5]:

$$\widetilde{S}_{\mathcal{X}_{qv}} = \min \sum_q \sum_v c_{qv} \hat{S}_{\mathbf{x}_{qv}} \text{ where } \hat{S}_{\mathbf{x}_{qv}} = \begin{cases} S_{\mathbf{x}_{qv}} & \text{if } S_{\mathbf{x}_{qv}} \leq \eta \\ \infty & \text{if } S_{\mathbf{x}_{qv}} > \eta \end{cases} \tag{3}$$

where $\eta = \frac{1}{n_s^q} \sum_q S_{\mathbf{x}_{qv}}$. As a complementary analysis, we will solve the same problem using Hungarian algorithm and refer readers to [9] (Table 1).

3   Experiments and Results

We compare our method against an atlas selection technique (baseline) similar to [1]. The performance of each algorithm is evaluated by MAS with joint label fusion employing [15]. Like [12], in our quantification, we use the Dice Similarity Coefficient (DSC) between manual ground truths and automated segmentation results. We also justify the need for our proposed ranking technique in MAS against deep learning segmentation methods and deploy multi-label V-net [6].

3.1   Datasets

We collected 43 cardiac CTA volumes with labels for 16 anatomical structures including sternum(ST), ascending(A-Ao)/descending aorta(D-Ao), left(L-PA)/right (R-PA)/trunk pulmonary artery(T-PA), aorta/arch(Ao-A)/root(Ao-R), vertebrae(Ve), left(L-At)/right atrium(R-At), left(LV)/right ventricle(RV), lLV myocardium(Myo), and superior(S-VC)/inferior vena cava(I-VC). Each image has isotropic in-plane resolution of $1\,mm^2$. The slice thickness varies from $0.8\,mm$ to $2\,mm$. All images are intensity equalized to eliminate intensity variations among patients and then resampled to voxel size of $1.5\,mm$ in all dimensions.

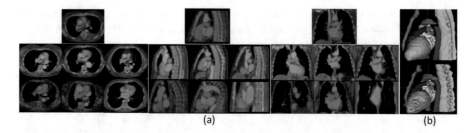

(a)   (b)

Fig. 3. The mHF-LP qualitative results. Query volume (top row) in axial, coronal, and sagittal views (from left to right) and corresponding retrieve volumes in corresponding views. The middle and bottom rows show the most similar and dissimilar cases (from left to right), respectively (a). The 3D visualization of segmentation results for the query volume (top) and corresponding manual ground truth (bottom) (b).

3.2   Validation Against Baseline

In this section, we validate the performance of the proposed hashing based atlas ranking selection strategies (mHF-LP, described in Sect. 2.3, and mHF-Hungarian (mHF-Hun)) on segmentation results against [1] where NMI is used as similarity metric for atlas selection and registration. We use $f_{s_{min}} = 50$ and resize each sampling voxel to 224×224 as an input to VGG network. We then extract $d = 4096$ features from FC7 layer for training the mHF. The forest comprises of 16 trees with depth of 4 to learn and generate 64 bits hashing codes.

We indicate that the NMI atlas selection method requires deformable registration whereas neither mHF-LP nor mHF-Hun does. Once atlases are ranked and selected using any approach, a global deformable registration is performed as part of MAS. We perform 43-fold leave-one-out cross validation and train models using all 16 labels (organs: $\iota = 1, \cdots, 16$). Figure 2(b) shows the average Dice values over all organs when N nearest atlases are selected using NMI, mHF-LP, and mHF-Hun algorithms. To speed up experiments, we introduced intervals while increasing N as the top similar cases weigh more in segmentation performance. As seen, the mHF-LP outperforms up to $N = 14$ where its performance equals the NMI (Dice = 80.66%). This is an optimal number of selected atlases where only 1.22% of performance is compromised in contrast to the case that we use all atlases ($N = 42$, Dice = 81.88%).

We performed an additional experiment by selecting atlases randomly and repeated the experiment five times. The averaged results are shown in Fig. 2 (cyan graph). This substantiates that the performance of our proposed techniques is solely depending on retrieval efficacy and not registration as part of MAS. Looking at qualitative results demonstrated in Fig. 3, we can justify the mHF-LP superior performance when a few atlases are selected ($N \leq 9$). As we can see, the top ranked atlases are the most similar ones to query and therefore they contribute to segmentation significantly. As we further retrieve and add more dissimilar atlases, the mHF-LP performance almost reaches a plateau.

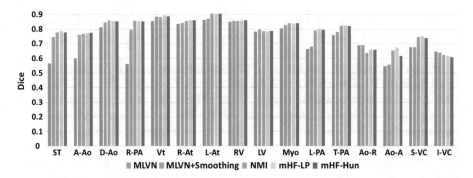

Fig. 4. The Dice segmentation results of all organs using MLVN with and without smoothing in contrast to MAS algorithm with proposed atlas selection techniques and NMI (baseline).

3.3 Validation Against Multi-label V-Net (MLVN)

We perform a comparative experiment to study the need for such atlas selection techniques as part of MAS process in contrast to CNN segmentation methods. We performed volumetric data augmentation through random non-rigid deformable registration during training. The ratio of augmented and non-augmented data was kept 1:1. Due to high memory requirements in 3D convolution, the input image is down-sampled to $2\,mm \times 2\,mm \times 3.5\,mm$, and a sub-image of size $128 \times 192 \times 64$ is cropped from the center of the original image and fed to the network. For segmentation, the output of the MLVN [6] is up-sampled to the original resolution padded into the original spatial space. We preserve the same network architecture as [6] and implemented the model in CAFFE.

Figure 4 demonstrates the results of MLVN segmentation with and without smoothing on 4-fold cross validation along with mHF-LP, mHF-Hun, and NMI. As expected, we obtained better results with smoothing. We performed the t-test and found significant difference between generated results by MLVN and the rest $(p > 0.05)$. The performance of MLVN is fairly comparable with the rest excluding the results for L-PA and Ao-A. Both are relatively small organs and may not be presented in all volumes, therefore, we could justify that the network has not seen enough examples during training despite augmentation.

3.4 Discussion Around Performance and Computational Speed

The MLVN is very fast at testing/deployment stage, particularly when performed on GPU. It takes less than $10\,s$ to segment a 3D volume on one TITAN X GPUs with $12\,GB$ of memory. However, The averaged segmentation performance $(\mathrm{Dice}_{\mathrm{MLVN+smoothing}} = 0.7663)$ was found to be smaller than the rest $(\mathrm{Dice}_{\mathrm{mHF\text{-}LP}} = 0.7969, \mathrm{Dice}_{\mathrm{mHF\text{-}Hun}} = 0.7909, \mathrm{Dice}_{\mathrm{NMI}} = 0.7921)$. The MAS generates more accurate results but at the cost of high computational burden due to the requirement for pairwise registrations and voxel-wise label fusion, of which the latter is not the focus of this work. We refer readers to [16] where the trade-off between computational cost and performance derived by registration has been thoroughly investigated.

We parallelized the pairwise registrations between atlases and deployed the MAS on Intel(R) Xeon(R) CPU E5-2620 v2 with frequency of 2.10 GHz. In the NMI based atlas selection technique, each deformable registration took about 55 s on $3\,mm^3$ resolution. In contrast, solving the LP problem took only 10 s. By looking at Fig. 2, using $N = 14$, where we achieve reasonbaly good segmentation performance (Dice $= 80.66\%$), we can save up to $14 \times 45 = 630$ s. The computational speed advantage of proposed method can be more appreciated in presence of large atlases especially when at least equal performance is achievable. Moreover, in the presence of limited data, we can achieve reasonably good segmentation performance using MAS algorithm with ranking, which seems very challenging for CNNs as they are greatly depending on availability of large amount of training data.

4   Conclusions

In this paper, for the first time, we proposed a hashing based atlas ranking and selection algorithm without the need for pairwise registration that is often required as a preprocessing step in existing MAS methods. We introduced the concept of *ensemble hashing* by extending mHF [3] for volumetric hashing and posed retrieval as an assignment problem that we solved through LP and Hungarian algorithm in Hamming space. The segmentation results were benchmarked against the NMI based atlas selection technique (baseline) and MLVN. We demonstrated that our retrieval solution in combination with MAS boosts up computational speed significantly without compromising the overall performance. Although the combination is still slower than CNN based segmentation at deployment stage it generates better results especially in presence of limited data. As future work, we will investigate the extension of the proposed technique for organ- or disease-specific MAS by confining the retrieval on local regions (organ level) rather global (whole volume level).

References

1. Aljabar, P., et al.: Multi-atlas based segmentation of brain images: atlas selection and its effect on accuracy. NeuroImage **46**(3), 726–738 (2009)
2. Artaechevarria, X., et al.: Combination strategies in multi-atlas image segmentation: application to brain MR data. IEEE Trans. Med. Imag. **28**(8), 1266–1277 (2009)
3. Conjeti, S., et al.: Metric hashing forests. Med. Image Anal. **34**, 13–29 (2016)
4. Jain, A.K., et al.: Matching and reconstruction of brachytherapy seeds using the Hungarian algorithm (MARSHAL). Med. Phys. **32**(11), 3475–3492 (2005)
5. Lee, J., et al.: Reduced dimensionality matching for prostate brachytherapy seed reconstruction. IEEE Tran. Med. Imaging **30**(1), 38–51 (2011)

6. Tang, H., et al.: Segmentation of anatomical structures in cardiac CTA using multi-label V-Net. In: Proceedings of the SPIE Medical Imaging (2018)
7. Jia, H., et al.: ABSORB: Atlas building by self-organized registration and bundling. NeuroImage **51**(3), 1057–1070 (2010)
8. Konukoglu, E., et al.: Neighbourhood approximation using randomized forests. Med. Image Anal. **17**(7), 790–804 (2013)
9. Kuhn, H.W., et al.: The Hungarian method for the assignment problem. Naval Res. Logist. Q. **2**, 83–97 (1955)
10. Lombaert, H., Zikic, D., Criminisi, A., Ayache, N.: Laplacian forests: semantic image segmentation by guided bagging. In: Golland, P., Hata, N., Barillot, C., Hornegger, J., Howe, R. (eds.) MICCAI 2014. LNCS, vol. 8674, pp. 496–504. Springer, Cham (2014). https://doi.org/10.1007/978-3-319-10470-6_62
11. Lotjonen, J.M.P., et al.: Fast and robust multi-atlas segmentation of brain magnetic resonance images. NeuroImage **99**, 2352–2365 (2010)
12. Sanroma, G.: Learning to rank atlases for multiple-atlas segmentation. IEEE Tran. Med. Imaging **33**(10), 1939–1953 (2014)
13. Schrijver, A., et al.: A Course in Combinational Optimization. TU Delft, Delft (2006)
14. Simonyan, K., et al.: Very deep convolutional networks for large-scale image recognition. arXiv:1409.1556 (2015)
15. Wang, H., et al.: Multi-atlas segmentation with joint label fusion. IEEE Tran. PAMI **35**(3), 611–623 (2013)
16. Wang, H., et al.: Fast anatomy segmentation by combining low resolution multi-atlas lebel fusion with high resolution corrective learning: an experimental study. In: Proceedings of the ISBI, pp. 223–226 (2017)
17. Wolz, R., et al.: LEAP: learning embeddings for atlas propagation. NeuroImage **49**(4), 1316–1325 (2010)

Corners Detection for Bioresorbable Vascular Scaffolds Segmentation in IVOCT Images

Linlin Yao[1,2], Yihui Cao[1,3], Qinhua Jin[4], Jing Jing[4], Yundai Chen[4(✉)], Jianan Li[1,3], and Rui Zhu[1,3]

[1] State Key Laboratory of Transient Optics and Photonics,
Xi'an Institute of Optics and Precision Mechanics, Chinese Academy of Sciences,
Xi'an, People's Republic of China
[2] University of Chinese Academy of Sciences, Beijing, People's Republic of China
[3] Shenzhen Vivolight Medical Device & Technology Co., Ltd.,
Shenzhen, People's Republic of China
[4] Department of Cardiology, Chinese PLA General Hospital,
Beijing, People's Republic of China
cyundai@vip.163.com

Abstract. Bioresorbable Vascular scaffold (BVS) is a promising type of stent in percutaneous coronary intervention. Struts apposition assessment is important to ensure the safety of implanted BVS. Currently, BVS struts apposition analysis in 2D IVOCT images still depends on manual delineation of struts, which is labor intensive and time consuming. Automatic struts segmentation is highly desired to simplify and speed up quantitative analysis. However, it is difficult to segment struts accurately based on the contour, due to the influence of fractures inside strut and blood artifacts around strut. In this paper, a novel framework of automatic struts segmentation based on four corners is introduced, in which prior knowledge is utilized that struts have obvious feature of box-shape. Firstly, a cascaded AdaBoost classifier based on enriched haar-like features is trained to detect struts corners. Then, segmentation result can be obtained based on the four detected corners of each strut. Tested on the same five pullbacks consisting of 480 images with strut, our novel method achieved an average Dice's coefficient of 0.85 for strut segmentation areas, which is increased by about 0.01 compared to the state-of-the-art. It concludes that our method can segment struts accurately and robustly and has better performance than the state-of-the-art. Furthermore, automatic struts malapposition analysis in clinical practice is feasible based on the segmentation results.

Keywords: Intravascular optical coherence tomography
Bioresorbable Vascular Scaffolds segmentation · Corners detection

© Springer Nature Switzerland AG 2018
A. F. Frangi et al. (Eds.): MICCAI 2018, LNCS 11073, pp. 552–560, 2018.
https://doi.org/10.1007/978-3-030-00937-3_63

1   Introduction

Nowadays, stenting after angioplasty has become one of the principal treatment options for coronary artery disease (CAD) [11]. Stents are tiny tube-like devices designed to support the vessel wall and are implanted in the coronary arteries by means of the percutaneous coronary intervention (PCI) procedure [12]. Among a series type of stents, Bioresorbable Vascular Scaffold (BVS) could offer temporary radial strength and be fully absorbed at a later stage [5]. However, malapposition which is defined as a separation of a stent strut from the vessel wall [6] may take place when BVS is implanted improperly and may potentially result in stent thrombosis. Therefore, it is crucial to analyze and evaluate BVS struts malapposition accurately.

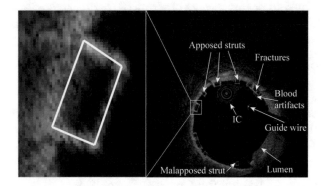

Fig. 1. An IVOCT image with immediately implanted BVS struts. One strut contour (white) can be segmented based on the four corners (green) labeled by expert.

Intravascular optical coherence tomography (IVOCT) is the most suitable imaging technique used for accurate BVS analysis due to its radial resolution of about $10\,\mu m$ [11]. An IVOCT image with immediately implanted BVS struts in the Cartesian coordinate system is shown in Fig. 1, in which apposed and malapposed BVS struts could be recognized obviously. However, the recognition is mainly conducted manually by experts. It is labor intensive and time consuming on account of large quantities of struts in IVOCT pullbacks. Thus, automatic analysis is highly desired.

Few articles about automatic BVS struts analysis has been published previously. Wang et al. proposed a method [11] of detecting the box-shape contour of strut based on gray and gradient features. It has limitation of poor generalization due to its a lot of empirical threshold setting. Lu et al. proposed a novel framework [13] of separating the whole work into two steps, which were machine learning based strut region of interest (ROI) detection and dynamic programming (DP) based strut contour segmentation. However, DP algorithm requires of searching all points in image to get the energy-minimizing active contour. On the energy-minimizing way, segmentation is sometimes influenced by fractures inside strut and blood artifacts around strut contour, which may cause inaccurate strut contour segmentation.

Stents are tiny tube-like devices designed manually and BVS struts have obvious feature of the box-shape in IVOCT image. As shown in the left part of Fig. 1, one strut can be represented by four corners in green color labeled by experts and strut contour represented by white rectangle can be segmented based on these four corners. Taking this prior knowledge into account, a novel corner based method of segmenting BVS struts using four corners is proposed in this paper, which transforms the problem of segmenting strut contour into detecting four corners of the strut. The advantage of this method is that it prevents the segmentation results from the influence of interference information, such as fractures inside strut and blood artifacts around strut contour, during the segmentation process. Specially, a cascaded AdaBoost classifier based on Haar-like features is trained to detect corners of struts. Experiment results illustrate that the corner detection method is accurate and contour segmentation is effective.

2   Method

The overview of this novel method is presented in Fig. 2. The segmentation method can be summarized as two main steps: (1) Training a classifier for corners detection; (2) Segmentation based on detected corners. Each step is described at length in the following subsections.

2.1   Training a Classifier for Corners Detection

A wide variety of detectors and descriptors have already been proposed in the literature [1, 4, 7–9]. Feature prototypes of simple haar-like, as described in proposed work [10], consist of edge, line and special diagonal line features and have been successfully applied to face detection. Haar-like features prove to be sensitive to corner structure. In our method, 11 feature prototypes of five kinds given in Fig. 2(b) are designed based on struts structure, consisting of two edge features, two line features, one diagonal line feature, four corner features and two T-junctions features. Those feature prototypes are combined to extract haar-like features which are capable of detecting corners effectively. However, the total number of haar-like features is very large associated with each image sliding window. High dimension of haar-like features need to be reduced. Due to the effective learning algorithm and strong bounds on generalization performance of AdaBoost [10], the classifier is trained using AdaBoost based on haar-like features.

During training, an image is transformed into polar coordinates shown as Fig. 2(a) based on lumen center. Samples are selected based on corners labeled by an expert, which are displayed as green points shown in Fig. 2(a). Bias about 1–3 pixels of labeling points is allowable, so the labeled corners is extended to its eight neighborhoods, which are shown as eight purple points around green center points. Positive samples are selected centered on each of the nine points

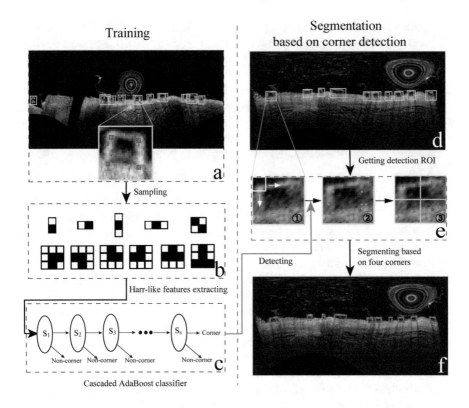

Fig. 2. The framework of our novel method of segmenting struts using four corners.

for one corner and negative samples are selected when those centers of sliding windows are not coincided with nine labeled points.

As shown in Fig. 2(c), s stages of strong classifiers are trained and cascaded to speed up the process of corners detection. The front stages of strong classifiers with simple structure are used to remove most sub-windows with obvious negative features. Then, strong classifiers with more complex structures are applied to remove false positives that are difficult to reject. Therefore, a cascaded AdaBoost classifier is constructed by gradually increasing complex strong classifiers at subsequent stages.

2.2 Segmentation Based on Detected Corners

As the right part of Fig. 2 presents, segmentation results are obtained based on four corners of each strut. This step consists of three main parts stated as follows.

(1) Image transformation and getting detection ROI. Cartesian IVOCT images are transformed into polar images using a previously developed method [2,3]. It can be seen that the shape of BVS struts in polar images are more

rectangular and approximately parallel to lumen since the lumen in polar coordinates is nearly horizontal. Detection ROI in polar images can be determined using the method in [13], which are represented as yellow rectangles in Fig. 2(d).

(2) Sliding on the ROI and getting candidate corners. As Fig. 2(e)① shows, a sliding window of size N is sliding on the ROI to detect corners and the step of sliding window is set as K. Each sliding window is classified utilizing the cascaded Adaboost classifier based on the selected haar-like features. Assuming that the cascaded classifiers have a total of s stages, the sum $\sum_{i=1}^{s} S_i$ can be seen as a score to measure how likely it is that an input sliding window's center can be a candidate corner, where S_i represents the score of $i_{th}, i = 1, 2, ...s$ stage. A sliding window's center is considered as a candidate corner when it passes through all s stages of cascaded classifier. The detection results are shown as orange points in Fig. 2(e)②, which are considered as candidate corners.

(3) Post-processing and segmentation. As shown in the Fig. 2(d), the upper and bottom sides of strut is approximately parallel to the lumen in polar coordinates. Considering the box-like shape of the strut, four corners to represent the strut should be located in four independent area. As shown in Fig. 2(e)③, the yellow rectangle of ROI is divided into four parts according to the center of the rectangle. Each candidate point has a score got from the cascaded AdaBoost classifier mentioned above. According to these scores, four points with top score of the four separated parts are chosen, which are considered as the four corners of the strut. As shown in Fig. 2(e)③, corners are displayed in red color.

After getting all four corners of struts in polar image shown as Fig. 2(f), the segmentation results are obtained by connecting these four corners in sequence, which are represented by rectangle in magenta color. Finally, the segmented contours are transformed back to Cartesian coordinate system as the final segmentation results.

3 Experiments

3.1 Materials and Parameter Settings

In our experiment, 15 pullbacks consisting of 3903 IVOCT images of baseline taken from 15 different patients were acquired using the FD-OCT system (C7-XR system, St. Jude, St. Paul, Minnesota). There were totally 1617 effective images containing struts. All BVS struts represented by four corners in effective images were manually labeled by an expert and the total number of struts was more than 4000. 10 pullbacks were used as training set which consisted of 1137 effective images and another 5 pullbacks of 480 effective images were used as test set.

During the experiment, all parameters mentioned above was set as follows: the size of sliding window was $N = 11$, which was near two-thirds of BVS strut's width (16 pixels) to ensure that there are only one corner in the sliding window. The sliding window step K was set as 3 pixels to ensure detected corners are in accurate positions. The stages of cascaded AdaBoost classifiers was $s = 23$ empirically, so that simple classifiers at early stages and complicated classifiers at late stages are both enough.

3.2 Evaluation Criteria

To quantitatively evaluate the performance of corners detection, the corner position error (CPE), defined as the distance between a detected corner and corresponding ground truth, is calculated as:

$$CPE = \sqrt{(x_D - x_G)^2 + (y_D - y_G)^2} \tag{1}$$

where (x_D, y_D) and (x_G, y_G) are the location of detected corner and corresponding ground truth, separately.

In order to assess the segmentation method quantitatively, Dice's coefficient was applied to measure the coincidence degree of the area between the ground truth and segmentation result. Dice's coefficient is defined as following in our experiment:

$$Dice = 2 \times \frac{\mid S_D \bigcap S_G \mid}{\mid S_D \mid + \mid S_G \mid} \tag{2}$$

where S_G and S_D represent the area of the ground truth and segmentation result, separately.

3.3 Results

To make a fair comparison between segmentation results of the proposed method and Lu et al. [13], both used the same data set. Specially, these two methods were tested on the same segmentation region, which was the detection rectangle described above. Qualitative and quantitatively evaluations were demonstrated based on the segmentation results.

Qualitative Results. The qualitative results demonstrated in Fig. 3 present some final segmentation results using the method of Lu et al. [13] in the first row and our proposed method in the second row. The green corners and white contour are the ground truth labeled by an expert. Red corners are the corners detection results and magenta contour refers to the segmentation result of our proposed method. Blood artifacts and fractures are indicated on the amplified white rectangle. The cyan contours are segmentation results using DP algorithm [13]. Figure $3a_2$–d_2 display some of segmentation results, as shown in the white rectangles, struts with special cases of fractures and blood artifacts, which fail to be segmented accurately using the DP method based on contour, whose segmentation results are displayed in Fig. $3a_1$–d_1, can be segmented well utilizing our proposed method. Qualitative results illustrate that our method has better performance and is more robust than the state-of-the-art.

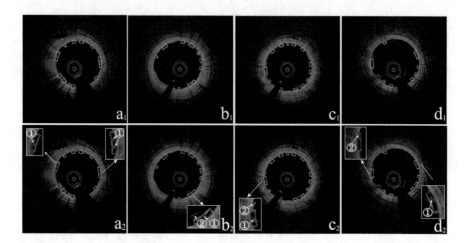

Fig. 3. The first row displays some segmentation results (cyan contour) using the method of Lu et al. The corresponding segmentation results of our proposed method (magenta contour) are shown in the second row. Contours of the ground truth labeled by an expert using corners are in white color. ① and ② in the a_2–d_2 represent fractures and blood artifacts respectively.

Quantitative Results. The quantitative statistic results are presented in Table 1. The 2th to 4th columns are the number of images, struts and corners evaluated in the 5 data sets respectively. It can be seen that the average corner position error (CPE) of 5 data sets in 5th column is $31.96 \pm 19.19\,\mu$m, namely about 3.20 ± 1.92 pixels, for immediately implanted struts. Considering the allowable bias of detected corners, this is reasonable. It proves that the detection method is accurate and effective. Average dice of Lu et al. and our proposed

Table 1. The quantitative evaluation results.

Data set	No.F	No.S	No.C	CPE (μm)	Dice	
					Lu et al.	Proposed
1	81	627	2508	28.83 ± 15.47	0.84	0.86
2	119	835	3340	30.25 ± 18.42	0.85	0.85
3	86	576	2304	32.76 ± 19.36	0.81	0.83
4	76	526	2104	30.37 ± 18.67	0.85	0.86
5	118	1077	4308	35.45 ± 22.12	0.83	0.83
Average	-	-	-	31.96 ± 19.19	0.84	0.85

No.F: Number of images evaluated; No.S: Number of struts evaluated; No.C: Number of corners evaluated; CPE: Corner position error between detected corners and ground truth; Dice: Dice's coefficient between ground truth and segmented contour.

work in 6*th* and 7*th* column of 5 data sets are 0.84 and 0.85 respectively. A rise of about 0.01 of average dice with our proposed method makes difference in clinical practice and this is difficult for small objection segmentation. It suggests that our proposed method is more accurate and robust compared to the DP method using by Lu et al. [13].

4   Conclusion

In this paper, we proposed a novel method of automatic BVS strut segmentation in 2D IVOCT image sequences. To our best knowledge, this was the first work that using the prior knowledge of struts' box-shape to segment strut contour based on four corners. Our presented work transforms the struts segmentation problem into corners detection, which avoids segmentation results from the influence of blood artifacts around strut contour and fractures inside strut. Specially, corners are detected using a cascaded AdaBoost classifier based on enriched haar-like features. Segmentation results are got based on the detected corners. Qualitative and quantitative evaluation results suggest that the corners detection method is accurate and our proposed segmentation method is more effective and robust than DP method. Automatic analysis of struts malapposition is feasible based on the segmentation results. Future work will mainly focus on further improving the current segmentation results by post-processing.

References

1. Bay, H., Ess, A., Tuytelaars, T., Van Gool, L.: Speeded-up robust features (SURF). Comput. Vis. Image Underst. **110**(3), 346–359 (2008)
2. Cao, Y., et al.: Automatic identification of side branch and main vascular measurements in intravascular optical coherence tomography images. In: 2017 IEEE 14th International Symposium on Biomedical Imaging (ISBI 2017), pp. 608–611. IEEE (2017)
3. Cao, Y., et al.: Automatic side branch ostium detection and main vascular segmentation in intravascular optical coherence tomography images. IEEE J. Biomed. Health Inf. **PP**(99) (2017). https://doi.org/10.1109/JBHI.2017.2771829
4. Dalal, N., Triggs, B.: Histograms of oriented gradients for human detection. In: IEEE Computer Society Conference on Computer Vision and Pattern Recognition, CVPR 2005, vol. 1, pp. 886–893. IEEE (2005)
5. Gogas, B.D., Farooq, V., Onuma, Y., Serruys, P.W.: The ABSORB bioresorbable vascular scaffold: an evolution or revolution in interventional cardiology. Hellenic J. Cardiol. **53**(4), 301–309 (2012)
6. Gonzalo, N., et al.: Optical coherence tomography patterns of stent restenosis. Am. Heart J. **158**(2), 284–293 (2009)
7. Lienhart, R., Maydt, J.: An extended set of Haar-like features for rapid object detection. In: Proceedings of 2002 International Conference on Image Processing, vol. 1, p. I. IEEE (2002)
8. Mikolajczyk, K., Schmid, C.: A performance evaluation of local descriptors. IEEE Trans. Pattern Anal. Mach. Intell. **27**(10), 1615–1630 (2005)

9. Ojala, T., Pietikäinen, M., Harwood, D.: A comparative study of texture measures with classification based on featured distributions. Pattern Recogn. **29**(1), 51–59 (1996)
10. Viola, P., Jones, M.J.: Robust real-time face detection. Int. J. Comput. Vis. **57**(2), 137–154 (2004)
11. Wang, A., et al.: Automatic detection of bioresorbable vascular scaffold struts in intravascular optical coherence tomography pullback runs. Biomed. Opt. Express **5**(10), 3589–3602 (2014)
12. Wang, Z., et al.: 3-D stent detection in intravascular OCT using a Bayesian network and graph search. IEEE Trans. Med. Imaging **34**(7), 1549–1561 (2015)
13. Yifeng, L., et al.: Adaboost-based detection and segmentation of bioresorbable vascular scaffolds struts in IVOCT images. In: 2017 IEEE International Conference on Image Processing (ICIP), pp. 4432–4436. IEEE (2017)

The Deep Poincaré Map: A Novel Approach for Left Ventricle Segmentation

Yuanhan Mo[1], Fangde Liu[1], Douglas McIlwraith[1], Guang Yang[2],
Jingqing Zhang[1], Taigang He[3], and Yike Guo[1(✉)]

[1] Data Science Institute, Imperial College London, London, UK
y.guo@imperial.ac.uk
[2] National Heart and Lung Institute, Imperial College London, London, UK
[3] St George's Hospital, University of London, London, UK

Abstract. Precise segmentation of the left ventricle (LV) within cardiac MRI images is a prerequisite for the quantitative measurement of heart function. However, this task is challenging due to the limited availability of labeled data and motion artifacts from cardiac imaging. In this work, we present an iterative segmentation algorithm for LV delineation. By coupling deep learning with a novel dynamic-based labeling scheme, we present a new methodology where a policy model is learned to guide an agent to travel over the image, tracing out a boundary of the ROI – using the magnitude difference of the Poincaré map as a stopping criterion. Our method is evaluated on two datasets, namely the Sunnybrook Cardiac Dataset (SCD) and data from the STACOM 2011 LV segmentation challenge. Our method outperforms the previous research over many metrics. In order to demonstrate the transferability of our method we present encouraging results over the STACOM 2011 data, when using a model trained on the SCD dataset.

1 Introduction

Automatic left ventricle (LV) segmentation from cardiac MRI images is a prerequisite to quantitatively measure cardiac output and perform functional analysis of the heart. However, this task is still challenging due to the requirement for relatively large manually delineated datasets when using statistical shape models or (multi-)atlas based methods. Moreover, as the heart and chest are constantly in motion the resulting images may contain motion artifacts with low signal to noise ratio. Such poor quality images can further complicate the subsequent LV segmentation.

Deep learning based methods have been proved effective for LV segmentation [1–3]. A detailed survey of the state-of-the-art lies outside the scope of this paper, but can be found elsewhere [4]. Such approaches are often based on, or extend image recognition research, and thus require large training datasets that are not always available for the cardiac MRI. To the best of our knowledge, there is very limited work using significant prior information to reduce the amount of training data required while maintaining a robust performance for LV segmentation.

© Springer Nature Switzerland AG 2018
A. F. Frangi et al. (Eds.): MICCAI 2018, LNCS 11073, pp. 561–568, 2018.
https://doi.org/10.1007/978-3-030-00937-3_64

In this paper, we propose a novel LV segmentation method called the Deep Poincaré Map (DPM). Our DPM method encapsulates prior information with a dynamical system employed for labeling. Deep learning is then used to learn a displacement policy for traversal around the region of interest (ROI). Given an image, a CNN-based policy model can navigate an agent over the cardiac MRI image, moving toward a path which outlines the LV. At each time step, a next step policy (a 2D displacement) is given by our trained policy model, taking into account the surrounding pixels in a local squared patch. In order to learn the displacement policy, the DPM requires a data transformation step which converts the labeled images into a customized dynamic capturing the prior information around the ROI. An important property of DPM is that no matter where the agent starts, it will finally travel around the ROI. This behavior is guaranteed by the existence of a limit cycle using our customized dynamic.

The main contributions of this work are as follows. (1) The DPM integrates prior information in the form of the context of the image surrounding the ROI. It does this by combining a dynamical system with a deep learning method for building a displacement policy model, and thus requires much less data that traditional deep learning methods. (2) The DPM is rotationally invariant. Because our next step policy predictor is trained with locally oriented patches, the orientation of the image with respect to the ROI is irrelevant. (3) The DPM is strongly transferable. Because the context of the segmentation boundary is considered, our method generalizes well to previously unseen images with the same or similar contexts.

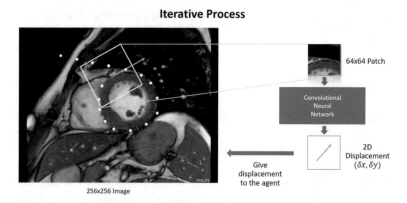

Iterative Process

Fig. 1. The red dot denotes the current position of the agent. In each time step, the DPM extracts a locally oriented patch from the original image. The extracted patch will be fed into a CNN to predict the next step displacement for the agent. After a finite number of iterations, a trajectory will be created by the agent. The magnitude of the Poincaré map is used to determine the final periodic orbit which is coincident with the boundary around the ROI.

2   Methodology

As shown in Fig. 1, the DPM uses a CNN-based policy model, trained on locally oriented patches from manually segmented data, to navigate an agent over a cardiac MRI image (256×256) using a locally oriented square patch (64×64) as its input. The agent creates a trajectory over the image tracing the boundary of the LV – no matter where the agent starts on the image. A crucial prerequisite of this methodology is the creation of a vector field whose limit cycle is equal to the boundary surrounding the ROI. This can be seen in Fig. 5b. In the following sections we will discuss the DPM methodology in detail, namely (1) the creation of a customized dynamic (i.e. a vector field) with a limit cycle around the ROI of the manually delineated images. (2) The creation of a patch-policy predictor. (3) The stopping criterion using the Poincaré map.

2.1   Generating a Customized Dynamic

A typical training dataset for segmentation consists of many image-to-label pairs. A label is a binary map that has the same resolution as its corresponding image. In each label, pixels of ground truth will be set to 1 while the background will be set to 0. Conversely, in our system, we firstly construct a customized dynamic (a vector field) for each labeled training instance. The constructed dynamic results in a unique limit cycle which is placed exactly on the boundary of the ROI.

To illustrate, let us consider an example indicated in Fig. 2. Consider a label of a training instance as a continuous 2D space $\mathbb{R}^2$ (a label with theoretical infinite resolution), we define the ground truth contour as a subspace $\Omega \subseteq \mathbb{R}^2$ as shown in step (a) in Fig. 2. To construct a dynamic in $\mathbb{R}^2$ where a limit cycle exists and is exactly the boundary $\partial\Omega$, we firstly introduce the distance function $S(p)$:

$$S(p) = \begin{cases} d(p, \partial\Omega) & \text{if } p \text{ is not on } \partial\Omega \\ 0 & \text{if } p \text{ is on } \partial\Omega \end{cases} \tag{1}$$

$d(p, \partial\Omega)$ denotes the infimum Euclidean distance from p to the boundary $\partial\Omega$. Equation 1 is used to create a scalar field from a binary image as shown in step (b) in Fig. 2. In order to build the customized dynamic, we need to create a vector field from this scalar field. A gradient operator is applied to create dynamic equivalent to the active contour [5] as shown in step (c) in Fig. 2. This gradient operator is expressed as Eq. 2.

$$\frac{dp}{dt} = \nabla_p S(p), \tag{2}$$

Our final step adds a limit cycle onto the system by gradually rotating the vectors according to the distance between each pixel and the boundary, as shown in Fig. 3b. The rotation function is given by $R(\theta)$,

$$R(\theta) = \begin{bmatrix} \cos\theta & -\sin\theta \\ \sin\theta & \cos\theta \end{bmatrix} \tag{3}$$

where θ is defined by Eq. 4.

$$\theta = \pi(1 - \mathbf{sigmoid}(S(p))) \tag{4}$$

Putting Eqs. 2 and 4 together, we obtain Eq. 5.

$$\frac{dp}{dt} = R(\theta)\nabla_p S(p), \tag{5}$$

Equation 5 has an important property: When $p \in \partial\Omega$, $S(p) = 0$ so that θ is equal to $\frac{\pi}{2}$ according to Eq. 3. This means on the boundary, the direction of $\frac{dp}{dt}$ is equal to the tangent of $p \in \partial\Omega$ as shown in step (d) in Fig. 2.

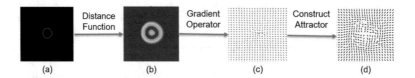

Fig. 2. Demonstrating customized dynamic creation from label data.

As opposed to active contour methods [5] where the dynamic is generated from images, we generate the discretized version of Eq. 5 for each label. Then, a vector field is generated from it for each training instance with the property that limit cycle of the field is the boundary of ROI. This process generates a set of tuples (image, label, dynamic). That is, for each cardiac image, we have its associated binary label image, and its corresponding vector field. In the next subsection, we introduce the methodology to learn a CNN which maps an image patch to a vector from our vector field (Fig. 3a). This allows us to create an agent which follows step-by-step displacement predictions.

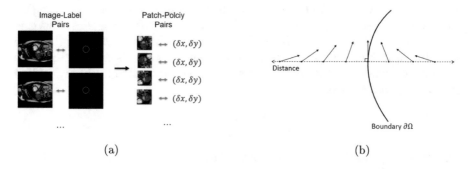

Fig. 3. (a) Transferring original dataset to patch-policy pairs. Patch-policy pairs are the training data for policy CNN. (b) The distance between a pixel and the boundary determines how much a vector will be rotated.

2.2   Creating a Patch-Policy Predictor Using a CNN

Training. Our CNN operates over patches which are oriented with respect to our created dynamic. In order to prepare data for training, for each training image, we randomly choose a pre-defined proportion of points acting as the center of a rectangular sampling patch. We define a sampling direction which is equal to the velocity vector of the associated point. For example, for a given position (x_0, y_0) on image, its velocity $(\delta x, \delta y)$ in the corresponding vector field is defined as the sampling direction, as shown in Fig. 4. In the training process, such vectors are easily accessible, however they must be predicted during inference (see next Subsect. 2.2). It is worth noting that a coordinate transformation is required to convert the velocity from the coordinate system of the dynamic to that of the patch, as illustrated in Fig. 4. In order to improve robustness, training data augmentation can be performed by adding symmetric offsets to the sampling directions (e.g. $(+45°, -45°)$). Our CNN is based on the AlexNet architecture [6] with two output neurons. During training we use Adam optimizer with the mean square error (MSE) loss.

Inference. At the inference stage, before the first time step $t = 0$, we determine an initial, rough, starting point using a basic LV detection module and a random sampling direction. This ensures that we don't start on an image boundary where there is insufficient input to create the first 64×64 pixel patch, and that we have an initial sampling direction. At each step, given an position p_t and a sampling direction s_t of the agent (which is unknown and is thus inferred as the difference between the current sampling direction and the last), a local patch is extracted and used as the input to the CNN-based policy model. The policy model then predicts the displacement for the agent to move, which in turn leads to the next local patch sample. This process iterates until the limit cycle is reached as illustrated earlier (Fig. 1).

2.3   Stopping Criterion: The Poincaré Map

Instead of identifying the periodic orbit (the limit cycle) from the trajectory itself, we introduce the Poincaré section [7] which is a hyperplane, Σ, transversal to the trajectory. This cuts through the trajectory of the vector field, as seen in Fig. 5a. The stability of a periodic orbit in the image can be reflected by the procession of corresponding points of intersection in Σ (a lower dimensional space). The Poincaré map is the function which maps successive intersection points with the previous point, and thus, when the mapping reaches a small enough value we may say that the procession of the agent in the image has converged to the boundary (the limit cycle). The convergence of customized dynamic has been studied using the Poincaré-Bendixson theorem [7], however the details are beyond the scope of this paper.

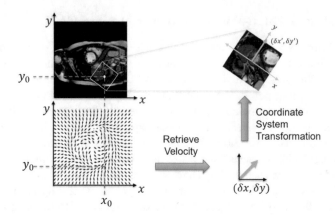

Fig. 4. A patch extracted from the original image with its corresponding velocity in a vector field. The sampling patch's orientation is determined by the corresponding velocity. The velocity should be transformed into the coordinate system of the patch to be used as ground truth in training.

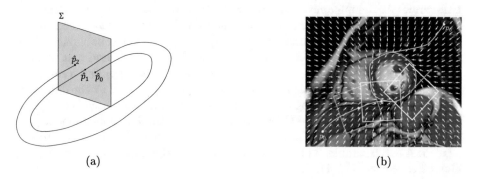

(a)   (b)

Fig. 5. (a) An agent in a 3D space starting at $\hat{p}_0$ intersects the hyperplane (the Poincaré section) Σ twice at $\hat{p}_1$ and $\hat{p}_2$. Performing analysis of the points on Σ is much simpler and more efficient than the analysis of the trajectory in 3D space. (b) An agent starts at initial point p_0 on a cardiac MRI image. After t iterations, the agent moves slowly toward the boundary of the object. Due to the underlying customized vector field, the DPM is able to guarantee that using different starting points we converge to the same unique periodic orbit (limit cycle).

3   Experimental Setting and Results

In this study, we evaluate our method on (1) the Sunnybrook Cardiac Dataset (SCD) [8], which contains 45 cases and (2) the STACOM 2011 LV Segmentation Challenge, which contains 100 cases.

SCD Dataset. The DPM was trained on the given training subset. We applied our trained model to the validation and online subsets (800 images from 30 cases in total) to provide a fair comparison with previous research, and we present our findings in Table 1. We report the dice score, average perpendicular distance (APD) (in millimeters) and 'good' contour rate (Good) for both the endocardium (i) and epicardium (o). We obtained a mean Dice score of 0.94 with a mean sensitivity of 0.95 and a mean specificity of 1.00.

Transferability to the STACOM2011 Dataset. To demonstrate the strong transferability of our method we train on the training subset of the SCD dataset and test on the STACOM 2011 dataset. We performed myocardium segmentation by segmenting the endocardium and epicardium separately, using 100 randomly selected MRI images from 100 cases. We report the Dice index, sensitivity, specificity, positive and negative predictive values (PPV and NPV) in Table 2. We obtained a mean Dice index of 0.74 with a mean sensitivity of 0.84 and a mean specificity of 0.99.

Table 1. Comparison of LV endocardium and epicardium segmentation performance between DPM and previous research using the Sunnybrook Cardiac Dataset. Number format: mean value (standard deviation).

Method	Dice(i)	Dice(o)	$APD(i)$	$APD(o)$	$Good(i)$	$Good(o)$
DPM	0.92 (0.02)	**0.95 (0.02)**	**1.75 (0.45)**	**1.78 (0.45)**	**97.5**	**97.7**
Av2016 [1]	**0.94 (0.02)**	-	1.81 (0.44)	-	96.69 (5.7)	-
Qs2014 [9]	0.90 (0.05)	0.94 (0.02)	1.76 (0.45)	1.80 (0.41)	92.70 (9.5)	95.40 (9.6)
Ngo2013 [10]	0.90 (0.03)	-	2.08 (0.40)	-	97.91 (6.2)	-
Hu2013 [11]	0.89 (0.03)	0.94 (0.02)	2.24 (0.40)	2.19 (0.49)	91.06 (9.4)	91.21 (8.5)

Table 2. Comparison of myocardium segmentation performance by training on SCD data and testing on the STACOM 2011 LVSC dataset. Number format: mean value (standard deviation).

Method	Dice	Sens.	Spec.	PPV	NPV
DPM	**0.74 (0.15)**	**0.84 (0.20)**	0.99 (0.01)	0.67 (0.21)	0.99 (0.01)
Jolly2012 [12]	0.66 (0.25)	0.62 (0.27)	0.99 (0.01)	**0.75 (0.23)**	0.99 (0.01)
Margeta2012 [13]	0.51 (0.25)	0.69 (0.31)	0.99 (0.01)	0.47 (0.21)	0.99 (0.01)

4 Conclusion

In this paper we have presented the Deep Poincaré Map as a novel method for LV segmentation and demonstrate its promising performance. The developed DPM method is robust for medical images, which have limited spatial resolution, low SNR and indistinct object boundaries. By encoding prior knowledge of a ROI as a customized dynamic, fine grained learning is achieved resulting in a displacement policy model for iterative segmentation. This approach requires much less training data than traditional methods. The strong transferability and rotational invariance of the DPM can be also attributed to this patch-based policy learning strategy. These two advantages are crucial for clinical applications.

Acknowledgement. Yuanhan Mo is sponsored by Sultan Bin Khalifa International Thalassemia Award. Guang Yang is supported by the British Heart Foundation Project Grant (PG/16/78/32402). Jingqing Zhang is supported by LexisNexis HPCC Systems Academic Program. Thanks to TensorLayer Community.

References

1. Avendi, M., Kheradvar, A., Jafarkhani, H.: A combined deep-learning and deformable-model approach to fully automatic segmentation of the left ventricle in cardiac MRI. Med. Image Anal. **30**, 108–119 (2016)
2. Tan, L.K., et al.: Convolutional neural network regression for short-axis left ventricle segmentation in cardiac cine MR sequences. Med. Image Anal. **39**, 78–86 (2017)
3. Ngo, T.A., Lu, Z., Carneiro, G.: Combining deep learning and level set for the automated segmentation of the left ventricle of the heart from cardiac cine magnetic resonance. Med. Image Anal. **35**, 159–171 (2017)
4. Xue, W., Brahm, G., Pandey, S., Leung, S., Li, S.: Full left ventricle quantification via deep multitask relationships learning. Med. Image Anal. **43**, 54–65 (2018)
5. Cootes, T.F., Edwards, G.J., Taylor, C.J.: Active appearance models
6. Krizhevsky, A., et al.: ImageNet classification with deep convolutional neural networks. In: Advances in Neural Information Processing Systems, pp. 1–9 (2012)
7. Parker, T.S., Chua, L.O.: Practical Numerical Algorithms for Chaotic Systems. Springer, New York (1989). https://doi.org/10.1007/978-1-4612-3486-9
8. Radau, P., Lu, Y., Connelly, K., Paul, G., Dick, A., Wright, G.: Evaluation framework for algorithms segmenting short axis cardiac MRI. MIDAS J. Card. MR Left Ventricle Segm. Chall. **49** (2009)
9. Queirós, S., et al.: Fast automatic myocardial segmentation in 4D cine CMR datasets. Med. Image Anal. **18**(7), 1115–1131 (2014)
10. Ngo, T.A., Carneiro, G.: Left ventricle segmentation from cardiac MRI combining level set methods with deep belief networks. In: 2013 20th IEEE International Conference on Image Processing (ICIP), pp. 695–699. IEEE (2013)
11. Hu, H., Liu, H., Gao, Z., Huang, L.: Hybrid segmentation of left ventricle in cardiac MRI using gaussian-mixture model and region restricted dynamic programming. Magn. Reson. Imaging **31**(4), 575–584 (2013)
12. Jolly, M.P., et al.: Automatic segmentation of the myocardium in cine MR images using deformable registration. In: Camara, O. (ed.) STACOM 2011. LNCS, vol. 7085, pp. 98–108. Springer, Heidelberg (2012). https://doi.org/10.1007/978-3-642-28326-0_10
13. Margeta, J., Geremia, E., Criminisi, A., Ayache, N.: Layered spatio-temporal forests for left ventricle segmentation from 4D cardiac MRI data. In: Camara, O. (ed.) STACOM 2011. LNCS, vol. 7085, pp. 109–119. Springer, Heidelberg (2012). https://doi.org/10.1007/978-3-642-28326-0_11

Bayesian VoxDRN: A Probabilistic Deep Voxelwise Dilated Residual Network for Whole Heart Segmentation from 3D MR Images

Zenglin Shi[1], Guodong Zeng[1], Le Zhang[2], Xiahai Zhuang[3], Lei Li[4],
Guang Yang[5], and Guoyan Zheng[1(✉)]

[1] Institute of Surgical Technology and Biomechanics, University of Bern,
Bern, Switzerland
guoyan.zheng@istb.unibe.ch
[2] Advanced Digital Sciences Center, Illinois at Singapore, Singapore, Singapore
[3] School of Data Science, Fudan University, Shanghai, China
[4] Department of Biomedical Engineering, Shanghai Jiao Tong University,
Shanghai, China
[5] National Heart and Lung Institute, Imperial College London, London, UK

Abstract. In this paper, we propose a probabilistic deep voxelwise dilated residual network, referred as *Bayesian VoxDRN*, to segment the whole heart from 3D MR images. Bayesian VoxDRN can predict voxelwise class labels with a measure of model uncertainty, which is achieved by a dropout-based Monte Carlo sampling during testing to generate a posterior distribution of the voxel class labels. Our method has three compelling advantages. First, the dropout mechanism encourages the model to learn a distribution of weights with better data-explanation ability and prevents over-fitting. Second, focal loss and Dice loss are well encapsulated into a complementary learning objective to segment both hard and easy classes. Third, an iterative switch training strategy is introduced to alternatively optimize a binary segmentation task and a multi-class segmentation task for a further accuracy improvement. Experiments on the MICCAI 2017 multi-modality whole heart segmentation challenge data corroborate the effectiveness of the proposed method.

1 Introduction

Whole heart segmentation from magnetic resonance (MR) imaging is a prerequisite for many clinical applications including disease diagnosis, surgical planning and computer assisted interventions. Manually delineating all the substructures (SS) of the whole heart from 3D MR images is labor-intensive, tedious and subject to intra- and inter-observer variations. This has motivated numerous research works on automated whole heart segmentation such as atlas-based approaches [1,2], deformable model-based approaches [3], patch-based approaches [2,4] and machine learning based approaches [5]. Although significant

© Springer Nature Switzerland AG 2018
A. F. Frangi et al. (Eds.): MICCAI 2018, LNCS 11073, pp. 569–577, 2018.
https://doi.org/10.1007/978-3-030-00937-3_65

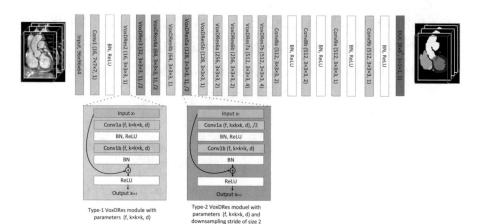

Fig. 1. The architecture of the proposed VoxDRN, consisting of BN layers, ReLU, and dilated convolutional layers N (ConvN) with parameters (**f**, **k** × **k** × **k**, **d**), where **f** is the number of channels, **k** × **k** × **k** is the filter size, and **d** is the dilation size. At the output, we use DUC layer to generate voxel-level prediction. We also illustrate two different types of VoxDRes modules: type-1 without stride downsampling and type-2 with downsampling stride of size 2.

progress has been achieved, automated whole heart segmentation remains to be a challenging task due to large anatomical variations among different subjects, ambiguous cardiac borders and similar or even identical intensity distributions between adjacent tissues or SS of the heart.

Recently, with the advance of deep convolutional neural network (CNN)-based techniques [6–10], many CNN-based approaches have been proposed as well for automated whole heart segmentation with superior performance [2,11]. These methods basically follow a fully convolutional downsample-upsample pathway and typically commit to a single prediction without estimating the model uncertainty. Moreover, different SS of the heart vary greatly in volume size, e.g., the left atrium blood cavity and the pulmonary artery often have smaller volume size than others. This can cause learning bias towards the majority class and poor generalization, i.e., the class-imbalance problem. To address such a concern, class-balanced loss functions have been proposed such as weighted cross entropy [2] and Dice loss [10].

This paper proposes a probabilistic deep voxelwise dilated residual network (VoxDRN), referred as *Bayesian VoxDRN*, which is able to predict voxelwise class labels with a measure of the model uncertainty. This involves following key innovations: (1) we extend the dilated residual network (DRN) of [12], previously limited to 2D image segmentation, to 3D volumetric segmentation; (2) inspired by the work of [13,14], we introduce novel architectures incorporating multiple dropout layers to estimate the model uncertainty, where units are randomly inactivated during training to avoid over-fitting. At testing, the posterior distribution of voxel labels is approximated by Monte Carlo sampling of multiple predictions with dropout; (3) we propose to combine focal loss with Dice loss, aiming for a complementary learning to address the class imbalance issue; and (4) we introduce an iterative switching training strategy to alternatively optimize a binary segmentation task and a multi-class segmentation task for a further accuracy improvement. We conduct ablation study to investigate the effectiveness of each proposed component in our method.

2   Methods

We first present our 3D extension to the 2D DRN of [12], referred as *VoxDRN*. Building on it, we then devise new architectures incorporating multiple dropout layers for model uncertainty estimation.

DRN. Dilated residual network [12] is a recently proposed method built on residual connections and dilated convolutions. The rationale behind DRN is to retain high spatial resolution and provide dense output to cover the input field such that back-propagation can learn to preserve detailed information about smaller and less salient objects. This is achieved by dilated convolutions which allow for exponential increase in the receptive field of the network without loss of spatial resolution. Building on the ResNet architecture of [6], Yu et al. [12] devised DRN architecture using dilated convolutions. Additional adaptations were used to eliminate gridding artifacts caused by dilated convolutions [12] via (a) removing max pooling operation from ResNet architecture; (b) adding 2 dilated residual blocks at the end of the network with progressively lower dilation; and (c) removing residual connections of the 2 newly added blocks. DRN works in a fully-convolutional manner to generate pixel-level prediction using bilinear interpolation of the output layer.

VoxDRN. We extend DRN to 3D by substituting 2D operators with 3D ones to create a deep voxelwise dilated residual network (VoxDRN) architecture as shown in Fig. 1. Our architecture consists of stacked voxelwise dilated residual (VoxDRes) modules. We introduce two different types of VoxDRes modules: type-1 without stride downsampling and type-2 with downsampling stride of size 2 as shown in Fig. 1. In each VoxDRes module, the input feature x_l and transformed feature $F_l(x_l, W_l)$ are added together with skip connection, and hence the information can be directly propagated to next layer in the forward and backward passes. There are three type-2 VoxDRes modules with downsampling stride of size 2, which reduce the resolution size of input volume by a factor of 8. We empirically find that such a resolution works well to preserve important information about smaller and less salient objects. The last VoxDRes module is followed by four convolutional layers with progressively reduced dilation to eliminate gridding artifacts. Batch normalization (BN) layers are inserted intermediately to accelerate the training process and improve the performance [15]. We use the rectified linear units (ReLU) as the activation function for non-linear transformation [16].

In order to achieve volumetric dense prediction, we need to recover full resolution at output. Conventional method such as bilinear upsampling [12] is

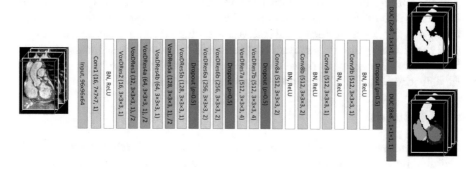

Fig. 2. The architecture of our Bayesian VoxDRN.

not attractive as the upsampling parameters are not learnable. Deconvolution could be an alternative but, unfortunately, it can easily lead to "uneven overlap", resulting in checkerboard artifacts. In this paper, we propose to use Dense Upsampling Convolution (DUC) of [17] to get the voxel-level prediction at the output where the final layer has Cr^3 channels, r being the upsampling rate and C being the number of classes. The DUC operation takes an input of shape $h \times w \times d \times Cr^3$ and remaps voxels from different channels into different spatial locations in the final output, producing a $rh \times rw \times rd \times C$ image, where h, w, and d denote height, width and depth. The mapping is done in 3D with $O(F)_{i,j,k,c} = F_{[i/r],[j/r],[k/r],r^3 \cdot c + \bmod (i,r) + r \cdot \bmod (j,r) + r^2 \cdot \bmod (k,r)}$ where F is the pre-mapped feature responses and O is the output image. DUC is equivalent to a learned interpolation that can capture and recover fine-detailed information with the advantages to avoid checkerboard artifacts of deconvolution.

Bayesian VoxDRN. Gal and Ghahramani [13] demonstrated that Bayesian CNN offered better robustness to over-fitting on small data than traditional approaches. Given our observed training data $\mathbf{X}$ and labels $\mathbf{Y}$, Bayesian CNN requires to find the posterior distribution $p(\mathbf{W}|\mathbf{X}, \mathbf{Y})$ over the convolutional weights, $\mathbf{W}$. In general, this posterior distribution is not tractable. Gal and Ghahramani [13] suggested to use variational dropout to tackle this problem for neural networks. Inspired by the work of [13,14], we devise a new architecture incorporating dropout layers as shown in Fig. 2, referred as *Bayesian VoxDRN*, to enable estimation of the model uncertainty, where subsets of units are inactivated with a dropout probability of 0.5 during training to avoid over-fitting. Applying dropout after each convolution layer may slow down the learning process. This is because the shallow layers of a CNN, which aims at extracting low-level features such as edges can be better modeled with deterministic weights [14]. We insert four dropout layers in the higher layers of VoxDRN to learn Bayesian weights on higher level features such as shape and contextual information. At testing, we sample the posterior distribution over the weights using dropout to obtain the posterior distribution of softmax class probabilities. The final segmentation is obtained by conducting majority voting on these samples. We use the variance to obtain model uncertainty for each class. In our experiments, following the suggestion in [13,14], we used 10 samples in majority voting to have a better accuracy and efficiency trade-off.

Hybrid Loss. We propose to combine weighted focal loss [18] with Dice loss [10] to solve class imbalance problem. The weighted focal loss is calculated as $L_{wFL} = \sum_{c\in C} -\alpha_c(1-p_c)^\lambda log(p_c)$, where $|X|$ and $|X_c|$ are the frequency of all classes and that of class c, respectively; $\alpha_c = 1 - \frac{|X_c|}{|X|}$ is designed to adaptively balance the importance of large and small SS of the heart; p_c is the probability of class c and $(1-p_c)^\lambda$ is the scaling factor to reduce the relative loss for well-classified examples such that we can put more focus on hard, misclassified examples. Focal loss often guides networks to preserve complex boundary details but could bring certain amount of noise, while Dice loss tends to generate smoother segmentation. Therefore, we propose to combine these two loss functions with equal weights for a complementary learning.

Iterative Switch Training. We propose a progressive learning strategy to train our Bayesian VoxDRN. The rationale and intuition behind such a strategy are that we would like to first separate foreground from background, and then further segment the foreground into a number of SS of the heart. By doing this, our network is alternatively trained to solve a simpler problem at each step than the original one. To achieve this, as shown in Fig. 2, the Bayesian VoxDRN is modified to have two branches after the last convolution layer: each branch, equipped with its own loss and operated only on images coming from the corresponding dataset, is responsible for estimating the segmentation map therein. During training, we alternatively optimize our network by using binary loss and multi-class loss supervised by binary labels and multi-class labels, respectively. Please note that at any moment of the training, only one branch is trained. More specifically, at each training epoch, we first train the binary branch to learn to separate the foreground from the background. We then train the multi-class branch to put the attention of our model to segment foreground into a few SS of the heart. While at testing, we are only interested in the output from the multi-class branch.

Implementation Details. The proposed method was implemented with Python using TensorFlow framework and trained on a workstation with a 3.6 GHz Intel i7 CPU and a GTX1080 Ti graphics card with 11 GB GPU memory. The network was trained using Adam optimizer with mini-batch size of 1. In total, we trained our network for 5'000 epochs. All weights were randomly initialized. We set initial momentum value to 0.9 and initial learning rate to 0.001. Randomly cropped $96 \times 96 \times 64$ sub-volumes serve as input to train our network. We adopted sliding window and overlap-tiling stitching strategies to generate predictions for the whole volume, and removed small isolated connected components in the final labeling results.

3   Experiments and Results

Data and Pre-processing. We conducted extensive experiments to evaluate our method on the 2017 MM-WHS challenge MR dataset [1,4][1]. There are in total 20 3D MR images for training and another 40 scans for testing. The training dataset contains annotations for seven SS of the heart including blood cavity for the left ventricle (LV), the right ventricle (RV), the left atrium (LA) and the right atrium (RA) as well as the myocardium of the LV (Myo), the ascending aorta (AA) and the pulmonary artery (PA). We resampled all the training data to isotropic resolution and normalized each image as zero mean and unit variance. Data augmentation was used to enlarge the training samples by rotating each image with a random angle in the range of $[-30°, 30°]$ around z axis.

Comparison with Other Methods. The quantitative comparison between our method and other approaches from the participating teams is shown in Table 1. According to the rules of the challenge, methods were ranked based on Dice score on the whole heart segmentation, not on each individual substructure. Although most of the methods are based on CNNs, Heinrich et al. [2] achieved impressive results using discrete nonlinear registration and fast non-local fusion.

Table 1. Comparison (Dice score) with different approaches on MM-WHS 2017 MR dataset. The best result for each category is highlighted with bold font.

Methods	LV	Myo	RV	LA	RA	AA	PA	Whole heart
Our method	0.914	**0.811**	**0.880**	0.856	0.873	0.857	0.794	**0.871**
Heinrich et al. [2]	**0.918**	0.781	0.871	**0.886**	0.873	**0.878**	**0.804**	0.870
Payer et al. [2]	0.916	0.778	0.868	0.855	**0.881**	0.838	0.731	0.863
Mortazi et al. [2]	0.871	0.747	0.830	0.811	0.759	0.839	0.715	0.818
Galisot et al. [2]	0.897	0.763	0.819	0.765	0.808	0.708	0.685	0.817
Yang et al. [2]	0.836	0.721	0.805	0.742	0.832	0.821	0.697	0.797
Wang et al. [2]	0.855	0.728	0.760	0.832	0.782	0.771	0.578	0.792
Yu et al. [2]	0.750	0.658	0.750	0.826	0.859	0.809	0.726	0.783
Liao et al. [2]	0.702	0.623	0.680	0.676	0.654	0.599	0.470	0.670

Table 2. Ablation study results [x 100%].

Methods	Dice		Jaccard		Specificity		Recall	
	WH	SS	WH	SS	WH	SS	WH	SS
HighRes3DNet [19]	88.17 ± 0.25	80.42 ± 0.29	79.21 ± 0.63	68.85 ± 0.48	93.96 ± 0.02	87.54 ± 0.20	83.37 ± 0.65	76.63 ± 0.58
3D U-net [9]	88.33 ± 0.35	81.67 ± 0.36	79.59 ± 0.84	70.91 ± 0.62	94.17 ± 0.02	89.04 ± 0.12	83.79 ± 0.91	78.16 ± 0.78
Bayesian VoxDRN+Dice	89.38 ± 0.09	82.58 ± 0.30	80.94 ± 0.25	71.25 ± 0.61	92.97 ± 0.06	85.84 ± 0.30	87.18 ± 0.42	81.13 ± 0.45
Bayesian VoxDRN+Hybrid	90.15 ± 0.10	83.12 ± 0.26	82.23 ± 0.29	72.27 ± 0.49	91.81 ± 0.08	85.53 ± 0.21	88.91 ± 0.43	82.92 ± 0.34
Our method	90.83 ± 0.06	84.39 ± 0.19	83.30 ± 0.19	73.75 ± 0.42	91.99 ± 0.06	85.62 ± 0.17	89.93 ± 0.28	89.93 ± 0.28

---

[1] One can find details about the MICCAI 2017 MM-WHS challenge at: http://www.sdspeople.fudan.edu.cn/zhuangxiahai/0/mmwhs/.

The other non-CNN approach was introduced by Galisot et al. [2], which was based on local probabilistic atlases and a posterior correction.

Ablation Analysis. In order to evaluate the effectiveness of different components in the proposed method, we performed a set of ablation experiments. Because the ground truth of the testing dataset is held out by the organizers and the challenge organizers only allow resubmission of substantially different methods, we conducted experiments via a standard 2-fold cross-validation study on the training dataset. We also implemented two other state-of-the-art 3D CNN approaches, 3D U-net [9] and HighRes3DNet [19], for comparison. We compared these two methods with following variants of the proposed method: (1) Bayesian VoxDRN trained with Dice loss (Bayesian VoxDRN+Dice); (2) Bayesian Vox-DRN trained with our hybrid loss but without using the iterative switch training strategy (Bayesian VoxDRN+Hybrid); and (3) Bayesian VoxDRN trained with our hybrid loss using the iterative switch training strategy (Our method). We evaluated these methods using Dice, Jaccard, specificity and recall for the whole heart (WH) segmentation as well as for segmentation of all SS. The quantitative comparison can be found in Table 2. As observed, our method and its variants achieved better performance than the other two methods under limited training data. Moreover, each component in our method helped to improve the performance. Qualitative results are shown in Fig. 3, where we (A) visually compared the results obtained by different methods; (B) visualized the uncertainty map; and (C) depicted the relationship between the segmentation accuracy and the uncertainty threshold. From Fig. 3(B), one can see that the model is uncertain at object boundaries and with difficult and ambiguous SS.

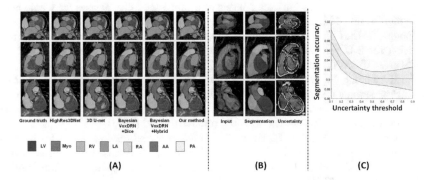

Fig. 3. Qualitative results. (A) qualitative comparison of different methods. Red circles highlight the major differences among various methods; (B) visualization of uncertainty, where the brighter the color, the higher the uncertainty; and (C) the relationship between the segmentation accuracy and the uncertainty threshold. The shaded area represents the standard errors.

4   Conclusion

In this study, we proposed the Bayesian VoxDRN, a probabilistic deep voxelwise dilated residual network with a measure of the model uncertainty, for automatic whole heart segmentation from 3D MR images. The proposed Bayesian Vox-DRN models uncertainty by incorporating variational dropouts for an approximated Bayesian inference. In addition, it works well in imbalanced dataset by using both focal loss and Dice loss. Finally, a further improvement on performance is achieved by employing an iterative switch training strategy to train the Bayesian VoxDRN. Comprehensive experiments on an open challenge dataset demonstrated the efficacy of our method in dealing with whole heart segmentation under limited training data. Our network architecture shows promising generalization and can be potentially extended to other applications.

Acknowlegement. The project is partially supported by the Swiss National Science Foundation Project 205321_169239.

References

1. Zhuang, X., Rhode, K., et al.: A registration-based propagation framework for automatic whole heart segmentation of cardiac MRI. IEEE Trans. Med. Imaging **29**, 1612–1625 (2010)
2. Pop, M., et al. (eds.): STACOM 2017. LNCS, vol. 10663. Springer, Cham (2018). https://doi.org/10.1007/978-3-319-75541-0
3. Peters, J., et al.: Optimizing boundary detection via simulated search with applications to multi-modal heart segmentation. Med. Image Anal. **14**, 70–84 (2009)
4. Zhuang, X., Shen, J.: Multi-scale patch and multi-modality atlases for whole heart segmentation of MRI. Med. Image Anal. **31**, 77–87 (2016)
5. Zheng, Y., Barbu, A., et al.: Four-chamber heart modeling and automatic segmentation for 3-D cardiac CT volumes using marginal space learning and steerable features. IEEE Trans. Med. Imaging **27**(11), 1668–1681 (2008)
6. He, K., Zhang, X., Ren, S., Sun, J.: Deep residual learning for image recognition. In: Proceedings CVPR, pp. 770–778 (2016)
7. Long, J., Shelhamer, E., Darrell, T.: Fully convolutional networks for semantic segmentation. In: Proceedings CVPR, pp. 3431–3440 (2015)
8. Ronneberger, O., Fischer, P., Brox, T.: U-Net: convolutional networks for biomedical image segmentation. In: Navab, N., Hornegger, J., Wells, W.M., Frangi, A.F. (eds.) MICCAI 2015. LNCS, vol. 9351, pp. 234–241. Springer, Cham (2015). https://doi.org/10.1007/978-3-319-24574-4_28
9. Çiçek, Ö., et al.: 3D U-Net: learning dense volumetric segmentation from sparse annotation. In: Ourselin, S., et al. (eds.) MICCAI 2016. LNCS, vol. 9901, pp. 424–432. Springer, Cham (2016). https://doi.org/10.1007/978-3-319-46723-8_49
10. Milletari, F., Navab, M., Ahmadi, S.A.: V-net: fully convolutional neural networks for volumetric medical image segmentation. arXiv:1606.04797 (2016)
11. Yu, L., et al.: Automatic 3D cardiovascular MR segmentation with densely-connected volumetric ConvNets. In: Descoteaux, M., et al. (eds.) MICCAI 2017. LNCS, vol. 10434, pp. 287–295. Springer, Cham (2017). https://doi.org/10.1007/978-3-319-66185-8_33

12. Yu, F., Koltun, V., Funkhouser, T.: Dilated residual networks. In: Proceedings CVPR, pp. 636–644 (2017)
13. Gal, Y., Ghahramani, Z.: Bayesian convolutional neural networks with bernoulli approximate variational inference. arXiv:1506.02158 (2015)
14. Kendall, A., Badrinarayanan, V., Cipolla, R.: Bayesian segnet: model uncertainty in deep convolutional encoder-decoder architectures for scene understanding. arXiv:1511.02680 (2016)
15. Ioffe, S., Szegedy, C.: Batch normalization: accelerating deep network training by reducing internal covariate shift. In: Proceedings ICML, pp. 448–456 (2015)
16. Krizhevsky, A., Ilya, S., Hinton, G.: Imagenet classification with deep convolutional neural networks. In: Proceedings of the NIPS, pp. 1097–1105 (2012)
17. Wang, P., Chen, P., et al.: Understanding convolution for semantic segmentation. arXiv:1702.08502 (2017)
18. Lin, T.Y., et al.: Focal loss for dense object detection. In: Proceedings ICCV (2017)
19. Li, W., et al.: On the compactness, efficiency, and representation of 3D convolutional networks: brain parcellation as a pretext task. In: Niethammer, M., et al. (eds.) IPMI 2017. LNCS, vol. 10265, pp. 348–360. Springer, Cham (2017). https://doi.org/10.1007/978-3-319-59050-9_28

Real-Time Prediction of Segmentation Quality

Robert Robinson[1]([✉]), Ozan Oktay[1], Wenjia Bai[1], Vanya V. Valindria[1],
Mihir M. Sanghvi[3,4], Nay Aung[3,4], José M. Paiva[3], Filip Zemrak[3,4],
Kenneth Fung[3,4], Elena Lukaschuk[5], Aaron M. Lee[3,4], Valentina Carapella[5],
Young Jin Kim[5,6], Bernhard Kainz[1], Stefan K. Piechnik[5], Stefan Neubauer[5],
Steffen E. Petersen[3,4], Chris Page[2], Daniel Rueckert[1], and Ben Glocker[1]

[1] BioMedIA Group, Department of Computing, Imperial College London,
London, UK
r.robinson16@imperial.ac.uk
[2] Research & Development, GlaxoSmithKline, Brentford, UK
[3] NIHR Barts Biomedical Research Centre, Queen Mary University London,
London, UK
[4] Barts Heart Centre, Barts Health NHS Trust, London, UK
[5] Radcliffe Department of Medicine, University of Oxford, Oxford, UK
[6] Severance Hospital, Yonsei University College of Medicine, Seoul, South Korea

Abstract. Recent advances in deep learning based image segmentation
methods have enabled real-time performance with human-level accuracy.
However, occasionally even the best method fails due to low image quality, artifacts or unexpected behaviour of black box algorithms. Being
able to predict segmentation quality in the absence of ground truth is of
paramount importance in clinical practice, but also in large-scale studies
to avoid the inclusion of invalid data in subsequent analysis.

In this work, we propose two approaches of real-time automated quality control for cardiovascular MR segmentations using deep learning.
First, we train a neural network on 12,880 samples to predict Dice Similarity Coefficients (DSC) on a per-case basis. We report a mean average
error (MAE) of 0.03 on 1,610 test samples and 97% binary classification
accuracy for separating low and high quality segmentations. Secondly,
in the scenario where no manually annotated data is available, we train
a network to predict DSC scores from estimated quality obtained via a
reverse testing strategy. We report an MAE = 0.14 and 91% binary classification accuracy for this case. Predictions are obtained in real-time
which, when combined with real-time segmentation methods, enables
instant feedback on whether an acquired scan is analysable while the
patient is still in the scanner. This further enables new applications of
optimising image acquisition towards best possible analysis results.

1 Introduction

Finding out that an acquired medical image is not usable for the intended purpose is not only costly but can be critical if image-derived quantitative measures

© Springer Nature Switzerland AG 2018
A. F. Frangi et al. (Eds.): MICCAI 2018, LNCS 11073, pp. 578–585, 2018.
https://doi.org/10.1007/978-3-030-00937-3_66

should have supported clinical decisions in diagnosis and treatment. Real-time assessment of the downstream analysis task, such as image segmentation, is highly desired. Ideally, such an assessment could be performed while the patient is still in the scanner, so that in the case an image is not analysable, a new scan could be obtained immediately (even automatically). Such a real-time assessment requires two components, a real-time analysis method and a real-time prediction of the quality of the analysis result. This paper proposes a solution to the latter with a particular focus on image segmentation as the analysis task.

Recent advances in deep learning based image segmentation have brought highly efficient and accurate methods, most of which are based on Convolutional Neural Networks (CNNs). However, even the best method will occasionally fail due to insufficient image quality (e,g., noise, artefacts, corruption) or show unexpected behaviour on new data. In clinical settings, it is of paramount importance to be able to detect such failure cases on a per-case basis. In clinical research, such as population studies, it is important to be able to detect failure cases in automated pipelines, so invalid data can be discarded in the subsequent statistical analysis.

Here, we focus on automatic quality control of image segmentation. Specifically, we assess the quality of automatically generated segmentations of cardiovascular MR (CMR) from the UK Biobank (UKBB) Imaging Study [1].

Automated quality control is dominated by research in the natural-image domain and is often referred to as image quality assessment (IQA). The literature proposes methodologies to quantify the technical characteristics of an image, such as the amount of blur, and more recently a way to assess the aesthetic quality of such images [2]. In the medical image domain, IQA is an important topic of research in the fields of image acquisition and reconstruction. An example is the work by Farzi et al. [3] proposing an unsupervised approach to detect artefacts. Where research is conducted into the quality or accuracy of image segmentations, it is almost entirely assumed that there is a manually annotated ground truth (GT) labelmap available for comparison. Our domain has seen little work on assessing the quality of generated segmentations particularly on a per-case basis and in the absence of GT.

Related Work: Some previous studies have attempted to deliver quality estimates of automatically generated segmentations when GT is unavailable. Most methods tend to rely on a reverse-testing strategy. Both Reverse Validation [4] and Reverse Testing [5] employ a form of cross-validation by training segmentation models on a dataset that are then evaluated either on a different fold of the data or a separate test-set. Both of these methods require a fully-labeled set of data for use in training. Additionally, these methods are limited to conclusions about the quality of the segmentation algorithms rather than the individual labelmaps as the same data is used for training and testing purposes.

Where work has been done in assessing individual segmentations, it often also requires large sets of labeled training data. In [6] a model was trained using numerous statistical and energy measures from segmentation algorithms. Although this model is able to give individual predictions of accuracy for a given

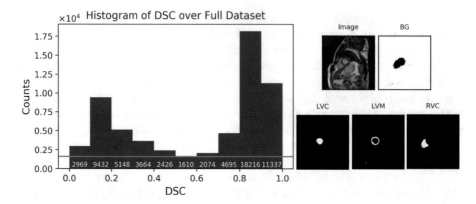

Fig. 1. (left) Histogram of Dice Similarity Coefficients (DSC) for 29,292 segmentations. Range is $[0, 1]$ with 10 equally spaced bins. Red line shows minimum counts (1,610) at DSC in the bin $[0.5, 0.6]$ used to balance scores. (right) 5 channels of the CNNs in both experiments: the image and one-hot-encoded labelmaps for background (BG), left-ventricular cavity (LV), left-ventricular myocardium (LVM) and right-ventricular cavity (RVC).

segmentation, it again requires the use of a fully-annotated dataset. Moving away from this limitation, [7,8] have shown that applying Reverse Classification Accuracy (RCA) gives accurate predictions of traditional quality metrics on a per-case basis. They accomplish this by comparing a set of reference images with manual segmentations to the test-segmentation, evaluating a quality metric between these, and then taking the best value as a prediction for segmentation quality. This is done using a set of only 100 reference images with verified labelmaps. However, the time taken to complete RCA on a single segmentation is prohibits real-time quality control frameworks: around 11 min.

Contributions: In this study, we show that applying a modern deep learning approach to the problem of automated quality control in deployed image-segmentation frameworks can decrease the per-case analysis time to the order of milliseconds whilst maintaining good accuracy. We predict Dice Similarity Coefficient (DSC) at large-scale analyzing over 16,000 segmentations of images from the UKBB. We also show that measures derived from RCA can be used to inform our network removing the need for a large, manually-annotated dataset. When pairing our proposed real-time quality assessment with real-time segmentation methods, one can envision new avenues of optimising image acquisition automatically toward best possible analysis results.

2   Method and Material

We use the Dice Similarity Coefficient (DSC) as a metric of quality for segmentations. It measures the overlap between a proposed segmentation and its ground truth (GT) (usually a manual reference). We aim to predict DSC for segmentations in the *absence* of GT. We perform two experiments in which CNNs are trained to predict DSC. First we describe our input data and the models.

Our initial dataset consists of 4,882 3D (2D-stacks) end-diastolic (ED) cardiovascular magnetic resonance (CMR) scans from the UK Biobank (UKBB) Imaging Study[1]. All images have a manual segmentation which is unprecedented at this scale. We take these labelmaps as reference GT. Each labelmap contains 3 classes: left-ventricular cavity (LVC), left-ventricular myocardium (LVM) and right-ventricular cavity (RVC) which are separate from the background class (BG). In this work, we also consider the segmentation as a single binary entity comprising all classes: whole-heart (WH).

A random forest (RF) of 350 trees and maximum Depth 40 is trained on 100 cardiac atlases from an in-house database and used to segment the 4,882 images at depths of 2, 4, 6, 8, 10, 15, 20, 24, 36 and 40. We calculate DSC from the GT for the 29,292 generated segmentations. The distribution is shown in Fig. 1. Due to the imbalance in DSC scores of this data, we choose to take a random subset of 1,610 segmentations from each DSC bin, equal to the minimum number of counts-per-bin across the distribution. Our final dataset comprises 16,100 score-balanced segmentations with reference GT.

From each segmentation we create 4 one-hot-encoded masks: masks 1 to 4 correspond to the classes BG, LVC, LVM and RVC respectively. The voxels of the ith mask are set at $[0, 0, 0, 0]$ when they do not belong to the mask's class and the ith element set to 1 otherwise. For example, the mask for LVC is $[0, 0, 0, 0]$ everywhere except for voxels of the LVC class which are given the value $[0, 1, 0, 0]$. This gives the network a greater chance to learn the relationships between the voxels' classes and their locations. An example of the segmentation masks is shown in Fig. 1.

At training time, our data-generator re-samples the UKBB images and our segmentations to have consistent shape of $[224, 224, 8, 5]$ making our network fully 3D with 5 data channels: the image and 4 segmentation masks. The images are also normalized such that the entire dataset falls in the range $[0.0, 1.0]$.

For comparison and consistency, we choose to use the same input data and network architecture for each of our experiments. We employ a 50-layer 3D residual network written in Python with the Keras library and trained on an 11 GB Nvidia GeForce GTX 1080 Ti GPU. Residual networks are advantageous as they allow the training of deeper networks by repeating smaller blocks. They benefit from skip connections that allow data to travel deeper into the network. We use the Adam optimizer with learning rate of $1e^{-5}$ and decay of 0.005. Batch sizes are kept constant at 46 samples per batch. We run validation at the end of each epoch for model-selection purposes.

Experiments

Can we take advantage of a CNN's inference speed to give fast and accurate predictions of segmentation quality? This is an important question for analysis

---

[1] UK Biobank Resource under Application Number 2964.

pipelines which could benefit from the increased confidence in segmentation quality without compromising processing time. To answer this question we conduct the following experiments.

Experiment 1: Directly Predicting DSC. Is it possible to directly predict the quality of a segmentation given only the image-segmentation pair? In this experiment we calculate, per class, the DSC between our segmentations and the GT. These are used as training labels. We have 5 nodes in the final layer of the network where the output X is $\{X \in \mathbb{R}^5 \mid X \in [0.0, 1.0]\}$. This vector represents the DSC per class including background and whole-heart. We use mean-squared-error loss and report mean-absolute-error between the output and GT DSC. We split our data 80:10:10 giving 12,880 training samples and 1,610 samples each for validation and testing. Performing this experiment is costly as it requires a large manually-labeled dataset which is not readily available in practice.

Experiment 2: Predicting RCA Scores. Considering the promising results of the RCA framework [7,8] in accurately predicting the quality of segmentations in the absence of large labeled datasets, can we use the predictions from RCA as training data to allow a network to give comparatively accurate predictions on a test-set? In this experiment, we perform RCA on all 16,100 segmentations. To ensure that we train on balanced scores, we again perform histogram binning on the RCA scores and take equal numbers from each class. We finish with a total of 5363 samples split into training, validation and test sets of 4787, 228 and 228 respectively. The predictions per-class are used as labels during training. Similar to Experiment 1, we obtain a single predicted DSC output for each class using the same network and hyper-parameters, but without the need for the large, often-unobtainable manually-labeled training set.

3 Results

Results from Experiment 1 are shown in Table 1. We report mean absolute error (MAE) and standard deviations per class between reference GT and predicted DSC. Our results show that our network can directly predict whole-heart DSC from the image-segmentation pair with MAE of 0.03 (SD = 0.04). We see similar performance on individual classes. Table 1 also shows MAE over the top and bottom halves of the GT DSC range. This suggests that the MAE is equally distributed over poor and good quality segmentations. For WH we report 72% of the data have MAE less than 0.05 with outliers (DSC ≥ 0.12) comprising only 6% of the data. Distributions of the MAEs for each class can be seen in Fig. 3. Examples of good and poor quality segmentations are shown in Fig. 2 with their GT and predictions. Results show excellent true (TPR) and false-positive rates (FPR) on a whole-heart binary classification task with DSC threshold of 0.70. The reported accuracy of 97% is better than the 95% reported with RCA in [8].

Our results for Experiment 2 are recorded in Table 1. It is expected that direct predictions of DSC from the RCA labels are less accurate than in Experiment 1.

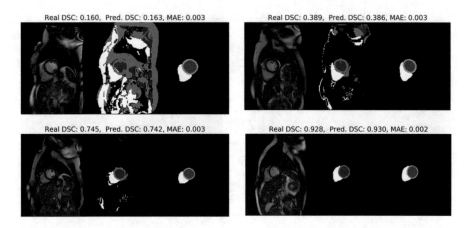

Fig. 2. Examples showing excellent prediction of Dice Similarity Coefficient (DSC) in Experiment 1. Quality increases from top-left to bottom-right. Each panel shows (left to right) the image, test-segmentation and reference GT.

The reasoning is two-fold: first, the RCA labels are themselves *predictions* and retain inherent uncertainty and second, the training set here is much smaller than in Experiment 1. However, we report MAE of 0.14 (SD $= 0.09$) for the WH case and 91% accuracy on the binary classification task. Distributions of the MAEs are shown in Fig. 3. LVM has a greater variance in MAE which is in line with previous results using RCA [8]. Thus, the network would be a valuable addition

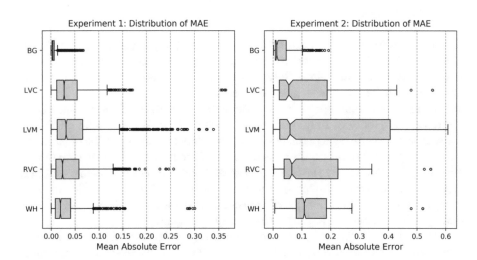

Fig. 3. Distribution of the mean absolute errors (MAE) for Experiments 1 (left) and 2 (right). Results are shown for each class: background (BG), left-ventricular cavity (LV), left-ventricular myocardium (LVM), right-ventricular cavity (RVC) and for the whole-heart (WH).

Table 1. For Experiments 1 and 2, Mean absolute error (MAE) for poor (DSC < 0.5) and good (DSC ≥ 0.5) quality segmentations over individual classes and whole-heart (WH). Standard deviations in brackets. (right) Statistics from binary classification (threshold DSC = 0.7 [8]): True (TRP) and false-positive (FPR) rates over full DSC range with classification accuracy (Acc).

Class	Mean Absolute Error (MAE)					
	Experiment 1			Experiment 2		
	$0 \leq \text{DSC} \leq 1$ $n = 1,610$	DSC < 0.5 $n = 817$	DSC ≥ 0.5 $n = 793$	$0 \leq \text{DSC} \leq 1$ $n = 288$	DSC < 0.5 $n = 160$	DSC ≥ 0.5 $n = 128$
BG	0.008 (0.011)	0.012 (0.014)	0.004 (0.002)	0.034 (0.042)	0.048 (0.046)	0.074 (0.002)
LV	0.038 (0.040)	0.025 (0.024)	0.053 (0.047)	0.120 (0.128)	0.069 (0.125)	0.213 (0.065)
LVM	0.055 (0.064)	0.027 (0.027)	0.083 (0.078)	0.191 (0.218)	0.042 (0.041)	0.473 (0.111)
RVC	0.039 (0.041)	0.021 (0.020)	0.058 (0.047)	0.127 (0.126)	0.076 (0.109)	0.223 (0.098)
WH	**0.031 (0.035)**	**0.018 (0.018)**	**0.043 (0.043)**	**0.139 (0.091)**	**0.112 (0.093)**	**0.188 (0.060)**
	TPR 0.975	FPR 0.060	**Acc. 0.965**	TPR 0.879	FPR 0.000	**Acc. 0.906**

to an analysis pipeline where operators can be informed of likely poor-quality segmentations, along with some confidence interval, in real-time.

On average, the inference time for each network was of the order 600 ms on CPU and 40 ms on GPU. This is over 10,000 times faster than with RCA (660 s) whilst maintaining good accuracy. In an automated image analysis pipeline, this method would deliver excellent performance at high-speed and at large-scale. When paired with a real-time segmentation method it would be possible provide real-time feedback during image acquisition whether an acquired image is of sufficient quality for the downstream segmentation task.

4   Conclusion

Ensuring the quality of a automatically generated segmentation in a deployed image analysis pipeline in real-time is challenging. We have shown that we can employ Convolutional Neural Networks to tackle this problem with great computational efficient and with good accuracy.

We recognize that our networks are prone to learning features specific to assessing the quality of Random Forest segmentations. We can build on this by training the network with segmentations generated from an ensemble of methods. However, we must reiterate that the purpose of the framework in this study is to give an indication of the *predicted quality* and not a direct one-to-one mapping to the reference DSC. Currently, these networks will correctly predict whether a segmentation is 'good' or 'poor' on some threshold, but will not confidently distinguish between two segmentations of similar quality.

Our trained CNNs are insensitive to small regional or boundary differences in labelmaps which are of good quality. Thus they cannot be used to assess quality of a segmentation at fine-scale. Again, this may be improved by a more diverse and granular training-sets. The labels for training the network in Experiment 1 are not easily available in most cases. However, by performing RCA, one can automatically obtain training labels for the network in Experiment 2 and this could be applied to segmentations generated with other algorithms. The cost of using data obtained with RCA is an increase in MAE. This is reasonable compared to the effort required to obtain a large, manually-labeled dataset.

Acknowledgements. RR is funded by KCL&Imperial EPSRC CDT in Medical Imaging (EP/L015226/1) and GlaxoSmithKline; VV by Indonesia Endowment for Education (LPDP) Indonesian Presidential PhD Scholarship; KF supported by The Medical College of Saint Bartholomew's Hospital Trust. AL and SEP acknowledge support from NIHR Barts Biomedical Research Centre and EPSRC program grant (EP/P001009/ 1). SN and SKP are supported by the Oxford NIHR BRC and the Oxford British Heart Foundation Centre of Research Excellence. This project supported by the MRC (grant number MR/L016311/1). NA is supported by a Wellcome Trust Research Training Fellowship (203553/Z/Z). The authors SEP, SN and SKP acknowledge the British Heart Foundation (BHF) (PG/14/89/31194). BG received funding from the ERC under Horizon 2020 (grant agreement No. 757173, project MIRA, ERC-2017-STG).

References

1. Petersen, S.E., et al.: Reference ranges for cardiac structure and function using cardiovascular magnetic resonance (CMR) in Caucasians from the UK Biobank population cohort. J. Cardiovasc. Magn. Reson. **19**(1), 18 (2017)
2. Bosse, S., Maniry, D., Müller, K.R., Wiegand, T., Samek, W.: Deep neural networks for no-reference and full-reference image quality assessment. **1**, 1–14 (2016)
3. Farzi, M., Pozo, J.M., McCloskey, E.V., Wilkinson, J.M., Frangi, A.F.: Automatic quality control for population imaging: a generic unsupervised approach. In: Ourselin, S., Joskowicz, L., Sabuncu, M.R., Unal, G., Wells, W. (eds.) MICCAI 2016. LNCS, vol. 9901, pp. 291–299. Springer, Cham (2016). https://doi.org/10. 1007/978-3-319-46723-8_34
4. Zhong, E., Fan, W., Yang, Q., Verscheure, O., Ren, J.: Cross validation framework to choose amongst models and datasets for transfer learning. In: Balcázar, J.L., Bonchi, F., Gionis, A., Sebag, M. (eds.) ECML PKDD 2010. LNCS (LNAI), vol. 6323, pp. 547–562. Springer, Heidelberg (2010). https://doi.org/10.1007/978-3-642-15939-8_35
5. Fan, W., Davidson, I.: Reverse testing. In: Proceedings of the 12th ACM SIGKDD International Conference on Knowledge Discovery and Data Mining - KDD 2006, p. 147. ACM Press, New York (2006)
6. Kohlberger, T., Singh, V., Alvino, C., Bahlmann, C., Grady, L.: Evaluating segmentation error without ground truth. In: Ayache, N., Delingette, H., Golland, P., Mori, K. (eds.) MICCAI 2012. LNCS, vol. 7510, pp. 528–536. Springer, Heidelberg (2012). https://doi.org/10.1007/978-3-642-33415-3_65
7. Valindria, V.V., et al.: Reverse classification accuracy: predicting segmentation performance in the absence of ground truth. IEEE Trans. Med. Imaging **36**, 1597–1606 (2017)
8. Robinson, R., et al.: Automatic quality control of cardiac MRI segmentation in large-scale population imaging. In: Descoteaux, M., Maier-Hein, L., Franz, A., Jannin, P., Collins, D.L., Duchesne, S. (eds.) MICCAI 2017. LNCS, vol. 10433, pp. 720–727. Springer, Cham (2017). https://doi.org/10.1007/978-3-319-66182-7_82

Recurrent Neural Networks for Aortic Image Sequence Segmentation with Sparse Annotations

Wenjia Bai[1(✉)], Hideaki Suzuki[2], Chen Qin[1], Giacomo Tarroni[1],
Ozan Oktay[1], Paul M. Matthews[2,3], and Daniel Rueckert[1]

[1] Biomedical Image Analysis Group, Department of Computing,
Imperial College London, London, UK
w.bai@imperial.ac.uk
[2] Division of Brain Sciences, Department of Medicine, Imperial College London,
London, UK
[3] UK Dementia Research Institute, Imperial College London,
London, UK

Abstract. Segmentation of image sequences is an important task in medical image analysis, which enables clinicians to assess the anatomy and function of moving organs. However, direct application of a segmentation algorithm to each time frame of a sequence may ignore the temporal continuity inherent in the sequence. In this work, we propose an image sequence segmentation algorithm by combining a fully convolutional network with a recurrent neural network, which incorporates both spatial and temporal information into the segmentation task. A key challenge in training this network is that the available manual annotations are temporally sparse, which forbids end-to-end training. We address this challenge by performing non-rigid label propagation on the annotations and introducing an exponentially weighted loss function for training. Experiments on aortic MR image sequences demonstrate that the proposed method significantly improves both accuracy and temporal smoothness of segmentation, compared to a baseline method that utilises spatial information only. It achieves an average Dice metric of 0.960 for the ascending aorta and 0.953 for the descending aorta.

1 Introduction

Segmentation is an important task in medical image analysis. It assigns a class label to each pixel/voxel in a medical image so that anatomical structures of interest can be quantified. Recent progress in machine learning has greatly improved the state-of-the-art in medical image segmentation and substantially increased accuracy. However, most of the research so far focuses on static image segmentation, whereas segmentation of temporal image sequences has received less attention. Image sequence segmentation plays an important role in assessing the anatomy and function of moving organs, such as the heart and vessels. In

© Springer Nature Switzerland AG 2018
A. F. Frangi et al. (Eds.): MICCAI 2018, LNCS 11073, pp. 586–594, 2018.
https://doi.org/10.1007/978-3-030-00937-3_67

this work, we propose a novel method for medical image sequence segmentation and demonstrate its performance on aortic MR image sequences.

There are two major contributions of this work. First, the proposed method combines a fully convolutional network (FCN) with a recurrent neural network (RNN) for image sequence segmentation. It is able to incorporate both spatial and temporal information into the task. Second, we address the challenge of training the network from temporally sparse annotations. An aortic MR image sequence typically consists of tens or hundreds of time frames. However, manual annotations may only be available for a few time frames. In order to train the proposed network end-to-end from temporally sparse annotations, we perform non-rigid label propagation on the annotations and introduce an exponentially weighted loss function for training.

We evaluated the proposed method on an aortic MR image set from 500 subjects. Experimental results show that the method improves both accuracy and temporal smoothness of segmentation, compared to a state-of-the-art method.

1.1 Related Works

FCN and RNN. The FCN was proposed to tackle pixel-wise classification problems, such as image segmentation [1]. Ronnerberger et al. proposed the U-Net, which is a type of FCN that has a symmetric U-shape architecture for feature analysis and synthesis paths [2]. It has demonstrated remarkable performance in static medical image segmentation. The RNN was designed for handling sequences. The long short-term memory (LSTM) network is a type of RNN that introduces self-loops to enable the gradient flow for long durations [3].

In the domain of medical image analysis, the combination of FCN with RNN has been explored recently [4–9]. In some works, RNN was used to model the spatial dependency in static images [4–6], such as the inter-slice dependency in anisotropic images [4,5]. In other works, RNN was used to model the temporal dependency in image sequences [7–9]. For example, Kong et al. used RNN to model the temporal dependency in cardiac MR image sequences and to predict the cardiac phase for each time frame [7]. Xue et al. used RNN to estimate the left ventricular areas and wall thicknesses across a cardiac cycle [8]. Huang et al. used RNN to estimate the location and orientation of the heart in ultrasound videos [9]. These works on medical image sequence analysis [7–9] mainly used RNN for image-level regression. The contribution of our work is that instead of performing regression, we integrate FCN and RNN to perform pixel-wise segmentation for medical image sequences.

Sparse Annotations. Manual annotation of medical images is time-consuming and tedious. It is normally performed by image analysts with clinical knowledge and not easy to outsource. Consequently, we often face small or sparse annotation sets, which is a challenge for training a machine learning algorithm, especially neural networks. To learn from spatially sparse annotations, Cicek et al. proposed to assign a zero weight to unlabelled voxels in the loss function [10]. In this work, we focus on learning from temporally sparse annotations and address the challenge by performing non-rigid label propagation and introducing an exponentially weighted loss function.

Aortic Image Segmentation. For aortic image sequence segmentation, a deformable model approach has been proposed [11], which requires a region of interest and the centre of aorta to be manually defined in initialisation. This work proposes a fully automated segmentation method.

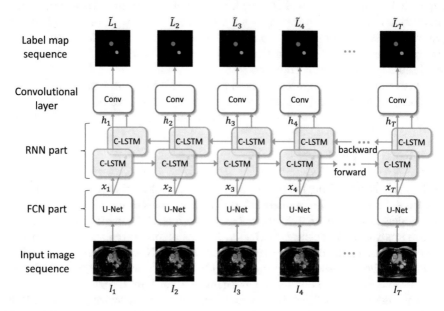

Fig. 1. The proposed method analyses spatial features in the input image sequence using U-Net, extracts the second last layer of U-Net as feature maps x_t, connects them using convolutional LSTM (C-LSTM) units across the temporal domain and finally predicts the label map sequence.

2   Methods

2.1   Network Architecture

Figure 1 shows the diagram of the method. The input is an image sequence $I = \{I_t | t = 1, 2, \ldots, T\}$ across time frames t and the output is the predicted label map sequence $\tilde{L} = \{\tilde{L}_t | t = 1, 2, \ldots, T\}$. The method consists of two main parts, FCN and RNN. The FCN part analyses spatial features in each input image I_t and extracts a feature map x_t. We use the U-Net architecture [2] for the FCN part, which has demonstrated good performance in extracting features for image segmentation.

The second last layer of the U-Net [2] is extracted as the feature map x_t and fed into the RNN part. For analysing temporal features, we use the convolutional LSTM (C-LSTM) [12]. Compared to the standard LSTM which analyses one-dimensional signals, C-LSTM is able to analyse multi-dimensional images across the temporal domain. Each C-LSTM unit is formulated as:

$$
\begin{aligned}
i_t &= \sigma(x_t * W_{xi} + h_{t-1} * W_{hi} + b_i) \\
f_t &= \sigma(x_t * W_{xf} + h_{t-1} * W_{hf} + b_f) \\
c_t &= c_{t-1} \odot f_t + i_t \odot \tanh(x_t * W_{xc} + h_{t-1} * W_{hc} + b_c) \\
o_t &= \sigma(x_t * W_{xo} + h_{t-1} * W_{ho} + b_o) \\
h_t &= o_t \odot tanh(c_t)
\end{aligned}
\tag{1}
$$

where $*$ denotes convolution[1], $\odot$ denotes element-wise multiplication, $\sigma(\cdot)$ denotes the sigmoid function, i_t, f_t, c_t and o_t are respectively the input gate (i), forget gate (f), memory cell (c) and output gate (o), W and b denote the convolution kernel and bias for each gate, x_t and h_t denote the input feature map and output feature map. The equation shows that output h_t at time point t is determined by both the current input x_t and the previous states c_{t-1} and h_{t-1}. In this way, C-LSTM utilises past information during prediction. In the proposed method, we use bi-directional C-LSTM, which consists of a forward stream and a backward stream, as shown in Fig. 1, so that the network can utilise both past and future information.

The output of C-LSTM is a pixel-wise feature map h_t at each time point t. To predict the probabilistic label map $\tilde{L}_t$, we concatenate the outputs from the forward and backward C-LSTMs and apply a convolution to it, followed by a softmax layer. The loss function at each time point is defined as the cross-entropy between the ground truth label map L_t and the prediction $\tilde{L}_t$.

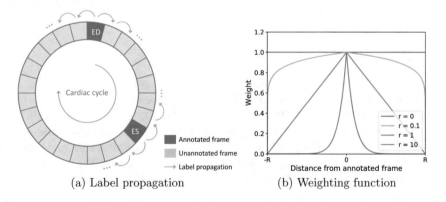

(a) Label propagation   (b) Weighting function

Fig. 2. Label propgation and the weighting function for propagated label maps.

2.2 Label Propagation and Weighted Loss

To train the network end-to-end, we require the ground truth label map sequence across the time frames. However, the typical manual annotation is temporally

---

[1] The standard LSTM performs multiplication instead of convolution here.

sparse. For example, in our dataset, we only have manual annotations at two time frames, end-diastole (ED) and end-systole (ES). In order to obtain the annotations at other time frames, we perform label propagation. Non-rigid image registration [13] is performed to estimate the motion between each pair of successive time frames. Based on the motion estimate, the label map at each time frame is propagated from either ED or ES annotations, whichever is closer, as shown in Fig. 2(a).

Registration error may accumulate during label propagation. The further a time frame is from the original annotation, the larger the registration error might be. To account for the potential error in propagated label maps, we introduce a weighted loss function for training,

$$E(\theta) = \sum_t w(t - s) \cdot f(L_t, \tilde{L}_t(\theta)) \tag{2}$$

where θ denotes the network parameters, $f(\cdot)$ denotes the cross-entropy between the propagated label map L_t and the predicted label map $\tilde{L}_t(\theta)$ by the network, s denotes the nearest annotated time frame to t and $w(\cdot)$ denotes an exponential weighting function depending on the distance between t and s,

$$w(t - s) = (1 - \frac{|t - s|}{R})^r \tag{3}$$

where R denotes the radius of the time window T for the unfolded RNN and the exponent r is a hyper-parameter which controls the shape of the weighting function. Some typical weighting functions are shown in Fig. 2(b). If $r = 0$, it treats all the time frames equally. If $r > 0$, it assigns a lower weight to time frames further from the original annotated frame.

2.3   Evaluation

We evaluate the method performance in two aspects, segmentation accuracy and temporal smoothness. For segmentation accuracy, we evaluate the Dice overlap metric and the mean contour distance between automated segmentation and manual annotation at ED and ES time frames. We also calculate the aortic area and report the difference between automated measurement and manual measurement. For evaluating temporal smoothness, we plot the curve of the aortic area $A(t)$ against time, as shown in Fig. 4, calculate the curvature of the time-area curve, $\kappa(t) = \frac{|A''(t)|}{(1+A'^2(t))^{1.5}}$, and report the mean curvature across time.

3   Experiments and Results

3.1   Data and Annotations

We performed experiments on an aortic MR image set of 500 subjects, acquired from the UK Biobank. The typical image size is 240×196 pixel with the spatial resolution of $1.6 \times 1.6\,\text{mm}^2$. Each image sequence consists of 100 time frames, covering the cardiac cycle. Two experienced image analysts manually annotated the ascending aorta (AAo) and descending aorta (DAo) at ED and ES time frames. The image set was randomly split into a training set of 400 subjects and a test set of 100 subjects. The performance is reported on the test set.

3.2   Implementation and Training

The method was implemented using Python and Tensorflow. The network was trained in two steps. In the first step, the U-Net part was trained for static image segmentation using the Adam optimiser for 20,000 iterations with a batch size of 5 subjects. The initial learning rate was 0.001 and it was divided by 10 after 5,000 iterations. In the second step, the pre-trained U-Net was connected with the RNN and trained together end-to-end using image and propagated label map sequences for 20,000 iterations with the same learning rate settings but a smaller batch size of 1 subject due to GPU memory limit. Data augmentation was performed online, which applied random translation, rotation and scaling to each input image sequence. Training took ~22 h on a Nvidia Titan Xp GPU. At test time, it took ~10 s to segment an aortic MR image sequence.

3.3   Network Parameters

There are a few parameters for the RNN, including the length of the time window T after unfolding the RNN and the exponent r for the weighting function. We investigated the impact of these parameters. Table 1 reports the average Dice metric when the parameters vary. It shows that a combination of time window $T = 9$ and exponent $r = 0.1$ achieves a good performance. When the time window increases to 21, the performance slightly decreases, possibly because the accumulative error of label propagation becomes larger. The exponent $r = 0.1$ outperforms $r = 0$, the latter treating the annotated frames and propagated frames equally, without considering the potential propagation error.

Table 1. Mean dice overlap metrics of the aortas when parameters vary.

(a) Varying T ($r = 0.1$)

T	AAo	DAo
5	0.959	0.952
9	**0.960**	**0.953**
13	0.959	0.950
17	0.959	0.952
21	0.958	0.951

(b) Varying r ($T = 9$)

r	AAo	DAo
0	0.955	0.949
0.1	**0.960**	**0.953**
1.0	0.959	0.951
10.0	0.959	0.948
100.0	**0.960**	0.949

Table 2. Quantitative comparison to U-Net. The columns list the mean dice metric, contour distance error, aortic area error and time-area curve curvature.

	Dice metric		Dist. error (mm)		Area error (mm²)		Curvature	
	AAo	DAo	AAo	DAo	AAo	DAo	AAo	DAo
U-Net	0.953	0.944	0.80	0.69	51.68	35.96	0.47	0.38
Proposed	**0.960**	**0.953**	**0.67**	**0.59**	**39.61**	**27.98**	**0.41**	**0.28**

3.4   Comparison to Baseline

We compared the proposed method to the U-Net [2], which is a strong baseline method. U-Net was applied to segment each time frame independently. Figure 3

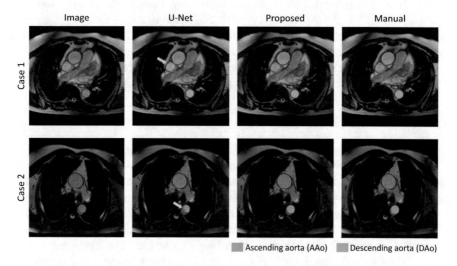

Fig. 3. Comparison of the segmentation results for U-Net and the proposed method. The yellow arrows indicate segmentation errors made by U-Net.

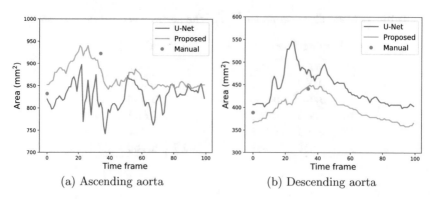

Fig. 4. Comparison of aortic time-area curves. The green dots indicate the manual measurements at ED and ES time frames.

compares the segmentation results on two exemplar cases. In Case 1, the U-Net misclassifies a neighbouring vessel as the ascending aorta. In Case 2, the U-Net under-segments the descending aorta. For both cases, the proposed method correctly segments the aortas. Figure 4 compares the time-area curves of the two methods on a exemplar subject. It shows that the curve produced by the proposed method is temporally smoother with less abrupt changes. Also, the curve agrees well with the manual measurements at ED and ES. Table 2 reports the quantitative evaluation results for segmentation accuracy and temporal smoothness. It shows that the proposed method outperforms the U-Net in segmentation accuracy, achieving a higher Dice metric, a lower contour distance error and a lower aortic area error (all with $p < 0.001$ in paired t-tests). In addition, the proposed method reduces the curvature of the time-area curve ($p < 0.001$), which indicates improved temporal smoothness.

4   Conclusions

In this paper, we propose a novel method which combines FCN and RNN for medical image sequence segmentation. To address the challenge of training the network with temporally sparse annotations, we perform non-rigid label propagation and introduce an exponentially weighted loss function for training, which accounts for potential errors in label propagation. We evaluated the method on aortic MR image sequences and demonstrated that by incorporating spatial and temporal information, the proposed method outperforms a state-of-the-art baseline method in both segmentation accuracy and temporal smoothness.

Acknowledgements. This research has been conducted using the UK Biobank Resource under Application Number 18545. This work is supported by the SmartHeart EPSRC Programme Grant (EP/P001009/1). We would like to acknowledge NVIDIA Corporation for donating a Titan Xp for this research. P.M.M. thanks the Edmond J. Safra Foundation, Lily Safra and the UK Dementia Research Institute for their generous support.

References

1. Long, J., et al.: Fully convolutional networks for semantic segmentation. In: CVPR, pp. 3431–3440 (2015)
2. Ronneberger, O., Fischer, P., Brox, T.: U-Net: convolutional networks for biomedical image segmentation. In: Navab, N., Hornegger, J., Wells, W.M., Frangi, A.F. (eds.) MICCAI 2015. LNCS, vol. 9351, pp. 234–241. Springer, Cham (2015). https://doi.org/10.1007/978-3-319-24574-4_28
3. Hochreiter, S., Schmidhuber, J.: Long short-term memory. Neural Comput. **9**(8), 1735–1780 (1997)
4. Chen, J., et al.: Combining fully convolutional and recurrent neural networks for 3D biomedical image segmentation. In: NIPS, pp. 3036–3044 (2016)

5. Poudel, R.P.K., Lamata, P., Montana, G.: Recurrent fully convolutional neural networks for multi-slice MRI cardiac segmentation. In: Zuluaga, M.A., Bhatia, K., Kainz, B., Moghari, M.H., Pace, D.F. (eds.) RAMBO/HVSMR -2016. LNCS, vol. 10129, pp. 83–94. Springer, Cham (2017). https://doi.org/10.1007/978-3-319-52280-7_8

6. Yang, X., et al.: Towards automatic semantic segmentation in volumetric ultrasound. In: Descoteaux, M., Maier-Hein, L., Franz, A., Jannin, P., Collins, D.L., Duchesne, S. (eds.) MICCAI 2017. LNCS, vol. 10433, pp. 711–719. Springer, Cham (2017). https://doi.org/10.1007/978-3-319-66182-7_81

7. Kong, B., Zhan, Y., Shin, M., Denny, T., Zhang, S.: Recognizing end-diastole and end-systole frames via deep temporal regression network. In: Ourselin, S., Joskowicz, L., Sabuncu, M.R., Unal, G., Wells, W. (eds.) MICCAI 2016. LNCS, vol. 9902, pp. 264–272. Springer, Cham (2016). https://doi.org/10.1007/978-3-319-46726-9_31

8. Xue, W., Lum, A., Mercado, A., Landis, M., Warrington, J., Li, S.: Full quantification of left ventricle via deep multitask learning network respecting intra- and inter-task relatedness. In: Descoteaux, M., Maier-Hein, L., Franz, A., Jannin, P., Collins, D.L., Duchesne, S. (eds.) MICCAI 2017. LNCS, vol. 10435, pp. 276–284. Springer, Cham (2017). https://doi.org/10.1007/978-3-319-66179-7_32

9. Huang, W., Bridge, C.P., Noble, J.A., Zisserman, A.: Temporal HeartNet: towards human-level automatic analysis of fetal cardiac screening video. In: Descoteaux, M., Maier-Hein, L., Franz, A., Jannin, P., Collins, D.L., Duchesne, S. (eds.) MICCAI 2017. LNCS, vol. 10434, pp. 341–349. Springer, Cham (2017). https://doi.org/10.1007/978-3-319-66185-8_39

10. Çiçek, Ö., Abdulkadir, A., Lienkamp, S.S., Brox, T., Ronneberger, O.: 3D U-Net: learning dense volumetric segmentation from sparse annotation. In: Ourselin, S., Joskowicz, L., Sabuncu, M.R., Unal, G., Wells, W. (eds.) MICCAI 2016. LNCS, vol. 9901, pp. 424–432. Springer, Cham (2016). https://doi.org/10.1007/978-3-319-46723-8_49

11. Herment, A., et al.: Automated segmentation of the aorta from phase contrast MR images: validation against expert tracing in healthy volunteers and in patients with a dilated aorta. J. Mag. Reson. Imag. 31(4), 881–888 (2010)

12. Stollenga, M.F., et al.: Parallel multi-dimensional LSTM, with application to fast biomedical volumetric image segmentation. In: NIPS, pp. 2998–3006 (2015)

13. Rueckert, D., et al.: Nonrigid registration using free-form deformations: application to breast MR images. IEEE Trans. Med. Imag. 18(8), 712–721 (1999)

Deep Nested Level Sets: Fully Automated Segmentation of Cardiac MR Images in Patients with Pulmonary Hypertension

Jinming Duan[1,2(✉)], Jo Schlemper[1], Wenjia Bai[1], Timothy J. W. Dawes[2], Ghalib Bello[2], Georgia Doumou[2], Antonio De Marvao[2], Declan P. O'Regan[2], and Daniel Rueckert[1]

[1] Biomedical Image Analysis Group, Imperial College London, London, UK
[2] MRC London Institute of Medical Sciences, Imperial College London, London, UK
j.duan@imperial.ac.uk

Abstract. In this paper we introduce a novel and accurate optimisation method for segmentation of cardiac MR (CMR) images in patients with pulmonary hypertension (PH). The proposed method explicitly takes into account the image features learned from a deep neural network. To this end, we estimate simultaneous probability maps over region and edge locations in CMR images using a fully convolutional network. Due to the distinct morphology of the heart in patients with PH, these probability maps can then be incorporated in a single nested level set optimisation framework to achieve multi-region segmentation with high efficiency. The proposed method uses an automatic way for level set initialisation and thus the whole optimisation is fully automated. We demonstrate that the proposed deep nested level set (DNLS) method outperforms existing state-of-the-art methods for CMR segmentation in PH patients.

1 Introduction

Pulmonary hypertension (PH) is a cardiorespiratory syndrome characterised by increased blood pressure in pulmonary arteries. It typically follows a rapidly progressive course. As such, early identification of PH patients with elevated risk of a deteriorating course is of paramount importance. For this, accurate segmentation of different functional regions of the heart in CMR images is critical.

Numerous methods for automatic and semi-automatic CMR image segmentation have been proposed, including deformable models [1], atlas-based image registration models [2] as well as statistical shape and appearance models [3]. More recently, deep learning-based methods have achieved state-of-the-art performance in the CMR domain [4]. However, the above approaches for CMR image segmentation have multiple drawbacks. First, they tend to focus on left ventricle (LV) [1]. However, the prognostic importance of the right ventricle (RV) is a broad range of cardiovascular disease and using the coupled biventricular motion of the heart enables more accurate cardiac assessment. Second, existing

© Springer Nature Switzerland AG 2018
A. F. Frangi et al. (Eds.): MICCAI 2018, LNCS 11073, pp. 595–603, 2018.
https://doi.org/10.1007/978-3-030-00937-3_68

approaches rely on manual initialisation of the image segmentation or definition of key anatomical landmarks [1–3]. This becomes less feasible in population-level applications involving hundreds or thousands of CMR images. Third, existing techniques have been mainly developed and validated using normal (healthy) hearts [1, 2, 4]. Few studies have focused on abnormal hearts in PH patients.

To address the aforementioned limitations of current approaches, in this paper we propose a deep nested level set (DNLS) method for automated biventricular segmentation of CMR images. More specifically, we make three distinct contributions to the area of CMR segmentation, particularly for PH patients: First, we introduce a deep fully convolutional network that effectively combines two loss functions, i.e. softmax cross-entropy and class-balanced sigmoid cross-entropy. As such, the neural network is able to simultaneously extract robust region and edge features from CMR images. Second, we introduce a novel implicit representation of PH hearts that utilises multiple nested level lines of a continuous level set function. This nested level set representation can be effectively deployed with the learned deep features from the proposed network. Furthermore, an initialisation of the level set function can be readily derived from the learned feature. Therefore, DNLS does not need user intervention (manual initialisation or landmark placement) and is fully automated. Finally, we apply the proposed DNLS method to clinical data acquired from 430 PH patients (approx. 12000 images), and compare its performance with state-of-the-art approaches.

2   Modelling Biventricular Anatomy in Patients with PH

To illustrate cardiac morphology in patients with PH, Fig. 1 shows the difference in CMR images from a representative healthy subject and a PH subject. In health, the RV is crescentic in short-axis views and triangular in long-axis views, wrapping around the thicker-walled LV. In PH, the initial hypertrophic response of the RV increases contractility but is followed invariably by progressive dilatation and failure heralding clinical deterioration and ultimately death. During this deterioration, the dilated RV pushes onto the LV to deform and lose its roundness. Moreover, in PH the myocardium around RV become much

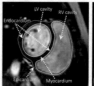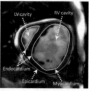

Fig. 1. Short-axis images of a healthy subject (left) and a PH subject (right), including the anatomical explanation of both LV and RV. The desired epicardial contours (red) and endocardial contours (yellow) from both ventricles are plotted.

thicker than a healthy one, allowing PH cardiac morphology to be modelled by a nested level set. Next, we incorporate the biventricular anatomy of PH hearts into our model for automated segmentation of LV and RV cavities and myocardium.

3   Methodology

Nested Level Set Approach: We view image segmentation in PH as a multi-region image segmentation problem. Let $I : \Omega \rightarrow \mathbb{R}^d$ denote an input image defined on the domain $\Omega \subset \mathbb{R}^2$. We segment the image into a set of n pairwise disjoint region Ω_i, with $\Omega = \cup_{i=1}^n \Omega_i$, $\Omega_i \cap \Omega_j = \emptyset \ \forall i \neq j$. The segmentation task can be solved by computing a labelling function $l(x) : \Omega \rightarrow \{1, \ldots, n\}$ that indicates which of the n regions each pixel belongs to: $\Omega_i = \{x \mid l(x) = i\}$. The problem is then formulated as an energy minimisation problem consisting of a data term and a regularisation term

$$\min_{\Omega_1, \ldots, \Omega_n} \left\{ \sum_{i=1}^n \int_{\Omega_i} f_i(x)\, dx + \lambda \sum_{i=1}^n \mathrm{Per}_g(\Omega_i, \Omega) \right\}. \tag{1}$$

The data term, $f_i : \Omega \rightarrow \mathbb{R}$ is associated with region that takes on smaller values if the respective pixel position has stronger response to region. In a Bayesian MAP inference framework, $f_i(x) = -\log P_i(I(x) \mid \Omega_i)$ corresponds to the negative logarithm of the conditional probability for a specific pixel color at the given location x within region Ω_i. Here we refer to f_i as region feature. The second term, $\mathrm{Per}_g(\Omega_i, \Omega)$ is the perimeter of the segmentation region Ω_i, weighted by the non-negative function g. This energy term alone is known as geodesic distance, the minimisation over which can be interpreted as finding a geodesic curve in a Riemannian space. The choice of g can be an edge detection function

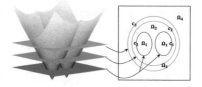

Fig. 2. An example of partitioning the domain Ω into 4 disjoint regions (right), using 3 nested level lines $\{x \mid \phi(x) = c_i, i = 1, 2, 3\}$ of the same function ϕ (left). The intersections between the 3D smooth surface ϕ and the 2D plans correspond to the three nested curves on the right.

which favours boundaries that have strong gradients of the input image I. Here we refer to g as edge feature.

We apply the variational level set method [5,6] to (1) in this study. Because a PH heart can be implicitly represented by two nested level lines of a continuous level set function ($\{x \mid \phi(x) = c_i, i = 1, 2\}$ in Fig. 2). Note that the nested level set idea present here is inspired from previous work [1,7]. Our approach uses features learned from many images while previous work only consider single image. With the idea, we are able to approximate the multi-region segmentation energy (1) by using only one continuous function. The computational cost is thus small. Now assume that the contours in the image I can be represented by level lines of the same Lipschitz continuous level set function $\phi : \Omega \rightarrow \mathbb{R}$. With $n-1$ distinct levels $\{c_1 < c_2 < \cdots < c_{n-1}\}$, the implicit function ϕ partitions the domain Ω into n disjoint regions, together with their boundaries (see Fig. 2 right). We can then define the characteristic function $\chi_i \phi$ for each region Ω_i as

$$\chi_i \phi(x) = \begin{cases} H\left(c_i - \phi(x)\right) & i = 1 \\ H\left(\phi(x) - c_{i-1}\right) H\left(c_i - \phi(x)\right) & 2 \leq i \leq n-1 \\ H\left(\phi(x) - c_{i-1}\right) & i = n \end{cases}, \tag{2}$$

where H is the one-dimensional Heaviside function that takes on either 0 or 1 over the whole domain Ω. Due to the non-differentiate nature of H it is usually approximated by its smooth version H_ϵ for numerical calculation [7]. Note that in (2) $\sum_{i=1}^{n} \chi_i \phi = 1$ is automatically satisfied, meaning that the resulting segmentation will not produce a vacuum or an overlap effect. That is, by using (2) $\Omega = \cup_{i=1}^{n} \Omega_i$ and $\Omega_i \cap \Omega_j = \emptyset$ hold all the time. With the definition of $\chi_i \phi$, we can readily reformulate (1) in the following new energy minimisation problem

$$\min_{\phi(x)} \left\{ \sum_{i=1}^{n} \int_{\Omega} f_i(x) \chi_i \phi(x) \, dx + \lambda \sum_{i=1}^{n-1} \int_{\Omega} g(x) \left| \nabla H\left(\phi(x) - c_i\right) \right| dx \right\}. \tag{3}$$

Note that (3) differs from (1) in multiple ways due to the use of the smooth function ϕ and characteristic function (2). First, the variable to be minimised is the n regions $\Omega_1, \ldots, \Omega_n$ in (1) while the smooth function ϕ in (3). Second, the minimisation domain is changing from over Ω_i in (1) to over Ω in (3). Third (1) uses an abstract $\mathrm{Per}_g\left(\Omega_i, \Omega\right)$ for the weighted length of the boundary between two adjacent regions, while (3) represents the weighted length with the co-area formula, i.e. $\int_{\Omega} g \left| \nabla H\left(\phi - c_i\right) \right| dx$. Finally, the upper limit of summation in the regularisation term of (1) is n while $n-1$ in that of (3). So far, the region features f_i and the edge feature g have not been defined. Next, we will tackle this problem.

Learning Deep Features Using Fully Convolutional Network: We propose a deep neural network that can effectively learn region and edge features from many labelled PH CMR images. Learned features are then incorporated to (3). Let us formulate the learning problem as follows: we denote the input training data set by $S = \{(U_p, R_p, E_p), p = 1, \ldots, N\}$, where sample $U_p = \{u_j^p, j = 1, \ldots, |U_p|\}$ is the raw input image, $R_p = \{r_j^p, j = 1, \ldots, |R_p|\}$, $r_j^p \in \{1, \ldots, n\}$ is the ground truth region labels (n regions) for image U_p, and $E_p = \{e_j^p, j = 1, \ldots, |E_p|\}$, $e_j^p \in \{0, 1\}$ is the ground truth binary edge map for U_p. We denote all network layer parameters as $\mathbf{W}$ and propose to minimise the following objective function via the (back-propagation) stochastic gradient descent

$$\mathbf{W}^* = \mathrm{argmin}(L_R(\mathbf{W}) + \alpha L_E(\mathbf{W})), \tag{4}$$

where $L_R(\mathbf{W})$ is the region associated cross-entropy loss that enables the network to learn region features, while $L_E(\mathbf{W})$ is the edge associated cross-entropy loss for learning edge features. The weight α balances the two losses. By minimising (4), the network is able to output joint region and edge probability maps simultaneously. In our image-to-image training, the loss function is computed over all pixels in a training image $U = \{u_j, j = 1, \ldots, |U|\}$, a region map $R = \{r_j, j = 1, \ldots, |R|\}$, $r_j \in \{1, \ldots, n\}$ and an edge map $E = \{e_j, j = 1, \ldots, |E|\}$, $e_j \in \{0, 1\}$. The definitions of $L_R(\mathbf{W})$ and $L_E(\mathbf{W})$ are given as follows.

$$L_R(\mathbf{W}) = -\sum_j \log P_{so}(r_j|U, \mathbf{W}), \tag{5}$$

where j denotes the pixel index, and $P_{so}(r_j|U, \mathbf{W})$ is the channel-wise softmax probability provided by the network at pixel j for image U. The edge loss is

$$L_E(\mathbf{W}) = -\beta \sum_{j \in Y_+} \log P_{si}(e_j = 1|U, \mathbf{W}) - (1 - \beta) \sum_{j \in Y_-} \log P_{si}(e_j = 0|U, \mathbf{W}). \tag{6}$$

For a typical CMR image, the distribution of edge and non-edge pixels is heavily biased. Therefore, we use the strategy [8] to automatically balance edge and non-edge classes. Specifically, we use a class-balancing weight β. Here, $\beta = |Y_-|/|Y|$ and $1-\beta = |Y_+|/|Y|$, where $|Y_-|$ and $|Y_+|$ respectively denote edge and non-edge ground truth label pixels. $P_{si}(e_j = 1|U, \mathbf{W})$ is the pixel-wise sigmoid probability provided by the network at non-edge pixel j for image U.

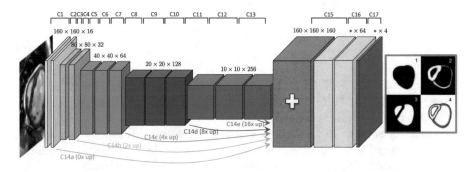

Fig. 3. The architecture of a fully convolutional network with 17 convolutional layers. The network takes the PH CMR image as input, applies a branch of convolutions, learns image features from fine to coarse levels, concatenates ('+' sign in the red layer) multi-scale features and finally predicts the region (1–3) and edge (4) probability maps simultaneously.

In Fig. 3, we show the network architecture for automatic feature extraction, which is a fully convolutional network (FCN) and adapted from the U-net architecture [9]. Batch-normalisation (BN) is used after each convolutional layer, and before a rectified linear unit (ReLU) activation. The last layer is however followed by the softmax and sigmoid functions. In the FCN, input images have pixel dimensions of 160×160. Every layer whose label is prefixed with 'C' performs the operation: convolution $\rightarrow$ BN $\rightarrow$ ReLU, except C17. The (filter size/stride) is $(3 \times 3/1)$ for layers from C1 to C16, excluding layers C3, C5, C8 and C11 which are $(3 \times 3/2)$. The arrows represent $(3 \times 3/1)$ convolutional layers (C14a−e) followed by a transpose convolutional (up) layer with a factor necessary to achieve feature map volumes with size $160 \times 160 \times 32$, all of which are concatenated into the red feature map volume. Finally, C17 applies a $(1 \times 1/1)$ convolution with a softmax activation and a sigmoid activation, producing the blue feature map volume with a depth $n + 1$, corresponding to n (3) region features and an edge feature of an image.

After the network is trained, we deploy it on the given image I in the validation set and obtain the joint region and edge probability maps from the last convolutional layer

$$(P_R, P_E) = \mathbf{CNN}(I, \mathbf{W}^*),\qquad(7)$$

where $\mathbf{CNN}(\cdot)$ denotes the trained network. P_R is a vector region probability map including n (number of regions) channels, while P_E is a scalar edge probability map. These probability maps are then fed to the energy (3), in which $f_i = -\log P_{Ri}, i = \{1, \ldots, n\}$ and $g = P_E$. With all necessary elements at hand, we are ready to minimise (3) next.

Optimisation: The minimisation process of (3) entails the *calculus of variations*, by which we obtain the resulting Euler-Lagrange (EL) equation with respect to the variable ϕ. A solution (ϕ^*) to the EL equation is then iteratively sought by the following gradient descent method

$$\frac{\partial \phi}{\partial t} = -\sum_{i=1}^{n} f_i \frac{\partial \chi_i \phi}{\partial \phi} + \lambda \kappa_g \sum_{i=1}^{n-1} \delta_\epsilon (\phi - c_i),\qquad(8)$$

where $\kappa_g = div\,(g \nabla \phi / |\nabla \phi|)$ is the weighted curvature that can be numerically implemented by the finite difference method on a half-point grid [10]. δ_ϵ is the derivative of H_ϵ, which is defined in [7].

At steady state of (8), a local or global minimiser of (3) can be found. Note that the energy (3) is nonconvex so it may have more than one global minimiser. To obtain a desirable segmentation result, we need a close initialisation of the level set function (ϕ^0) such that the algorithm converges to the solution we want. We tackle this problem by thresholding the region probability map P_{R3} and then computing the signed distance function (SDF) from the binary image using the fast sweeping algorithm. The resulting SDF is then used as ϕ^0 for (8). In this way, the whole optimisation process is fully automated.

4   Experimental Results

Data: Experiments were performed using short-axis CMR images from 430 PH patients. For each patient 10 to 16 short-axis slices were acquired roughly covering the whole heart. Each short-axis image has resolution of $1.5 \times 1.5 \times 8.0$ mm^3. Due to the large slice thickness of the short-axis slices and the inter-slice shift caused by respiratory motion, we train the FCN in a 2D fashion and apply the DNLS method to segment each slice separately. The ground truth region labels were generated using a semi-automatic process which included a manual correction step by an experienced clinical expert. Region labels for each subject contain the left and right ventricular blood pools and myocardial walls for all 430 subjects at end-diastolic (ED) and end-systolic (ES) frames. The ground truth edge labels are derived from the region label maps by identifying pixels with label transitions. The dataset was randomly split into training datasets (400 subjects) and validation datasets (30 subjects). For image pre-processing, all training images were reshaped to the same size of 160×160 with zero-padding, and image intensity was normalised to the range of $[0, 1]$ before training.

Parameters: The following parameters were used for the experiments in this work: First, there are six parameters associated with finding a desirable solution to (3). They are the weighting parameter λ (1), regularisation parameter ϵ (1.5), two levels c_1 (0) and c_2 (8), time step t (0.1), and iteration number (200). Second, for training the network, we use Adam SGD with learning rate (0.001) and batch size (two subjects) for each of 50000 iterations. The weight α in (4) is set to 1. We perform data augmentation on-the-fly, which includes random translation, rotation, scaling and intensity rescaling of the input images and labels at each iteration. In this way, the network is robust against new images as it has seen millions of different inputs by the end of training. Note that data augmentation is crucial to obtain better results. Training took approx. 10 h (50000 iterations) on a Nvidia Titan XP GPU, while testing took 5s in order to segment all the images for one subject at ED and ES.

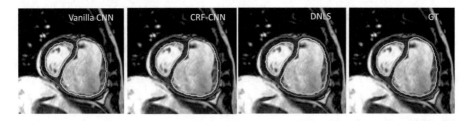

Fig. 4. Visual comparison of segmentation results from the vanilla CNN, CRF-CNN and proposed method. LV & RV cavities and myocardium are delineated using yellow and red contours. GT stands for ground truth.

Table 1. Quantitative comparison of segmentation results from the vanilla CNN, CRF-CNN and proposed method, in terms of Dice metric (mean±standard deviation) and computation time at testing stage.

Methods	LV & RV Cavities	Myocardium	Time
Vanilla CNN [4]	0.902 ± 0.047	0.703 ± 0.091	$\sim$**0.06**s
CRF-CNN [11]	0.911 ± 0.045	0.712 ± 0.082	$\sim$2s
Proposed DNLS	$\mathbf{0.925 \pm 0.032}$	$\mathbf{0.772 \pm 0.058}$	$\sim$5s

Comparsion: The segmentation performance was evaluated by computing the Dice overlap metric between the automated and ground truth segmentations for LV & RV cavities and myocardium. We compared our method with the vanilla CNN proposed in [4], the code of which is publicly available. DNLS was also compared with the vanilla CNN with a conditional random field (CRF) [11] refinement (CRF-CNN). In Fig. 4, visual comparison suggests that DNLS provides significant segmentation improvements over CNN and CRF-CNN. For example, at the base of the right ventricle both CNN and CRF-CNN fail to retain the correct anatomical relationship between endocardium and epicardium portraying the endocardial border outside the epicardium. CRF-CNN by contrast retains the endocardial border within the epicardium, as described in the ground truth. In Table 1, we report their Dice metric of ED and ES time frames in the validation dataset and show that our DNLS method outperforms the other two methods for all the anatomical structures, especially for the myocardium. CNN is the fastest method as it was deployed with GPU, and DNLS is the most computationally expensive method due to its complex optimisation processes.

5   Conclusion

In this paper, we proposed the deep nested level set (DNLS) approach for segmentation of CMR images in patients with pulmonary hypertension. The main contribution is that we combined the classical level set method with the prevalent fully convolutional network to address the problem of pathological image segmentation, which is a major challenge in medical image segmentation. The DNLS inherits advantages of both level set method and neural network, the former being able to model complex geometries of cardiac morphology and the latter providing robust features. We have shown the derivation of DNLS in detail and demonstrated that DNLS outperforms two state-of-the-art methods.

Acknowledgements. The research was supported by the British Heart Foundation (NH/17/1/32725, RE/13/4/30184); National Institute for Health Research (NIHR) Biomedical Research Centre based at Imperial College Healthcare NHS Trust and Imperial College London; and the Medical Research Council, UK. We would like to thank Dr Simon Gibbs, Dr Luke Howard and Prof Martin Wilkins for providing the CMR image data. The TITAN Xp GPU used for this research was kindly donated by the NVIDIA Corporation.

References

1. Feng, C., Li, C., Zhao, D., Davatzikos, C., Litt, H.: Segmentation of the left ventricle using distance regularized two-layer level set approach. In: Mori, K., Sakuma, I., Sato, Y., Barillot, C., Navab, N. (eds.) MICCAI 2013. LNCS, vol. 8149, pp. 477–484. Springer, Heidelberg (2013). https://doi.org/10.1007/978-3-642-40811-3_60
2. Bai, W., Shi, W., O'Regan, D.P., Tong, T., Wang, H., Jamil-Copley, S., Peters, N.S., Rueckert, D.: A probabilistic patch-based label fusion model for multi-atlas segmentation with registration refinement: application to cardiac MR images. IEEE Trans. Med. Imaging **32**(7), 1302–1315 (2013)
3. Albà, X., Pereañez, M., Hoogendoorn, C.: An algorithm for the segmentation of highly abnormal hearts using a generic statistical shape model. IEEE Trans. Med. Imaging **35**(3), 845–859 (2016)

4. Bai, W., Sinclair, M., Tarroni, G., et al.: Human-level CMR image analysis with deep fully convolutional networks. J. Cardiovasc. Magn. (2018)

5. Duan, J., Pan, Z., Yin, X., Wei, W., Wang, G.: Some fast projection methods based on Chan-Vese model for image segmentation. EURASIP J. Image Video Process. **7**, 1–16 (2014)

6. Tan, L., Pan, Z., Liu, W., Duan, J., Wei, W., Wang, G.: Image segmentation with depth information via simplified variational level set formulation. J. Math. Imaging Vis. **60**(1), 1–17 (2018)

7. Chung, G., Vese, L.A.: Image segmentation using a multilayer level-set approach. Comput. Vis. Sci. **12**(6), 267–285 (2009)

8. Xie, S., Tu, Z.: Holistically-nested edge detection. In: ECCV, pp. 1395–1403 (2015)

9. Simonyan, K., Zisserman, A.: Very deep convolutional networks for large-scale image recognition. CoRR abs/1409.1556 (2014)

10. Duan, J., Haines, B., Ward, W.O.C., Bai, L.: Surface reconstruction from point clouds using a novel variational model. In: Bramer, M., Petridis, M. (eds.) Research and Development in Intelligent Systems XXXII, pp. 135–146. Springer, Cham (2015). https://doi.org/10.1007/978-3-319-25032-8_9

11. Krähenbühl, P., Koltun, V.: Efficient inference in fully connected CRFs with Gaussian edge potentials. In: NIPS, pp. 109–117 (2011)

Atrial Fibrosis Quantification Based on Maximum Likelihood Estimator of Multivariate Images

Fuping Wu[1], Lei Li[2], Guang Yang[3], Tom Wong[3], Raad Mohiaddin[3], David Firmin[3], Jennifer Keegan[3], Lingchao Xu[2], and Xiahai Zhuang[1(✉)]

[1] School of Data Science, Fudan University, Shanghai, China
zxh@fudan.edu.cn
[2] School of BME and School of NAOCE, Shanghai Jiao Tong University, Shanghai, China
[3] National Heart and Lung Institute, Imperial College London, London, UK

Abstract. We present a fully-automated segmentation and quantification of the left atrial (LA) fibrosis and scars combining two cardiac MRIs, one is the target late gadolinium-enhanced (LGE) image, and the other is an anatomical MRI from the same acquisition session. We formulate the joint distribution of images using a multivariate mixture model (MvMM), and employ the maximum likelihood estimator (MLE) for texture classification of the images simultaneously. The MvMM can also embed transformations assigned to the images to correct the misregistration. The iterated conditional mode algorithm is adopted for optimization. This method first extracts the anatomical shape of the LA, and then estimates a prior probability map. It projects the resulting segmentation onto the LA surface, for quantification and analysis of scarring. We applied the proposed method to 36 clinical data sets and obtained promising results (Accuracy: $0.809 \pm .150$, Dice: $0.556 \pm .187$). We compared the method with the conventional algorithms and showed an evidently and statistically better performance ($p < 0.03$).

1 Introduction

Atrial fibrillation (AF) is the most common arrhythmia of clinical significance. It is associated with structural remodelling, including fibrotic changes in the left atrium (LA) and can increase morbidity. Radio frequency ablation treatment aims to eliminate AF, which requires LA scar segmentation and quantification. There are well-validated imaging methods for fibrosis detection and assessment in the myocardium of the ventricles such as the late gadolinium-enhanced (LGE)

X. Zhuang—This work was supported by Science and Technology Commission of Shanghai Municipality (17JC1401600).

Electronic supplementary material The online version of this chapter (https://doi.org/10.1007/978-3-030-00937-3_69) contains supplementary material, which is available to authorized users.

© Springer Nature Switzerland AG 2018
A. F. Frangi et al. (Eds.): MICCAI 2018, LNCS 11073, pp. 604–612, 2018.
https://doi.org/10.1007/978-3-030-00937-3_69

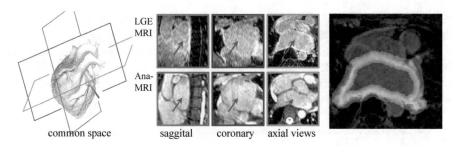

common space   saggital   coronary   axial views

Fig. 1. Illustration of the common space, MRI images, and LA wall probability map.

MRI. And recently there is a growing interest in imaging the thin LA walls for the identification of native fibrosis and ablation induced scarring of the AF patients [1].

Visualisation and quantification of atrial scarring require the segmentation from the LGE MRI images. Essentially, there are two segmentations required: one showing the cardiac anatomy, particularly the LA and pulmonary veins, and the other delineating the scars. The former segmentation is required to rule out confounding enhanced tissues from other substructures of the heart, while the latter is a prerequisite for analysis and quantification of the LA scarring. While manual delineation can be subjective and labour-intensive, automating this segmentation is desired but remains challenging mainly due to two reasons. First, the LA wall, including the scar, is thin and sometimes hard to distinguish even by experienced cardiologists. Second, the respiratory motion and varying heart rates can result in poor quality of the LGE MRI images. Also, artifactually enhanced signal from surrounding tissues can confuse the algorithms.

Limited number of studies have been reported in the literature to develop fully automatic LA segmentation and quantification of scarring. Directly segmenting the scars has been the focus of a number of works [2], which generally require delineation of the LA walls manually [3,4], thus some researchers directly dedicated to the automated segmentation of the walls [5,6]. Tobon-Gomez et al. organized a grand challenge evaluating and benchmarking LA blood pool segmentation with promising outcomes [7]. In MICCAI 2016, Karim et al. organized a LA wall challenge on 3D CT and T2 cardiac MRI [8]. Due to the difficulty of this segmentation task, only two of the three participants contributed to automatically segmenting the CT data, and no work on the MRI data has been reported.

In this study, we present a fully automated LA wall segmentation and scar delineation method combining two cardiac MRI modalities, one is the target LGE MRI, and the other is an anatomical 3D MRI, referred to as Ana-MRI, based on the balanced-Steady State Free Precession (bSSFP) sequence, which provides clear whole heart structures. The two images are aligned into a commons space, defined by the coordinate of the patient, as Fig. 1 illustrates. Then, a multivariate mixture model (MvMM) and the maximum likelihood estimator (MLE) are used for label classification. In addition, the MvMM can embed transformations assigned to each image, and the transformations and model parameters can be optimized by the iterated conditional modes (ICM) algorithm within the framework of MLE. In this framework, the clear anatomical information from the Ana-MRI provides a global guidance for the segmentation of the LGE MRI, and the enhanced LA scarring in the LGE MRI enables the segmentation of fibrosis which is invisible in Ana-MRI.

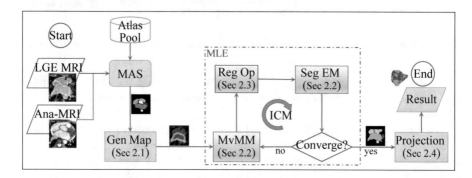

Fig. 2. Flowchart of the proposed LA wall segmentation combining two MRI sequences.

2 Method

The goal of this work is to obtain a fully automatic segmentation of LA wall and scars, combining the complementary information from the LGE MRI and Ana-MRI. Figure 2 presents the flowchart of the method, which includes three steps: (1) A multi-atlas segmentation (MAS) approach is used to extract the anatomy of the LA, based on which the probability map is generated. (2) The MLE and MvMM-based algorithm is performed to classify the labels and register the images. (3) Projection of the resulting segmentation onto the LA surface for quantification and analysis.

2.1 MAS for Generating LA Anatomy and Probability Map

The MAS consists of two major steps: (1) atlas propagation based on image registration and (2) label fusion. Directly registering the atlases to the target LGE MRI can introduce large errors, as the LGE MRI has relative poor quality in general, and consequently results in inaccurate probability map for the thin LA walls. We therefore propose to use atlases constructed from a set of Ana-MRI images and register these Ana-MRI atlases to the target space of the subject, where both the Ana-MRI and LGE MRI have been acquired. The inter-subject (atlas-to-patient) registration of Ana-MRI has been well developed [9], and the Ana-MRI to LGE MRI from the same subject can be reliably obtained by conventional registration techniques, since there only exists small misalignment between them. For the label fusion, the challenge comes from the fact that the target LGE MRI and the Ana-MRI atlases have very different texture patterns, sometimes referred to as different-modality images even though they are both obtained from cardiac MRI. We hence use the multi-modality label fusion algorithm based on the conditional intensity of images [10].

Having done the MAS, one can estimate a probability map of the LA wall by applying a Gaussian function, e.g. with zero mean and 2 mm standard deviation, to the boundary of the LA segmentation results assuming a fixed wall thickness for initialization [1]. The probability of background can be computed by normalizing the two labels. Figure 1 displays a slice of the LA wall probability map superimposed onto the LGE MRI.

2.2   MvMM and MLE for Multivariate Image Segmentation

Let $\hat{I} = \{I_1 = I_{LGE}, I_2 = I_{Ana}\}$ be the two MRI images. We denote the spatial domain of the region of interest (ROI) of the subject as Ω, referred to as *the common space*. Figure 1 demonstrates the common space and images. For a location $x \in \Omega$, the label of x, i.e. LA wall or none LA wall (background), is determined regardless the appearance of the MRI images. We denote the label of x using $s(x) = k, k \in K$. Provided that the two images are both aligned to the common space, the label information of them should be the same. For the LA wall in LGE MRI, the intensity values are distinctly different for the fibrosis and normal myocardium. We denote the subtype of a tissue k in image I_i as $z_i(x) = c, c \in C_{ik}$ and use the multi-component Gaussian mixture to model the intensity of the LA walls in LGE MRI.

The likelihood (LH) of the model parameters θ in MvMM is given by $LH(\theta; \hat{I}) = p(\hat{I}|\theta)$, similar to the conventional Gaussian mixture model (GMM) [11]. Assuming independence of the locations (pixels), one has $LH(\theta; \hat{I}) = \prod_{x \in \Omega} p(\hat{I}(x)|\theta)$. In the EM framework, the label and component information are considered as hidden data. Let Θ denotes the set of both hidden data and model parameters, the likelihood of the complete data is then given by,

$$p(\hat{I}(x)|\Theta) = \sum_{k \in K} \pi_{kx} p(\hat{I}(x)|s(x) = k, \Theta), \tag{1}$$

where, $\pi_{kx} = p(s(x) = k|\Theta) = \frac{p_A(s(x)=k)\pi_k}{NF}$, $p_A(s(x) = k)$ is the prior probability map, π_k is the label proportion, and NF is the normalization factor.

When the tissue type of a position is known, *the intensity values from different images then become independent*,

$$p(\hat{I}(x)|s(x) = k, \Theta) = \prod_{i=1,2} p(I_i(x)|s(x) = k, \Theta). \tag{2}$$

Here, the intensity PDF of an image is given by the conventional GMM. To estimate the Gaussian model parameters and then segmentation variables, one can employ the EM to solve the log-likelihood (LL) by rewriting it as follows,

$$LL = \sum_x \sum_k \delta_{s(x),k} \left(\log \pi_{kx} + \sum_i \sum_{c_{ik}} \delta_{z_i(x),c_{ik}} (\log \tau_{ikc} + \log \Phi_{ikc}(I_i(x))) \right), \tag{3}$$

where $\delta_{a,b}$ is the Kronecker delta function, τ_{ikc} is the component proportion and $\Phi_{ikc}(\cdot)$ is the Gaussian function to model the intensity PDF of a tissue subtype c belonging to a tissue k in the image I_i. The model parameters and segmentation variables can be estimated using the EM algorithm and related derivation. Readers are referred to the supplementary materials for details of the derivation.

2.3   Optimization Strategy for Registration in MvMM

The proposed MvMM can embed transformations for the images ($\{F_i\}$) and map (F_m), such as $p(I_i(x)|c_{ik}, \theta, F_i) = \Phi_{ikc}(I_i(F_i(x)))$, and $p_A(s(x) = k|F_a) = A_k(F_a(x)), k = [l_{bk}, l_{la}]$, where $\{A_k(\cdot)\}$ are the probabilistic atlas image. With the deformation embedded prior $\pi_{kx|F_m} = p(s(x) = k|F_m)$, the LL becomes,

$$LL = \sum_{x \in \Omega} \log LH(x) = \sum_{x \in \Omega} \log \left\{ \sum_k \pi_{kx|F_m} \prod_i \sum_{c_{ik}} \tau_{ikc}\Phi_{ikc}(I_i(F_i(x))) \right\}. \quad (4)$$

Here, the short form $LH(x)$ is introduced for convenience.

There is no closed form solution for the minimization of (4). Since the Gaussian parameters depend on the values of the transformation parameters, and vice versa, one can use the ICM approach to solve this optimization problem, which optimizes one group of parameters while keeping the others unchanged at each iteration. The two groups of parameters are alternately optimized and this alternation process iterates until a local optimum is found. The MvMM parameters and the hidden data are updated using the EM approach, and the transformations are optimized using the gradient ascent method. The derivatives of LL with respect to the transformations of the MRI images and probability map are respectively given by,

$$\frac{\partial LL}{\partial F_i} = \sum_x \frac{1}{LH(x)} \sum_k \pi_{kx} \prod_{j \neq i} \left\{ p(I_j(x)|k_x, \theta, F_j) \sum_c \tau_{ikc}\Phi'_{ikc}\nabla I_i(y) \times \nabla F_i(x) \right\}$$
$$\text{and } \frac{\partial LL}{\partial F_m} = \sum_x \frac{1}{LH(x)} \sum_k \frac{\partial \pi_{kx|F_m}}{\partial F_m} p(\mathbf{I}(x)|k_x, \theta, \{F_i\}), \quad (5)$$

where $y = F_i(x)$. The computation of $\frac{\partial \pi_{kx|F_m}}{\partial F_m}$ is related to $\frac{\partial A_k(F_m(x))}{\partial F_m}$, which equals $\nabla A_k(F_m(x)) \times \nabla F_m(x)$. Both F_m and $\{F_i\}$ are based on the free-form deformation (FFD) model concatenated with an affine transformation, which can be denoted as $F = G(D(x))$, where G and D are respectively the affine and FFD transformations [12].

2.4   Projection of the Segmentation onto the LA Surface

The fibrosis is commonly visualized and quantified on the surface of the LA, focusing on the area and position of the scarring similar to the usage of EAM system [13]. Following the clinical routines, we project the classification result of scarring onto the LA surface extracted from the MAS, based on which the quantitative analysis is performed.

3 Experiments

3.1 Materials

Data Acquisition: Cardiac MR data were acquired on a Siemens Magnetom Avanto 1.5T scanner (Siemens Medical Systems, Erlangen, Germany). Data were acquired during free-breathing using a crossed-pairs navigator positioned over the dome of the right hemi-diaphragm with navigator acceptance window size of 5 mm and CLAWS respiratory motion control [14]. The LGE MRI were acquired with resolution $1.5 \times 1.5 \times 4$ mm and reconstructed to $.75 \times .75 \times 2$ mm, the Ana-MRI were acquired with $1.6 \times 1.6 \times 3.2$ mm, and reconstructed to $0.8 \times 0.8 \times 1.6$ mm. Figure 1 provides an example of the images within the ROI.

Patient Information: In agreement with the local regional ethics committee, cardiac MRI was performed in longstanding persistent AF patients. Thirty-six cases had been retrospectively entered into this study.

Ground truth and Evaluation: The 36 LGE-MRI images were all manually segmented by experienced radiologists specialized in cardiac MRI to label the enhanced atrial scarring regions, which were considered as the ground truth for evaluation of the automatic methods. Since, the clinical quantification of the LA fibrosis is made with the EAM system which only focuses on the surface area of atrial fibrosis, both the manual and automatic segmentation results were projected onto the LA surface mesh [13]. The Dice score of the two areas in the projected surface was then computed as the accuracy of the scar quantification. The Accuracy, Sensitivity and Specificity measurements between the two classification results were also evaluated.

Atlases for MAS and Probability Map: First we obtained 30 Ana-MRI images from the KCL LA segmentation grand challenge, together with manual segmentations of the left atrium, pulmonary veins and appendages [7]. In these data, we further labelled the left and right ventricles, the right atrium, the aorta and the pulmonary artery, to generate 30 whole heart atlases for target-to-image registration. These 30 images were employed only for building an independent multi-atlas data set, which will then be used for registering to the Ana-MRI data that linked with the LGE MRI scans of the AF patients.

Table 1. Quantitative evaluation results of the five schemes.

Method	Accuracy	Sensitivity	Specificity	Dice
OSTU$^{+AnaMRI}$	0.395 ± 0.181	0.731 ± 0.165	0212 ± 0.115	0.281 ± 0.129
GMM$^{+AnaMRI}$	0.569 ± 0.132	0.950 ± 0.164	0.347 ± 0.133	0.464 ± 0.133
MvMM	0.809 ± 0.150	0.905 ± 0.080	0.698 ± 0.238	0.556 ± 0.187

3.2   Result

For comparisons, we included the results using OSTU threshold [15] and conventional GMM [11]. Both the two schemes however could not generate scar segmentation directly from the LGE MRI. Therefore, we employed the whole heart segmentation results from combination of Ana-MRI and LGE MRI. We generated a mask of the LA wall for OSTU threshold and used the same probability map of LA wall for GMM. Therefore, the two methods are indicated as OSTU$^{+\text{AnaMRI}}$ and GMM$^{+\text{AnaMRI}}$, respectively.

Table 1 presents the quantitative statistical results of three methods, and Fig. 3 (left) provides the corresponding box plots. Here, the proposed method is denoted as MvMM. The proposed method performed evidently better than the two compared methods with statistical significance ($p < 0.03$), even though both OSTU and GMM used the initial segmentation of LA wall or probabilistic map computed from MAS of the combined LGE MRI and Ana-MRI. It should be noted that without Ana-MRI, the direct segmentation of the LA wall from LGE MRI could fail, which results in a failure of the LA scar segmentation or quantification by the OSTU or GMM.

Figure 3 (right) visualizes three examples for illustrating the segmentation and quantification of scarring for clinical usages. These three cases were selected from the first quarter, median, third quarter cases of the test subjects according to their Dice scores by the proposed MvMM method. The figure presents both the results from the manual delineation and the automatic segmentation by MvMM for comparisons. Even though the first quarter case has much better Dice score, the accuracy of the localizing and quantifying the scarring can be similar to that of the other two cases. This is confirmed by the comparable results using the other measurements as indicators of quantification performance, 0.932 VS 0.962 VS 0.805 (Accuracy), 0.960 VS 0.973 VS 0.794 (Sensitivity) and 0.746 VS 0.772

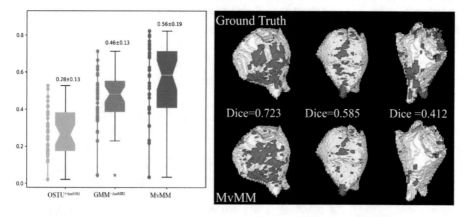

Fig. 3. Left: the box plots of the three results. Right: the 3D visualization of the three cases from the first quarter, median and third quarter of MvMM segmentation in terms of Dice with the ground truth.

VS 0.983 (Specificity) for the three cases. This is because when the scarring area is small, the Dice score of the results tends to be low. Note that for all the pre-ablation scans of our AF patients, the scars may be relatively rare to see.

4 Conclusion

We have presented a new method, based on the maximum likelihood estimator of multivariate images, for LA wall segmentation and scar quantification, combining the complementary information of two cardiac MRI modalities. The two images of the same subject are aligned to a common space and the segmentation of them is performed simultaneously. To compensate the deformations of the images to the common space, we formulate the MvMM with transformations and propose to use ICM to optimize the different groups of parameters. We evaluated the proposed techniques using 36 data sets acquired from AF patients. The combined segmentation and quantification of LA scarring yielded promising results, Accuracy: 0.809, Sensitivity: 0.905, Specificity: 0.698, Dice: 0.556, which is difficult to achieve for the methods solely based on single-sequence cardiac MRI. In conclusion, the proposed MvMM is a generic, novel and useful model for multivariate image analysis. It has the potential of achieving good performance in other applications where multiple images from the same subject are available for complementary and simultaneous segmentation.

References

1. Akcakaya, M., et al.: Accelerated late gadolinium enhancement cardiac MR imaging with isotropic spatial resolution using compressed sensing: initial experience. Radiology **264**(3), 691–699 (2012)
2. Karim, R., et al.: Evaluation of current algorithms for segmentation of scar tissue from late gadolinium enhancement cardiovascular magnetic resonance of the left atrium: an open-access grand challenge. J. Card. Mag. Res. **15**(1), 105–121 (2013)
3. Oakes, R.S., et al.: Detection and quantification of left atrial structural remodeling with delayed-enhancement magnetic resonance imaging in patients with atrial fibrillation. Circulation **119**, 1758–1767 (2009)
4. Perry, D., et al.: Automatic classification of scar tissue in late gadolinium enhancement cardiac MRI for the assessment of left-atrial wall injury after radiofrequency ablation. In: Proceedings of SPIE, vol. 8315, pp. 83151D–83151D-9 (2012)
5. Veni, G., et al.: Proper ordered meshing of complex shapes and optimal graph cuts applied to atrial-wall segmentation from DE-MRI. ISB **I**, 1296–1299 (2013)
6. Veni, G., et al.: A Bayesian formulation of graph-cut surface estimation with global shape priors. ISB **I**, 368–371 (2015)
7. Tobon-Gomez, C., et al.: Benchmark for algorithms segmenting the left atrium from 3D CT and MRI datasets. IEEE Trans. Med. Image **34**(7), 1460–1473 (2015)
8. Karim, R., et al.: Segmentation challenge on the quantification of left atrial wall thickness. In: Mansi, T., McLeod, K., Pop, M., Rhode, K., Sermesant, M., Young, A. (eds.) STACOM 2016. LNCS, vol. 10124, pp. 193–200. Springer, Cham (2017). https://doi.org/10.1007/978-3-319-52718-5_21

9. Zhuang, X., et al.: A registration-based propagation framework for automatic whole heart segmentation of cardiac MRI. IEEE Trans. Med. Image **29**(9), 1612–1625 (2010)
10. Zhuang, X., Shen, J.: Multi-scale patch and multi-modality atlases for whole heart segmentation of MRI. Med. Image Ana. **31**, 77–87 (2016)
11. Leemput, K.V., et al.: Automated model-based tissue classification of MR images of the brain. IEEE Trans. Med. Image **18**(10), 897–908 (1999)
12. Rueckert, D., et al.: Nonrigid registration using free-form deformations: application to breast MR images. IEEE Trans. Med. Image **18**, 712–721 (1999)
13. Williams, S.E., et al.: Standardized unfold mapping: a technique to permit left atrial regional data display and analysis. J. Int. Card. Electrophysiol. **50**(1), 125–131 (2017)
14. Keegan, J., et al.: Navigator artifact reduction in three-dimensional late gadolinium enhancement imaging of the atria. Mag. Res. Med. **72**(3), 779–785 (2014)
15. Otsu, N.: A threshold selection method from gray-level histograms. IEEE Trans. Syst. Man Cybern. SMC **9**(1), 62–66 (1979)

Left Ventricle Segmentation via Optical-Flow-Net from Short-Axis Cine MRI: Preserving the Temporal Coherence of Cardiac Motion

Wenjun Yan[1], Yuanyuan Wang[1(✉)], Zeju Li[1], Rob J. van der Geest[2], and Qian Tao[2(✉)]

[1] Department of Electrical Engineering, Fudan University, Shanghai, China
yywang@fudan.edu.cn
[2] Department of Radiology, Leiden University Medical Center,
Leiden, The Netherlands
Q.Tao@lumc.nl

Abstract. Quantitative assessment of left ventricle (LV) function from cine MRI has significant diagnostic and prognostic value for cardiovascular disease patients. The temporal movement of LV provides essential information on the contracting/relaxing pattern of heart, which is keenly evaluated by clinical experts in clinical practice. Inspired by the expert way of viewing Cine MRI, we propose a new CNN module that is able to incorporate the temporal information into LV segmentation from cine MRI. In the proposed CNN, the optical flow (OF) between neighboring frames is integrated and aggregated at feature level, such that temporal coherence in cardiac motion can be taken into account during segmentation. The proposed module is integrated into the U-net architecture without need of additional training. Furthermore, dilated convolution is introduced to improve the spatial accuracy of segmentation. Trained and tested on the Cardiac Atlas database, the proposed network resulted in a Dice index of 95% and an average perpendicular distance of 0.9 pixels for the middle LV contour, significantly outperforming the original U-net that processes each frame individually. Notably, the proposed method improved the temporal coherence of LV segmentation results, especially at the LV apex and base where the cardiac motion is difficult to follow.

Keywords: Cine MRI · Optical flow · U-net · Feature aggregation

1 Introduction

1.1 Left Ventricle Segmentation

Cardiovascular disease is a major cause of mortality and morbidity worldwide. Accurate assessment of cardiac function is very important for diagnosis and prognosis of cardiovascular disease patients. Cine magnetic resonance imaging (MRI) is the current gold standard to assess the cardiac function [1], covering different imaging planes (around 10) and cardiac phases (ranging from 20 to 40).

The large number of total images (200–400) poses significant challenges for manual analysis in clinical practice, therefore computer-aided analysis of cine MRI has

© Springer Nature Switzerland AG 2018
A. F. Frangi et al. (Eds.): MICCAI 2018, LNCS 11073, pp. 613–621, 2018.
https://doi.org/10.1007/978-3-030-00937-3_70

been actively studied for decades. Most traditional methods in literature are based on dedicated mathematical models of shape and intensity [2]. However, the substantial variations in the cine images, including the acquisition parameters, image quality, heart morphology/pathology, etc., all make it too challenging, if not impossible, for traditional image analysis methods to reach a clinically acceptable balance of accuracy, robustness, and generalizability. As such, in current practice, the analysis of cine images still involves significant manual work, including contour tracing, or initialization and correction to aid semi-automated computer methods.

Current development of deep Convolutional Neural Networks (CNN) has made revolutionary improvement on many medical image analysis problems, including automated cine MRI analysis [3, 4]. In most of the CNN-based framework for cine MRI, nevertheless, the segmentation problem is still formulated as learning a label image from a given cine image, i.e. each frame is individually processed and there is no guarantee of temporal coherence in the segmentation results.

1.2   Our Motivation and Contribution

This is in contrast to what we have observed in clinical practice, as clinical experts always view the cine MRI as a temporal sequence instead of individual frames, paying close attention to the temporally-resolving motion of the heart. Inspired by the expert way of view cine MRI, we aim to integrate the temporal information to guide and regulate LV segmentation, in an easily interpretable manner.

Between temporally neighboring frames, there are two types of useful information: (1) *Difference*: the relative movement of the object between neighboring frames, providing clues of object location and motion. (2) *Similarity*: sufficient coherence exists between temporally neighboring frames, with the temporal resolution of cine set to follow cardiac motion. In this work, we proposed to use optical flow to extract the object location and motion information, while aggregating such information over a moving time window to enforce temporal coherence. Both difference and similarity measures were formulated into one module, named "optical flow feature aggregation sub-network", which is integrated into the U-net architecture. Compared to the prevailing recurrent neural network (RNN) applied to temporal sequences [4], our method eliminates the need of introducing massive learnable RNN parameters, while preserving the simplicity and elegancy of U-net. In relatively simple scenarios like cine MRI, our proposed method has high interpretability and low computation cost.

2   Method

2.1   Optical Flow in Cine MRI

Given two neighboring temporal frames in cine MRI, the optical flow field can be calculated to infer the horizontal and vertical motion of objects in image [4], by the following equation and constraint:

$$I(x, y, t) = I(x + \Delta x, y + \Delta y, t + \Delta t) \tag{1}$$

$$\frac{\partial I}{\partial x} V_x + \frac{\partial I}{\partial y} V_y + \frac{\partial I}{\partial t} = 0 \tag{2}$$

where V_x, V_y are the velocity components of the pixel at location x and y in image I. As the major moving object in the field of view, the optical flow provides essential information on the location of LV, as well as its mode of motion, as illustrated in Fig. 1, in which the background is clearly suppressed.

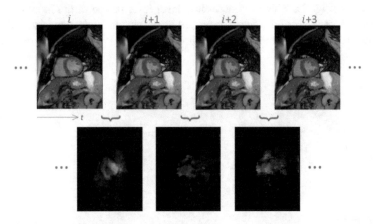

Fig. 1. Illustration of optical flow in cine MRI between temporal frames. The flow field (lower panel) reflects the local displacement between two frames (upper panel).

2.2 Optical Flow Feature Aggregation

We propose to integrate the optical flow into the feature maps, which are extracted by convolutional kernels:

$$m_{j \to i} = I(m_i, O_{j \to i}) \tag{3}$$

where $I(\cdot)$ is the bilinear interpolation function as is often used as a warp function in computer vision for motion compensation [5], m_i represents the feature maps of frame i, $O_{j \to i}$ is the optical flow field from frame j to frame i, and $m_{j \to i}$ represents the motion-compensated feature maps.

We further aggregated the optical flow information over a longer time span in the cardiac cycle. The aggregated feature map is defined as follows:

$$\bar{m}_i = \sum_{j=i-k}^{j=i+k} w_{j \to i} m_{j \to i} \tag{4}$$

where k denotes the number of temporal frames before and after the target frame. Larger k indicates higher capability to follow temporal movement but heavier computation load. We used $k = 2$ as an empirical choice to balance computation load and capture range. The weight map $w_{j\rightarrow i}$ measures the cosine similarity between feature maps m_j and m_i at all x and y locations, defined as:

$$w_{j\rightarrow i} = \frac{m_j \cdot m_i}{|m_j||m_i|} \tag{5}$$

The feature map m_i and m_j contain all channels of features extracted by convolutional kernels (Fig. 2), which represent low-level information of the input image, such as location, intensity, and edge. Computed over all channels, $w_{j\rightarrow i}$ describes local similarity between two temporally neighboring frames. By introducing the weighted

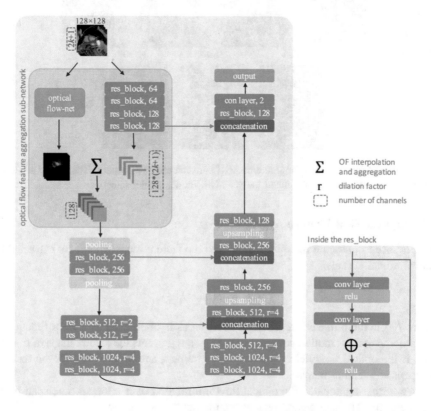

Fig. 2. The proposed OF-net, including three new characteristics: (1) the optical flow feature aggregation sub-network, (2) res-block, and (3) dilated convolution.

feature map, we assign higher weights on locations with little temporal movement for coherent segmentation, while lower weights on locations with larger movement to allow changes.

2.3   Optical Flow Net (OF-net)

The proposed optical flow feature aggregation is integrated into the U-net architect, which we name as optical flow net (OF-net). The OF-net consists of the following new characteristics compared to the original U-net:

Optical Flow Feature Aggregation Sub-network: The first part of the contracting path is made of a sub-network of optical flow feature aggregation described in Sects. 2.1 and 2.2. With this sub-network embedded, the segmentation of an individual frame takes into consideration information from neighboring frames, both before and after it, and the aggregation acts as a "memory" as well as a prediction. The aggregated feature maps are then fed into the subsequent path, as shown in Fig. 2.

Dilated Convolution: The max-pooling operation reduces the image size to enlarge the receptive field, causing loss of resolution. Unlike in the classification problem, resolution can be important for segmentation performance. To improve the LV segmentation accuracy, we propose to use dilated convolution [6] to replace part of the max-pooling operation. As illustrated in Fig. 3, dilated convolution enlarges the receptive field by increasing the size of convolution kernels. We replaced max-pooling with dilated convolution in 8 deep layers as shown in Fig. 2.

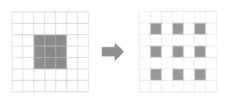

Fig. 3. Dilated convolution by a factor of 2. Left: the normal convolutional kernel, right: the dilated convolution kernel, which expands the receptive field by a factor of 2 without adding more parameters. Blue indicates active parameters of the kernel while white are inactivated, i.e. set to zero.

Res-Block: To mitigate the vanishing gradient problem in deep CNNs, all blocks in the U-net (i.e. a convolutional layer, a batch normalization layer, and a ReLU unit) were updated to res-block [7], as illustrated in Fig. 2.

The proposed OF-net preserves the U-shape architecture, and its training can be performed the same way as U-net without need of joint-training, as optical flow between MRI frames only need to be computed once. Simplified algorithm is summarized in Algorithm 1. $N_{feature}$, $N_{segment}$ are sub-networks of feature extractor and segmentation, respectively. $P(\cdot)$ denotes computation of optical flow.

Algorithm 1: the proposed OF-net.

input: n cine MR frames $\{f_i\}$, aggregation parameter k

for $j = 1:n$ **do**

    $m_j = N_{feature}(f_j)$

end for

for $i = 1:n$ **do**

    for $j = max(1, i - k): min(n, i + k)$ **do**

        $O_{j \to i} = P(f_j, f_i)$

        $m_{j \to i} = I(m_j, O_{j \to i})$

        $m_{j \to i}^n = softmax(m_{j \to i})$

        $w_{j \to i} = \frac{m_j^n \cdot m_i^n}{|m_j^n| \, ||m_i^n|}$

    end for

    $\bar{m}_i = \sum_{j=max\,(1,i-k)}^{j=min\,(n,i+k)} w_{j \to i} \, m_{j \to i}$

    $p_i = N_{segment}(\bar{m}_i)$

end for

output: predicted segmentation $\{p_i\}$

---

3 Experiments and Results

3.1 Data and Ground Truth

Experiments were performed on the short-axis steady-state free precession (SSFP) cine MR images of 100 patients with coronary artery disease and prior myocardial infarction from the Cardiac Atlas database [8]. A large variability exists in the dataset: the MRI scanner systems included GE Medical Systems (Signa 1.5T), Philips Medical Systems (Achieva 1.5T, 3.0T, and Intera 1.5T), and Siemens (Avanto 1.5T, Espree 1.5T and Symphony 1.5T); image size varied from 138×192 to 512×512 pixels; and the number of frames per cardiac cycle ranged from 19 to 30.

Ground truth annotations of the LV myocardium and blood pool in every image were a consensus result of various raters including two fully-automated raters and three semi-automated raters demanding initial manual input. We randomly selected 66 subjects out of 100 for training (12,720 images) and the rest for testing (6,646 images). All cine MR and label images were cropped at the center to a size of 128×128. To suppress the variability in intensity range, each cine scan was normalized to a uniform signal intensity range of $[0, 255]$. Data augmentation was performed by random rotation within $[-30°, 30°]$, resulting in 50,880 training images.

3.2   Network Parameters and Performance Evaluation

We used stochastic gradient descent optimization with an exponentially-decaying learning rate of 10^{-4} and a mini-batch size of 10. The number of epochs was 30. Using the same training parameters, 3 CNNs were trained: (1) the original U-net, (2) the OF-net with max-pooling, (3) the OF-net with dilated convolution. The performance of LV segmentation was evaluated in terms of Dice overlap index and average perpendicular distance (APD) between the ground truth and CNN segmentation results. Since LV segmentation is known to have different degree of difficulty at apex, middle, and base, we evaluated the performance in the three segments separately.

3.3   Results

The Dice and APD of the three CNNs are reported in Table 1. It can be seen that the proposed OF-net outperformed the original U-net at all segments of LV ($p < 0.001$), and with the dilated convolution introduced, the performance is further enhanced ($p < 0.001$).

Some examples of the LV segmentation results at apex, middle, and base of LV are shown in Fig. 4. It can be observed from (a)–(c) that the proposed method is able to detect a very small myocardium ring at the apex which may be missed by the original U-net. From (g)–(i) it is seen that the OF-net eliminates localization failure at the base. In the middle slices (d)–(f), the OF-net also produced smoother outcome than the original U-net which processes each slice individually. The effect of integrating temporal information is better illustrated in Fig. 5, in which we plotted the myocardium (upper panel) and blood pool (lower panel) area, as determined by the resulting endocardial and epicardial contours, against frame index in a cardiac cycle. It can be observed that the results produced by OF-net is smoother and closer to the ground truth than those produced by U-net, showing improved temporal coherence of segmentation.

In Fig. 6, we illustrate the mechanism how aggregated feature map can help preserve the temporal coherence: the 14th channel in the sub-network is a localizer of LV. While localization of LV in one frame can be missed, the aggregated information from neighboring frames can correct for it and lead to coherent segmentation.

Table 1. Comparison of performance of the three CNNs: (1) the original U-net, (2) the OF-net with max-pooling, (3) the OF-net with dilated convolution. Performance is differentiated at apex, middle, and base of LV. Paired t-test is done comparing (2) and (1), (3) and (2).

	Apex			Middle			Base		
	Dice (%)	APD (pixel)	p value	Dice (%)	APD (pixel)	p value	Dice (%)	APD (pixel)	p value
U-net	73.3 ± 4.3	1.67 ± 0.25		91.2 ± 4.0	1.21 ± 0.16		82.4 ± 4.6	1.41 ± 0.19	
OF-net (max-pooling)	81.9 ± 3.2	1.19 ± 0.18	<0.0001	92.3 ± 3.6	0.95 ± 0.11	<0.0001	86.3 ± 2.9	0.99 ± 0.14	<0.0001
OF-net (dilated conv)	**84.5 ± 3.7**	**1.04 ± 0.11**	**<0.0001**	**94.8 ± 3.2**	**0.90 ± 0.09**	**<0.0001**	**89.3 ± 2.5**	**0.94 ± 0.12**	**<0.0001**

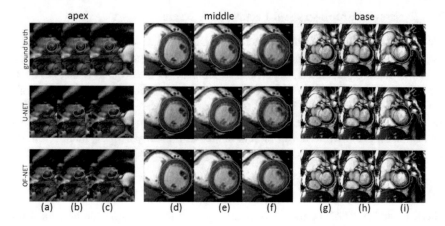

Fig. 4. Examples of temporal frames at different locations: apex (a)–(c), middle (d)–(f), and base (g)–(i). From top to bottom, the contours are delineated from the ground truth, U-net, and the proposed OF-net, respectively.

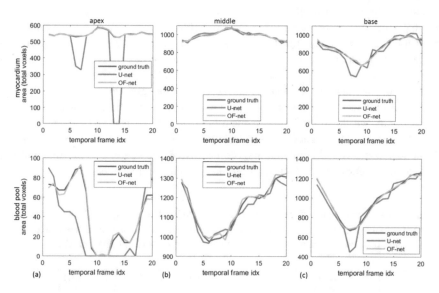

Fig. 5. Examples of myocardium (upper) and blood pool (lower) area in a cardiac cycle, estimated from the ground truth, U-net, and OF-net, at apex, middle, and base.

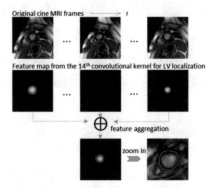

Fig. 6. Effect of feature aggregation. In the middle frame, the feature map related to "LV location" did not activate. The proposed feature aggregation could retrieve the location of LV based on temporally neighboring slices.

4 Conclusion

We have proposed an OF-net for fully automated segmentation of LV from cine MRI. The network integrates temporal information to imitate the expert way of viewing cine. Evaluated on the Cardiac Atlas database, the method outperformed the original U-net, producing more accurate and temporally-coherent LV segmentation.

Acknowledgements. This work was supported by National Key Research and Development Program of China (No. 2018YFC0116303).

References

1. de Roos, A., Higgins, C.B.: Cardiac radiology: centenary review. Radiology **273**(2S), S142–S159 (2014)
2. Peng, P., Lekadir, K., Gooya, A., Shao, L., Petersen, S.E., Frangi, A.F.: A review of heart chamber segmentation for structural and functional analysis using cardiac magnetic resonance imaging. Magma **29**, 155–195 (2016)
3. Litjens, G., et al.: A survey on deep learning in medical image analysis. Med. Image Anal. **42**, 60–88 (2017)
4. Xue, W., Lum, A., Mercado, A., Landis, M., Warrington, J., Li, S.: Full quantification of left ventricle via deep multitask learning network respecting intra- and inter-task relatedness. In: Descoteaux, M., Maier-Hein, L., Franz, A., Jannin, P., Collins, D.L., Duchesne, S. (eds.) MICCAI 2017. LNCS, vol. 10435, pp. 276–284. Springer, Cham (2017). https://doi.org/10.1007/978-3-319-66179-7_32
5. Zhu, X., Wang, Y., Dai, J., Yuan, L., Wei, Y.: Flow-guided feature aggregation for video object detection. In: ICCV, pp. 408–417, October 2017
6. Yu, F., Koltun, V.: Multi-scale context aggregation by dilated convolutions. In: ICLR, May 2016
7. He, K., Zhang, X., Ren, S., Sun, J.: Deep residual learning for image recognition. In: CVPR, pp. 770–778, June 2016
8. Fonseca, C.G., et al.: The cardiac atlas project–an imaging database for computational modeling and statistical atlases of the heart. Bioinformatics **27**(16), 2288–2295 (2011)

VoxelAtlasGAN: 3D Left Ventricle Segmentation on Echocardiography with Atlas Guided Generation and Voxel-to-Voxel Discrimination

Suyu Dong[1], Gongning Luo[1], Kuanquan Wang[1], Shaodong Cao[2],
Ashley Mercado[3,4], Olga Shmuilovich[3,4], Henggui Zhang[1,5(✉)], and Shuo Li[3,4]

[1] Harbin Institute of Technology, Harbin, China
[2] Department of Radiology, The Fourth Hospital of Harbin Medical University,
Harbin, China
[3] Department of Medical Imaging, Western University, London, ON, Canada
[4] Digital Image Group (DIG), London, ON N6A 3K7, Canada
[5] University of Manchester, Manchester, UK
henggui.zhang@manchester.ac.uk

Abstract. 3D left ventricle (LV) segmentation on echocardiography is very important for diagnosis and treatment of cardiac disease. It is not only because of that echocardiography is a real-time imaging technology and widespread in clinical application, but also because of that LV segmentation on 3D echocardiography can provide more full volume information of heart than LV segmentation on 2D echocardiography. However, 3D LV segmentation on echocardiography is still an open and challenging task owing to the lower contrast, higher noise and data dimensionality, limited annotation of 3D echocardiography. In this paper, we proposed a novel real-time framework, i.e., VoxelAtlasGAN, for 3D LV segmentation on 3D echocardiography. This framework has three contributions: (1) It is based on voxel-to-voxel conditional generative adversarial nets (cGAN). For the first time, cGAN is used for 3D LV segmentation on echocardiography. And cGAN advantageously fuses substantial 3D spatial context information from 3D echocardiography by self-learning structured loss; (2) For the first time, it embeds the atlas into an end-to-end optimization framework, which uses 3D LV atlas as a powerful prior knowledge to improve the inference speed, address the lower contrast and the limited annotation problems of 3D echocardiography; (3) It combines traditional discrimination loss and the new proposed consistent constraint, which further improves the generalization of the proposed framework. VoxelAtlasGAN was validated on 60 subjects on 3D echocardiography and it achieved satisfactory segmentation results and high inference speed. The mean surface distance is 1.85 mm, the mean hausdorff surface distance is 7.26 mm, mean dice is 0.953, the correlation of EF is 0.918, and the mean inference speed is 0.1 s. These results have demonstrated that our proposed method has great potential for clinical application.

Keywords: Voxel-to-voxel conditional generative adversarial nets
Atlas · 3D left ventricle segmentation · Echocardiography

© Springer Nature Switzerland AG 2018
A. F. Frangi et al. (Eds.): MICCAI 2018, LNCS 11073, pp. 622–629, 2018.
https://doi.org/10.1007/978-3-030-00937-3_71

1 Introduction

3D left ventricle segmentation on echocardiography, which directly uses full volume as input, is very important for diagnosis and treatment of cardiac disease. This is because of echocardiography now is the most widely used imaging modality by clinician [1], and 3D LV segmentation on echocardiography has an inherent advantage on 3D spatial context information, which is capable of providing more anatomical structure information for clinician. For example, it is possible that there is no LV boundary in some 2D echocardiography slices. While 3D echocardiography combines the full context information, so we can infer the disappeared boundary based on context information. Hence, 3D left ventricle segmentation on echocardiography, compared to the traditional 2D LV segmentation on echocardiography, has more clinical value and has become a hot topic nowadays.

However, 3D LV segmentation on echocardiography is still an open and challenging task owing to the following intrinsic limitations: lower contrast, higher noise and data dimensionality, limited annotation of 3D echocardiography. (1) 3D echocardiography has a lower contrast between the LV borders and surrounding tissue than 2D echocardiography [2], so that 3D LV segmentation will be more likely to have leakage and shrinkage. (2) 3D echocardiography has the higher dimensionality and is more complex than 2D echocardiography, so obtaining better expressive features to achieve accurate segmentation with high processing speed is difficult. (3) Up to now, annotated 3D echocardiography are limited, so it is difficult to train a model to achieve high generalization on 3D LV segmentation task based on the limited annotation 3D echocardiography. Hence, how to utilize 3D echocardiography's advantages and overcome its difficulties to get more accurate 3D LV segmentation results is an urgent problem.

Although some methods have been proposed to segment 3D LV on echocardiography [3], these methods are still difficult to overcome the above challenging completely [4]. Deformable models and statistical models are widely used for the LV segmentation in echocardiography [5]. However, these methods are sensitive to the large variations of intensity and unable to deal with the low contrast images. Machine learning methods, which use handcrafted features usually, also have been used to segment 3D LV [6], yet they have limited representation capability to represent the higher dimensionality 3D echocardiography data, complex structure and appearance variations between different subjects. Recently, deep convolutional neural networks (CNNs) [7] have been implemented for 3D LV segmentation and it improve the accuracy [8], yet they need large computation depending on the complex 3D CNNs's structure.

In this paper, we proposed a novel automated framework (VoxelAtlasGAN) for 3D LV segmentation on echocardiography. The proposed framework has three contributions: **(1) It uses conditional generative adversarial nets (cGAN) [9] on voxel-to-voxel mode, which is used for 3D LV segmentation on echocardiography for the first time. Hence, the proposed framework advantageously fuses substantial 3D spatial context information from 3D echocardiography by self-learning structured loss;**

624   S. Dong et al.

**(2) For the first time, based on cGAN, it embeds the atlas segmenta-
tion problem into an end-to-end optimization framework and which
uses 3D LV atlas as powerful prior knowledge. In this way, it not only
improves the inference speed but also addresses the lower contrast and
the limited annotation problems of 3D echocardiography; (3) It combines the traditional discrimination loss and new proposed consistent
constraint, which further improves the generalization of the proposed
framework.** Experiment results have demonstrated that our proposed method
can obtain satisfactory segmentation accuracy and has the potential for clinical
application.

2   Methods

VoxelAtlasGAN is demonstrated in Fig. 1. Different from usual cGAN, VoxelAtlasGAN adopts a voxel-to-voxel cGAN for high-quality 3D LV segmentation on
echocardiography. It uses atlas to provide prior knowledge for 3D generator to
guide segmentation, and it combines consistent constraint with discrimination
loss as the final optimization object to improve the generalization.

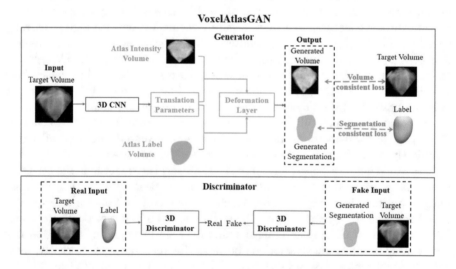

Fig. 1. Framework of the proposed VoxelAtlasGAN.

2.1   Voxel-to-Voxel cGAN for High-Quality 3D LV Segmentation

Voxel-to-voxel cGAN is designed to automatically achieve high-quality 3D LV
segmentation on echocardiography. It adopts full volume as the input which is
useful to acquire and exploit substantial 3D spatial context information in 3D
echocardiography, hence we call it 'voxel-to-voxel' cGAN.

Advantages of cGAN Compared with CNNs: (1) The recently proposed cGAN can automatically learn loss function which satisfyingly adapts to data. For segmentation problem, cGAN learns a loss that tries to discriminate the output which is ground truth label or segmentation result from generator, and this loss is minimized by training a generative model. (2) cGAN learns a structured loss, which considers each output pixel depending on the other pixels from the input image, to penalize any possible structure differences between output and target. Hence, the proposed method is based on cGAN for high-quality 3D LV segmentation.

Structure of VoxelAtlasGAN: Based on the above advantages of cGAN, we designed novel networks for VoxelAtlasGAN. To address the lower contrast and the limited annotation problems of 3D echocardiography, the proposed method combines atlas prior knowledge, i.e., we formulate the traditional atlas segmentation procedure into the proposed end-to-end deep learning framework (which will be detailed in Sect. 2.2). The specific structure of VoxelAtlasGAN is following. **Generator:** it has five 3D convolution layers, one fully connected layer, and one atlas deformation layer. Specially, the fully connected layer has w nodes, and the w is the number of parameters for translation function of atlas. Besides, the atlas deformation layer models the deformation registration procedure of atlas segmentation. And 3D echocardiography volumes are directly used as the input of the generator. **Discriminator:** the proposed discriminator also has five 3D convolution layers and one fully connected layer with two nodes (to classify real or fake). And we use 3D echocardiography volume with the corresponding label and 3D echocardiography volume with the corresponding segmentation result as the input of discriminator. **The optimization object:** the proposed VoxelAtlasGAN combines discrimination loss and the new proposed consistent constraint (consistent segmentation constraint and consistent intensity volume constraint) as the optimization object, which will be detailed in Sect. 2.3.

2.2 Atlas Guided Generation

Advantages of Atlas Guided Generation: Atlas prior knowledge is able to provide basic anatomical shape information of LV, and incorporating such prior knowledge is crucial for the improvement of LV segmentation performance. Hence, the proposed method embeds the atlas into end-to-end optimization of cGAN framework to provide powerful prior knowledge to overcome some problems. (1) Embedding the atlas prior into cGAN addresses the lower contrast problem of 3D echocardiography through direct registration segmentation method. (2) Embedding the atlas prior into cGAN addresses the limited annotation data problem, due to the proposed method no longer depends on the large numbers of training data to model the shape prior. (3) Embedding the atlas prior into cGAN avoids the complex and time-consuming computation of traditional atlas-based methods, because of that the proposed method formulates the transformation parameters optimization problem into the end-to-end deep learning framework (cGAN), which is based on the differentiability of transformation parameters on atlas segmentation procedure. (4) Embedding the atlas segmentation procedure into cGAN enhances the interpretability of cGAN.

Atlas Deformation Layer: Specifically, the transformation function of atlas segmentation includes global rigid transformation T_{global} using affine transformation and local non-rigid transformation T_{local} using free-form deformations (FFD) method [10]. Hence, we model the atlas deformation layer as following:

$$T(X) = T_{local}(T_{global}(X)), X \in \{Atlas_{label\_volume}, Atlas_{intensity\_volume}\} \quad (1)$$

$$T_{global}(X) = \begin{bmatrix} \theta_1, \theta_2, \theta_3 \\ \theta_4, \theta_5, \theta_6 \\ \theta_7, \theta_8, \theta_9 \end{bmatrix} * X + \begin{bmatrix} \theta_{10} \\ \theta_{11} \\ \theta_{12} \end{bmatrix} \quad (2)$$

$$T_{local}(T_{global}(X)) = B_\phi(T_{global}(X)) \quad (3)$$

where T denotes the final deformation function for atlas transformation, X denotes the 3D LV atlas including atlas label volume $Atlas_{label\_volume}$ and atlas intensity volume $Atlas_{intensity\_volume}$, θ is rigid affine transformation parameter set including 12 parameters, B is the B-spline function, and ϕ is the control point set (which is the parameter set of non-rigid FFD transformation). Specially, B-spline FFD is initialized by 1000 equidistant control points with 3000 parameters to control deformation. To embed the 3012 transformation parameters into end-to-end cGAN, we make the output of the fully connected layer (which in the generator network of cGAN) has 3012 nodes. Hence, 3012 deformation parameters of transformation function are formulated as corresponding 3012 latent variables, which are solved by unified deep learning optimization framework. Besides, in this way, model's interpretability is strong compared with common deep learning methods, because the 3012 deformation parameters are inherently clear for transformation function for atlas deformation layer.

Additionally, in this work, atlas was built from the mean space of a set of 3D echocardiography. To avoid segmentation biases to specific noise and artifacts, we employed 3D echocardiographies which were acquired using two devices to construct atlas. They were registered to mean space. Atlas intensity volume and atlas label volume were computed from this set of registered 3D echocardiography and corresponding registered segmentation results respectively. In the test stage, based on atlas and the learned translation parameters, we obtained the final 3D LV segmentation results through the generator of VoxelAtlasGAN.

2.3   Voxel-to-Voxel Discrimination with Consistent Constraint

Based on the shared deformation layer, the consistent constraint, including segmentation consistent constraint and volume consistent constraint, is proposed as a part of cGAN's loss function to naturally guarantee the generalization of the proposed framework and further improve the segmentation accuracy. The segmentation consistent constraint measures the similarity between the ground truth labels and the generated segmentation results. Analogously, the volume consistent constraint measures the similarity between the input volumes and the generated intensity volumes. Hence, the final optimization object of the proposed VoxelAtlasGAN is:

$$\arg \min_{G} \max_{D} L_{VoxelAtlasGAN} = L_{cGAN}(G, D) + \alpha L_{label}(G) + \beta L_{intensity}(G) \quad (4)$$

where G denotes the generator of VoxelAtlasGAN, D denotes the discriminator of VoxelAtlasGAN, $L_{cGAN}(G, D)$ denotes the cGAN loss, $L_{label}(G)$ and $L_{intensity}(G)$ denote the segmentation consistent constraint and volume consistent constraint with weights α and β respectively. The cGAN loss is:

$$L_{cGan}(G, D) = \log D(x, y) + \log(1 - D(x, G_{label\_volume})) \quad (5)$$

where G and D have the same denotations with above equations (4), x denotes the target volume, y denotes the ground truth label, and G_{label_volume} is the generated segmentation result from generator. Specially, segmentation consistent constraint is modeled by L1 norm:

$$L_{label}(G) = \|y - G_{label\_volume}\|_1 \quad (6)$$

Because the 3D echocardiography exist large random noisy and high intensity variability, the volume consistent constraint is modeled through normalized mutual information method [11], which has high robustness on similarity measurement. The volume consistent constraint is:

$$L_{intensity}(G) = -(H(x) + H(G_{intensity\_volume}))/H(x, G_{intensity\_volume}) \quad (7)$$

where $G_{intensity\_volume}$ denotes the intensity volume from generator, $H(x)$ and $H(G_{intensity\_volume})$ denote the marginal entropies of x and $G_{intensity\_volume}$ respectively, and $H(x, G_{intensity\_volume})$ denotes the joint entropies of x and $G_{intensity\_volume}$.

3   Dataset and Setting

VoxelAtlasGAN is validated on 3D echocardiography with 25 training subjects and 35 validation subjects. Each subject includes two labeled volumes in the end-systole (ES) and end-diastole (ED) frames. The labels are obtained by three clinicians and the final labels are mutually authenticated. We adopt the same cGAN training mode with [9]. We use SGD solver, the learning rate is 0.0002, the momentum is 0.5, and the batch size is 1. At inference time, we run the generator net in the same manner as the training phase. The weights α and β for segmentation consistent constraint and volume consistent constraint are 0.6 and 0.4 respectively. The proposed VoxelAtlasGAN was implemented based on the widely used pytorch framework and the whole experiment was performed on NVIDIA Titan X GPU.

We adopt the evaluation criterions in [12] to evaluate our proposed method, which include mean surface distance (MSD), mean hausdorff surface distance (HSD), mean dice index (D), and correlation (corr) of ejection fractions (EF).

4   Results and Analysis

VoxelAtlasGAN's segmentation performance is powerfully supported in Table 1. (1) In the aspect of segmentation accuracy, we find that VoxelAtlasGAN achieves the best segmentation results. The mean surface distance, hausdorff surface distance and dice are 1.85 mm, 7.26 mm and 0.953 respectively. And the correlation of EF (between the segmentation results and the ground truth) is 0.918 and the corresponding standard deviation is 0.016. These results prove the superiority of the proposed VoxelAtlasGAN compared with the existing methods. (2) In the aspect of segmentation efficiency, the proposed method achieves the best segmentation speed, it only needs 0.1 s for segmentation of every volume, which is crucial for real-time clinical application.

We also evaluated the importance of atlas prior and the proposed consistent constraint by ablation experiments (in the last three rows of Table 1), which replace or remove a single component from our framework. The results showed that atlas prior improved the segmentation accuracy apparently, and the proposed consistent constraint also brought important improvement for segmentation. What's more, compared to the 3D CNN method, which adopts 3D full convolution network (V-net [13]) to segment 3D LV on echocardiography, the proposed voxel-to-voxel cGAN is superior even without the atlas and the proposed consistent constraint.

Table 1. The segmentation performance comparison among existing methods and the proposed VoxelAtlasGAN under different configurations. (3D cGAN denotes the VoxelAtlasGAN without atlas prior and consistent constraint, VoxelGANWA denotes VoxelAtlasGAN without consistent constraint.)

Methods	D	MSD (mm)	HSD (mm)	Corr of EF	Speed (s)
3D Atlas [14]	0.88 ± 0.03	2.26 ± 0.74	9.92 ± 2.16	0.836 ± 0.079	2000
V-net [13]	0.89 ± 0.035	2.1 ± 0.71	9.79 ± 8.9	0.86 ± 0.053	20
3D cGAN	0.914 ± 0.028	1.98 ± 0.65	8.91 ± 7.3	0.89 ± 0.032	10
VoxelGANWA	0.939 ± 0.021	1.93 ± 0.52	8.35 ± 4.57	0.907 ± 0.029	0.1
VoxelAtlasGAN	$\mathbf{0.953 \pm 0.019}$	$\mathbf{1.85 \pm 0.43}$	$\mathbf{7.26 \pm 2.3}$	$\mathbf{0.918 \pm 0.016}$	**0.1**

5   Conclusions

In this paper, we proposed a novel automated framework VoxelAtlasGAN for high-quality 3D LV segmentation on echocardiography. The proposed framework used voxel-to-voxel cGAN to advantageously fuse substantial 3D spatial context information from 3D echocardiography for the first time. Besides, it embedded the powerful atlas prior knowledge into end-to-end optimization framework for the first time. It also combined the new proposed consistent constraint and traditional discrimination loss as the final optimization object to further improve the generalization of the proposed framework. Experiment results have demonstrated that our proposed method obtained satisfactory segmentation accuracy and has potential of clinical application.

Acknowledgments. This work was supported by the Natural Science Foundation of China under Grant No. 61572152 and 61571165.

References

1. Pedrosa, J., Barbosa, D., et al.: Cardiac chamber volumetric assessment using 3D ultrasound-a review. Curr. Pharm. Des. **22**(1), 105–121 (2016)
2. Lang, R.M., Badano, L.P., et al.: EAE/ASE recommendations for image acquisition and display using three-dimensional echocardiography. J. Am. Soc. Echocardiogr. **25**(1), 3–46 (2012)
3. Leung, K.E., Bosch, J.G.: Automated border detection in three-dimensional echocardiography: principles and promises. Eur. J. Echocardiogr. **11**(2), 97–108 (2010)
4. Dong, S., Luo, G., Sun, G., Wang, K., Zhang, H.: A left ventricular segmentation method on 3D echocardiography using deep learning and snake. In: Computing in Cardiology Conference (CinC), pp. 473–476. IEEE (2016)
5. Barbosa, D., Dietenbeck, T., et al.: Fast and fully automatic 3-D echocardiographic segmentation using B-spline explicit active surfaces: feasibility study and validation in a clinical setting. Ultrasound Med. Biol. **39**(1), 89–101 (2013)
6. Yang, L., Georgescu, B., et al.: Prediction based collaborative trackers (PCT): a robust and accurate approach toward 3D medical object tracking. IEEE Trans. Med. Imaging **30**(11), 1921–1932 (2011)
7. Luo, G., Dong, S., Wang, K., Zuo, W., Cao, S., Zhang, H.: Multi-views fusion CNN for left ventricular volumes estimation on cardiac MR images. IEEE Trans. Biomed. Eng. **65**(9), 1924–1934 (2018)
8. Oktay, O., et al.: Anatomically constrained neural networks (ACNNs): application to cardiac image enhancement and segmentation. IEEE Trans. Med. Imaging **37**(2), 384–395 (2018)
9. Mirza, M., Osindero, S.: Conditional generative adversarial nets. arXiv preprint arXiv:1411.1784 (2014)
10. Rueckert, D., Sonoda, L.I., Hayes, C., Hill, D.L., Leach, M.O., Hawkes, D.J.: Non-rigid registration using free-form deformations: application to breast MR images. IEEE Trans. Med. imaging **18**(8), 712–721 (1999)
11. Zhuang, X., Rhode, K.S., Razavi, R.S., Hawkes, D.J., Ourselin, S.: A registration-based propagation framework for automatic whole heart segmentation of cardiac MRI. IEEE Trans. Med. Imaging **29**(9), 1612–1625 (2010)
12. Bernard, O., et al.: Standardized evaluation system for left ventricular segmentation algorithms in 3D echocardiography. IEEE Trans. Med. Imaging **35**(4), 967–977 (2016)
13. Milletari, F., Navab, N., Ahmadi, S.A.: V-net: fully convolutional neural networks for volumetric medical image segmentation. In: 2016 Fourth International Conference on 3D Vision (3DV), pp. 565–571. IEEE (2016)
14. Oktay, O., Shi, W., Keraudren, K., Caballero, J., Rueckert, D., Hajnal, J.: Learning shape representations for multi-atlas endocardium segmentation in 3D echo images. In: Proceedings MICCAI Challenge on Echocardiographic Three-Dimensional Ultrasound Segmentation (CETUS), Boston, MIDAS Journal, pp. 57–64 (2014)

Domain and Geometry Agnostic CNNs for Left Atrium Segmentation in 3D Ultrasound

Markus A. Degel[1,2(✉)], Nassir Navab[1,3], and Shadi Albarqouni[1]

[1] Computer Aided Medical Procedures (CAMP), Technische Universität München, Munich, Germany
{markus.degel,shadi.albarqouni}@tum.de
[2] TOMTEC Imaging Systems GmbH, Unterschleissheim, Germany
[3] Whiting School of Engineering, Johns Hopkins University, Baltimore, USA

Abstract. Segmentation of the left atrium and deriving its size can help to predict and detect various cardiovascular conditions. Automation of this process in 3D Ultrasound image data is desirable, since manual delineations are time-consuming, challenging and observer-dependent. Convolutional neural networks have made improvements in computer vision and in medical image analysis. They have successfully been applied to segmentation tasks and were extended to work on volumetric data. In this paper we introduce a combined deep-learning based approach on volumetric segmentation in Ultrasound acquisitions with incorporation of prior knowledge about left atrial shape and imaging device. The results show, that including a shape prior helps the domain adaptation and the accuracy of segmentation is further increased with adversarial learning.

1 Introduction

Quantification of cardiac chambers and their functions stay the most important objective of cardiac imaging [7]. Left atrium (LA) physiology and function have an impact on the whole heart performance and its size is a valuable indicator for various cardiovascular conditions, such as atrial fibrillation (AF), stroke and diastolic dysfunction [7]. Compared to cardiac computed tomography (CCT) and cardiac magnetic resonance (CMR), as modalities to examine the heart, echocardiography provides wide availability, safety and good spatial and temporal resolution, without exposing the patients to harmful radiation. Volumetric measurements consider changes in all spatial dimensions, however, to obtain reproducible and accurate three-dimensional (3D) measurements, requires expert experience and is time consuming [4]. Automated segmentation and quantification could help to reduce inter/intra-observer variabilities and might also save costs and time in echocardiographic laboratories [4].

Previous automatic and semi-automatic approaches for LA segmentation have focused CCT and CMR as a planning and guidance tool for LA catheter interventions [1]. For 3D Ultrasound (US), the left ventricle (LV) was the

© Springer Nature Switzerland AG 2018
A. F. Frangi et al. (Eds.): MICCAI 2018, LNCS 11073, pp. 630–637, 2018.
https://doi.org/10.1007/978-3-030-00937-3_72

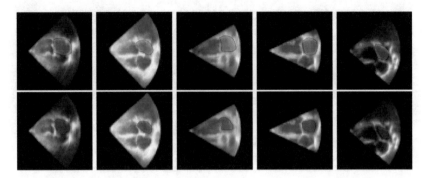

Fig. 1. Row 1: ground truth segmentation of LA, Row 2: prediction by *DGA* architecture (Table 3), Column 1 & 2: device EPIQ 7C (trained on Vivid E9), Column 3 & 4: device Vivid E9 (trained on EPIQ 7C), Column 5: device iE33 (trained on Vivid E9).

segmentation target, since its size and function remain the most important indication for a cardiac study [6]. LA segmentation in 3D US has not received much attention, apart from commercially available methods, which were also successfully validated against the gold standard CMR and CCT [3,10]. Almeida *et al.* [1] adapted a segmentation framework for LV, based on B-spline explicit active surfaces. Those methods, however, require more or less manual interaction. Recently, fully automatic segmentation of the left heart was validated against 2D and 3D echocardiography, as well as CCT [4].

Convolutional neural networks (CNN) and their special architectures of fully convolutional networks (FCN) have successfully been applied to the problem of medical image segmentation. Those networks are trained end-to-end, process the whole image and perform pixel-wise classification. The *V-Net* extends this idea to volumetric image data and enables 3D segmentation with the help of spatial convolutions, instead of processing the volumes slice-wise [8].

Automated segmentation in cardiac US images is challenging, due to artifacts caused by respiratory motion, shadows or signal-dropouts. Including shape priors in this task can help algorithms to yield more accurate and anatomically plausible results. Oktay *et al.* [9] introduced a way to incorporate such a prior with the help of an autoencoder network, that leads segmentation masks to follow an underlying shape representation.

Image data might be different (*e.g* with respect to resolution, contrast), due to varying imaging protocols and device manufacturers [2,5]. Although the segmentation task is equivalent, neural networks perform poorly when applied to data that was not available during training. Generating ground truth maps and retraining a new model for each domain is not a scalable solution. The problem of models to generalize to new image data can be approached by domain adaptation. Kamnitsas *et al.* [5] successfully introduced the application of unsupervised domain adaptation for different MRI databases, when an adversarial neural network was influencing the feature maps of a CNN, which was employed for a segmentation task.

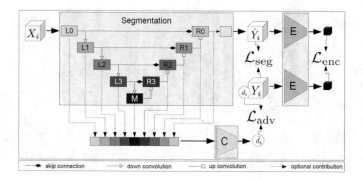

Fig. 2. Overview of the combined architecture: Image data X_i is processed by *V-Net* [8]. $\mathcal{L}_{seg}$ is calculated from the resulting segmentation $\hat{Y}_i$ and the ground truth Y_i. Additionally, $\hat{Y}_i$ and Y_i are encoded (E) to get the shape constraint. An optional number of feature maps, based on X_i are extracted from *V-Net* to be processed in the classifier (C), which predicts a domain $\hat{d}_i$. Cross-entropy between $\hat{d}_i$ and the real domain d_i determines the adversarial loss.

In this work, LA segmentation in 3D US volumes is performed with the help of neural networks. For the volumetric segmentation, *V-Net* will be trained, combined with additional losses, taking into account the geometrical constraint introduced by the shape of the LA and the desired ability to generalize to different US devices and settings.

2   Methodology

Our framework, as depicted in Fig. 2, consists of three existing methods; 3D Fully Convolutional Segmentation Network [8], Anatomic Constraint [9], and Domain Adaptation [5]. Nevertheless, it is a novelty to model the solution in a single framework, enabling analysis on the contribution of each element on the primary segmentation task. Further, the domain adaptation method has been leveraged to a 3D FCN segmentation framework, and applied successfully to the LA, showing a statistical significant improvement, as reported in Sect. 3.

Segmentation. For the segmentation task, we employ *V-Net* [8] as a 3D FCN, which processes an image volume of size n, $X_i = \{x_1, ..., x_n\}$, $x_i \in \mathcal{X}$ and yields a segmentation mask $\hat{Y}_i = \{\hat{y}_1, ..., \hat{y}_n\}$, $\hat{y}_i \in \hat{\mathcal{Y}}$ in the original resolution. $\mathcal{X}$ represents the feature space of US acquisitions and $\hat{\mathcal{Y}}$ describes the probability of a voxel belonging to the segmentation.

The objective function of *V-Net* is adapted to the segmentation task. It is based on the Dice coefficient (Eq. 1), taking into account the possible imbalance of foreground to background, alleviating the need to re-weight samples.

$$\mathcal{L}_{seg} = 1 - \frac{2 \cdot \sum_i y_i \cdot \hat{y}_i}{\sum_i y_i^2 + \sum_i \hat{y}_i^2}, \tag{1}$$

with $\hat{y}_i$ being the prediction and y_i the voxels of the ground truth Y_i from the binary distribution $\mathcal{Y}$.

Shape Prior. Incorporation of the shape prior to help the segmentation task is realized by training an autoencoder network on the segmentation ground truth masks $\mathbf{Y}$. The encoder reduces the label to a latent, low resolution representation $E(Y_i)$ and the decoder tries to retrieve the original volume Y_i. Due to the resolution reduction of the encoder, the shape information is encoded in a compact fashion [9].

During training, the output of the segmentation network $\hat{Y}_i$ is passed to the encoder, along with the ground truth label Y_i. Based on a distance metric $d(\cdot,\cdot)$, a loss between the latent codes of both inputs is calculated as

$$\mathcal{L}_{enc} = d(E(Y_i), E(\hat{Y}_i)). \tag{2}$$

The gradient is then back-propagated to the segmentation network.

Domain Adaptation. When a network is trained on one type of data $\mathcal{X}_S$ (source domain) and evaluated on another $\mathcal{X}_T$ (target domain), the performance is poor in most cases. Domain invariant features are desired to make the segmentation network perform well on different data sets. Kamnitsas *et al.* [5] propose an approach to generate domain invariant features to increase a networks generalization capability.

Processing an image volume in a CNN yields a latent representation $h_l(X_i)$ after convolutional layer l. If the network is not domain invariant, those feature maps contain information about the data type (source or target domain). The idea to solve this issue, is to train a classifier C, which takes feature maps of the segmentation network as input and returns whether the input data was from source (X_S) or target (X_T) domain: $C(h_l(X_i)) = \hat{d}_i \in \{S, T\}$. The accuracy of this classifier is an indicator of how domain invariant the features are.

Combination. The ideas introduced in the previous sections are combined to exploit the advantages of the individual approaches (Fig. 2). The loss of the domain classifier is used as an adversarial loss term, since the goal of the segmentation network is to lower the classification accuracy (*i.e* maximize its loss). The inability of the classifier to tell, which type of data was segmented means that the feature maps are domain invariant. At the same time, $\mathcal{L}_{seg}$ and $\mathcal{L}_{enc}$ should be minimized. With $\mathcal{L}_{adv}$ as the binary cross entropy loss of the classifier C, this yields the following combined loss function:

$$\mathcal{L} = \mathcal{L}_{seg} + \lambda_{enc} \cdot \mathcal{L}_{enc} - \lambda_{adv} \cdot \mathcal{L}_{adv} \tag{3}$$

3   Experiments and Results

To evaluate the influence of different loss terms, we apply it to 3D Ultrasound data to perform end-systolic LA segmentation. The network is trained with images and labels from one device and tested on different devices.

Table 1. Data device and set distribution. iE33 datasets are only used for evaluation. Resolutions are equidistant. Resolution and opening angles of Ultrasound devices (azimuth & elevation) shown as: mean ± standard deviation.

Property	EPIQ 7C	Vivid E9	iE33
Train/val/test	33/7/27	39/8/32	0/0/15
Resolution (mm/voxel)	0.95 ± 0.10	0.95 ± 0.10	0.96 ± 0.11
Azimuth (deg)	87.1 ± 4.7	47.3 ± 10.4	80.2 ± 0.0
Elevation (deg)	78.2 ± 0.1	47.4 ± 10.5	91.6 ± 0.0

Dataset. The data available for this work are 3D transthoracic echocardiography (TTE) examinations taken from clinical routine, which brings variations from differences in US imaging devices, protocols (resolution, opening angle) and patients (healthy, abnormal), raising the necessity of our proposed framework (Table 1). Multiple international centers contributed to a pool of 161 datasets, containing the LA ground truth segmentation in the entire recorded heart cycle, with the relevant phases for LA functionality (end-diastole, end-systole and pre-atrial contraction) identified.

Acquisition was performed with systems from GE (Vivid E9, GE Vingmed Ultrasound) and Philips (EPIQ 7C and iE33, Philips Medical Systems), each equipped with a matrix array transducer. Since there are only 15 datasets for device iE33, those examinations are not used for training, only for evaluation. The data is down-sampled, preserving angles and ratios, by zero padding (*cf.* Fig. 1), to enable processing of the entire volumes.

Implementation. Network architectures are implemented using the Tensor-Flow[1] library (version 1.4) with GPU support. For our approach, the *V-Net* architecture is adapted, such that volumes of size 64 × 64 × 64 can be processed. The autoencoder network architecture is inspired from the one proposed in [9]. Feature maps from different levels and sizes are extracted from *V-Net* to be processed in the classifier (Fig. 2). By (repeated) application of convolutions of filter size 2 with stride 2, the feature maps are brought to the *V-Net* valley size (4 × 4 × 4), so they can be concatenated along the channel dimension.

Training Details. The autoencoder network is trained before the combined training procedure, to obtain a meaningful latent representation for the shape prior. In the following training stages, the parameters of this network are frozen. The segmentation network is shortly pre-trained, as well as the classifier to introduce stability in the combined training and it can focus on realizing the scenario defined by the settings of λ_{enc} and λ_{adv}. Feature maps L0, L2, M, R2 and R0 of the segmentation network are extracted for the classifier.

---

[1] https://www.tensorflow.org/.

Table 2. Training procedure details. Each training uses a learning rate decay of 0.99 after each epoch and a batch size of 4. $X = X_S \cup X_T$, d: domain labels.

#	Name (parameters)	Optimizer	Learning rate	Weight reg.	Epochs	Data	Label
1	Autoencoder (θ_{ae})	Momentum β:0.9	$5 \cdot 10^{-4}$	0.1	100	Y_S	Y_S
2	Segmentation (θ_{seg})	Adam β_1: 0.99, β_2: 0.999	$1 \cdot 10^{-5}$	$5 \cdot 10^{-4}$	50	X_S	Y_S
3	Classifier (θ_{adv})	SGD	$5 \cdot 10^{-5}$	$1 \cdot 10^{-5}$	15	X	d
4	Combination 3 (θ_{seg})	Momentum β:0.99	$1 \cdot 10^{-5}$	$5 \cdot 10^{-4}$	100	X_S	Y_S,d
	Classifier (θ_{adv})	SGD	$5 \cdot 10^{-5}$	$1 \cdot 10^{-5}$		X	d

The combined training procedure starts by adding $\mathcal{L}_{enc}$, for incorporation of the shape prior to the segmentation loss $\mathcal{L}_{seg}$. Adversarial influence begins after 10 epochs of combined training, linearly increasing λ_{adv} until it reaches its maximum of 0.001 after another 10 epochs. While the combined training exclusively adjusts the parameters of the segmentation network θ_{seg}, the classifier parameters θ_{adv} are continued to be trained in parallel to retain a potent adversarial loss term. A training overview is given in Table 2.

Evaluation. The segmentation network returns a volume $\hat{Y}_i$ of probabilities for the voxels to belong to the foreground, *i.e* the segmentation of the LA. The threshold for the cutoff probability to obtain a binary segmentation mask is determined by the best Dice coefficient on the validation set, from which the biggest connected component is selected as the final LA segmentation.

Segmentation metrics [1,9] are reported in Table 3 for the recommended phase of LA segmentation (end-systole ES [7]). We refer to the *V-Net* architecture with the additional loss term $\mathcal{L}_{enc}$, calculated from the L2-distance $(d(p,q) \doteq \|p - q\|_2^2)$, as geometry agnostic CNN *GAL2*. To investigate the influence of a different distance metric, *GAACD* uses the angular cosine distance, as it was proposed in [2] (ACD, $d(p,q) = 1 - \frac{\sum_i p_i \cdot q_i}{\|p\|_2 \cdot \|q\|_2}$). Our domain and geometry agnostic CNN *DGA* leverages the better performing distance metric (ACD, based on test results) with the adversarial loss $\mathcal{L}_{adv}$. We define statistical significance based on the paired two-sample t-test on a 5% significance level.

When training on EPIQ 7C, *V-Net* performs better than the other architectures on the same device. However, those margins are not statistically significant (MSD: $p = 0.65$, HD: $p = 0.24$, DC: $P = 0.66$), compared to *DGA*. The increased performance of *DGA* compared to *V-Net* and *ACNN* is significant with respect to all metrics. Vivid E9 training yields *V-Net* with the best performance on the same device, with statistical significance on all metrics. *DGA* is significantly outperforming *V-Net* on EPIQ 7C in terms of MSD and HD. No significant differences are observable on the evaluation of device iE33. Independent of the distance metric utilized, an improvement in generalizability is observable compared to *V-Net* when the shape prior is included (*GAL2* & *GAACD*).

Table 3. Results for ES LA segmentation. Baseline *ACNN* and *V-Net* results are reported. *GAL2*: $\lambda_{adv} = 0$, *d*: L2-distance. *GAACD*: $\lambda_{adv} = 0$, *d*: ACD. *DGA*: $\lambda_{adv} = 0.001$, *d*: ACD. *GAL2,GAACD* & *DGA*: $\lambda_{enc} = 0.001$. Format: mean $\pm$ std.

Training	Test	V-Net [8]	ACNN[9]	GAL2	GAACD	DGA
Mean Surface Distance (MSD)						
EPIQ 7C	EPIQ 7C	**1.16±0.88**	1.35 ± 1.19	1.26 ± 0.69	1.27 ± 0.69	1.21 ± 0.60
	Vivid E9	3.56 ± 1.71	10.67 ± 7.29	3.87 ± 3.06	2.42 ± 1.32	**2.01±1.63**
	iE33	1.44 ± 0.77	**1.38±0.40**	2.33 ± 2.38	1.94 ± 1.49	1.44 ± 0.35
Vivid E9	EPIQ 7C	2.87 ± 1.53	4.39 ± 1.33	2.12 ± 0.96	1.87 ± 0.96	**1.59±1.04**
	Vivid E9	**0.94±0.59**	1.57 ± 0.87	1.18 ± 0.38	1.12 ± 0.37	1.18 ± 0.37
	iE33	4.72 ± 4.86	3.28 ± 2.22	4.18 ± 3.36	3.18 ± 2.88	**2.62±1.46**
Hausdorff Distance (HD)						
EPIQ 7C	EPIQ 7C	**4.46±2.73**	5.52 ± 3.15	5.51 ± 2.31	5.33 ± 2.07	4.92 ± 1.60
	Vivid E9	7.66 ± 2.94	16.87 ± 8.92	8.21 ± 5.06	5.79 ± 2.21	**5.46±3.36**
	iE33	**4.06±1.21**	5.03 ± 1.39	5.60 ± 2.86	4.98 ± 2.02	4.70 ± 0.91
Vivid E9	EPIQ 7C	10.82 ± 3.80	13.63 ± 2.87	8.09 ± 2.88	7.31 ± 2.51	**5.47±2.45**
	Vivid E9	**3.67±2.29**	7.09 ± 3.21	5.41 ± 1.84	5.05 ± 1.70	5.14 ± 1.26
	iE33	9.52 ± 6.44	11.60 ± 3.72	9.08 ± 3.64	7.13 ± 3.49	**6.63±2.25**
Dice Coefficient (DC)						
EPIQ 7C	EPIQ 7C	**0.75±0.17**	0.69 ± 0.20	0.74 ± 0.10	0.73 ± 0.11	0.74 ± 0.10
	Vivid E9	0.10 ± 0.21	0.15 ± 0.25	0.33 ± 0.27	0.32 ± 0.26	**0.55±0.23**
	iE33	0.57 ± 0.31	0.64 ± 0.11	0.55 ± 0.19	0.59 ± 0.19	**0.67±0.08**
Vivid E9	EPIQ 7C	0.56 ± 0.15	0.32 ± 0.18	0.59 ± 0.14	0.62 ± 0.17	**0.63±0.17**
	Vivid E9	**0.80±0.08**	0.69 ± 0.11	0.73 ± 0.07	0.74 ± 0.08	0.73 ± 0.09
	iE33	0.49 ± 0.37	**0.50±0.16**	0.38 ± 0.25	0.46 ± 0.27	0.46 ± 0.19

4   Discussion and Conclusion

While *V-Net* performs well on the task of LA segmentation, the ability to generalize to new domains is achieved by the introduction of a shape prior and the adversarial loss, as shown in the results. Including the shape prior boosts the segmentation performance on unseen devices and theoretically leads to a geometrically plausible segmentation in case of image artifacts. We ensure a potent classifier by training it in parallel to the *DGA* architecture. Thus, it can detect domain-specific features throughout the training procedure. The distance metric for the geometrical constraint is an interesting subject to further investigate, as well as extracting different *V-Net*-layers for processing in the classifier network.

Acknowledgment. We would like to thank Ozan Oktay for sharing his implementation of the *ACNN* architecture as a baseline of our project. Further, we thank Georg Schummers and Matthias Friedrichs from TOMTEC Imaging Systems GmbH for their support and helpful discussions.

References

1. Almeida, N., et al.: Left-atrial segmentation from 3-D ultrasound using B-spline explicit active surfaces with scale uncoupling. IEEE UFFC-S **63**(2), 212–221 (2016)
2. Baur, C., Albarqouni, S., Navab, N.: Semi-supervised deep learning for fully convolutional networks. In: Descoteaux, M., Maier-Hein, L., Franz, A., Jannin, P., Collins, D.L., Duchesne, S. (eds.) MICCAI 2017. LNCS, vol. 10435, pp. 311–319. Springer, Cham (2017). https://doi.org/10.1007/978-3-319-66179-7_36
3. Buechel, R.R., et al.: Assessment of left atrial functional parameters using a novel dedicated analysis tool for real-time three-dimensional echocardiography: validation in comparison to magnetic resonance imaging. Int. J. Cardiovas Imag. **29**(3), 601–608 (2013)
4. van den Hoven, A.T., et al.: Transthoracic 3D echocardiographic left heart chamber quantification in patients with bicuspid aortic valve disease. Int. J. Cardiovas Imag. **33**(12), 1895–1903 (2017)
5. Kamnitsas, K., et al.: Unsupervised domain adaptation in brain lesion segmentation with adversarial networks. In: Niethammer, M., et al. (eds.) IPMI 2017. LNCS, vol. 10265, pp. 597–609. Springer, Cham (2017). https://doi.org/10.1007/978-3-319-59050-9_47
6. Knackstedt, C., et al.: Fully automated versus standard tracking of left ventricular ejection fraction and longitudinal strain: the FAST-EFs multicenter study. JACC **66**(13), 1456–1466 (2015)
7. Lang, R.M., et al.: Recommendations for cardiac chamber quantification by echocardiography in adults: an update from the american society of echocardiography and the european association of cardiovascular imaging. Eur. Heart J. **16**(3), 233–271 (2015)
8. Milletari, F., Navab, N., Ahmadi, S.: V-net: fully convolutional neural networks for volumetric medical image segmentation. In: 2016 Fourth International Conference on 3D Vision (3DV), pp. 565–571 (2016)
9. Oktay, O., et al.: Anatomically constrained neural networks (ACNNs): application to cardiac image enhancement and segmentation. IEEE TMI **37**(2), 384–395 (2018)
10. Rohner, A., et al.: Functional assessment of the left atrium by real-time three-dimensional echocardiography using a novel dedicated analysis tool: initial validation studies in comparison with computed tomography. Eur. J. Echocardiogr. **12**(7), 497–505 (2011)

Image Segmentation Methods: Chest, Lung and Spine Segmentation

Densely Deep Supervised Networks with Threshold Loss for Cancer Detection in Automated Breast Ultrasound

Na Wang[1], Cheng Bian[1], Yi Wang[1,2], Min Xu[3], Chenchen Qin[1], Xin Yang[4], Tianfu Wang[1], Anhua Li[3], Dinggang Shen[5], and Dong Ni[1,2(✉)]

[1] National-Regional Key Technology Engineering Laboratory for Medical Ultrasound, School of Biomedical Engineering, Health Science Center, Shenzhen University, Shenzhen, China
nidong@szu.edu.cn
[2] Medical UltraSound Image Computing (MUSIC) Lab, Shenzhen, China
[3] Department of Ultrasound, Sun Yat-Sen University Cancer Center, State Key Laboratory of Oncology in South China, Collaborative Innovation Center for Cancer Medicine, Guangzhou, China
[4] Department of Computer Science and Engineering, The Chinese University of Hong Kong, Hong Kong, China
[5] Department of Radiology and BRIC, University of North Carolina at Chapel Hill, Chapel Hill, NC 27599, USA

Abstract. Automated breast ultrasound (ABUS) is a new and promising tool for diagnosing breast cancer. However, reviewing ABUS images is extremely time-consuming and oversight errors could happen. We propose a novel 3D convolutional network for automatic cancer detection in ABUS. Our contribution is twofold. First, we propose a threshold loss function to provide voxel-level adaptive threshold for discriminating cancer and non-cancer, thus achieving high sensitivity with low FPs. Second, we propose a densely deep supervision (DDS) mechanism to improve the sensitivity significantly by utilizing multi-scale discriminative features of all layers. Both class-balanced cross entropy loss and overlap loss are employed to enhance DDS performance. The efficacy of the proposed network is validated on a dataset of 196 patients with 661 cancer regions. The 4-fold cross-validation experiments show our network obtains a sensitivity of 93% with 2.2 FPs per ABUS volume. Our proposed novel network can provide an accurate and automatic cancer detection tool for breast cancer screening by maintaining high sensitivity with low FPs.

1 Introduction

Recently, automated breast ultrasound (ABUS) has been developed as a new and promising tool for diagnosing breast cancer. ABUS can provide 3D views of the breast by automatically scanning the whole breast. It also has a number of advantages over traditional 2D handheld ultrasound: higher reproducibility, less operator dependence, and less image acquisition time [8]. However, reviewing ABUS images is extremely time-consuming, because a typical exam often

© Springer Nature Switzerland AG 2018
A. F. Frangi et al. (Eds.): MICCAI 2018, LNCS 11073, pp. 641–648, 2018.
https://doi.org/10.1007/978-3-030-00937-3_73

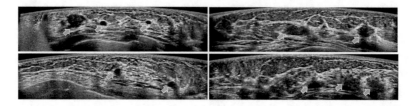

Fig. 1. Example ABUS images. Blue arrows indicate biopsy-proven cancer regions, and orange arrows indicate cancer mimicry with very similar appearance to cancer regions.

consists of three volumes of each breast in order to cover the whole breast. Furthermore, the large size of the ABUS volumes may cause oversight errors in some malignancies. Therefore, automated cancer detection in ABUS is highly expected to assist clinicians in facilitating the identification of breast cancer.

As shown in Fig. 1, computer-aided detection (CADe) of cancer from ABUS images remains very challenging. First, cancers often possess high intraclass appearance variation caused by various factors like imaging artifacts of acoustic shadows and speckles, deformation of soft tissues and large difference in lesion size. Second, malignant lesions may possibly appear similar to other structures, such as benign lesions and normal hypoechoic structures. Third, small cancers are mostly likely to be missed even by clinical experts because of the relatively low quality of ultrasound imaging, the existence of similar normal structures and the oversight errors. Finally, the severe class imbalance between cancer and non-cancer voxels is another challenge because of the extremely small size of the cancer relative to the large ABUS volume. In this situation, the predictive model developed based on machine learning methods could be biased and inaccurate.

To better assist clinician with cancer screening, a number of CADe approaches have been developed. Moon *et al.* developed a CADe system based on a two-stage multi-scale blob analysis method [5]. The system showed sensitivities of 100%, 90% and 70% with false positives (FPs) per volume of 17.4, 8.8, and 2.7, respectively. Tan *et al.* proposed a multi-stage system using an ensemble of neural networks to classify cancers [9]. Although the FPs per volume could be controlled at 1, the sensitivity was only 64%. Lo *et al.* employed watershed segmentation to extract potential abnormalities in ABUS and reduced FPs using various quantitative features [3]. The sensitivities were 100%, 90% and 80% with FPs per volume of 9.44, 5.42, and 3.33, respectively. Generally, maintaining high sensitivity with low FPs remains a vital problem in ABUS CADe.

Recently, a surge of deep learning is becoming dominant over traditional CADe methods [7]. We propose a novel 3D convolutional neural network (CNN) for automatic cancer detection in ABUS. We believe we are the first to employ deep learning based techniques for this problem. Our contribution is twofold. First, we propose a threshold loss function by adding a threshold map (TM) layer in the CNN. The proposed method provides voxel-level adaptive threshold to classify voxels into cancer or non-cancer, thus achieving high sensitivity with low FPs. Second, we propose a densely deep supervision (DDS) mechanism

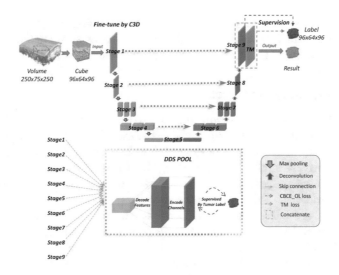

Fig. 2. The illustration of the proposed network for cancer detection in ABUS.

to improve the sensitivity significantly by utilizing multi-scale discriminative features of all layers [2]. We employ two loss functions to enhance DDS performance. Specifically, class-balanced cross entropy is employed to tackle the issue of limited positive training samples; overlap loss is for selecting discriminative cancer representations. The proposed network was extensively evaluated on a 196-patient dataset, with 661 cancer regions.

2   Methods

Figure 2 illustrates the proposed network, which leverages the DDS to learn more discriminative cancer representations for the improvement of detection sensitivity, and utilizes the proposed TM to adaptively refine the probability map for the FPs reduction while maintaining high sensitivity.

2.1   Network Architecture

We choose the most successful segmentation net 3D U-net [6], [11] as our backbone architecture but make the following modifications (Fig. 2): (a) we employ the pre-trained C3D model [10] to fine-tune our network parameters to restrain the over-fitting issue induced by limited ABUS training samples; (b) we design a DDS mechanism to effectively learn discriminative features for cancer identification and meanwhile boost the gradient flow of the whole network; (c) we add a TM layer to provide voxel-level adaptive threshold for optimizing the probability map, thus achieving high sensitivity with low FPs. Specifically, the TM is automatically learned from the complementary information of learned features, label information and predicted probability map. (d) other customizations: each convolutional layer is connected with a batch normalization (BN) layer and a rectified linear unit (ReLU); each of the stages 3–7 uses 3 convolutional layers to increase receptive fields for using more global information.

2.2 Densely Deep Supervision

Deep neural networks are powerful to generate abundant multi-scale features for object detection in natural images. Nevertheless, this is challenging in ABUS images, because breast cancers possess high intraclass appearance variation and some are relatively subtle. Furthermore, due to gradient vanishing issue, the parameter tuning processes of the 3D CNN may encounter low efficiency and overfitting problems. Taking advantages of deeply supervised nets (DSN) [2], we implement the DDS into our 3D U-net to alleviate above problems by fully exploiting the multi-scale features from all stages. Specifically, we input each of the stages 1-9 and the concatenation of all stages into DDS pool (thus totally 10 DSNs), and introduce a DDS loss function to supervise the generation of cancer probability map. The DDS loss function is defined as

$$\mathcal{L}_{dds}(X, Y; \mathcal{W}, \omega) = \sum_{t=1}^{T-1} \left(\theta_t * \left(\mathcal{L}_{cbce}^{(t)}(X, Y; \mathcal{W}, \omega^{(t)}) + \mathcal{L}_{ol}^{(t)}(X, Y; \mathcal{W}, \omega^{(t)}) \right) \right), \quad (1)$$

where X is training image and Y is corresponding label image, $\mathcal{W}$ is the weight of main network, $\omega = (\omega^{(1)}, \omega^{(2)}, \cdots, \omega^{(T)})$ where $(\omega^{(1)}, \omega^{(2)}, \cdots, \omega^{(T-1)})$ are the weights of each DSN and $\omega^{(T=11)}$ is the weight of TM layer, $\theta = (\theta_1, \theta_2, \cdots, \theta_T)$ are the coefficients to weight each DSN loss and threshold loss in total loss, respectively. The class-balanced cross entropy (CBCE) loss $\mathcal{L}_{cbce}$ and overlap (OL) loss $\mathcal{L}_{ol}$ in Eq. (1) will be explained in the following paragraphs.

Class-Balanced Cross Entropy Loss. Considering lots of breast cancers are relatively subtle, the distribution of cancer/non-cancer regions in a large ABUS volume is heavily biased. We employ a CBCE loss to tackle the issue of limited positive training samples. Specifically, we introduce a class-balancing weight α to offset the imbalance between cancer and non-cancer voxels and define the CBCE loss function as

$$\mathcal{L}_{cbce}^{(t)}(\mathcal{W}, \omega^{(t)}) = -\alpha \sum_{i \in Y_+} \log Ps(y_i = 1 | X; \mathcal{W}, \omega^{(t)})$$
$$-(1 - \alpha) \sum_{i \in Y_-} \log Ps(y_i = 0 | X; \mathcal{W}, \omega^{(t)}), \quad (2)$$

where $y_i \in \{0, 1\}$ represents the label of Y at location i. $\alpha = sum(Y_-)/sum(Y)$ and $1 - \alpha = sum(Y_+)/sum(Y)$, where Y_- and Y_+ are non-cancer and cancer label sets. $Ps(y_i | X; \mathcal{W}, \omega^{(t)}) = e^{z_j} / \sum_k e^{z_k} \in (0, 1)$ denotes the feature map obtained by *softmax* function, where z_j is the score of class j and $k = 2$.

Overlap Loss. To further improve the detection sensitivity, especially for better identification of subtle cancers, we design a new loss function, i.e. overlap loss, to learn more discriminative features for cancer representations. The OL loss function is defined as

$$\mathcal{L}_{ol}^{(t)}(\mathcal{W}, \omega^{(t)}) = \sum_{i=1}^{|X|} (Ps(y_i = 1 | X; \mathcal{W}, \omega^{(t)}) * Ps(y_i = 0 | X; \mathcal{W}, \omega^{(t)})). \quad (3)$$

The purpose of this loss is to ensure that cancer regions should have little overlap with non-cancer regions, thus the optimal overlapped region should be zero. By minimizing the overlap loss, we attempt to learn more discriminative features to distinguish cancer and non-cancer regions.

2.3   Threshold Map

Although the probability map generated by the proposed DDS mechanism can indicate cancer locations with high sensitivity, it may still have some high probability regions which are actually normal tissues. Thus the further post-processing of the probability map is essential to obtain a better detection. However, conventional methods often fail in simultaneously achieving high sensitivity and low FPs, for example, fixed threshold is sensitive to the selected value; softmax method often achieves high FPs when coping with challenging problems; directly performing conditional random field tends to lower the sensitivity.

To address the above issues, we concatenate and train a threshold map (TM) layer in our network to adaptively refine the probability map for better detection. The proposed TM can provide voxel-level adaptive threshold to classify voxels into cancer or non-cancer by making use of all the information from learned features, label information and probability map, thus achieving a good balance between high sensitivity and low FPs. To train the TM, we design a new loss function, i.e. threshold loss, which can be calculated as follow:

$$\mathcal{L}_{threshold}(\mathcal{W}, \omega^{(t)}) = 1 - \frac{2 * \left| Mask(y_i = 1 | X; \mathcal{W}, \omega^{(t)}) * Y \right|}{\left| Mask(y_i; \mathcal{W}, \omega^{(t)}) \right| + |Y|}, \quad (4)$$

$$Mask(y_i; \mathcal{W}, \omega^{(t)}) = 1/(1 + e^{-tmp}), \quad (5)$$

$$tmp = \begin{cases} Ps(y_i = 1 | X; \mathcal{W}, \omega^{(t)}), & Ps(y_i) > Threshold\_Map(y_i) \\ -e^{10}, & else \end{cases}. \quad (6)$$

The objective of this threshold loss is to learn a voxel-wise threshold map, which can be further employed to adaptively refine the probability map by suppressing non-cancer regions and meanwhile maintaining cancer regions. To the best of our knowledge, we are the first to design a threshold map to adaptively optimize the probability map. The efficacy of the proposed TM is shown in our experiments.

We summarize the total loss function for our cancer detection as

$$\mathcal{L}_{total} = \mathcal{L}_{dds} + \theta_T * \mathcal{L}_{threshold}. \quad (7)$$

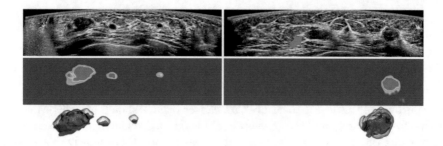

Fig. 3. Example results of cancer detection in ABUS. Top row: ABUS images with annotated cancer locations (red contours) and purple arrow indicates cancer mimicry. Middle row: refined cancer probability maps by the proposed threshold map. Bottom row: 3D visualization of our detected cancers (gray) and ground truth (red).

3   Experiments

Materials. Experiments were carried on the dataset obtained using Invenia ABUS system (GE, USA) in Sun Yat-Sen University Cancer Center. Informed consent for this retrospective study was obtained from our institutional review board. To cover the whole breast, three volumes including anterior-posterior, medial and lateral passes were obtained for each breast. Thus for each patient, six ABUS volumes were acquired. The voxel resolutions of the acquired 3D ABUS volumes were 0.511 mm, 0.082 mm and 0.200 mm in the transverse, sagittal and coronal direction, respectively.

In this study, ABUS data from 196 women (age range: 30–75 years, mean 49 years) with biopsy-proven breast cancers were collected. From these ABUS data, 559 volumes were annotated by an experienced clinician, which included 661 cancer regions (volume: 0.01–86.54 cm^3, mean: 2.84 cm^3). Four-fold cross-validation was conducted to evaluate the detection performance. As a control, 119 ABUS volumes with no abnormal findings were also included for evaluations.

Implementation Details. Our proposed framework was implemented with the popular library Keras for Tensorflow. To tackle the issues of limited cancer samples and demanding 3D computational cost, we divided ABUS volume into multiple 96 × 64 × 96 cubes and adopted data augmentation (i.e., translation, rotation, cropping, flipping) for training, and further combine the predicted cube into a volume as detection result. The framework was trained on a 8x NVIDIA Tesla GPU. Adaptive moment estimation was used to train the whole framework. We set the learning rate as 1e−4 and learning stopped after 30000 iterations.

Detection Performance. We extensively compared our method with state of the art, including SegNet [1], FCN [4], U-net [11]. To illustrate the efficacy of the proposed triplet loss, we further evaluated the proposed network with different loss functions, including dice loss (DL), cross entropy (CE) loss, CBCE loss, CBCE-OL loss, and the triplet CBCE-OL-TM loss.

Figure 3 visualizes the cancer detection results by our network. By utilizing the proposed DDS and threshold map, our network can output accurate cancer probability maps even when cancers were subtle or cancer mimicry existed.

Table 1. Sensitivities and corresponding FPs per volume for different methods

Method	Sensitivity (%)	FPs per volume		
		Cancer	Normal	All
3D-SegNet [1]	63.75	1.69	2.42	1.82
3D-FCN [4]	66.47	1.84	2.77	2.00
3D-Unet [11]	79.61	0.56	1.04	0.65
3D-Unet-DDS-DL	84.21	3.56	3.06	3.47
3D-Unet-DDS-CE	76.16	4.77	4.90	4.79
3D-Unet-DDS-CBCE	88.69	3.60	4.48	3.75
3D-Unet-DDS-CBCE-OL	100.00	9.81	8.62	9.60
3D-Unet-DDS-CBCE-OL-TM	93.04	2.23	2.19	2.22

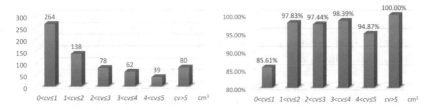

Fig. 4. Left: the cancer volume (cv) distribution of all 661 cancer regions. Right: the detection sensitivities for different ranges of cancer volume.

Table 1 lists the sensitivities and corresponding FPs per volume for different methods. Our network obtained a sensitivity of 93% with 2.2 FPs per ABUS volume. Compared to SegNet and FCN, our network significantly improved detection sensitivity meanwhile still controlled FPs at about 2. Although U-net obtained a FP value less than 1, its sensitivity is less than 80%. By observing the results of our network with different loss functions in Table 1, the designed DDS and TM contributed to the improvement of detection performance. Specifically, the DDS with CBCE-OL loss contributed to select discriminative cancer representations and the TM loss helped to adaptively optimize probability map for the FPs reduction while maintaining high sensitivity. Table 1 also records the difference between FPs in cancer and normal volumes. Our network got the number of FPs for normal volumes slightly lower than that for abnormal volumes.

Figure 4 further illustrates the volume distribution of all 661 cancer regions, as well as the corresponding detection sensitivities for different ranges of cancer volume. It can be observed that our network achieved a sensitivity above 85% even when cancer volume was smaller than $1\,cm^3$, and when cancer volume was larger than $5\,cm^3$, we got a sensitivity of 100%.

4   Conclusion

In this paper, we propose a novel 3D convolutional network for automatic cancer detection in ABUS. To the best of our knowledge, we are the first to employ deep learning techniques for this problem. In the proposed network, a novel threshold map is designed to provide voxel-level adaptive threshold to classify voxels into cancer or non-cancer, thus achieving high sensitivity with low FPs. Furthermore, a densely deep supervision mechanism is employed to improve the sensitivity greatly by utilizing multi-scale discriminative features of all layers. Experiments show our network obtains a sensitivity of 93% with 2.2 FPs per ABUS volume. Our method can provide an accurate and automatic cancer detection tool for breast cancer screening by maintaining high sensitivity and low FPs.

Acknowledgments. This work was supported in part by the National Natural Science Foundation of China under Grant 61571304, Grant 61701312, and in part by the Shenzhen Peacock Plan under Grant KQTD2016053112051497.

References

1. Badrinarayanan, V., Kendall, A., Cipolla, R.: SegNet: a deep convolutional encoder-decoder architecture for image segmentation. IEEE Trans. Pattern Anal. Mach. Intell. **39**(12), 2481–2495 (2017)
2. Lee, C.Y., Xie, S., Gallagher, P., Zhang, Z., Tu, Z.: Deeply-supervised nets. In: Artificial Intelligence and Statistics, pp. 562–570 (2015)
3. Lo, C.M., et al.: Multi-dimensional tumor detection in automated whole breast ultrasound using topographic watershed. IEEE Trans. Med. Imaging **33**(7), 1503–1511 (2014)
4. Long, J., Shelhamer, E., Darrell, T.: Fully convolutional networks for semantic segmentation. In: CVPR, pp. 3431–3440 (2015)
5. Moon, W.K., Shen, Y.W., Bae, M.S., Huang, C.S., Chen, J.H., Chang, R.F.: Computer-aided tumor detection based on multi-scale blob detection algorithm in automated breast ultrasound images. IEEE Trans. Med. Imaging **32**(7), 1191–1200 (2013)
6. Ronneberger, O., Fischer, P., Brox, T.: U-Net: convolutional networks for biomedical image segmentation. In: Navab, N., Hornegger, J., Wells, W.M., Frangi, A.F. (eds.) MICCAI 2015. LNCS, vol. 9351, pp. 234–241. Springer, Cham (2015). https://doi.org/10.1007/978-3-319-24574-4_28
7. Shen, D., Wu, G., Suk, H.I.: Deep learning in medical image analysis. Annu. Rev. Biomed. Eng. **19**, 221–248 (2017)
8. Shin, H.J., Kim, H.H., Cha, J.H.: Current status of automated breast ultrasonography. Ultrasonography **34**(3), 165 (2015)
9. Tan, T., Platel, B., Mus, R., Tabar, L., Mann, R.M., Karssemeijer, N.: Computer-aided detection of cancer in automated 3-D breast ultrasound. IEEE Trans. Med. Imaging **32**(9), 1698–1706 (2013)
10. Tran, D., Bourdev, L., Fergus, R., Torresani, L., Paluri, M.: Learning spatiotemporal features with 3D convolutional networks. In: ICCV, pp. 4489–4497. IEEE (2015)
11. Yang, X.: Towards automatic semantic segmentation in volumetric ultrasound. In: Descoteaux, M., Maier-Hein, L., Franz, A., Jannin, P., Collins, D.L., Duchesne, S. (eds.) MICCAI 2017. LNCS, vol. 10433, pp. 711–719. Springer, Cham (2017). https://doi.org/10.1007/978-3-319-66182-7_81

Btrfly Net: Vertebrae Labelling with Energy-Based Adversarial Learning of Local Spine Prior

Anjany Sekuboyina[1,2(✉)], Markus Rempfler[1], Jan Kukačka[1,2], Giles Tetteh[1],
Alexander Valentinitsch[2], Jan S. Kirschke[2], and Bjoern H. Menze[1]

[1] Department of Informatics, Technical University of Munich, Munich, Germany
[2] Department of Neuroradiology, Klinikum rechts der Isar, Munich, Germany
anjany.sekuboyina@tum.de

Abstract. Robust localisation and identification of vertebrae is essential for automated spine analysis. The contribution of this work to the task is two-fold: (1) Inspired by the human expert, we hypothesise that a sagittal and coronal reformation of the spine contain sufficient information for labelling the vertebrae. Thereby, we propose a butterfly-shaped network architecture (termed Btrfly Net) that efficiently combines the information across reformations. (2) Underpinning the Btrfly net, we present an energy-based adversarial training regime that encodes local spine structure as an anatomical prior into the network, thereby enabling it to achieve state-of-art performance in all standard metrics on a benchmark dataset of 302 scans without any post-processing during inference.

1 Introduction

The localisation and identification of anatomical structures is a significant part of any medical image analysis routine. In spine's context, labelling of vertebrae has immediate diagnostic and modelling significance, e.g.: localised vertebrae are used as markers for detecting kyphosis or scoliosis, vertebral fractures, in surgical planning, or for follow-up analysis tasks such as vertebral segmentation or their bio-mechanical modelling for load analysis.

Vertebrae Labelling. Like several analysis approaches off-late, vertebrae labelling has seen successful utilisation of machine learning. One of the incipient and notable works by Glocker et al. [2], followed by [3] used context-based features with regression forests and Markov models for labelling. In spite of their intuitive motivation, these approaches suffer a setback due to limited FOVs or presence of metal insertions. On a similar footing, [7] proposed a deep multi-layer perceptron using long-range context features. With the emergence of convolutional neural networks (CNN), Chen et al. [1] proposed a joint-CNN as a combination of a random forest for initial candidate selection followed by a

---

J. S. Kirschke and B. H. Menze—Joint supervising authors.

© Springer Nature Switzerland AG 2018
A. F. Frangi et al. (Eds.): MICCAI 2018, LNCS 11073, pp. 649–657, 2018.
https://doi.org/10.1007/978-3-030-00937-3_74

CNN trained to identify the vertebra based on its appearance and a conditional dependency on its neighbours. Without hand-crafting features this approach performed remarkably well. However, since the CNN works on a limited region around the vertebra, it results in a high variability of the localisation distance. Recently, Yang et al. with [8,9], proposed a deep, volumetric, fully-convolutional 3D network (FCN) called DI2IN with deep-supervision. The output of DI2IN is improved in subsequent stages that employ either message-passing across channels or a convolutional LSTM followed by further tuning with a shape dictionary.

Owing to equivariance of the convolutional operator and limited receptive field, an FCN doesn't always learn the anatomy of the region-of-interest. This is a severe limitation as human-equivalent learning utilises anatomical details aided with prior knowledge. An immediate remedy is to increase the receptive field by going deeper. However, this comes at the cost of higher model complexity or is just unfeasible due to memory constraints when working with volumetric data.

Prior and Adversarial Learning in CNNs. Recent work in [5] and [4] propose encoding (anatomical) segmentation priors into an FCN by learning the shape representation using an auto encoder (AE). The segmentation is expressed in terms of a pre-learnt latent space for evaluating a prior-oriented loss, which is then used to guide the FCN into predicting an anatomically sound segmentation. Our approach shares similarities with this approach with certain fundamental differences: (1) Our approach is aimed at localisation, which requires a redefinition of the notion of anatomical *shape*. (2) We employ an AE for shape regularisation, but do not 'pre-train' it to learn the latent space. We train the AE adversarially in tandem with the FCN. Parallels can be drawn between end-to-end learning of priors and learning the distribution of priors using generative adversarial networks (GANs). Both have two networks, a predictor (generator) and an auxiliary network which works on the 'goodness' of the prediction. In medical image analysis where scan sizes are large and data are few, inspired from an energy-based adversarial generation framework (Zhao et al. [11]), it is preferable to employ an adversary providing an anatomically-inspired supervision instead of the usual binary adversarial supervision (vanilla GAN).

Our Contribution. In this work, we propose an end-to-end solution for vertebrae labelling by adversarially training an FCN, thereby encoding the local spine structure into it. More precisely, relying on the sufficiency of information in certain 2D projections of 3D data, we propose: (1) A butterfly-shaped network that operates on 2D sagittal and coronal reformations, combining information across these views at a large receptive field, (2) Encoding the spine's structure into the Btrfly net using an energy-based, fully-convolutional, adversarial auto encoder acting as a discriminator. Our approach attains identification rates above 85% without any post-processing stages, achieving state-of-art performance.

2   Methodology

We present our approach in two stages. First, we describe the Btrfly network tasked with the labelling of the vertebrae. Then we present the adversarial

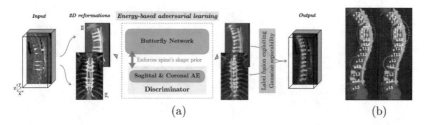

Fig. 1. (a) Overview of our approach. (b) Label correcting capability of the AE when trained as a denoising convolutional auto-encoder (red: corrupted, green: corrected). This motivates the discriminator in our adversarial framework.

learning of the local spine shape with an energy-based auto-encoder acting as the discriminator. Figure 1a gives an overview of the proposed approach and the motivation for prior-encoding is illustrated in Fig. 1b.

2.1 Btrfly Network

Working with 3D volumetric data is computationally restrictive, more so for localisation and identification that rely on a large context so as to capture spatially distant landmarks. Consequently, there is a trade-off between working with low-resolution data or resorting to shallow networks. Therefore, we propose working in 2D with *sufficiently–representative* projections of the volumetric data. The choice of projection is application dependant. Since we are working with bone, we work on sagittal and coronal maximum intensity projections (MIP). The former captures the spine's curve and the latter captures the rib-vertebrae joints, both of which are crucial markers for labelling. Note that a naive MIP might not always be the optimal choice of projection, eg. in full-body scans where spine is not spatially centred or is obstructed by the ribcage in a MIP. Such cases are handled with a pre-processing stage detecting the occluded spine in the MIP.

Annotations. We formulate the problem of learning the vertebrae labels as a multi-variate regression. The ground-truth annotation $\mathbf{Y} \in \mathbb{R}^{(h \times w \times d \times 25)}$ is a 25-channeled, 3D volume with each channel corresponding to each of the 24 vertebrae (C1 to L5), and one for the background. Each channel i is constructed as a Gaussian heat map of the form $\mathbf{y}_i = e^{-||x-\mu_i||^2/2\sigma^2}$, $x \in \mathbb{R}^3$ where μ_i is the location of the ith vertebra and σ controls the spread. The background channel is constructed as, $\mathbf{y}_0 = 1 - \max_i(\mathbf{y}_i)$. The sagittal and coronal MIPs of $\mathbf{Y}$ are denoted by $\mathbf{Y}_{\text{sag}} \in \mathbb{R}^{(h \times w \times 25)}$ and $\mathbf{Y}_{\text{cor}} \in \mathbb{R}^{(h \times d \times 25)}$, respectively.

Architecture. We employ an FCN to perform the task of labelling. Since essential information is contained in both the sagittal and coronal reformations, and since the spine is approximately spatially centred in both, fusing this information across views leads to an improved identification. We propose a butterfly-like network (cf. Fig. 2) with two arms (xz- and yz-arms) each concerned with one of the views. The feature maps of both the views are combined after a certain depth in order to learn their inter-dependency.

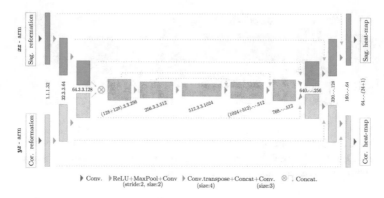

Fig. 2. The Btrfly architecture. The xz- (blue) and the yz-arms (yellow) correspond to the sagittal and coronal views. The kernel's shape resulting in each of the blocks is indicated as: {input channels} · {kern. height} · {kern. width} · {output channels}

Loss. We choose an ℓ_2 distance as the primary loss supported by a cross-entropy loss over the softmax excitation of the ground truth and the prediction. The total loss is expressed as:

$$\mathcal{L}_{b,sag} = ||\mathbf{Y}_{sag} - \tilde{\mathbf{Y}}_{sag}||^2 + \omega H(\mathbf{Y}^{\sigma}_{sag}, \tilde{\mathbf{Y}}^{\sigma}_{sag}), \tag{1}$$

where $\tilde{\mathbf{Y}}_{sag}$ is the prediction of the net's xz-arm, H is the cross-entropy function, and $\mathbf{Y}^{\sigma}_{sag} = \sigma(\mathbf{Y}_{sag})$, the softmax excitation. ω is the median frequency weighing map (described in [6]), boosting the learning of less frequent classes. The loss for the yz-arm is constructed in a similar fashion and the total loss of the Btrfly net is given by $\mathcal{L}_b = \mathcal{L}_{b,sag} + \mathcal{L}_{b,cor}$.

2.2   Energy-Based Adversary for Encoding Prior

Since the Btrfly net is fully-convolutional, its predictions across voxels are independent of each other owing to the spatial invariance of convolutions. Whatever information it encodes is solely due to its receptive field, which may not be anatomically consistent across the image. We propose to impose the anatomical prior of the spine's shape onto the Btrfly net with *adversarial* learning.

Denoting the projected annotation as $\mathbf{Y}_{view}$, where view $\in$ {sag, cor}, a sample annotation consists of a 2D Gaussian at the vertebral location in each channel (except $\mathbf{y}_0$). Looking at $\mathbf{Y}_{view}$ as a 3D volume enables us in learning the spread of Gaussians across channels and consequently the vertebral labels. However, owing to the extreme variability of FOVs and scan sizes, it is preferable to learn the spread of the vertebrae in parts. Therefore, we employ a fully-convolutional, 3D auto encoder (AE) with a receptive field covering a part of the spine at a time. The absence of fully-connected layers in the AE also removes the necessity to resize the data, making it end-to-end trainable with the Btrfly net. Figure 3a shows the arrangement of the AEs as adversaries w.r.t the Btrfly net. In an adversarial framework, the Btrfly net acts as the generator (G), and the local manifolds learnt from $\mathbf{Y}_{\text{view}}$ influence $\tilde{\mathbf{Y}}_{\text{view}}$ and vice versa.

Discriminator. We devise the 3D adversary $(D,$ cf. Fig. 3b) consisting of the AE as a functional predicting the ℓ_2 distance between the input $\mathbf{Y}_{\text{view}}$ and its reconstruction by the AE, $rec(\mathbf{Y}_{\text{view}})$: $D(\mathbf{Y}_{\text{view}}) = E = ||\mathbf{Y}_{\text{view}} - rec(\mathbf{Y}_{\text{view}})||^2$. This energy, E is fed back into G for adversarial supervision, as in [11]. As it is an energy-based functional, we interchangeably refer to the discriminator as EB-D. Since $\mathbf{Y}_{\text{view}}$ consists of Gaussians, it is less informative than an image. Therefore, we avoid using max-pooling by resorting to average pooling. In order to have a receptive field covering multiple vertebrae without using pooling operations, we employ spatially dilated convolution kernels [10] of size $(5 \times 5 \times 5)$ with a dilation rate of 2 (only in image plane), resulting in a receptive field of 76×76 pixels. At 1 mm isotropic resolution, this covers 2 to 3 vertebrae in the lumbar region and more elsewhere.

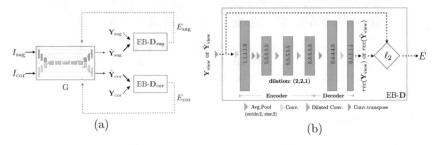

(a)   (b)

Fig. 3. (a) A overview of adversarial training showing the input to, and the energy-based supervision signal from, the discriminators. (b) The composition of the energy-based discriminator (EB-D). It gives the ℓ_2 reconstruction error as output.

Losses. As in any adversarial setup, EB-D is shown real $(\mathbf{Y}_x (\equiv \mathbf{Y}_{\text{view}}))$ and generated annotations $(\mathbf{Y}_g (\equiv \hat{\mathbf{Y}}_{\text{view}}))$, and it learns to discriminate between both by predicting a low E for real annotations, while G learns to generate annotations that would trick D. For a given positive, scalar margin m, the following generator and discriminator losses are optimised:

$$\mathcal{L}_D = D(\mathbf{Y}_x) + \max(0, m - D(\mathbf{Y}_g)), \text{ and} \tag{2}$$

$$\mathcal{L}_G = D(\mathbf{Y}_g) + \mathcal{L}_{\text{b,view}}. \tag{3}$$

The joint optimisation of (2) and (3) for both the EB-Ds results in a G that performs vertebrae labelling while respecting the spatial distribution of the vertebrae across channels. We refer to this prior-encoded G as the 'Btrfly$_{\text{pe}}$' net.

2.3   Inference

Once trained, an inference for a given input scan of size $(h \times w \times d)$ proceeds as: the desired sagittal and coronal MIP reformations are obtained and given as input to the xz- and yz-arms of the Btrfly net, resulting in a $(h \times w \times 25)$ sagittal heatmap and $(h \times d \times 25)$ coronal heatmap. The values below a threshold $(T,$ selected on validation set) are ignored in order to remove noisy predictions. As the Gaussian kernel is separable, an outer product of the predictions results in the final heat map as $\tilde{\mathbf{Y}} = \tilde{\mathbf{Y}}_{\text{sag}} \otimes \tilde{\mathbf{Y}}_{\text{cor}}$, where $\otimes$ denotes the outer product. The 3D location of the vertebral centroids are obtained as the maxima in their corresponding channels. Note that the EB-D is no longer required during inference as its role in encoding the prior ends with the convergence of the Btrfly$_{\text{pe}}$ net.

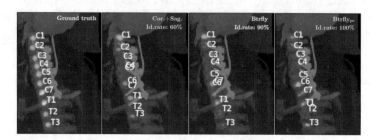

Fig. 4. Effect of prior encoding: the prior-encoded Btrfly$_{\text{pe}}$ net successfully performs its task of prevent overlapping labels (C6 & C7), consequently reordering all the vertebral labels. The reported id. rates are per volume.

3   Experiments

The evaluation is performed using a dataset introduced in [3] with a total of 302 CT scans (242 for training and 60 for testing) including various challenges such as scoliotic spines, metal insertions, and highly restrictive FOVs. However, these are cropped to a region around the spine which excludes the ribcage. Thus, a naive sagittal and coronal MIP, without any pre-processing, suffices to obtain the input images for our approach. In order to enhance the net's robustness, 10 MIPs are obtained from one 3D scan, each time randomly choosing half the slices of interest. This leads to a total of 2420 reformations per view for training (incl. a validation split of 100). We present the experiments with the Btrfly net trained as stand-alone as well as with the prior-encoding discriminator EB-D. Batch-normalisation is used after every convolution layer, along with 20% dropout in the fused layers of Btrfly. Additionally, so as to validate the necessity of the combination of views, we compare the Btrfly net's performance with that of two networks working individually on the views (denoted as Cor.+Sag. nets). The architecture of each of these networks is similar to one arm of the Btrfly net. The optimiser's setup in all the three cases is similar: an Adam optimiser is employed with an initial learning rate of $\lambda = 1 \times 10^{-3}$, working on data resampled to a 1 mm isotropic resolution. λ is decayed by a factor of $3/4th$ every 10k iterations to 0.2×10^{-3}. Convergence of all the networks is tested on the validation set.

Evaluation and Discussion. For evaluating the performance of our network with prior work, we use two metrics defined in [2] namely, the *identification rates*

Table 1. Performance comparison of our approach (setting $T = 0$, for a fair comparison) with Glocker et al. [3], Chen et al. [1] and Yang et al. [8]. DI2IN refers to stand-alone FCN, while DI2IN* includes use of message passing and shape dictionary. We do not compare with experiments in [8] that use additional undisclosed data.

Measures	[3]	[1]	DI2IN[8]	DI2IN*[8]	Cor.+Sag.	Btrfly	Btrfly$_{pe}$
Id.rate	74.0	84.2	76.0	85.0	78.1	81.8	**86.1**
d_{mean}	13.2	8.8	13.6	8.6	9.3	7.5	**7.4**
d_{std}	17.8	13.0	37.5	7.8	8.0	**5.4**	9.3

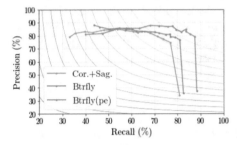

Table 2. The optimal P and R values based on F1 score, along with the optimal T. R at optimal-F1 of Btrfly$_{pe}$ is comparable to state-of-art.

Approach	P	R	F1
Cor.+Sag.$_{(T=0.05)}$	74.7	77.0	75.8
Btrfly$_{(T=0.1)}$	78.7	79.1	78.9
Btrfly$_{pe}$ $(T=0.2)$	**84.6**	**83.7**	**84.1**

Fig. 5. A precision-recall curve with F1 isolines, illustrating the effect of the T during inference. For any T, Btrfly$_{pe}$ offers a better trade-off between P and R.

(id. rate, in %) and *localisation distances* (d_{mean} & d_{std}, in mm). We report the measures in Table 1. It lists the performance of three variants of our network and compares them with several recent approaches. We address three main questions through our experiments: *(1) Why the butterfly shape?* Compared to Cor.+Sag. nets, performance improves with the Btrfly net. This is because the combination of views causes the predictions of the Btrfly net to be spatially consistent across views. We also observe a 6% improvement in the id.rate over a naive 3D FCN (DI2IN). *(2) Why the adversarial prior-encoding?* In addition to the advantages of the Btrfly net, the Btrfly$_{pe}$ net possesses adversarially encoded spatial distribution of the vertebrae. This results in about a 4% increase in the id. rate. Compared to the prior work, Btrfly$_{pe}$ net achieves state-of-art measures in both the metrics, and it does so by being a single network trained end-to-end. (cf. Fig. 4) *(3) Relation to latent-space learning?* EB-D is more flexible than the AEs in [4,5] as it learns from scratch and converges to a latent manifold best representing the true as well as generated data. The reconstruction capability of the AE for a generated sample is of interest. Using the output of the AE instead of Btrfly$_{pe}$, we achieve an id.rate of 75% with a d_{mean} of 19 mm, indicating the AEs' capability of transferring the learning from true to contrastive samples.

Precision and Recall. Localisation distance and id.rate capture the ability of the network in accurately labelling a vertebra. However, both the measures are agnostic to false positive predictions. Accounting for spurious predictions becomes important especially when dealing with FCNs, as the predictions depend on a locally constrained receptive field. In our case, the false positives are controlled by the threshold T as described in Sect. 2.3. Accounting for these, we define two measures, *precision* (P) and *recall* (R) as: $P = \#\text{hits}/\#\text{predicted}$ and $R = \#\text{hits}/\#\text{actual}$, where #hits is the number of vertebrae satisfying the condition of identification as defined for id.rate, #predicted is the vertebrae in the prediction, and #actual is the vertebrae actually present in the image. Observe that id. rate is measured over all vertebrae in the test set while R is measured *per scan* and averaged over test scans. Figure 5 shows a precision-recall curve generated by varying T between 0 to 0.8 in steps of 0.05, while Table 2 shows the performance at the F1-optimal threshold. In spite of not choosing an recall-optimistic threshold, our networks perform comparably well. Notice the over-arcing nature of Btrfly over Cor.+Sag. nets and that of Btrfly$_{pe}$ over others.

4   Conclusions

We validate the sufficiency of 2D orthogonal projections of the spine for localising and identifying the vertebrae by combining information across the projections using a butterfly-like architecture. In addition to looking at a local receptive field like any FCN, our approach considers the local structure of the spine thanks to an adversarial energy-based prior encoding, thereby outperforming the state-of-art approaches as a stand-alone network without any post-processing stages.

Acknowledgements. This work is supported by the European Research Council (ERC) under the European Union's 'Horizon 2020' research & innovation programme (GA637164–iBack–ERC–2014–STG). We acknowledge NVIDIA Corporation's support with the donation of the Quadro P5000 used for this research.

References

1. Chen, H., et al.: Automatic localization and identification of vertebrae in spine ct via a joint learning model with deep neural networks. In: MICCAI, pp. 515–522 (2015)
2. Glocker, B., et al.: Automatic localization and identification of vertebrae in arbitrary field-of-view ct scans. In: MICCAI, pp. 590–598 (2012)
3. Glocker, B., et al.: Vertebrae localization in pathological spine ct via dense classification from sparse annotations. In: MICCAI, pp. 262–270 (2013)
4. Oktay, O., et al.: Anatomically constrained neural networks (ACNN): application to cardiac image enhancement and segmentation. CoRR abs/1705.08302 (2017)
5. Ravishankar, H., et al.: Learning and incorporating shape models for semantic segmentation. In: MICCAI, pp. 203–211 (2017)
6. Roy, A.G., et al.: Error corrective boosting for learning fully convolutional networks with limited data. In: MICCAI, pp. 231–239 (2017)
7. Suzani, A., et al.: Fast automatic vertebrae detection and localization in pathological ct scans - a deep learning approach. In: MICCAI, pp. 678–686 (2015)

8. Yang, D., et al.: Automatic vertebra labeling in large-scale 3D CT using deep image-to-image network with message passing and sparsity regularization. In: IPMI, pp. 633–644 (2017)
9. Yang, D., et al.: Deep image-to-image recurrent network with shape basis learning for automatic vertebra labeling in large-scale 3D CT volumes. In: MICCAI, pp. 498–506 (2017)
10. Yu, F., Koltun, V.: Multi-scale context aggregation by dilated convolutions. In: ICLR (2016)
11. Zhao, J.J., et al.: Energy-based generative adversarial network. CoRR abs/1609.03126 (2016)

AtlasNet: Multi-atlas Non-linear Deep Networks for Medical Image Segmentation

M. Vakalopoulou[1(✉)], G. Chassagnon[1,2], N. Bus[4], R. Marini[4],
E. I. Zacharaki[3], M.-P. Revel[2], and N. Paragios[1,4]

[1] CVN, CentraleSupélec, Université Paris-Saclay, Paris, France
maria.vakalopoulou@centralesupelec.fr
[2] Groupe Hospitalier Cochin-Hotel Dieu, Université Paris Descartes, Paris, France
[3] University of Patras, Patras, Greece
[4] TheraPanacea, Paris, France

Abstract. Deep learning methods have gained increasing attention in addressing segmentation problems for medical images analysis despite the challenges inherited from the medical domain, such as limited data availability, lack of consistent textural or salient patterns, and high dimensionality of the data. In this paper, we introduce a novel multi-network architecture that exploits domain knowledge to address those challenges. The proposed architecture consists of multiple deep neural networks that are trained after co-aligning multiple anatomies through multi-metric deformable registration. This multi-network architecture can be trained with fewer examples and leads to better performance, robustness and generalization through consensus. Comparable to human accuracy, highly promising results on the challenging task of interstitial lung disease segmentation demonstrate the potential of our approach.

1 Introduction

Image segmentation is one of the most well studied problems in medical image analysis [6,8]. Segmentation seeks to group together voxels corresponding to the same organ, or to the same tissue type (healthy or pathological). Existing literature can be classified into two distinct categories, model-free and model-based methods. Model-based methods assume the manifold of the solution space can be expressed in the form of a prior distribution, with sub-space approaches (e.g. active shapes), probabilistic or graphical models and atlas-based approaches being some representatives in this category. Model-free approaches on the other hand rely purely on the observation space combining image likelihoods with different classification techniques.

The emergence of deep learning as disruptive innovation method in the field of computer vision has impacted significantly the medical imaging community [13].

M. Vakalopoulou and G. Chassagnon—Authors with equal contribution.

© Springer Nature Switzerland AG 2018
A. F. Frangi et al. (Eds.): MICCAI 2018, LNCS 11073, pp. 658–666, 2018.
https://doi.org/10.1007/978-3-030-00937-3_75

Numerous architectures have been proposed to address task-specific segmentation problems with the currently most successful technique being the Fully Convolutional Network (FCN) [11]. Additionally, FCNs have been combined with upsampling layers, creating a variety of networks [2,9], and have been extended to 3D [7], boosting even more the accuracy of semantic segmentation.

The main challenges for deep learning in medical imaging arise from the limited availability of training samples – that is amplified when targeting 3D architectures –, the lack of discriminant visual properties and the three-dimensional nature of observations (high dimensional data). In this paper, we propose a novel multi-network architecture that copes with the above limitations. The central idea is to train multiple redundant networks fusing training samples mapped to various anatomical configurations. These configurations correspond to a representative set of anatomies and are used as reference spaces (frequently referred to as atlases). The mapping corresponds to a non-linear transformer. Elastic registration based on a robust, multi-metric, multi-modal graph-based framework is used within the non-linear transformer of the network. Training is performed on the sub-space and back-projected to the original space through a de-transformer that applies an inverse nonlinear mapping. The responses of the redundant networks are then combined to determine the optimal response to the problem.

The proposed framework relates also to the multitask learning paradigm (MTL), where disparate sources of experimental data across multiple targets are combined in order to increase predictive power. The idea behind this paradigm is that by sharing representations between related tasks, we can improve generalization. Even though an inductive bias is plausible in such paradigms, the implicit data augmentation helps reducing the effect of the data-dependent noise. The idea of MTL for image segmentation has been incorporated before, such as in deep networks [10] where soft or hard parameter sharing of hidden layers is performed, or in multi-atlas segmentation [6], where multiple pre-segmented atlases are utilized in order to better capture anatomical variation. As in most ensemble methods, the concept is that the combination of solutions by probabilistic inference procedures can offer superior segmentation accuracy.

AtlasNet differs from previous methods with respect to both scope and applicability. In (single or multi) atlas segmentation, the aim is to map a presegmented region of interest from a reference image to the test image, therefore applicability is limited to normal structures (e.g. organs of the body or healthy tissue) that exist in both images. Exploitability is further reduced in the case of multi-atlas segmentation due to the rareness of multiple atlases. The proposed strategy on the contrary is suitable also for semantic labeling of voxels (as part of healthy or pathological tissue) without the requirement of spatial correspondence between those voxels in atlas and test image.

AtlasNet uses multiple forward non-linear transformers that map all training images to common subspaces to reduce biological variability and a backward detransformer to relax the effect of possible artificial local deformations. In fact, due to the ill-posedness of inter-subject image registration, regularization constraints are applied to derive smooth solutions and maintain topological relation-

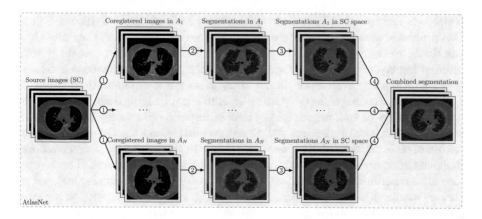

Fig. 1. The proposed AtlasNet framework. A_i indicates atlas i.

ships among anatomical structures. Consequently, image registration does not always produce a perfectly conforming diffeomorphism due to the nonexistence of a single atlas that matches all anatomies. The use of multiple spaces comes to reduce the atlas selection bias, while the backward transformation aims to balance the effect of possible alterations in local image texture due to the non-linearity in the transformation. Highly promising results comparable to human accuracy on the challenging task of interstitial lung disease (ILD) segmentation demonstrate the potential benefits of our approach. Furthermore, the obtained performance outreached redundant conventional networks.

Finally, the proposed approach (Fig. 1) addresses most of the limitations of existing neural network approaches. First, it requires fairly small number of training examples due to the reduced diversity of observations once mapped to a common anatomy. Second, it performs data augmentation in a natural manner thanks to the elastic mapping between observations and representative anatomies. Third, it inherits robustness, stability and better generalization properties for two reasons: the limited complexity of observations after mapping, and the "anatomically" consistent redundancy of the networks.

2   Methodology

The method consists of two main parts, a transformer and a de-transformer part. The former maps a sample S to N different atlases $A_i, i \in \{1, \ldots, N\}$, constructs their warped versions, and trains N different networks, while the latter projects back the N predictions to the initial space. These projections are then combined to obtain the final segmentation. The transformer part consists of a non-linear deformable operator (transformer T_i) and a segmentation network C_i while the de-transformer part uses the inverse deformable operator (de-transformer T_i^{-1}) to map everything back to the initial space of a sample S. The framework is flexible, enables any suitable transformation operator (with an existing inverse) to be coupled with a classifier.

2.1   Multimetric Deformable Operator

The multimetric deformable operator, responsible for mapping samples to different anatomies (atlases) therefore reducing variance and producing anatomically meaningful results, is an elastic image registration method that follows a context-driven metric aggregation approach [4] which aims to find the optimal combination of different similarity metrics. The operator is implemented using a deformable mapping from a source image S to a given atlas A_i. Let us consider that a number of metric functions ρ_j, $j \in \{1, \ldots, k\}$, can be used to compare the deformed source image and the target A_i. The non-linear transformer T corresponds to the operator that optimizes in the domain Ω the following energy:

$$E(\hat{T}; S, A_i) = \iint_{\Omega} \sum_{j=1}^{k} w_j \rho_j (S \circ \hat{T}, A_i) d\Omega + \alpha \iint_{\Omega} \psi(\hat{T}) d\Omega$$

where w_j are linear constraints factorizing the importance of the different metric functions, and $\psi()$ is a penalty function acting on the spatial derivatives of the transformation as regularization to impose smoothness. Such a formalism can be considered either in the continuous setting that requires differentiable functions with respect to the metric functions ρ_j or in a discrete setting. The advantage of a discrete variant is that it can integrate an arbitrary number and nature of metric functions as well as regularizers while offering good guarantees concerning the optimality properties of the obtained objective function. Inspired by the work done in [5] we express the non-linear operator as a discrete optimization problem acting on a quantized version of the deformation space.

We used free form deformations as an interpolation strategy, invariant to intensity image metrics, pyramidal implementation approach for the optimization and belief propagation for the estimation of the optimal displacement field in the discrete setting. Details on the implementation can be found in [5].

2.2   Segmentation Networks

The segmentation networks C_i operate on the mapped image, $T_i(S)$, to produce a segmentation map and can be the same or different depending on the task and the application and are completely independent of the exact classifier. After defining the optimal deformations $T_i, i = 1 \ldots N$, between the source image and the different atlases in the transformer part, AtlasNet uses the inverse transformations to project back to the initial space of the source image S the predicted segmentation maps: $S_i^{seg} = T_i^{-1}(C_i(T_i(S)))$.

In this work, motivated by the state-of-the-art performance of FCNs in several problems we adapted them for dense labeling. We use the SegNet deep learning network [2] which performs pixelwise classification and is composed of an encoder and a decoder architecture and follows the example of U-net [9]. It consists of repetitive blocks of convolutional, batch normalization, rectified-linear units (ReLU) and indexed max-pooling layers, similar to the ones of the VGG16 network. For more details we refer to the original publication.

Different fusion strategies can be used for the combination of the segmentations. We used the probabilistic output of the classifiers (before hard decision) and fused the output of the different networks based on majority voting.

3   Implementation Details

For the registration, we used the same parameters for all images and all atlases. Three different similarity metrics have been used, namely, mutual information, normalized cross correlation and discrete wavelet metric. For the mutual information 16 bins were used, in the range of -900 to 100.

We used the same parameters for training all SegNet networks (initial learning rate $= 0.01$, decrease of learning rate $= 2.5 \cdot 10^{-3}$ every 10 epochs, momentum $= 0.9$, weight decay $= 5 \cdot 10^{-4}$). The training of a single network required around 16 hours on a GeForce GTX 1080 GPU, while the prediction for a single (volumetric) subject lasted only a few seconds. For data augmentation we performed only random rotations (between -10 and $10°$) and translations (between 0 and 20 pixels per axis) avoiding local deformations since the anatomy should not artificially change. Moreover, for training, we performed median frequency balancing [2] to balance the data, as the samples with disease are considerably fewer than the rest of the samples.

4   Experimental Results and Dataset

We used as case study to evaluate our method the ILD segmentation in CT images because it is a challenging problem; boundaries are hard to detect and delineation suffers from poor-to-moderate interobserver agreement [3]. Moreover, although several visual scoring systems have been proposed for the disease, they only allow basic quantification of ILD severity. The dataset includes 17 (volumetric) CT images consisting of 6000 slices in total, each being of 512×512 dimension, and annotations of lung and disease. The ILD annotation was performed by a medical expert by tracing the disease boundaries in axial view over all slices and used for training the classification model. Assessment of the method was performed on images from 29 additional patients being fully annotated only on selected CT slices ($n = 20$) by three different observers. Note that the data was multi-vendor (GE & Siemens) and corresponds to the same moment of the respiratory cycle.

Table 1. Evaluation metrics for the testing dataset for the scleroderma disease.

Method	Sensitivity	Precision	Hausdorff dist.	Average dist.	Dice
SegNet [2]	0.348	**0.623**	4.984	1.891	0.533
Augmentation & SegNet [2]	0.534	0.567	4.077	1.309	0.619
Inter-observer	**0.693**	0.522	4.005	1.317	0.662
AtlasNet	0.682	0.545	**3.981**	**1.274**	**0.677**

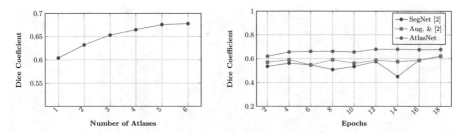

(a) Dice coefficient for different number of atlases.

(b) Dice coefficient evolution for the different methods in the test dataset.

Fig. 2. Quantitative evaluation of the dice coefficient for varying parameters.

For all experiments we used 6 different atlases and registered both training and testing images to them. The choice of atlases was made by a radiologist towards integrating important variability of the considered anatomies. Our experimental evaluation has two objectives: (i) to show that AtlasNet provides more robust and accurate solutions compared to conventional networks and (ii) to examine whether the proposed methodology can truly be trained with fewer examples while leading to good performance. We used five metrics, namely sensitivity, precision, Hausdorff, average contour distance and dice coefficient (over the number of epochs), to evaluate the performance of the proposed method.

On the Number of Atlases: Figure 2a presents the behavior of our method using different number of atlases. It can be observed that the dice initially increases and tends to stabilize for more than 5 templates. Note that, even with the use of only one atlas the deformable operator of AtlasNet helps to increase the dice coefficient (from 0.533 to 0.604), as indicated by Fig. 2b and achieves the highest values of dice compared to conventional networks and usual data augmentation techniques.

On the Number of Training Samples: To evaluate the performance of our architecture with less samples we used a reduced number of samples (30%, 50% and 70% respectively) for the same number of epochs (18) and compare the performance with the one in [2]. The obtained mean dice coefficient values in [2] were 0.434, 0.462, 0.487, while for AtlasNet were 0.613, 0.646 and 0.672 respectively, indicating the robustness of AtlasNet with a significantly lower number of samples. In simple words, the proposed architecture produces better or similar results with 30% of the samples compared to the state-of-the-art architecture [2] with and without data augmentation.

Comparison with the State-of-Art: Although results on different datasets are not directly comparable, we compare our method with works related to ILD segmentation. Anthimopoulos *et al.* [1] classified CT image patches with ILD patterns using a CNN and obtained 0.856 accuracy for 6 disease classes. By extracting patches on our data (where different patterns are annotated as

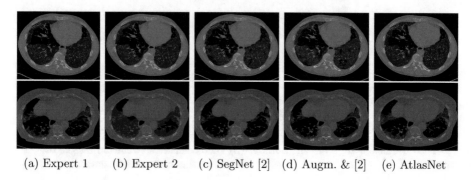

(a) Expert 1   (b) Expert 2   (c) SegNet [2]   (d) Augm. & [2]   (e) AtlasNet

Fig. 3. Interstitial lung disease segmentation (depicted with red color) on two testing subjects using the different employed strategies.

a single class) in the same way as in [1] we obtained 0.916 accuracy. In [12] a patch-based CNN was augmented with a deep encoder-decoder to exploit partial annotations. By applying AtlasNet on the same dataset as in [12], we increased the mean dice from 0.671 to 0.725.

Moreover we compared AtlasNet with respect to disease segmentation with standard frameworks (without registration and with or without data augmentation) for the same number of epochs (18) and illustrate results in Table 1 and Fig. 2b. For equal comparison, we assessed accuracies using the same classification strategy [2] trained on the initial CT slices, and after performing data augmentation as described earlier. The proposed method reports the best accuracy with respect to Hausdorff distance, average contour distance and dice, indicating that the disease segmentation is much more accurate than by the conventional frameworks with or without data augmentation. This can be inferred also from Fig. 3 where axial slices of two different subjects are depicted. It is clear that the proposed approach segments accurately the boundaries of the disease.

For a more complete evaluation, we compare AtlasNet also with inter-observer agreement using the annotations of three different medical experts. In particular, the annotations of one observer have been used as ground truth to evaluate the rest. From Table 1 and Fig. 3, it can be observed that Atlas-Net demonstrates more robust performance than manual segmentation. Finally, it is worth mentioning that even if the network operates on 2D slices, without accounting for out-of-slice connections, the fusion of the different atlases' predictions makes the final segmentation smooth across all three axes.

Concerning the computational resources, we use a single segmentation network [2] for each of the N atlases, therefore the time and memory usage for one atlas is that of the CNN, while we also showed that a small N (such as 6) suffices. For segmentation of one volumetric CT on a single GPU the total testing time (using 6 atlases) is 3–4 min, including the registration step while the registration cost is negligible since a graph-based GPU algorithm is used taking 3–5 s per subject. This cost drops linearly with the number and computing power of GPUs. Thus, we believe that the additional complexity of AtlasNet is fully justified, since it improves performance by more than 20% and also maintains it stable with only 30% of the training data compared to conventional single networks.

5   Conclusion

In this paper, we present a novel multi-network architecture for (healthy or pathological) tissue or organ segmentation that maximizes consistency by exploiting diversity. Evaluation of the method on interstitial lung disease segmentation highlighted its advantages over previous competing approaches as well as inter-observer agreement. The investigation of techniques for soft parameter sharing of hidden layers, and information transfer between the different networks and atlases is our direction for future work. Finally, the extension to multi-organ segmentation including multiple classes and loss functions is one of the potential directions of our method.

References

1. Anthimopoulos, M., Christodoulidis, S., Ebner, L., Christe, A., Mougiakakou, S.: Lung pattern classification for interstitial lung diseases using a deep convolutional neural network. IEEE Trans. Med. Imaging **35**(5), 1207–1216 (2016)
2. Badrinarayanan, V., Kendall, A., Cipolla, R.: SegNet: a deep convolutional encoder-decoder architecture for image segmentation. IEEE PAMI (2017)
3. Camiciottoli, G., et al.: Lung CT densitometry in systemic sclerosis: correlation with lung function, exercise testing, and quality of life. Chest **131**(3), 672–681 (2007)
4. Ferrante, E., Dokania, P.K., Marini, R., Paragios, N.: Deformable registration through learning of context-specific metric aggregation. In: Wang, Q., Shi, Y., Suk, H.-I., Suzuki, K. (eds.) MLMI 2017. LNCS, vol. 10541, pp. 256–265. Springer, Cham (2017). https://doi.org/10.1007/978-3-319-67389-9_30
5. Glocker, B., Komodakis, N., Tziritas, G., Navab, N., Paragios, N.: Dense image registration through MRFs and efficient linear programming. Med. Image Anal. **12**(6), 731–741 (2008)
6. Iglesias, J.E., Sabuncu, M.R.: Multi-atlas segmentation of biomedical images: a survey. Med. Image Anal. **24**(1), 205–219 (2015)
7. Milletari, F., Navab, N., Ahmadi, S.A.: V-net: fully convolutional neural networks for volumetric medical image segmentation. In: 2016 Fourth International Conference on 3D Vision (3DV), pp. 565–571. IEEE (2016)
8. Paragios, N., Ferrante, E., Glocker, B., Komodakis, N., Parisot, S., Zacharaki, E.I.: (Hyper)-graphical models in biomedical image analysis. Med. Image Anal. **33**, 102–106 (2016)
9. Ronneberger, O., Fischer, P., Brox, T.: U-net: convolutional networks for biomedical image segmentation. In: Navab, N., Hornegger, J., Wells, W.M., Frangi, A.F. (eds.) MICCAI 2015. LNCS, vol. 9351, pp. 234–241. Springer, Cham (2015). https://doi.org/10.1007/978-3-319-24574-4_28
10. Ruder, S.: An overview of multi-task learning in deep neural networks. CoRR abs/1706.05098 (2017)

11. Shelhamer, E., Long, J., Darrell, T.: Fully convolutional networks for semantic segmentation. IEEE Trans. Pattern Anal. Mach. Intell. **39**(4), 640–651 (2017)
12. Vakalopoulou, M., Chassagnon, G., Paragios, N., Revel, M., Zacharaki, E.: Deep patch-based priors under a fully convolutional encoder-decoder architecture for interstitial lung disease segmentation. In: 2018 IEEE International Symposium on Biomedical Imaging (ISBI) (2018)
13. Zhou, S., Greenspan, H., Shen, D.: Deep Learning for Medical Image Analysis. Academic Press, Cambridge (2017)

CFCM: Segmentation via Coarse to Fine Context Memory

Fausto Milletari[1]([✉]), Nicola Rieke[1,2], Maximilian Baust[2], Marco Esposito[2], and Nassir Navab[2]

[1] NVIDIA, Santa Clara, USA
fmilletari@nvidia.com
[2] Technische Universität München, Munich, Germany

Abstract. Recent neural-network-based architectures for image segmentation make extensive usage of feature forwarding mechanisms to integrate information from multiple scales. Although yielding good results, even deeper architectures and alternative methods for feature fusion at different resolutions have been scarcely investigated for medical applications. In this work we propose to implement segmentation via an encoder-decoder architecture which differs from any other previously published method since (i) it employs a very deep architecture based on residual learning and (ii) combines features via a convolutional Long Short Term Memory (LSTM), instead of concatenation or summation. The intuition is that the memory mechanism implemented by LSTMs can better integrate features from different scales through a coarse-to-fine strategy; hence the name Coarse-to-Fine Context Memory (CFCM). We demonstrate the remarkable advantages of this approach on two datasets: the Montgomery county lung segmentation dataset, and the EndoVis 2015 challenge dataset for surgical instrument segmentation.

1 Introduction and Previous Work

The usefulness of multi-scale feature representations has been acknowledged by the computer vision community for decades, c.f. Burt and Adelson [2] or Koenderink and van Doorn [13] for instance, and both traditional and modern approaches for image segmentation, registration or stereo rely on the integration of features from multiple scales. In recent years, convolutional neural networks (CNNs) have advanced the state of art in image segmentation tremendously as this technique allows to learn rich feature representations over multiple scales. However, the integration of these representations for obtaining full-resolution segmentations is not straightforward and it is an active field of research.

Besides applying CNNs in a patch-based fashion as proposed by [6], which is still common practice for very large data such as whole slide images in digital pathology, FCNNs making use of whole-image information, originally suggested by Long et al. [16], have turned out to be powerful tools. Based on this work,

---

Maximilian Baust is now working for Konica Minolta Laboratory Europe.

© Springer Nature Switzerland AG 2018
A. F. Frangi et al. (Eds.): MICCAI 2018, LNCS 11073, pp. 667–674, 2018.
https://doi.org/10.1007/978-3-030-00937-3_76

Ronneberger *et al.* [19] extended the idea of feature forwarding and proposed a symmetrical architecture. In this work the expanding or decoding path takes advantage of fine-grained features from the compressing path that are forwarded via skip connections. Feature forwarding has also turned out to be a very successful concept for 3D volumetric segmentation as demonstrated by Milletari *et al.* [17] and Çiçek *et al.* [5]. Further achievements to these architectures have then been accomplished by improved up-sampling, e.g. [1], improved training strategies, e.g. [10], integration of random fields and àtrous convolutions [4], and particularly the application of residual learning [8], e.g. [3,14]. For a more complete review of related works, we refer the interested reader to the recent review of Litjens *et al.* [15]. In summary, it can be said that most state-of-the-art segmentation architectures use skip connections for feature forwarding and multi-scale context integration. However, most current approach resort to simple feature fusion schemes, based on concatenation or summation. An exception is represented by the gated feedback refinement network by Islam *et al.* [11] which comprise gate units to control the information flow and filter out ambiguity.

In this work, we present an alternative approach to multi-scale feature integration based on Long-Short-Term-Memory-units (LSTMs) initially proposed by Hochreiter and Schmidhuber [9], wich we term Coarse-to-Fine Context Memory (CFCM). The rationale behind this approach is that LSTMs implement a memory mechanism in which information can be maintained through different steps and only be updated with new information when necessary. We employ this idea to manage features extracted at different resolutions from the compressing path of the network. To demonstrate the potential of this approach, we compare our method to established architectures on two different datasets.

2   Method

Our segmentation approach is based on a fully convolutional architecture consisting of an encoding and a decoding part, c.f. Fig. 1. While encoding is based on a standard ResNet architecture, decoding is implemented using convolutional LSTMs. The core idea of this approach is to use a memory mechanism, implemented via convolutional LSTMs, for fusing features extracted from different layers of the encoder. Thereby, the convolutional LSTMs take the role of a coarse-to-fine focusing mechanism which first perceives the global context of the input data, as the deepest activations are fed to the inputs of the LSTM, and later processes fine-grained details. This happens when shallower, high-resolution features are considered. Code available on http://github.com/faustomilletari/CFCM-2D.

2.1   Encoder

Recent works [5,17,19] have proven that forwarding features extracted by the layers of the encoding path to the corresponding layers of the decoding path greatly improves performance: At training time, convergence can be achieved within a smaller number of epochs, and at testing time the segmentation

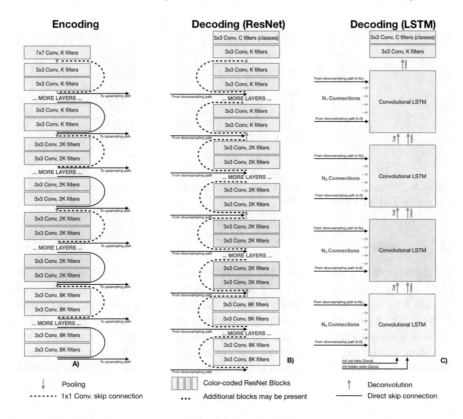

Fig. 1. Graphical Representation of the ResNet+Skip connection architecture and the proposed Coarse to Fine Context Memory (CFCM) based on LSTM. The number of layers in each block of the ResNet varies according to the architecture (ResNet-18, -34, -50, -101). The number of skip connection follows accordingly.

performance is better. To this end, feature fusion strategies based on concatenation and summation have been employed by various authors [5,14,16,19], but alternatives have been rarely investigated, which constitutes one of the motivations for this work. Our aim is to model the hierarchical nature of the features we extract from the encoding path explicitly in order to build a principled and more effective way of fusing them.

As shown in Fig. 1, we employ a ResNet architecture and we derive features at each residual block. These features are interpreted as a coarse-to-fine scale sequence, starting from the bottom of the ResNet up to its top. The deepest features are characterized by low resolution but high receptive field. As shown by Zeiler *et al.* [21] as well as other recent works, these features are taking into account global image information and high-level, complex patterns. Due to their coarse resolution, however, they do not yield information about fine-grained details. The uppermost features, on the other hand, refer to much more low-level, and fine-grained details, which is due to their high resolution and their limited receptive field.

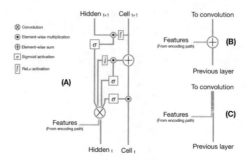

Fig. 2. Schematic Comparison of convolutional LSTMs (A) and feature fusion by summation (B) and concatenation (C).

2.2 Decoder

Our decoder treats each block of the ResNet encoder as a single time-step. As shown in Fig. 1 we forward the outputs of these blocks to our decoder, where the features are processed through LSTM cells. To this end, we employ convolutional LSTMs [20], which have the capability of selectively updating their internal states at each step depending on the result of a convolution. As shown in Fig. 2 each time step makes use of three feature sets: inputs, hidden and cell state. Inputs are concatenated with the hidden state. A convolution is performed and its result is used to (1) pass a part of the information stored in the cell state through the forget gate; (2) compute new activations which contribute to the cell state after being (3) decimated; (4) compute a new hidden state.

The initial hidden and cell states of the first LSTM are set to zero. The states of all other LSTM blocks in the decoder are initialized to be the up-sampled versions of the hidden and cell activations of the cell below. Intuitively, this mechanism can be understood as a coarse-to-fine context integration mechanism. The whole context of the picture is perceived first and, gradually, fine-grained details are added as the feature receptive fields decrease. Compared to other strategies, depicted also in Fig. 2, this architecture allows global context to be kept in memory while details are gradually being added. This aims at imitating the mechanism allowing humans to focus on details of an object while keeping in mind its global appearance. The hidden state of the last LSTM cell of the decoder constitutes the output of the memory mechanism and the last two convolutional layers produce the final segmentation.

3 Experimental Evaluation

To demonstrate the advantages and general applicability of the proposed technique, we evaluate the segmentation performance on two different datasets. First, we compare CFCM against to two baselines, U-Net and ResNet+Skip, on the Montgomery Country X-ray Dataset. In the second experiment, we focus on the general applicability and test the performance regarding segmentation of surgical instruments in endoscopic surgery sequences. To show the superior performance of the method, we compare to state-of-the-art networks that are specialized on instrument tracking.

Implementation Details. Our networks are initialized with the same set of parameters, trained with batch-size 16 with a learning rate of 0.00001 optimizing for the dice coefficient [17]. When learning to segment the Montgomery county X-Ray we train for 150 epochs. When dealing with EndoVis we train for 30 epochs. The images are scaled to an input size of 256 × 256 pixels. Our ResNet+Skip connection is depicted in Fig. 1. Its decoder is a mirrored version of the encoder with skip connections at each block. Our method CFCM is implemented in tensorflow and will be made publicly available upon paper publication.

Montgomery County X-ray Set. This dataset comprises 138 annotated posterior-anterior chest x-rays and has been acquired from the tuberculosis control program of the Department of Health and Human Services of Montgomery County, MD, USA [12]. The set contains 80 normal cases and 58 abnormal cases with manifestations of tuberculosis including effusions and miliary patterns. For testing, we perform a three fold cross evaluation for binary lung segmentation and report the mean scores in Table 1. As shown in Fig. 3, U-Net and ResNet tend to misclassify the air-filled upper trachea or fractions of the shoulder as part of the lung, while the proposed CFCM is successful in capturing the global shape and fine outlines of the anatomy. Especially the leakage to the region of the shoulder is reduced. The improved performance is also reflected in consistent better quantitative results (see Table 1). It can be observed that the performance of CFCM improves with depth while the ResNet with simple skip connections starts to overfit due to high number of parameters.

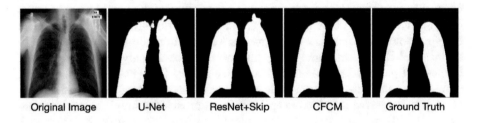

Original Image   U-Net   ResNet+Skip   CFCM   Ground Truth

Fig. 3. Qualitative results on the Montgomery county X-Ray dataset.

EndoVis 2015[1]. The dataset covers in total 6 *ex-vivo* endoscopic surgery sequences of image resolution 720 × 576 pixels. The training data contains four 45s sequences. The remaining 15s of the same sequence together with two new 60s

---

[1] MICCAI 2015 Endoscopic Vision Challenge Instrument Segmentation and Tracking Sub-challenge http://endovissub-instrument.grand-challenge.org.

Table 1. Results for Montgomery county X-Ray set. Abbreviations: $DICE$ = Dice coefficient, MAD = Mean Absolute Distance, RMS = Root-Mean-Square distance, HD = Hausdorff Distance

Architecture	DICE	MAD	RMS	HD
U-Net	0.961 ± 0.020	0.160 ± 0.288	$0.960 \pm \mathbf{1.207}$	20.463 ± 15.607
ResNet18+Skip	0.966 ± 0.0239	0.228 ± 0.475	1.265 ± 1.865	21.670 ± 19.529
ResNet34+Skip	0.969 ± 0.0217	0.189 ± 0.400	1.034 ± 1.664	16.335 ± 14.959
ResNet50+Skip	0.969 ± 0.0225	0.201 ± 0.456	1.072 ± 1.809	17.015 ± 16.651
ResNet101+Skip	0.969 ± 0.0222	0.198 ± 0.414	1.120 ± 1.766	17.340 ± 16.807
CFCM18	0.967 ± 0.019	0.151 ± 0.298	0.907 ± 1.324	15.838 ± 14.853
CFCM34	0.969 ± 0.0189	0.145 ± 0.328	0.844 ± 1.414	14.984 ± 15.078
CFCM50	0.970 ± 0.0188	0.144 ± 0.311	0.863 ± 1.414	14.848 ± 15.151
CFCM101	$\mathbf{0.972 \pm 0.0181}$	$\mathbf{0.143 \pm 0.307}$	$\mathbf{0.821} \pm 1.379$	$\mathbf{14.238 \pm 15.011}$

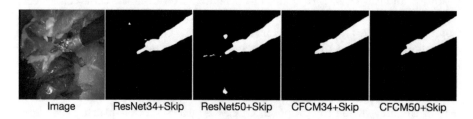

Image   ResNet34+Skip   ResNet50+Skip   CFCM34+Skip   CFCM50+Skip

Fig. 4. Qualitative results on the EndoVis dataset.

videos form the testing dataset. There are three semantic classes (manipulator, shaft and background). As specified in the guidelines, we preformed a cross-validation by leaving one surgery out of the training data. The segmentation result was compared to generic methods as well as algorithms that were explicitly published for this task [7,14,18]. García-Peraza-Herrera *et al.* [7] proposed a Fully convolutional network for segmentation in minimally invasive surgery. To achieve real-time performance, they applied the network only on every couple of frames and propagated the information with optical flow (FCN+OF). DLR [18] represents a deep residual network with dilated convolutions. Laina and Rieke *et al.* [14] suggested a unified deep learning approach for simultaneous segmentation and 2D pose estimation using Fully Convolutional Residual Network with skip connections. As depicted in Table 2, we outperform state of the art for both binary segmentation as well as multi-class segmentation. The major advantage of the proposed method over alternative approaches can be seen in the robustness to specular noise and the precision for the grasper (Table 2, Fig. 4). While the other methods have problems with the most flexible part of the instrument, CFCM can still recover the fine segmentation by the deep feature integration with LSTMs.

Table 2. Results for EndoVis. Abbreviations: *B.Acc* = Balanced Accuracy, *Rec* = Recall, *Spec* = Specificity, *DICE* = Dice coefficient

Method	Binary				Shaft				Grasper			
	B.Acc.	Rec.	Spec.	DICE	Prec.	Rec.	Spec.	DICE	Prec.	Rec.	Spec.	DICE
FCN [7]	83.7	72.2	95.2	-	-	-	-	-	-	-	-	-
FCN+OF [7]	88.3	87.8	88.7	-	-	-	-	-	-	-	-	-
DRL [18]	92.3	85.7	98.8	-	-	-	-	-	-	-	-	-
CSL [14]	92.6	86.2	**99.0**	88.9	92.4	**83.8**	**99.3**	**87.7**	79.1	77.4	99.2	77.7
ResNet18+Skip	97.3	86.0	98.9	87.5	97.5	82.7	98.8	83.5	98.4	70.2	99.3	73.1
ResNet34+Skip	97.4	84.9	98.9	87.2	83.6	82.4	98.9	83.0	**98.6**	74.2	**99.4**	75.8
ResNet50+Skip	97.2	85.3	98.8	86.8	97.5	82.0	97.6	83.5	98.5	75.9	99.3	76.0
ResNet101+Skip	97.0	84.9	98.7	86.0	-	-	-	-	-	-	-	-
CFCM18	97.7	88.0	98.9	89.3	97.4	81.3	99.1	81.5	98.3	73.6	99.2	75.0
CFCM34	**97.8**	**88.8**	98.8	**89.5**	**97.6**	82.1	99.1	84.0	**98.6**	77.0	99.3	**78.3**
CFCM50	97.5	87.7	98.8	88.8	**97.6**	81.4	99.0	83.9	98.5	**77.8**	99.2	78.1
CFCM101	97.2	81.1	**99.0**	85.5	-	-	-	-	-	-	-	-

4 Conclusion

We presented a novel approach for CNN-based image segmentation that achieves multi-scale feature integration via LSTMs which we term Coarse-to-Fine Context Memory (CFCM). This approach has been evaluated on two challenging segmentation databases of chest radiographs and video data showing surgical instruments during an intervention in endoscopy. The experiments demonstrate that the proposed method achieves superior performance and can outperform generic as well as application-specific networks. Future research might include the extension of this concept to 3D and the exploration of different memory mechanisms.

References

1. Badrinarayanan, V., Kendall, A., Cipolla, R.: SegNet: a deep convolutional encoder-decoder architecture for image segmentation. IEEE Trans. Pattern Anal. Mach. Intell. **39**(12), 2481–2495 (2017)
2. Burt, P.J., Adelson, E.H.: The laplacian pyramid as a compact image code. In: Readings in Computer Vision, pp. 671–679. Elsevier (1987)
3. Chen, H., Dou, Q., Yu, L., Qin, J., Heng, P.A.: VoxresNet: deep voxelwise residual networks for brain segmentation from 3D MR images. NeuroImage (2017)
4. Chen, L.C., Papandreou, G., Kokkinos, I., Murphy, K., Yuille, A.L.: DeepLab: semantic image segmentation with deep convolutional nets, atrous convolution, and fully connected CRFs. arXiv preprint arXiv:1606.00915 (2016)
5. Çiçek, Ö., Abdulkadir, A., Lienkamp, S.S., Brox, T., Ronneberger, O.: 3D U-net: learning dense volumetric segmentation from sparse annotation. In: Ourselin, S., Joskowicz, L., Sabuncu, M.R., Unal, G., Wells, W. (eds.) MICCAI 2016. LNCS, vol. 9901, pp. 424–432. Springer, Cham (2016). https://doi.org/10.1007/978-3-319-46723-8_49

6. Ciresan, D., Giusti, A., Gambardella, L.M., Schmidhuber, J.: Deep neural networks segment neuronal membranes in electron microscopy images. In: Advances in Neural Information Processing Systems, pp. 2843–2851 (2012)

7. García-Peraza-Herrera, L.C., et al.: Real-time segmentation of non-rigid surgical tools based on deep learning and tracking. In: Peters, T., et al. (eds.) CARE 2016. LNCS, vol. 10170, pp. 84–95. Springer, Cham (2017). https://doi.org/10.1007/978-3-319-54057-3_8

8. He, K., Zhang, X., Ren, S., Sun, J.: Deep residual learning for image recognition. In: Proceedings of the IEEE Conference on Computer Vision and Pattern Recognition, pp. 770–778 (2016)

9. Hochreiter, S., Schmidhuber, J.: Long short-term memory. Neural comput. **9**(8), 1735–1780 (1997)

10. Hwang, S., Kim, H.-E.: Self-transfer learning for weakly supervised lesion localization. In: Ourselin, S., Joskowicz, L., Sabuncu, M.R., Unal, G., Wells, W. (eds.) MICCAI 2016. LNCS, vol. 9901, pp. 239–246. Springer, Cham (2016). https://doi.org/10.1007/978-3-319-46723-8_28

11. Islam, M.A., Rochan, M., Bruce, N.D., Wang, Y.: Gated feedback refinement network for dense image labeling. In: 2017 IEEE Conference on Computer Vision and Pattern Recognition (CVPR), pp. 4877–4885. IEEE (2017)

12. Jaeger, S., Candemir, S., Antani, S., Wáng, Y.X.J., Lu, P.X., Thoma, G.: Two public chest x-ray datasets for computer-aided screening of pulmonary diseases. Quant. Imaging Med. Surg. **4**(6), 475 (2014)

13. Koenderink, J.J., van Doorn, A.J.: Representation of local geometry in the visual system. Biol. Cybern. **55**(6), 367–375 (1987)

14. Laina, I., et al.: Concurrent segmentation and localization for tracking of surgical instruments. In: Descoteaux, M., Maier-Hein, L., Franz, A., Jannin, P., Collins, D.L., Duchesne, S. (eds.) MICCAI 2017. LNCS, vol. 10434, pp. 664–672. Springer, Cham (2017). https://doi.org/10.1007/978-3-319-66185-8_75

15. Litjens, G., et al.: A survey on deep learning in medical image analysis. Med. Image Anal. **42**, 60–88 (2017)

16. Long, J., Shelhamer, E., Darrell, T.: Fully convolutional networks for semantic segmentation. In: Proceedings of the IEEE Conference on Computer Vision and Pattern Recognition, pp. 3431–3440 (2015)

17. Milletari, F., Navab, N., Ahmadi, S.A.: V-net: Fully convolutional neural networks for volumetric medical image segmentation. In: 2016 Fourth International Conference on 3D Vision (3DV), pp. 565–571. IEEE (2016)

18. Pakhomov, D., Premachandran, V., Allan, M., Azizian, M., Navab, N.: Deep residual learning for instrument segmentation in robotic surgery. arXiv preprint arXiv:1703.08580 (2017)

19. Ronneberger, O., Fischer, P., Brox, T.: U-net: convolutional networks for biomedical image segmentation. In: Navab, N., Hornegger, J., Wells, W.M., Frangi, A.F. (eds.) MICCAI 2015. LNCS, vol. 9351, pp. 234–241. Springer, Cham (2015). https://doi.org/10.1007/978-3-319-24574-4_28

20. Xingjian, S., Chen, Z., Wang, H., Yeung, D.Y., Wong, W.K., Woo, W.C.: Convolutional LSTM network: a machine learning approach for precipitation nowcasting. In: Advances in Neural Information Processing Systems, pp. 802–810 (2015)

21. Zeiler, M.D., Fergus, R.: Visualizing and understanding convolutional networks. In: Fleet, D., Pajdla, T., Schiele, B., Tuytelaars, T. (eds.) ECCV 2014. LNCS, vol. 8689, pp. 818–833. Springer, Cham (2014). https://doi.org/10.1007/978-3-319-10590-1_53

Image Segmentation Methods: Other Segmentation Applications

Pyramid-Based Fully Convolutional Networks for Cell Segmentation

Tianyi Zhao and Zhaozheng Yin[✉]

Department of Computer Science,
Missouri University of Science and Technology, Rolla, MO, USA
yinz@mst.edu

Abstract. The low contrast and irregular cell shapes in microscopy images cause difficulties to obtain the accurate cell segmentation. We propose pyramid-based fully convolutional networks (FCN) to segment cells in a cascaded refinement manner. The higher-level FCNs generate coarse cell segmentation masks, attacking the challenge of low contrast between cell inner regions and the background. The lower-level FCNs generate segmentation masks focusing more on cell details, attacking the challenge of irregular cell shapes. The FCNs in the pyramid are trained in a cascaded way such that the residual error between the ground truth and upper-level segmentation is propagated to the lower-level and draws the attention of the lower-level FCNs to find the cell details missed from the upper-levels. The fine cell details from lower-level FCNs are gradually fused into the coarse segmentation from upper-level FCNs so as to obtain a final precise cell segmentation mask. On the ISBI cell segmentation challenge dataset and a newly collected dataset with high-quality ground truth, our method outperforms the state-of-the-art methods.

1 Introduction

Cell segmentation in microscopy images, as a cornerstone of many cell image analysis tasks, has been researched for years [12]. There are still a few unsolved major challenges: (1) the contrast between cells and their background is low in the microscopy images (e.g., in Fig. 1(a), the appearance of the inner region of the cell is quite similar to its surrounding culturing medium); and (2) cells exhibit irregular shapes during their growth process (e.g., Fig. 1(b)), yielding difficulties to segment the precise boundaries of cells.

1.1 Related Work

Recently, deep learning has demonstrated its superior performance on object segmentation in images. Long *et al.* [2] proposed a fully convolutional network for semantic segmentation, which is modified from the Alexnet [3] (a seminal convolutional neural network for large-scale image classification). He *et al.* [4] proposed a Mask R-CNN approach that detects objects in an image while simultaneously generating a segmentation mask for each object. Ronneberger *et al.* [1]

© Springer Nature Switzerland AG 2018
A. F. Frangi et al. (Eds.): MICCAI 2018, LNCS 11073, pp. 677–685, 2018.
https://doi.org/10.1007/978-3-030-00937-3_77

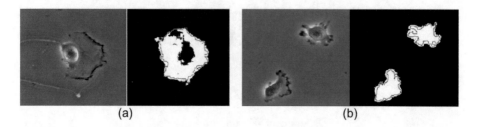

(a)   (b)

Fig. 1. Two major challenges in cell segmentation: (a) low contrast between cells and background and (b) irregular shapes of cells. Red contour: the ground truth cell boundary; white mask: cell segmentation by U-Net [1]. Images are from the ISBI cell segmentation challenge [9].

proposed a U-Net that consists of convolutional layers and deconvolutional layers with skip connection techniques. The U-Net won the ISBI cell segmentation challenge in Phase Contrast Microscopy Images in 2015. When checking the failure cases of U-Net, we found the two challenges (low contrast and irregular shapes) are the major causes, as shown in Fig. 1.

1.2   Motivation

There are some research studies about combining the Laplacian pyramid with deep neural networks. Ghiasi *et al.* [7] describes a multi-resolution reconstruction architecture for semantic segmentation which uses skip connections between different levels of a pyramid. Denton *et al.* [6] deploys the Laplacian Pyramid for a generative image model to generate images in a coarse-to-fine fashion. In a pyramid of gradu-

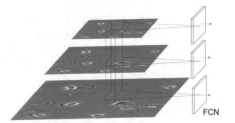

Fig. 2. Receptive field of each level.

ally downsized images, the receptive field (red rectangles in Fig. 2) analyzes the image content at different scales. The top-level receptive field perceives objects at the global level, which could attack the low contrast challenge, and the bottom-level receptive field perceives more on fine object details which could attack the irregular shape challenge. This motivated us to design a series of fully convolutional networks (FCN) to extract information from different sizes of image regions, which can enable us to compute a precise cell segmentation mask in a coarse-to-fine manner.

1.3   Our Proposal

We propose a pyramid-based fully convolutional network approach to segment cells in a cascaded refinement manner. The higher-level FCNs generate coarse cell segmentation masks, attacking the challenge of low contrast between cell inner regions and background. The lower-level FCNs generate segmentation masks focusing more on cell details, attacking the challenge of irregular cell shapes. There are a few novelties on the proposed method: (1) The input to the series of FCNs is a Gaussian pyramid, but fusing the output from FCNs is achieved in a way similar to the sequential image reconstruction in the Laplacian pyramid so the fine details on cells can be gradually collected into the final cell segmentation mask; (2) The FCNs in the pyramid are trained in a cascaded way. The highest level FCN is first trained to achieve the coarse mask. Then, the residual error (difference between the coarse mask and ground truth) is propagated to the lower-level FCNs, so the lower-level FCNs try to find cell details missed by the upper-level; and (3) At each level of the pyramid, we derive a residual mask to reflect different types of segmentation errors from the upper-level FCN, which draws the attention of the FCN at the current level.

2 Preliminaries

2.1 Fully Convolutional Networks (FCN)

The fully convolutional neural network only contains convolutional layers to generate the segmentation mask from the input image, as shown in Fig. 3. The fully convolutional neural network does not require a fixed-size input. The objective function could be pixel-wise such as the cross-entropy or mask-wise such as the dice-coefficient.

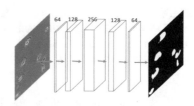

Fig. 3. A typical FCN architecture.

2.2 Gaussian Pyramid and Laplacian Pyramid

Let I be the original image, the Gaussian pyramid is denoted as $\mathcal{G}(I) = \{I_1, \ldots, I_k, \ldots, I_K\}$, where K is the number of levels in the pyramid. I_1 is the original image I and I_k at level k is downsized from the previous image I_{k-1}. The Laplacian pyramid [5] is denoted as $\mathcal{L}(I) = \{l_1, \ldots, l_k, \ldots, l_{K-1}, I_K\}$, representing a set of difference images (except the smallest level). The I_K from Gaussian pyramid $\mathcal{G}(I)$ and Laplacian pyramid $\mathcal{L}(I)$ are the same, which is a downsized image with the smallest scale. l_k at level k of Laplacian pyramid is a difference image so that the image I_k in Gaussian pyramid can be reconstructed by Eq. 1:

$$I_k = l_k + u(I_{k+1}) \tag{1}$$

$$= l_k + u(d(I_k)), \tag{2}$$

where $u(\cdot)$ is an up-sampling function, and $d(\cdot)$ is a down-sampling function. After down-sampling and up-sampling in Eq. 2, the image I_k is blurred and smoothed, thus some content information is lost, which is recorded in the difference image l_k. In the Laplacian pyramid, the original image can be sequentially reconstructed from level K to level 1 by applying Eq. 1 recursively.

3   Methodology

3.1   Pyramid-Based FCNs

Given the original input image I_1, we build a Gaussian pyramid $\mathcal{G}(I) = \{I_1, \ldots, I_k, \ldots, I_K\}$. Figure 4 demonstrates our work-flow using K = 3 as an example. At each level k, there is a fully convolutional network (FCN_k) which segments image I_k into mask image M_k. The FCNs will be trained sequentially following the coarse-to-fine fashion (to be described in Sect. 3.2) rather than independently.

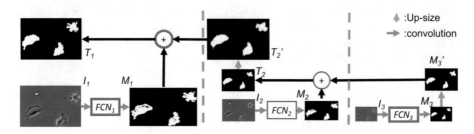

Fig. 4. Overview of the framework. This is an example of a pyramid with 3 levels. Each level is separated by the pink dashed line. Each fully convolutional network (FCN) has the input I_k on the left and the output M_k on the right. The up-sampled map is denoted by $'$. We use $\oplus$ symbol to represent the combination by Eq. 3.

To fuse the segmentation results from all levels in the pyramid, we propose a recursive method similar to the reconstruction procedure in the Laplacian pyramid. First, the segmentation mask M_K at the top/smallest level K is up-sampled to M_K' whose size matches the image size at level $K - 1$ (i.e., $M_K' = u(M_K)$). Then, mask M_K' is combined with mask M_{K-1} at level $K - 1$ by an alpha-fusion (Eq. 3), with the combination result denoted as T_{K-1}. The second iteration is to up-sample T_{K-1} and combine it with mask M_{K-2}. The recursive combination procedure stops until reaching the level 1.

$$T_k = \begin{cases} \alpha \cdot M_k + (1 - \alpha) \cdot u(T_{k+1}), & if\ k < K - 1 \\ \alpha \cdot M_k + (1 - \alpha) \cdot u(M_{k+1}), & if\ k = K - 1. \end{cases} \tag{3}$$

where α $(0 < \alpha < 1)$ is a parameter learned from cross-validation.

Using a 3-level pyramid as an example, Fig. 5 demonstrates the effect of our cascaded-trained FCNs and recursive segmentation fusion. M_3, M_2, M_1 represent the probability maps (soft segmentation, $M_{k,i}$ is the probability of pixel i being a cell pixel, i.e., $M_{k,i} \in [0, 1]$) generated by the fully convolutional networks FCN_3, FCN_2, FCN_1, respectively. FCN_3 is trained to generate a coarse segmentation (M_3). FCN_2 and FCN_1 are trained to focus more on cell details that are missed in the upper-levels, as shown in M_2 and M_1. Note that, M_2 and M_1 may be imperfect (e.g., the inner regions of cells are missed) but they contain the cell boundary details that are complement to the segmentation of

Fine ◄━━━━━━━━━━━━━━━━━━━━━━━━━━━━━━━━━━━ Coarse

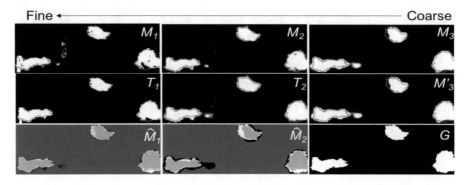

Fig. 5. Comparison between the generated mask M_k, the combined mask T_k and the residual mast $\hat{M}_k$ for a 3-level pyramid. Red contour: the boundary of ground truth segmentation.

upper-levels. M'_3, T_2, T_1 represent the recursively fused segmentation masks at each level, from which we can observe the segmentation mask is refined gradually. To better visualize the refinement process, we compute the residual mask defined as:

$$\hat{M}_k = \frac{G_k - (1 - \alpha) \cdot u(T_{k+1})}{\alpha} \tag{4}$$

The residual mask at level k ($\hat{M}_k$) computes the weighted residual error between the ground truth at level k (G_k) and the segmentation result from the upper-level ($u(T_{k+1})$). There are four classes of pixels in the residual mask: (1) black pixels ($\hat{M}_{k,i} < 0$, i is the pixel location): false positives from the upper level segmentation $u(T_{k+1})$ (the background pixels that are incorrectly classified in the upper level); (2) white pixels ($\hat{M}_{k,i} > 1$): false negative from the upper level (the foreground cell pixels that are missed in the upper level); (3) light gray pixels ($\hat{M}_{k,i} = 1$): the correctly classified cell pixels in the upper level; and (4) dark gray ($\hat{M}_{k,i} = 0$): the correctly classified cell pixels in the upper level.

From the residual masks, we can observe that the lower level FCN focuses more on the mistakes (false positive and false negative) made in the upper level. Thus, the sequentially fused segmentation masks (T_k) are refined gradually (i.e., the number of black and white pixels in the residual mask decreases gradually). The cascaded refinement is also verified in the following mathematical derivation.

3.2 Objective Function and Optimization

The objective function for level k in a Gaussian pyramid without cascaded refinement is the cross-entropy function:

$$L_k = \sum_i \sum_y G_{k,i,y} log(M_{k,i,y}), \tag{5}$$

where i is the pixel location and y denotes the class in segmentation masks ($y \in \{0,1\}$, representing cell or background). The gradient over $M_{k,i,y}$ is:

$$\frac{\partial L_k}{\partial M_{k,i,y}} = \frac{G_{k,i,y}}{M_{k,i,y}}, \tag{6}$$

which will be transferred backward in FCN to calculate the gradient over the parameters of the FCN through back-propagation process [11].

In our pyramid based FCNs, the objective function at the top/smallest level is Eq. 5 with k = K. The objective function of lower levels ($1 \leq k < K$) is:

$$L_k = \sum_i \sum_y G_{k,i,y} log(T_{k,i,y}). \tag{7}$$

Since T_k is the combined mask of M_k and T'_{k+1}, the gradient over $M_{k,i,y}$ is:

$$\frac{\partial L_k}{\partial M_{k,i,y}} = \frac{\partial L_k}{\partial T_{k,i,y}} \cdot \frac{\partial T_{k,i,y}}{\partial M_{k,i,y}} = \frac{G_{k,i,y}}{\alpha \cdot M_{k,i,y} + (1-\alpha) \cdot (T'_{k+1,i,y})} \cdot \alpha, \tag{8}$$

which will be transferred backward in the FCN for training. The last term α does not effect the training precess with a proper learning rate. Denote the denominator in Eq. 8 as β for shorthand, when $T'_{k+1,i,y} > M_{k,i,y}$, we have $\alpha M_{k,i,y} + (1-\alpha)T'_{k+1,i,y} > \alpha M_{k,i,y} + (1-\alpha)M_{k,i,y}$ (i.e., $\beta > M_{k,i,y}$), which means our gradient in Eq. 8 is smaller than that in Eq. 6. In other words, when the upper level FCN achieves good segmentation at pixel i, the lower level FCN will pay less attention on pixel i. On the other hand, when $T'_{k+1,i,y} < M_{k,i,y}$, we have $\beta < M_{k,i,y}$, which means the gradient in Eq. 8 is increased compared to Eq. 6 without cascaded refinement. In other words, when the upper level FCN does not generate good segmentation on pixel i, the lower level FCN will focus more on pixel i.

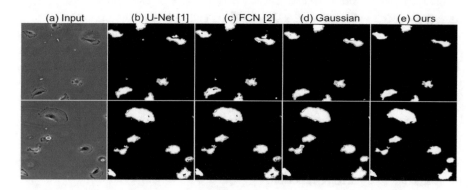

Fig. 6. Segmentation results on dataset PHC [9]. Red contour: the boundary of ground truth segmentation.

4   Experiments

In this section, we validate our approach on two datasets. The first dataset (PHC) is the phase-contrast dataset "PhC-U373" from the ISBI cell segmentation challenge in 2015 [8,9]. The dataset contains 34 partially annotated images for training. The images are resized to 512×512. We collect the second dataset (Phase100) consisting of 100 images (512×512) in total. 40 images are used for training. 20 images are used for cross-validation.

Neural Network Structures and Experimental Settings: the fully convolutional network at each level has 11 convolutional layers with batch-normalization on the first 9 layers. The filter size is fixed as 3 for each convolutional layer. The number of kernels in each layer is: $64, 64, 128, 128, 256, 256, 128, 128, 64, 64, 2$. Since the input images at different levels have different sizes, the fixed-size receptive field (3×3) extracts image content information from different scales. The learning rate is set as 10^{-3}, then divided by 10 when the loss nearly stops decreasing. After obtaining the final probability map (soft segmentation) by cascaded fusing the output from FCNs, we threshold it to get the bitmap. The threshold is 0.47 and the α in fusion is 0.5, learned from the cross-validation. We use shift, scale and rotation operations for data augmentation.

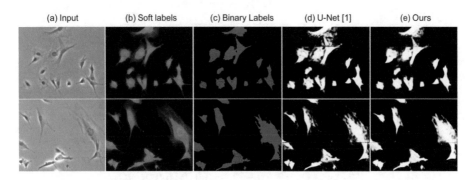

Fig. 7. Sample images in Phase100 dataset and segmentation results.

Evaluation: We perform sensitivity study on the number of pyramid levels (K) and compare our method with three methods: U-Net [1], FCN [2] (a fully convolutional network on the original image without pyramid), and Gaussian (A 3-level Gaussian pyramid is built. For each level of the pyramid, the fully convolutional network is trained independently. Then all the results from different levels are combined by the cascaded fusion as Eq. 3). Figure 6 shows some qualitative results on the comparison. We summarize the sensitivity study and quantitative comparison in Table 1 in terms of three metrics: F-score, IOU (pixel-wise intersection over union, between the segmentation and ground truth) and area-under-curve (the curve of precision vs. recall). The performance of our pyramid-based method increases when the number of pyramid levels increases from $K = 2$ to $K = 3$, and slightly drops with more levels. Our method outperforms the U-Net by about 2 % points on the ISBI segmentation challenge phase-contrast dataset (PHC). Our method with cascaded training beats the 'Gaussian' method with independent training by a large margin, which validates that in our method the lower level FCNs focus more on mistakes made from upper-level FCNs such that the fused segmentation mask is gradually refined.

When checking the quality of human-labeled ground truth in the ISBI segmentation challenge dataset, we notice that some cell labels are missed (e.g., 2nd row of Fig. 6). We collect a new Phase100 dataset by staining the cells and capturing their images with both phase contrast and fluorescent microscopy, as shown in Fig. 7(a) and (b). The fluorescent image (Fig. 7(b)) shows a high quality soft segmentation without human errors, which can be thresholded to a bitmap (Fig. 7(c)). (Note, for long-term cell monitoring, cells cannot be stained to damage their viability. The staining here is only for the purpose of collecting ground-truth.) The probability maps generated by U-Net and our method are shown in Fig. 7(d) and Fig. 7(e), respectively. The quantitative comparison in the bottom of Table 1 shows that our method outperforms U-Net on the Phase100 dataset. **The high quality dataset with soft segmentation ground truth will be publicized along with the codes.**

Table 1. Experiment result

Dataset	Method	F1 score	IOU	Area-under-curve
PHC	U-Net [1]	-	0.920	-
	FCN [2]	0.867	0.864	0.883
	Gaussian	0.865	0.862	0.881
	Ours ($K = 2$)	0.929	0.926	0.940
	Ours ($K = 3$)	**0.940**	**0.938**	**0.963**
	Ours ($K = 4$)	0.939	0.937	0.939
Phase100	U-Net [1]	0.855	0.844	0.932
	Ours ($K = 3$)	**0.923**	**0.912**	**0.970**

5   Conclusion

In this paper, we present pyramid-based fully convolutional networks (FCN) to attack the challenges in cell segmentation such as low contrast and irregular cell shapes. The accurate segmentation mask is achieved by fusing the segmentation outputs of all FCNs at different levels, in a cascaded refinement manner. The effectiveness of our method is validated on two datasets, which outperforms state-of-the-art methods.

Acknowledgement. This project was supported by NSF CAREER award IIS-1351049 and NSF EPSCoR grant IIA-1355406.

References

1. Ronneberger, O., Fischer, P., Brox, T.: U-net: convolutional networks for biomedical image segmentation. In: Navab, N., Hornegger, J., Wells, W.M., Frangi, A.F. (eds.) MICCAI 2015. LNCS, vol. 9351, pp. 234–241. Springer, Cham (2015). https://doi.org/10.1007/978-3-319-24574-4_28
2. Long, J., Shelhamer, E., Darrell, T.: Fully convolutional networks for semantic segmentation. In: CVPR (2015)
3. Krizhevsky, A., Sutskever, I., Hinton, G.E.: ImageNet classification with deep convolutional neural networks. In: NIPS (2012)
4. He, K., et al.: Mask R-CNN. In: ICCV (2017)
5. Burt, P.J., Adelson, E.H.: The Laplacian pyramid as a compact image code. In: Readings in Computer Vision, pp. 671–679 (1987)
6. Denton, E.L., Chintala, S., Fergus, R.: Deep generative image models using a Laplacian pyramid of adversarial networks. In: NIPS (2015)
7. Ghiasi, G., Fowlkes, C.C.: Laplacian pyramid reconstruction and refinement for semantic segmentation. In: Leibe, B., Matas, J., Sebe, N., Welling, M. (eds.) ECCV 2016. LNCS, vol. 9907, pp. 519–534. Springer, Cham (2016). https://doi.org/10.1007/978-3-319-46487-9_32
8. WWW: Web page of the ISBI cell tracking challenge. http://www.celltrackingchallenge.net
9. Maka, M., et al.: A benchmark for comparison of cell tracking algorithms. Bioinformatics $30(11)$, 1609–1617 (2014)
10. Ciresan, D., et al.: Deep neural networks segment neuronal membranes in electron microscopy images. In: NIPS (2012)
11. LeCun, Y., et al.: Handwritten digit recognition with a back-propagation network. In: NIPS (1990)
12. Meijering, E.: Cell segmentation: 50 years down the road [life sciences]. IEEE Sig. Process. Mag. $29(5)$, 140–145 (2012)

Automated Object Tracing
for Biomedical Image Segmentation
Using a Deep Convolutional
Neural Network

Erica M. Rutter$^{(\boxtimes)}$, John H. Lagergren, and Kevin B. Flores

Center for Research in Scientific Computation, Department of Mathematics,
North Carolina State University, Raleigh, USA
{erutter,jhlagerg,kbflores}@ncsu.edu

Abstract. Convolutional neural networks (CNNs) have been used for fast and accurate segmentation of medical images. In this paper, we present a novel methodology that uses CNNs for segmentation by mimicking the human task of tracing object boundaries. The architecture takes as input a patch of an image with an overlay of previously traced pixels and the output predicts the coordinates of the next m pixels to be traced. We also consider a CNN architecture that leverages the output from another semantic segmentation CNN, e.g., U-net, as an auxiliary image channel. To initialize the trace path in an image, we use either locations identified as object boundaries with high confidence from a semantic segmentation CNN or a short manually traced path. By iterating the CNN output, our method continues the trace until it intersects with the beginning of the path. We show that our network is more accurate than the state-of-the-art semantic segmentation CNN on microscopy images from the ISBI cell tracking challenge. Moreover, our methodology provides a natural platform for performing human-in-the-loop segmentation that is more accurate than CNNs alone and orders of magnitude faster than manual segmentation.

1 Introduction

Deep convolutional neural networks (CNNs) have recently attained state-of-the-art performance on many important biomedical imaging tasks [4,7–9]. CNNs have been increasingly applied to automated digital pathology and microscopy image analysis [4,9]. An advantage to using automated analysis is that the output can be less heterogeneous than manual annotation results from different observers, which could be variable due to differences in opinion [2,5].

Supported by the National Science Foundation under grant number DMS-1514929.

Electronic supplementary material The online version of this chapter (https://doi.org/10.1007/978-3-030-00937-3_78) contains supplementary material, which is available to authorized users.

© Springer Nature Switzerland AG 2018
A. F. Frangi et al. (Eds.): MICCAI 2018, LNCS 11073, pp. 686–694, 2018.
https://doi.org/10.1007/978-3-030-00937-3_78

An application where machine learning models, and in particular CNNs, have seen wider recent adoption in biomedical image analysis is cell segmentation [4], i.e., delineating the boundary of each cell in an image [12]. Developing methods for implementing CNNs for segmentation is an active research area, since no one method currently outperforms all others on every data set [10]. One of the first methods using CNNs for segmentation was one in which the input to the network is a square patch from the image and the output is a prediction for the class of the center pixel, i.e., either inside, outside, or on the boundary of an object [1,11]. This method requires the user to input one square patch per pixel in order to classify all pixels in the image, making it computationally restrictive. Recent improvements to this method include fully convolutional neural network architectures [4,9]. These networks take as input a large tile of the image and use deconvolution layers to output another image tile containing classification probabilities for every pixel in the output tile. Since the output tile size can be large, this method is orders of magnitude more efficient than using a CNN architecture that outputs class predictions for a single pixel at a time.

A current challenge in using CNNs, including fully convolutional networks, for segmentation of cell microscopy images is that they do not ensure that one contiguous region is generated for each cell. For example, we have observed that CNNs may produce segmentation predictions with holes or several separate regions in each cell. Many possible factors could contribute to these "patchy" segmentation patterns, such as local differences in contrast or sharpness that make the cell boundaries appear more diffuse. In such regions, low segmentation accuracy may reflect that the CNN produces ambiguous class prediction probabilities, i.e., low certainty between whether a pixel is in the interior, exterior, or boundary of a cell (see Supplementary Figure S1 for such an example).

Here, we propose a novel method using CNNs to improve segmentation accuracy that specifically focuses on tracing the boundaries of the cell, mimicking the human task of tracing the boundary of an object. By formulating segmentation as a tracing task, our method constrains the segmentation problem to better ensure continuity of segmented regions. We found that our tracing method can outperform the state-of-the-art segmentation method on an ISBI cell microscopy tracking challenge data set. Since our methodology is formulated for the general task of segmentation, it can be applied to many different segmentation tasks. We exemplify the use of our automated tracing methodology for "human-in-the-loop" segmentation by simulating a scenario in which the user first defines a short 8-pixel long initial trace, and then our CNN completes the tracing path. Thereby, our method provides a platform for which minimal user supervision can enable increased accuracy over CNNs alone, while still leveraging CNNs to be orders of magnitude more efficient than completely manual segmentation.

2   Data and Methods

2.1   Data

We used benchmark data from the ISBI cell tracking challenge [6, 10] to evaluate the performance of our methodology. We used a data set consisting of 34 fully annotated 2D grayscale light microscopy images of Glioblastoma-astrocytoma U373 cells on a polyacrylimide substrate. Each image is normalized by the pixel-wise mean and standard deviation across all 34 images. The normalized images are then randomly split into 20 training, 6 validation, and 8 testing images. The results we report here are averages from 10 random train/validation/test splits.

2.2   Network Architectures

A Convolutional Neural Network for Tracing Object Boundaries. Our tracing network takes as input a 64×64 image patch with an overlay of an 8-pixel long contour of the previously traced path ending at the center of the patch. The contour helped provide context for predicting the tracing direction. Ground truth masks were used to create the 8-pixel long contour in each training patch. An input patch generation example is shown in Fig. 1. We note that patch size needs to be tuned and we attempted smaller and larger patch sizes, but found that 64×64 provided adequate context for the prediction task on our considered data set. In general, we recommend using a patch size of the same order of magnitude as the mean object diameter, as previously suggested [11].

We also tested a tracing network whose input included an additional channel containing the output probabilities of a trained U-net, however, predictions from any segmentation method (e.g., Mask-RCNN [3]) could be used as additional data channels. A U-net prediction channel was concatenated with each full image and our $64 \times 64 \times 2$ patches were sampled from this 2 channel image.

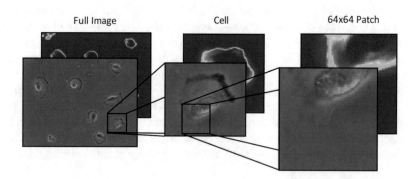

Fig. 1. Generating training data patches. Left: A full image from the microscopy data set. Middle: A cell within the image. Right: A 64×64 patch with the previous 8 pixels traced, shown in green. The U-net probability scores can be concatenated to the image to make a second channel, i.e., a $64 \times 64 \times 2$ patch.

The network architecture is comprised of 3 blocks of repeating layers followed by a final convolution layer (Supplementary Table S1). The repeating layers consist of 3 3×3 convolutional layers followed by a 2×2 max pooling layer with 32, 64, and 128 filters, respectively. The final layer is an 8×8 convolution with $2 \times m$ filters. The network output is a $2 \times m$ array consisting of predictions for the next m pixel locations along the cell border, i.e., the predicted horizontal and vertical pixel displacements of the next m steps along the tracing path. The training data for the output were extracted from the m pixels succeeding the center pixel in the input patch using the ground truth contours. We trained the network for 10 epochs using a mean squared error regression loss, the Adam optimizer, and a batch size of 32. Data augmentations were performed on full-size training images, including random rotations between $15\,°$ and $75\,°$, random shears between $10\,°$ and $30\,°$, vertical and horizontal flips, and Gaussian blur. Full-sized images were symmetrically-reflected with 32 pixels to ensure that pixels on the edge of the image could be used as the center of a 64×64 image patch.

U-net. We used a U-net architecture to create a second channel for the tracing network inputs, to propose candidate locations to initialize the tracing path, and as a baseline for comparing segmentation accuracy. We trained U-net on the same set of training images used to train the tracing network by following the overlap-tiling strategy for seamless segmentation outlined in [9]. The size of the input image tile for the network was 572×572 and the output is a 388×388 tile of probability scores for being in the interior of a cell. Input and output tiles were created from full-size training images and ground truth segmentation masks. Training data were augmented as described in the previous paragraph. For training, we used the pixel-wise soft-max cross entropy loss function described in [9] without the weighting scheme, since the data used in this work did not contain cells that touch.

2.3   Tracing Algorithm

We developed a tracing algorithm to create contours by iterating the output of our trained tracer network. The traced contours outline the boundary of cells and are used to define segmentation masks. The algorithm starts with an initial 64×64 patch with an 8-pixel long trace ending at the center pixel. Methods for generating the initial 8-pixel trace are discussed below. The patch is input to the tracer network, which then predicts the location of the next m pixel coordinates relative to the center pixel in the patch. We aggregate the information from the m pixel predictions by allowing each pixel to vote for one of the 8 directions to move the trace, corresponding to the 8 pixels adjacent to the center pixel of the patch. The vote for each pixel corresponds to the angle (θ) of the vector made by its coordinate relative to the center pixel. For example, if $\theta \in [\frac{-\pi}{8}, \frac{\pi}{8}]$, the vote is for the pixel adjacent to the right, and $\theta \in [\frac{\pi}{8}, \frac{3\pi}{8}]$ corresponds to the upper right adjacent pixel, etc. (Fig. 2). Pixel votes are weighted according to their distance (x) from the center pixel according to an exponential function $w(x) = e^{-\alpha x}$, where α is a hyper-parameter. The next pixel of the contour is drawn in the direction with the largest vote. The newly drawn pixel is used as the center of a new image patch and we iterate the process until the distance between the new pixel and the first 100 pixels in the trace is less than 5. Similar to the tracer network training, padded images were used for the tracing algorithm. The trace was not allowed to enter the padded region. If the trace was predicted to enter the padded region, it was instead automatically routed in a direction parallel to the boundary of the padded region that was most congruent to its previous path. Psuedo-code for our tracing algorithm is provided in the Supplementary Material.

To generate the initial 8-pixel trace, we used a segment of the contour for the ground truth mask to simulate a human-in-the-loop scenario. To implement a fully automated algorithm, the initial trace was generated by U-net. Because results may be sensitive to initial starting conditions, we want to ensure that the initial contour we choose from U-net is where U-net is most sure a boundary exists. Therefore, we determined the 8-pixel start path by calculating the laplacian of the U-net probability scores and the U-net generated masks. We calculated the 8 contiguous pixels that generated the highest U-net probability derivatives, within ± 4 pixels of contours found for U-net.

2.4   Training and Testing Procedure

U-net was used as a baseline for comparison, since it is currently the top performing segmentation method for the data set we use here. The augmented training and validation data sets were used for training U-net for 50 epochs, and the model from the epoch with the lowest validation loss was used for downstream procedures. The validation set was used to optimize the probability threshold for segmentation, where segmentation accuracy was quantified by the mean Jaccard score over the entire set of validation images.

We trained the tracer network with patches from the augmented training images, or 2-channel patches from the augmented training images concatenated with their corresponding U-net probability maps. Due to heavy data augmentation, 10 epochs were sufficient for training the network. The combined non-augmented set of training and validation data were used to optimize the hyper-parameter α with respect to the mean Jaccard score for the tracing algorithm.

We assessed the accuracy of each segmentation method, i.e., the fully automated or the ground-truth initialized tracing algorithm, each with one or two channel inputs, with the test set. To ensure robustness with respect to the randomly chosen training/validation/test split, we validated our results over 10 random data splits.

3   Results

We evaluated the segmentation accuracy of our tracer CNN method for several models corresponding to choices of whether we (1) used an 8-pixel initial trace generated by U-net gradients or the ground truth mask, (2) used the U-net probability scores as a second channel for patches input to the tracer CNN, and (3) set the number of pixels ahead predicted by the tracer CNN to $m = 10$ or 20. The Jaccard scores (intersection over union) over the full images in the testing set were used to quantify segmentation accuracy and U-net was used as a baseline for comparison. We note that, for the ISBI cell tracking challenge [10] and in the U-net paper [9], segmentation accuracy is averaged over all manually segmented objects and not on the full images as we calculate here. Importantly, this only quantifies accuracy for predicted segmentations that overlap with segmented objects in the ground truth, and hence ignores any false positives that do not overlap with ground truth objects. The Jaccard score calculation we perform here is over each entire test image, and thus better accounts for the

Table 1. Jaccard scores on the testing set averaged over ten train/val./test data splits for the current state-of-the-art segmentation algorithm (U-net) and our tracing network. Jaccard scores higher than state-of-the-art are in bold font.

Method	Ground truth Initialized	U-net channel	# pixels predicted	Jaccard score (mean ± std)	Jaccard score (median)
Tracer	No	No	10	0.8091 (0.04216)	0.8443
	No	No	20	0.8268 (0.03749)	0.8579
	No	Yes	10	**0.8407** (0.03873)	**0.8742**
	No	Yes	20	**0.8460** (0.04764)	**0.8841**
	Yes	No	10	**0.8479** (0.03485)	**0.8776**
	Yes	No	20	**0.8626** (0.01497)	**0.8942**
	Yes	Yes	10	**0.8621** (0.02785)	**0.9070**
	Yes	Yes	20	**0.8611** (0.02414)	**0.9044**
	Yes (retraced)	Yes	10	**0.8629** (0.0244)	**0.9074**
	Yes (retraced)	Yes	20	**0.8797** (0.0171)	**0.9054**
U-net [9]	-	-	-	0.8370 (0.03329)	0.8624

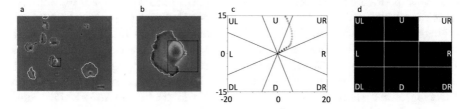

Fig. 2. (a) An example of an image in the process of being segmented. Ground truth contours in white, our traced contours in green. (b) A zoom of the current cell being traced. The black square in (a) and (b) is the current 64×64 patch input to the CNN to predict the location of the next pixel. (c) The predicted location of the next 20 pixels relative to the center pixel of the patch. (d) The score map used by the tracing algorithm to determine the location of the next pixel in the trace, e.g., the upper left (UR).

possibility of false positives. The results in Table 1 show the average scores over 10 train/validation/testing data splits. For a full table of results for each individual train/validation/testing data split, see Supplementary Table S2.

We found that our tracer method was more accurate than U-net when using either a ground truth initialization or the U-net prediction scores as a second channel to the tracer CNN. Using U-net for tracing initialization and to make a second data channel for the tracer CNN that predicts 20 pixels ahead resulted in higher mean (+0.9%) and median (+2.17%) Jaccard scores. When using ground truth initialization without a U-net channel, our method performed even better (+2.58% mean and +3.18% median jaccard score change for the 20-pixel predictions). The highest improvements in mean or median Jaccard score were achieved by the ground truth initialized tracer using a U-net channel (+2.51% mean and +4.46% median jaccard score change for the 10-pixel predictions). These findings suggest that a human-in-the-loop tracing system requiring minimal user input, combined with U-net to provide an additional data channel, could be more accurate than using U-net alone. Figure 2 shows the results of an example image from a testing set, with ground truth contours in white and our traced contours in green. An example video of our cell tracing algorithm is shown in Supplementary Video 1.

We observed that the margin for the median Jaccard scores between our tracer method and U-net were larger than the margin for the mean. For example, when using the 20-pixel tracer CNN with ground truth initialization and the U-net channel, the margin for the median was +4.20%, but the margin for the mean was +2.41%. This suggests that there may be outlier images for which the ground truth initialization performs poorly. Since the goal of testing the ground truth initialized method was to assess the potential increase in accuracy of a human-in-the-loop system, we hypothesized that the accuracy could be further increased by attempting several ground truth initializations for the 8-pixel trace if the Jaccard score was especially low for a given cell. This would emulate a system for which the user observes a poorly drawn trace, and then attempts to reinitialize the trace at a different location on the cell boundary. To investigate this, we implemented a check in the tracing algorithm to determine if the Jaccard score for a given cell was less than 0.8. We note that this condition was met on average <1 cell per image. If this condition was met, we reinitialized the 8-pixel trace at a random location in the ground truth cell boundary up to 10 times. The retraced contour with the maximum Jaccard score for that cell is then used when creating the segmentation mask for the image. We found that allowing for retracing of cell contours increased the margin for the mean to +4.27% when using the 20-pixel tracer CNN (Table 1).

4   Conclusions

We showed that the tracing CNN methodology presented here is able to increase segmentation accuracy over U-net when evaluating the Jaccard score over the entire image. Our tracing algorithm is fast, taking <1 s per cell to complete a trace initialized with an 8-pixel contour on an NVidia GTX 1080Ti (11 GB). This speed makes our methodology practical for implementation within a human-in-the-loop system that is orders of magnitude faster than completely manual segmentation. Moreover, although our fully automated results showed improvement over U-net, we found that the largest gains in accuracy came when we used ground truth initialization for the trace, which is representative of a human-in-the-loop system. For medical imaging applications of CNNs that currently require an expert to verify the CNN segmentation predictions, we envision that initial traces for our algorithm could be provided without much extra effort. We expect our method to benefit data sets with objects containing diffuse looking regions, which are common in biomedical data, e.g., brain tumor MRIs.

In future work we will test our methodology in settings such as brain tumor segmentation for which even small differences in accuracy could be detrimental and currently require human verification. We will also test whether our retracing strategy can be used with U-net initialized traces to handle inaccurate segmentations that arise from the rare occurrence if the trace deviates from the object boundary. For example, we can aggregate the results from 10 U-net initialized traces per object by majority vote.

References

1. Ciresan, D., et al.: Deep neural networks segment neuronal membranes in electron microscopy images. In: Pereira, F., Burges, C.J.C., Bottou, L., Weinberger, K.Q. (eds.) NIPS, pp. 2843–2851. Curran Associates, Inc. (2012)
2. Foran, D.J., et al.: Imageminer: a software system for comparative analysis of tissue microarrays using content-based image retrieval, high-performance computing, and grid technology. J. Am. Med. Inf. Assoc. **18**(4), 403–415 (2011). https://doi.org/10.1136/amiajnl-2011-000170
3. He, K., Gkioxari, G., Dollár, P., Girshick, R.: Mask R-CNN. In: IEEE ICCV, pp. 2980–2988. IEEE (2017)
4. Litjens, G., et al.: A survey on deep learning in medical image analysis. Med. Image Anal. **42**, 60–88 (2017)
5. López, C., et al.: Digital image analysis in breast cancer: an example of an automated methodology and the effects of image compression. St. Heal. T. **179**, 155–71 (2012)
6. Maška, M., et al.: A benchmark for comparison of cell tracking algorithms. Bioinformatics **30**(11), 1609–1617 (2014)
7. Milletari, F., Navab, N., Ahmadi, S.A.: V-net: fully convolutional neural networks for volumetric medical image segmentation. In: Fourth International Conference on 3D Vision (3DV), pp. 565–571 (2016). https://doi.org/10.1109/3DV.2016.79
8. Rodríguez Colmeiro, R.G., Verrastro, C.A., Grosges, T.: Multimodal brain tumor segmentation using 3D convolutional networks. In: Crimi, A., et al. (eds.) BrainLes 2017. LNCS, vol. 10670, pp. 226–240. Springer, Cham (2018). https://doi.org/10.1007/978-3-319-75238-9_20
9. Ronneberger, O., Fischer, P., Brox, T.: U-net: convolutional networks for biomedical image segmentation. In: Navab, N., Hornegger, J., Wells, W.M., Frangi, A.F. (eds.) MICCAI 2015. LNCS, vol. 9351, pp. 234–241. Springer, Cham (2015). https://doi.org/10.1007/978-3-319-24574-4_28

10. Ulman, V., et al.: An objective comparison of cell-tracking algorithms. Nat. Methods **14**, 1141 (2017). https://doi.org/10.1038/nmeth.4473
11. Valen, V., et al.: Deep learning automates the quantitative analysis of individual cells in live-cell imaging experiments. PLoS Comput. Biol. **12**(11), 1–24 (2016). https://doi.org/10.1371/journal.pcbi.1005177
12. Xing, F., Yang, L.: Robust nucleus/cell detection and segmentation in digital pathology and microscopy images: a comprehensive review. IEEE Rev. Biomed. Eng. **9**, 234–263 (2016)

RBC Semantic Segmentation for Sickle Cell Disease Based on Deformable U-Net

Mo Zhang[1], Xiang Li[2], Mengjia Xu[3], and Quanzheng Li[2,4,5(✉)]

[1] Center for Data Science, Peking University, Beijing 100871, China
[2] MGH/BWH Center for Clinical Data Science, Boston, MA 02115, USA
[3] Beijing International Center for Mathematical Research, Peking University,
Beijing 100871, China
[4] Center for Data Science in Health and Medicine, Peking University,
Beijing 100871, China
[5] Laboratory for Biomedical Image Analysis, Beijing Institute of Big Data Research,
Beijing 100871, China
li.quanzheng@mgh.harvard.edu

Abstract. Reliable cell segmentation and classification from biomedical images is a crucial step for both scientific research and clinical practice. A major challenge for more robust segmentation and classification methods is the large variations in the size, shape and viewpoint of the cells, combining with the low image quality caused by noise and artifacts. To address this issue, in this work we propose a learning-based, simultaneous cell segmentation and classification method based on the U-Net structure with deformable convolution layers. The U-Net architecture has been shown to offer a precise localization for image semantic segmentation. Moreover, deformable convolution enables the free form deformation of the feature learning process, thus making the whole network more robust to various cell morphologies and image settings. The proposed method is tested on microscopic red blood cell images from patients with sickle cell disease. The results show that U-Net with deformable convolution achieves the highest accuracy for both segmentation and classification tasks, compared with the original U-Net structure and unsupervised methods.

Keywords: RBC semantic segmentation · Sickle cell disease · U-Net
Deformable convolution

1   Introduction

Sickle cell disease (SCD) is an inherited blood disorder, where SCD patients have abnormal hemoglobin that can cause normal disc-shaped red blood cells (RBCs) to distort and generate heterogeneous shapes. The differences in cell morphology between healthy and pathological cells make it possible to perform image-based

---

M. Zhang, X. Li and M. Xu—Joint first authors.

© Springer Nature Switzerland AG 2018
A. F. Frangi et al. (Eds.): MICCAI 2018, LNCS 11073, pp. 695–702, 2018.
https://doi.org/10.1007/978-3-030-00937-3_79

diagnosis using image processing techniques, which is very important for faster and more accurate diagnosis of potential SCD crises. Various methods have been developed to perform RBC segmentation and/or classification, such as thresholding, region growing [1], watershed transform [2], deformable models [3], and clustering [4]. However, traditional image processing models such as thresholding and region growing are susceptible to the noisy image background and blurred cell boundaries, which are common in microscopy images. Moreover, deformable models like active contour [3] needs good initialization and relies on relatively clear cell morphology. In addition, due to the heterogeneous shapes and touching RBCs in SCD, recent open source cell detection tools, such as CellProfiler [5], CellTrack [6] or Fiji [7] are not readily used to accurately detect and classify the SCD RBCs. Hence, an effective SCD cell segmentation and classification method is still an open problem for the field.

Recently, deep learning methods with convolutional neural networks (CNN) have achieved remarkable success in the field of both natural image [8] and medical image analysis [9]. Among these methods, the fully convolutional network (FCN) has shown state-of-the-art performance in various real-world applications [10]. Specifically, FCN has been applied in the cell segmentation problems [11,12] and obtained good results. U-Net was developed based on FCN and takes skip connection between encoder and decoder into consideration [13], which has also been applied on medical images. On the other hand, one of the major challenges in capturing the most discriminative shape and texture features of the RBCs is that cells can be imaged in various poses and sizes, thus a spatial-invariant scheme is needed to overcome those variations. For example, the work applies dense transformer network based on thin-plate spline, and has achieved superior performance on brain electron microscopy image segmentation problems [14]. In this work, we apply deformable convolution [15] to the U-Net architecture and develop the deformable U-Net framework for semantic cell segmentation. Deformable convolution accommodates geometric variations in the images by learning and applying adaptive receptive fields driven by data [15], in contrast to standard CNNs where the receptive field is constant. Therefore, it can be more robust to the spatial variations of the RBCs.

The proposed framework is trained and tested on a large, multi-institutional RBC microscopic image base with manual annotations, consisting of both healthy and pathological populations. We perform the simultaneous segmentation and classification of the RBCs using the trained network based on various experimental settings. The supreme accuracy for both segmentation and classification indicates that the proposed framework is an effective solution for the automatic detection of SCD RBCs. To the best of our knowledge, this work is the first attempt of solving the SCD detection problem in an end-to-end semantic segmentation approach.

2   Materials and Methods

Since the traditional U-Net is inherently limited to deal with object shape transformations due to its regular square receptive field, in this work, we propose deformable U-Net replacing the convolution kernel with deformable convolution throughout the U-Net. In the classic CNN architecture, convolution kernel is defined with fixed shape and size by sampling the input feature map on a regular grid. For example, the grid $\mathcal{R}$ for a 3×3 kernel is $\mathcal{R} = \{(-1,-1), (-1,0), \cdots, (0,1), (1,1)\}$. For each pixel $\mathbf{p}_0$ on the output feature map $\mathbf{y}$, the standard convolution can be expressed as:

$$\mathbf{y}(\mathbf{p}_0) = \sum_{\mathbf{p}_n \in \mathcal{R}} \mathbf{w}(\mathbf{p}_n) \cdot \mathbf{x}(\mathbf{p}_0 + \mathbf{p}_n), \tag{1}$$

where $\mathbf{y}(\mathbf{p}_0)$ denotes the value of pixel $\mathbf{p}_0$ on the output feature map, $\mathbf{x}(\mathbf{p}_0 + \mathbf{p}_n)$ denotes the value of pixel $\mathbf{p}_0 + \mathbf{p}_n$ on the input feature map, and $\mathbf{w}(\mathbf{p}_n)$ is the weight parameter. In contrast, deformable convolution adds 2D offsets to the regular sampling grid $\mathcal{R}$, thus Eq. (1) becomes:

$$\mathbf{y}(\mathbf{p}_0) = \sum_{\mathbf{p}_n \in \mathcal{R}} \mathbf{w}(\mathbf{p}_n) \cdot \mathbf{x}(\mathbf{p}_0 + \mathbf{p}_n + \Delta\mathbf{p}_n). \tag{2}$$

As offset $\Delta\mathbf{p}_n$ is probably fractional, Eq. (2) is implemented by bilinear interpolation as:

$$\mathbf{x}(\mathbf{p}) = \sum_{\mathbf{q}} max(0, 1 - |q_x - p_x|) \cdot max(0, 1 - |q_y - p_y|) \cdot \mathbf{x}(\mathbf{q}), \tag{3}$$

where $\mathbf{p}$ enumerates an arbitrary fractional location on the input feature map, $\mathbf{q}$ denotes all integer locations on the input feature map, and p_x (p_y) denotes the x-coordinate (y-coordinate) of $\mathbf{p}$. Equation (3) is easy to compute as it is only related with the four nearest integer coordinates $\mathbf{q}_i, i = [1,2,3,4]$ of $\mathbf{p}$. Equation (3) is also equivalent to:

$$\mathbf{x}(\mathbf{p}) = \sum_{i=1}^{n} \mathbf{x}(\mathbf{q}_i) \cdot S_i, \tag{4}$$

where $S_i, i = [1,2,3,4]$ is the area of the assigned rectangle generated by $\mathbf{q}_i, i = [1,2,3,4]$ and $\mathbf{p}$, and the illustration is shown in Fig. 1.

The detailed procedure of deformable convolution is described in Fig. 1. First, we implement an additional classic convolution with activation function TANH to learn offset field from the input feature map, which is normalized to $[-1,1]$. The offset field has the same height and width with input feature map while its number of channels is $2N (N = |\mathcal{R}|)$. The offset field is then multiplied by parameter s (which is used to adjust the scope of receptive field) and added by the regular grid $\mathcal{R}$ to obtain the sampling locations (every coordinate on offset field has N pairs of values corresponding to the regular grid $\mathcal{R}$). Finally, values of the irregular sampling coordinates are computed via bilinear interpolation, then the original convolution kernel samples the deformed feature map to get the new feature map. In this work, we set deformable kernel works in the same way across different channels, rather than learning a separate kernel for each channel

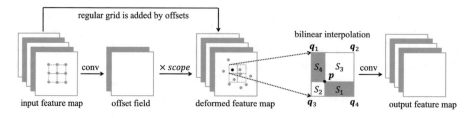

Fig. 1. Illustration of the deformable convolution, showing how the fixed sampling locations are adaptively deformed.

to improve the learning efficiency. Deformable convolution can sample the input feature map in a local and dense way, and be adaptive to the localization for objects with different shapes [15], which is exactly what we need in SCD RBC semantic segmentation.

The main architecture of the deformable U-Net is shown in Fig. 2. It includes two parts: encoder path and decoder path. In the encoder path, each layer has two 3×3 deformable convolutions followed by a 2×2 max pooling operation with stride of 2, which doubles the number of channels and halves the resolution of input feature map for down-sampling. The encoder is followed by two 3×3 deformable convolutions called bottom layers. Each step in the decoder path contains a 3×3 deconvolution with stride 2 followed by two 3×3 deformable convolutions. The skip connection between encoder and decoder helps to preserve more contextual information for better localization [13]. The proposed deformable U-Net can be easily trained end-to-end (from the input image to the label map) through back propagation in the same way with the U-Net architecture.

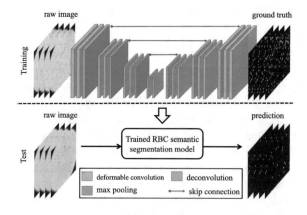

Fig. 2. Architecture of the deformable U-Net in this work.

3   Results

In this section, to evaluate the performance of the proposed deformable U-Net in dealing with RBC semantic segmentation for SCD, we perform experiments from two different aspects: (1) single-class RBC semantic segmentation, which aims at differentiating cells from background, and (2) multi-class RBC semantic segmentation, which aims at differentiating various sub-types of SCD RBC. The experimental data and implementation details are presented below.

Data and Implementation Details. In terms of the latest public SCD RBC image dataset from MIT, refer to [16], we use 266 raw microscopy images of 4 different SCD patients as our experimental data. The original blood sample is collected from UPMC (University of Pittsburgh Medical Center) and MGH (Massachusetts General Hospital). In the dataset, raw microscopy images are acquired using a Zeiss inverted Axiovert 200 microscope under 63× oil objective lens using an industrial camera (Sony Exmor CMOS color sensor, 1080p resolution), the image resolution is 1920 × 1080. Additionally, RBC areas and RBC categories are manually annotated as ground truths by the data provider. Based on the coarse RBC labeling strategy in previous work [16], three SCD RBC categories are employed in our experiments: (1) Dic+Ovl, (2) El+Sk, and (3) others. During the implementation, we initially pre-process the collected raw image data by removing two-side margins and resize them into same size 512 × 512.The network is implemented in TensorFlow 1.2.1, and we use RELU as activation function with scope of 2 and batch normalization for convolution operations. Furthermore, we employ the Adam algorithm for training with learning rate 10^{-3}, weight decay 10^{-8}, batch size (2) and epoch (30000).Our code can be accessed on GitHub[1].

Evaluation of Single-Class RBC Semantic Segmentation Performance. To demonstrate the performance of our method in single-class RBC semantic segmentation, we compare the proposed method with the prevalent U-Net and region growing methods.The preliminary SCD RBC dataset are divided into two parts: 166 random samples for training, and the rest 100 samples for testing. As it can be seen from Fig. 3, the proposed method improves the performance of U-Net in SCD RBC semantic segmentation significantly. First, it can effectively separate touching RBCs as shown in A and D (yellow circles) of Fig. 3; Second, for the cases of heterogeneous shapes SCD RBC segmentation, deformable U-Net obtains more accurate results than the other two methods, see C and D (blue circles) of Fig. 3; Third, regarding the RBC segmentation under blur boundary, our method receives a clearly high accuracy, see purple circles in C of Fig. 3. Moreover, Fig. 3 indicates that the proposed method has a better generalization ability for shaded cell segmentation at the edge. Furthermore, deformable U-Net can effectively avoid the disturbance of various noises (e.g. dirties, halos, etc.)

---

[1] https://github.com/moliqingcha/Deformable-U-Net.

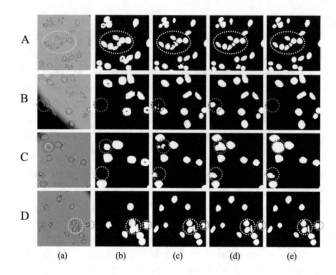

Fig. 3. Representative comparisons of different RBC semantic segmentation methods. (a) patch images, (b) region growing results, (c) U-Net results, (d) proposed method, (e) ground truth.

Table 1. Quantitative performance analysis of different methods in single-class SCD RBC segmentation.

	Accuracy	Precision	F1
Region growing	0.9680 ± 0.0013	0.7223 ± 0.0008	0.7036 ± 0.0020
U-Net	0.9942 ± 0.0002	0.9548 ± 0.0085	0.9566 ± 0.0005
Proposed	$\mathbf{0.9960 \pm 0.0003}$	$\mathbf{0.9614 \pm 0.0076}$	$\mathbf{0.9604 \pm 0.0006}$

in the RBC semantic segmentation procedure. To quantify the comprehensive performance of our method, three main indices are calculated, see Table 1. The proposed network outperforms the other two approaches in terms of accuracy, precision and F1 score.

Evaluation of Multi-class RBC Semantic Segmentation Performance. In addition to single-class segmentation evaluation for the proposed network, we also conduct an experiment on multi-class RBC semantic segmentation for SCD based on the same dataset division schema as above. The corresponding segmentation results is shown in Fig. 4, different colors indicate different RBC types: red (Dic+Ovl), blue (El+Sk) and green (others).Specifically,the proposed deformable U-Net gains better capability of predicting an integrated RBC without any shape prior than the standard U-Net method, as certain cells are segmented out yet identified as two classes simultaneously in the U-Net prediction, the yellow square region in Fig. 4. Additionally, deformable U-Net is more robust to the background noise presented in the microscopic images, e.g. the baseline

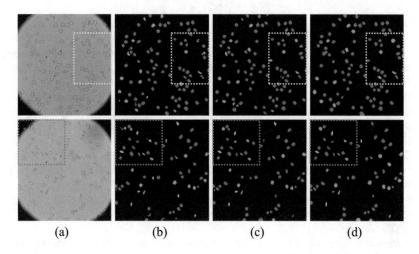

(a)   (b)   (c)   (d)

Fig. 4. Comparisons of multi-class RBC semantic segmentation results. (a) original images, (b) U-Net results, (c) proposed method results, (d) ground truth.

Table 2. Quantitative performance analysis of different methods in multi-class SCD RBC segmentation.

	Loss	Accuracy	Mean-IoU
U-Net	0.0664 ± 0.0003	0.9892 ± 0.0006	0.4173 ± 0.0034
Proposed	$\mathbf{0.0428 \pm 0.0007}$	$\mathbf{0.9912 \pm 0.0002}$	$\mathbf{0.4415 \pm 0.0050}$

U-Net predict background objects as RBCs in the blue square of Fig. 4, while deformable U-Net predict the accurate negative label. Furthermore, we perform the quantitative analysis for our trained model by three statistic metrics: loss, accuracy, and mean IoU (Intersection over Union). The evaluation results in Table 2 indicate that deformable U-Net possess a superior performance than the standard U-Net.

4   Conclusion

In this work, we present an improved U-Net framework (deformable U-Net) for automated SCD RBC semantic segmentation. Experimental results demonstrate that the proposed approach obtains an obvious superior performance than the baseline U-Net, especially for the key problems, e.g. background noise discrimination, heterogeneous shapes of RBC segmentation, touching RBC separation, blurred RBC segmentation. Moreover, it has high consistency in performing the prediction on cell boundaries.

Acknowledgments. Quanzheng Li is supported in part by the National Institutes of Health under Grant R01AG052653.

References

1. Chassery, J.-M., Garbay, C.: An iterative segmentation method based on a contextual color and shape criterion. IEEE Trans. Pattern Anal. Mach. Intell. **6**, 794–800 (1984)
2. Plissiti, M.E., Nikou, C., Charchanti, A.: Watershed-based segmentation of cell nuclei boundaries in pap smear images. In: 2010 10th IEEE International Conference on Information Technology and Applications in Biomedicine (ITAB), pp. 1–4. IEEE (2010)
3. Zamani, F., Safabakhsh, R.: An unsupervised GVF snake approach for white blood cell segmentation based on nucleus. In: 2006 8th International Conference on Signal Processing, vol. 2. IEEE (2006)
4. Savkare, S.S., Narote, S.P.: Blood cell segmentation from microscopic blood images. In: 2015 International Conference on Information Processing (ICIP), pp. 502–505. IEEE (2015)
5. Carpenter, A.E., et al.: CellProfiler: image analysis software for identifying and quantifying cell phenotypes. Genome Biol. **7**(10), R100 (2006)
6. Sacan, A., Ferhatosmanoglu, H., Coskun, H.: CellTrack: an open-source software for cell tracking and motility analysis. Bioinformatics **24**(14), 1647–1649 (2008)
7. Schindelin, J., et al.: Fiji: an open-source platform for biological-image analysis. Nat. Methods **9**(7), 676 (2012)
8. LeCun, Y., Bengio, Y., Hinton, G.: Deep learning. Nature **521**(7553), 436 (2015)
9. Shen, D., Guorong, W., Suk, H.-I.: Deep learning in medical image analysis. Ann. Rev. Biomed. Eng. **19**, 221–248 (2017)
10. Long, J., Shelhamer, E., Darrell, T.: Fully convolutional networks for semantic segmentation. In: Proceedings of the IEEE Conference on Computer Vision and Pattern Recognition, pp. 3431–3440 (2015)
11. Yang, L., Zhang, Y., Guldner, I.H., Zhang, S., Chen, D.Z.: 3D segmentation of glial cells using fully convolutional networks and k-terminal Cut. In: Ourselin, S., Joskowicz, L., Sabuncu, M.R., Unal, G., Wells, W. (eds.) MICCAI 2016 Part II. LNCS, vol. 9901, pp. 658–666. Springer, Cham (2016). https://doi.org/10.1007/978-3-319-46723-8_76
12. Aydin, A.S., Dubey, A., Dovrat, D., Aharoni, A., Shilkrot, R.: CNN based yeast cell segmentation in multi-modal fluorescent microscopy data. In: Proceedings of IEEE Conference on Computer Vision and Pattern Recognition (CVPR), pp. 753–759 (2017)
13. Ronneberger, O., Fischer, P., Brox, T.: U-Net: convolutional networks for biomedical image segmentation. In: Navab, N., Hornegger, J., Wells, W.M., Frangi, A.F. (eds.) MICCAI 2015 Part III. LNCS, vol. 9351, pp. 234–241. Springer, Cham (2015). https://doi.org/10.1007/978-3-319-24574-4_28
14. Li, J., Chen, Y., Cai, L., Davidson, I., Ji, S.: Dense transformer networks. arXiv preprint arXiv:1705.08881 (2017)
15. Dai, J., et al.: Deformable convolutional networks. CoRR, abs/1703.06211, vol. 1, no. 2, p. 3 (2017)
16. Xu, M., Papageorgiou, D.P., Abidi, S.Z., Dao, M., Zhao, H., Karniadakis, G.E.: A deep convolutional neural network for classification of red blood cells in sickle cell anemia. PLoS Comput. Biol. **13**(10), e1005746 (2017)

Accurate Detection of Inner Ears in Head CTs Using a Deep Volume-to-Volume Regression Network with False Positive Suppression and a Shape-Based Constraint

Dongqing Zhang[(✉)], Jianing Wang, Jack H. Noble,
and Benoit M. Dawant

Department of Electrical Engineering and Computer Science,
Vanderbilt University, Nashville, TN 37235, USA
dongqing.zhang@vanderbilt.edu

Abstract. Cochlear implants (CIs) are neural prosthetics which are used to treat patients with hearing loss. CIs use an array of electrodes which are surgically inserted into the cochlea to stimulate the auditory nerve endings. After surgery, CIs need to be programmed. Studies have shown that the spatial relationship between the intra-cochlear anatomy and electrodes derived from medical images can guide CI programming and lead to significant improvement in hearing outcomes. However, clinical head CT images are usually obtained from scanners of different brands with different protocols. The field of view thus varies greatly and visual inspection is needed to document their content prior to applying algorithms for electrode localization and intra-cochlear anatomy segmentation. In this work, to determine the presence/absence of inner ears and to accurately localize them in head CTs, we use a volume-to-volume convolutional neural network which can be trained end-to-end to map a raw CT volume to probability maps which indicate inner ear positions. We incorporate a false positive suppression strategy in training and apply a shape-based constraint. We achieve a labeling accuracy of 98.59% and a localization error of 2.45 mm. The localization error is significantly smaller than a random forest-based approach that has been proposed recently to perform the same task.

Keywords: Cochlear implants · Landmark localization · 3D U-Net

1 Introduction

Cochlear implants (CIs) have been one of the most successful neural prosthetics in the past few decades [1]. They are used to treat patients with severe to profound hearing loss. During a cochlear implantation surgery, an array of electrodes is threaded into the cochlea to replace the natural signal transduction mechanism in human hearing. After surgery, the CI needs to be programmed to adjust the implant for the recipient. The programming includes the assignment of a frequency range to each individual contact in the array so it will be activated when the incoming sound includes frequency components in this range. Traditionally, the programming is done by an audiologist

© Springer Nature Switzerland AG 2018
A. F. Frangi et al. (Eds.): MICCAI 2018, LNCS 11073, pp. 703–711, 2018.
https://doi.org/10.1007/978-3-030-00937-3_80

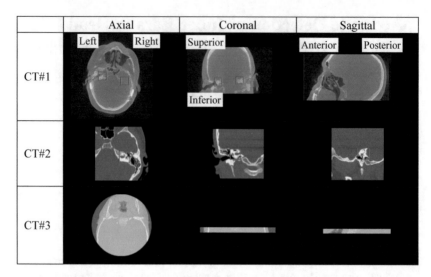

Fig. 1. Three exemplar CTs from our dataset. The inner ears are shown in red boxes if they are present in the volume and visible in the slice

who can only rely on the recipients' subjective response to certain stimuli, e.g., whether they can hear a signal or rank pitches, without other clues. Accurately localizing electrodes in CI relative to the intra-cochlear anatomy can provide useful guidance to audiologists to adjust the CI programming. Recently, technology has emerged that permits accurate segmentation of intra-cochlear anatomy and localization of CI electrodes using clinical head CTs in works such as [2, 3]. Studies have shown that the use of such image guidance to program the CI leads to a significant improvement in hearing outcomes [4].

However, currently the image guidance technology based on the techniques above cannot be fully automated. One hurdle is the heterogeneity of the clinical head CTs. The patients' CT volumes could be obtained from multiple sites. They are acquired using CT scanners of different brands without a standardized imaging protocol and the field of view of the CT volumes varies greatly. Figure 1 shows three representative examples. Here, CT#1 includes both inner ears. In CT#2, though the right half and a large portion of the left half of the head are present, only the right inner ear is included. In CT#3, only a narrow horizontal portion of the head is imaged and neither inner ear is present.

Because of this heterogeneity, when a new CT volume is received, manual image content documentation, i.e., what ear(s) is/are shown in the volume, and labelling, i.e., where is/are the ear(s) is needed to initialize the subsequent processing steps. Specifically, a technician needs to manually label which inner ear(s) is/are included in the volume and locate it (them). There are several factors that make automating this task challenging: images acquired from different scanners usually have different intensity characteristics and some images have really low quality. Also, the implants could cause serious beam-hardening imaging artifacts. In this paper, we solve this problem using a deep volume-to-volume regression network to directly relate images to probability maps which indicate inner ear positions. We further improve the detection performance by incorporating a false positive suppression strategy at the time of training and applying a post-processing shape-based constraint.

2 Methods

2.1 Data

The data we use in this study include head CTs from 322 patients. Since acquisitions were obtained both pre-operatively and post-operatively, and multiple reconstructions could be performed for one acquisition, one patient could have several CT volumes. In total, we have 1,593 CT volumes. The CTs are also obtained from both conventional and Xoran xCAT® (denoted as "Xoran") scanners. Xoran scanners are flat-panel, low-dose scanners and images acquired with such scanners typically have a lower quality than those acquired with conventional ones. We label the CT volumes according to the scanner type. The volumes we have also include regions of different sizes and resolutions. The size ranges from 10 mm to 256 mm in the left-right and anterior-posterior directions and from 52 mm to 195 mm in the inferior-superior direction. The resolution varies from 0.14 mm to 2 mm in the left-right and anterior-posterior directions and from 0.14 mm to 5 mm in the inferior-superior direction. We randomly split the data into a training set and a testing set. We make sure one patient's data is not split into different sets. The numbers of CTs in the training set and the testing set are 798 and 795, respectively. For each volume, we visually check the presence of inner ears. For each visible inner ear, a pre-defined landmark point close to the cochlea is manually selected. As we have mentioned, scans could include both inner ears, only one (left/right), or neither. However, the number of image volumes in each of these four categories is not balanced. Indeed, in our current data set about 80% of the volumes include both ears. About 20% include one inner ear. Image volumes that include neither inner ear are rare. To solve this issue, we augment each set by cropping sub volumes from volumes that include both ears to create artificial samples for the other three categories. After cropping, substantial but reasonable deformation, including isotropic scaling, rotation and skewing are applied to increase data variance. All image volumes are resampled to $2.25 \times 2.25 \times 2.25$ mm³/voxel and symmetrically cropped or padded to $96 \times 96 \times 96$ voxels. In Table 1, we list the number of CT volumes with (w/CI) and without (w/o CI) implant. We also specify the number of volumes acquired with a conventional scanner and with a Xoran scanner. In the test set, there are 625, 625, 625 and 611 CTs that includes both, left, right and neither ear(s), respectively.

Table 1. Distributions of our CT data w.r.t. presence of CI and w.r.t. scanner type

	Training data			Test data		
	w/CI	w/o CI	Total	w/CI	w/o CI	Total
Number	466	2136	2602	389	2097	2486
	Conventional	Xoran		Conventional	Xoran	
Number	2022	580		1935	551	

2.2   3D U-Net with False Positive Suppression and a Shape Constraint

In recent years, methods including [5, 6] have been proposed to localize organs in CTs using 2D CNNs as a classification tool. These authors use 2D slices in three orthogonal planes extracted from 3-D images volumes to train the CNNs. The location of the organs in the test image is inferred by testing each slice and aggregating them. These models require one forward propagation for each image slice thus requiring hundreds of forward propagations for one volume. Also, the 3-D contextual information is not leveraged. More recently, dense image-to-image or volume-to-volume networks have been favored. In [7], an image-to-image network is proposed to localize landmarks in cardiac and obstetric ultrasound images. The raw 2D image is used as the input and the output is designed to be an action map. In the action map, two vertical lines are drawn which intersect at the position of the landmark, dividing the image into four regions. For a new image, the landmark position can be inferred by aggregating the output action map. This approach only deals with 2D images. In [8], Yang et al. proposed a neural network that can use a whole 3-D CT volume as the input to find a set of vertebra points. However, the unique distribution of many closely-spaced, chain-shaped vertebra points provides far more supervision information in training than what is available in our application.

In this paper, we propose to use a 3D U-Net [9] to map a whole 3-D image volume to two probability maps that have the same dimensionality as the input volumes. As is shown in Fig. 2, the 3D U-Net requires a 3-D volume as input. It consists of multiple convolution-pooling layers which encode the raw input image into low-resolution, highly-abstracted feature maps. Following them are multiple convolution-upsampling layers, which decode the abstracted feature maps into output with the same resolution as the input, in a symmetrical way as the encoding layers. In our first attempt, at the training stage, for each inner ear, we design the probability map as a 3-D Gaussian function centered at the manually labeled landmark position. The standard deviation of the Gaussian is chosen as $\sigma = 3$. The maximum is scaled to 1. Any value below 0.05 is set to 0. If the inner ear is not present in the image, all values in the corresponding probability map are set to 0. We treat this volume-to-volume mapping as a regression problem. The weighted mean of voxel-wise squared errors between the output probability maps and the probability maps generated with manually labeled inner ear landmarks is used as the loss function. Larger weights are assigned to voxels with non-zero probabilities. They are sparse but are very important for detection. Specifically, in the output probability map, suppose the number of non-zero entries and zero entries are N_{none} and N_{zero}, respectively, the weights associated with none-zero entries and zero entries are w_{none} and w_{zero} defined as follows:

$$\begin{cases} w_{none} = \frac{N_{zero}}{N_{none} + N_{zero}} \\ w_{zero} = \frac{N_{none}}{N_{none} + N_{zero}} \end{cases} \tag{1}$$

For each new volume, using the trained network, we generate two probability maps, one for the left ear, the other for the right ear. For each probability map, we find its maximum. If it is larger than $p_{thres} = 0.5$, we predict that the corresponding inner ear is present. Otherwise, we predict that it is absent.

Results we obtained with this approach were not satisfactory because it led to a large number of false positives. We observed that the response map associated with one inner ear could have a very high response at the location of the other ear, possibly due to their similar intensity characteristics. In turn, this led to a substantial number of wrong detections. To solve this problem, we incorporate a false positive suppression strategy during training. Specifically, for the probability map associated with one ear, if the ear on the other side of the head is included in the image, we force the values around this second ear to be negative rather than zero to penalize the detection of the erroneous ear. The negative values that are used are the same Gaussian-distributed values that are used for the correct ear but centered on the incorrect ear and multiplied by minus one. By penalizing the network in such a way, we effectively suppress the number of false positives as will be shown in the results section. We train the neural network using stochastic gradient descent (SGD) with 0.9 momentum and an initial learning rate of 0.0001. The batch size is set to 1. The code is written in Keras [10] on a Nvidia Titan X GPU. The training takes ∼2 days. Figure 2 shows our final network architecture. The response maps of a test image with a left inner ear before and after using false positive suppression are shown in Fig. 3. This figure shows that the false positive caused by the right ear is effectively suppressed.

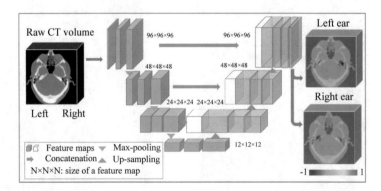

Fig. 2. Network architecture, input, and output for our approach

Even though the aforementioned method suppresses false positives caused by the contralateral ear, other false positives remain present at other random locations, e.g., the location of the CI transmitters in some post-operative CTs, as shown in Fig. 4. Here, we capture the spatial relationship between inner ear pairs using a low-dimension shape model and use this *a-priori* information to further evaluate the plausibility of the detected inner ear pairs. Specifically, in the training set, we collect the coordinates of the inner ear pairs. For the ith pair, these are denoted as $l_{left}^i = \left(x_{left}^i, y_{left}^i, z_{left}^i \right)$ and $l_{right}^i = \left(x_{right}^i, y_{right}^i, z_{right}^i \right)$ for the left and right ear, respectively. We subtract from each point the center of the two and stack the coordinate vectors to create a 6-d shape vector s^i. The mean shape is computed as

$$\bar{s} = \sum_{i=1}^{N} s^i. \tag{2}$$

Here, N is the number of inner ear pairs in the training set. The modes of variation of the shapes are computed as the k eigenvectors $\{\vec{u_j}, j = 1, 2, \ldots, k\}$ of the covariance matrix of $\{s^i, i = 1, 2, \ldots, N\}$. The k (in our case, $k = 3$ because ears come in pairs) non-zero eigenvalues associated with these are $\{\lambda_j, j = 1, 2, \ldots, k\}$. Suppose the projections of $s^i - \bar{s}$ onto $\{\vec{u_j}, j = 1, 2, \ldots, k\}$ are $\{b_j^i, j = 1, 2, \ldots, k\}$. The Mahalanobis distance between s^i and the mean shape $\bar{s}$ is thus

$$M(s^i, \bar{s}) = \sqrt{\frac{\sum_{j=1}^{k} b_j^{i2}}{\lambda_j}}. \tag{3}$$

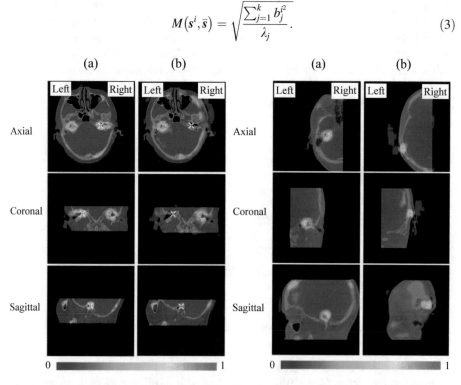

Fig. 3. The response maps of an input image containing a left ear. Column (a): before applying false positive suppression: the response at the right ear is also very high, (b): after applying false positive suppression, the false positive is eliminated (the location of the right ear is marked).

Fig. 4. The response maps of an input image that includes the left half of the head. Column (a): the response map associated with the left ear, (b): the response map associated with the right ear. The response at the location of the CI transmitter is so high that it is detected as an ear. It can be eliminated by the shape-based constraint.

It measures how much the spatial distribution of the ear pair deviates from the most 'common' ear pair distribution. We record the maximal Mahalanobis distance of the training shapes as M_{max}. For each test volume, when two inner ears are detected from the probability maps, the position vectors of the left and right inner ears, i.e., $l_{left}^{test} = \left(x_{left}^{test}, y_{left}^{test}, z_{left}^{test} \right)$ and $l_{right}^{test} = \left(x_{right}^{test}, y_{right}^{test}, z_{right}^{test} \right)$, are stacked and demeaned to create a shape vector s^{test}. If $M(s^{test}, \bar{s}) > M_{max}$, we reject the detected inner with the smallest response.

3   Results

In Table 2, we show the confusion matrix we have obtained with our testing set. In the upper part of Table 3, we show results with and without the false positive suppression training method and the shape-based constraint. We successfully improve the accuracy by $\sim 7\%$ by using the suppression and the shape-based constraint.

For the test image volumes that are correctly classified, we calculate the localization error, which is shown in the lower part of Table 3. The localization error is computed as the distance between the manually labeled inner ear position and the automatic localization. For comparison purpose, we use a Random Forest (RF)-based approach [11] developed for head CT landmark localization to find the same landmark in our current dataset and we report the localization accuracy obtained with this method. A number in bold indicates that the localization error generated by the method in this row is lower and significantly different from the other method. The results show that the proposed method produces substantially lower localization errors for all image groups. All differences for the five groups of comparisons are statistically different using a paired t-test ($p < 0.01$).

Table 2. Confusion matrix for each category with 'B', 'L', 'R', 'N' indicating volumes including both, left, right and neither ears, respectively.

Truth	Predict			
	B	L	R	N
B	618	5	1	1
L	0	619	2	4
R	0	4	613	8
N	1	4	5	601

Table 3. Categorization of error rate before and after the false positive suppression and shape-based constraint (denoted as FP reduction), and localization error using our proposed method and the baseline RF-based method.

Categorization of error rate					Overall
	Classified by presence of CI		Classified by scanner		
	w/CI	w/o CI	Conventional	Xoran	
Before FP reduction	14.65%	7.39%	4.65%	22.14%	8.53%
After FP reduction	0.77%	1.53%	1.50%	1.09%	1.41%
Localization error (in mm)					
Proposed	**2.32 ± 2.34**	**2.48 ± 2.35**	**2.41 ± 1.13**	**2.57 ± 4.49**	**2.45 ± 2.35**
RF-based	6.80 ± 18.14	5.39 ± 11.80	5.01 ± 11.14	8.17 ± 19.61	5.87 ± 13.57

4 Conclusions

In this paper, to detect the inner ears in head CTs, we have proposed to use the 3D U-Net to regress the image volume directly to probability maps associated with each inner ear. By incorporating a novel false positive suppression strategy at the time of training and applying a shape-based constraint, we achieve a 98.51% detection accuracy. We achieve a localization error of 2.45 mm, which is much better than an RF-based method that has been proposed recently to achieve the same.

Acknowledgments. This work has been supported by NIH grants R01DC014037, R01DC008408, R01DC014462 and Advanced Computing Center for Research and Education (ACCRE) of Vanderbilt University. The content is solely the responsibility of the authors and does not necessarily represent the official views of this institute.

References

1. NIDCD Fact Sheet: Cochlear Implants. NIH Publ. No. 11-4798, pp. 1–4 (2011)
2. Noble, J.H., Labadie, R.F., Majdani, O., Dawant, B.M.: Automatic segmentation of intracochlear anatomy in conventional CT. IEEE Trans. Biomed. Eng. **58**(9), 2625–2632 (2011)
3. Zhao, Y., Dawant, B.M., Labadie, R.F., Noble, J.H.: Automatic localization of cochlear implant electrodes in CT. In: Golland, P., Hata, N., Barillot, C., Hornegger, J., Howe, R. (eds.) MICCAI 2014. LNCS, vol. 8673, pp. 331–338. Springer, Cham (2014). https://doi.org/10.1007/978-3-319-10404-1_42
4. Noble, J.H., Gifford, R.H., Hedley-Williams, A.J., Dawant, B.M., Labadie, R.F.: Clinical evaluation of an image-guided cochlear implant programming strategy. Audiol. Neurotol. **19**(6), 400–411 (2014)
5. Mamani, G.E.H., Setio, A.A.A., van Ginneken, B., Jacobs, C.: Organ detection in thorax abdomen CT using multi-label convolutional neural networks. In: SPIE Conference on Medical Imaging, p. 1013416 (2017)

6. de Vos, B.D., Wolterink, J.M., de Jong, P.A., Leiner, T., Viergever, M.A., Isgum, I.: ConvNet-based localization of anatomical structures in 3-D medical images. IEEE Trans. Med. Imaging **36**(7), 1470–1481 (2017)
7. Xu, Z., et al.: Supervised action classifier: approaching landmark detection as image partitioning. In: Descoteaux, M., Maier-Hein, L., Franz, A., Jannin, P., Collins, D.L., Duchesne, S. (eds.) MICCAI 2017. LNCS, vol. 10435, pp. 338–346. Springer, Cham (2017). https://doi.org/10.1007/978-3-319-66179-7_39
8. Yang, D., et al.: Automatic vertebra labeling in large-scale 3D CT using deep image-to-image network with message passing and sparsity regularization. In: Niethammer, M., et al. (eds.) IPMI 2017. LNCS, vol. 10265, pp. 633–644. Springer, Cham (2017). https://doi.org/10.1007/978-3-319-59050-9_50
9. Çiçek, Ö., Abdulkadir, A., Lienkamp, S.S., Brox, T., Ronneberger, O.: 3D U-Net: learning dense volumetric segmentation from sparse annotation. In: Ourselin, S., Joskowicz, L., Sabuncu, M.R., Unal, G., Wells, W. (eds.) MICCAI 2016. LNCS, vol. 9901, pp. 424–432. Springer, Cham (2016). https://doi.org/10.1007/978-3-319-46723-8_49
10. Chollet, F.: Keras (2015)
11. Zhang, D., Liu, Y., Noble, J.H., Dawant, B.M.: Localizing landmark sets in head CTs using random forests and a heuristic search algorithm for registration initialization. J. Med. Imaging **4**(4) (2017). https://doi.org/10.1117/1.JMI.4.4.044007

Automatic Teeth Segmentation in Panoramic X-Ray Images Using a Coupled Shape Model in Combination with a Neural Network

Andreas Wirtz$^{(\boxtimes)}$, Sudesh Ganapati Mirashi, and Stefan Wesarg

Fraunhofer IGD, Fraunhoferstr. 5, 64283 Darmstadt, Germany
{Andreas.Wirtz,Stefan.Wesarg}@igd.fraunhofer.de

Abstract. Dental panoramic radiographs depict the full set of teeth in a single image and are used by dentists as a popular first tool for diagnosis. In order to provide the dentist with automatic diagnostic support, a robust and accurate segmentation of the individual teeth is required. However, poor image quality of panoramic x-ray images like low contrast or noise as well as teeth variations in between patients make this task difficult. In this paper, a fully automatic approach is presented that uses a coupled shape model in conjunction with a neural network to overcome these challenges. The network provides a preliminary segmentation of the teeth region which is used to initialize the coupled shape model in terms of position and scale. Then the 28 individual teeth (excluding wisdom teeth) are segmented and labeled using gradient image features in combination with the model's statistical knowledge about their shape variation and spatial relation. The segmentation quality of the approach is assessed by comparing the generated results to manually created gold-standard segmentations of the individual teeth. Experimental results on a set of 14 test images show average precision and recall values of 0.790 and 0.827, respectively and a DICE overlap of 0.744.

Keywords: Coupled shape model · Automatic segmentation
Panoramic dental x-ray image · Deep learning

1 Introduction

Radiographic images are a common tool used in dentistry for diagnosis. They help the dentist to identify many teeth related problems like caries, infections and bone abnormalities, which would be hard or impossible to detect during visual inspection only. This allows the dentist to choose the optimal treatment plan for the patient. Dental radiographs can be divided into two categories: Intra-oral and extra-oral [13]. Intra-oral images like bitewing, periapical or occlusal are obtained inside the patient's mouth. They only show specific regions of the set of teeth or individual teeth and are mostly used to get more detailed information. Extra-oral images like cephalometic or panoramic, also known as orthopantomographic

© Springer Nature Switzerland AG 2018
A. F. Frangi et al. (Eds.): MICCAI 2018, LNCS 11073, pp. 712–719, 2018.
https://doi.org/10.1007/978-3-030-00937-3_81

images, capture the entire teeth region as well as the surrounding areas and provide fundamental information about the teeth of a patient (cf. Fig. 1).

The analysis of these images is still done manually since automated tools that provide support for this procedure are not available. Therefore, the evaluation of these images and the design of the patient's treatment plan heavily relies on the dentist's experience and visual perception [13]. The lack of automated tools results from difficulties when dealing with dental X-Ray images. These include but are not limited to gaps caused by missing teeth, poor image quality like intensity variation, noise or low contrast, artifacts due to restorations, caries, and variations of the teeth in between patients [1]. An (automatic) segmentation of the individual teeth in a radiograpic image is an essential step for providing tools for an automatic analysis of such images [9]. Automatic analysis can not only be helpful for automatic diagnosis in dentistry but could also be used for forensic procures (i.e. postmortem identification).

Several methods have been proposed in the past to extract information form panoramic radiographs. Lira et al. [6] have used quadtree decomposition, morphological operators and snake models to segment individual teeth. They also employed shape models but use them only for teeth recognition. Amer and Aqel [1] have segmented only the wisdom teeth. They have used otsu-thresholding and morphological dilation to extract the region of interest (ROI) and have then applied masks at the end of the ROI to extract the wisdom teeth. Hasan et al. [3] have used clustering, thresholding and GVF snakes to segment the jaws in panoramic images. Recently, Silva et al. [10] reviewed state of the art methods for teeth segmentation in dental radiographs. They separated relevant works into different categories like threshold-based, region-based or boundary-based methods and also grouped them by the type of image these methods can be applied to. The majority are threshold-based approaches (54%) followed by boundary-based methods (34%). More importantly, the reviewed papers focused mostly on intra-oral X-Ray images (80%). To close this scientific gap, Jader et al. propose a novel data set featuring 1500 panoramic radiographic images. Additionally, they compared 10 different segmentation methods on their data set with the goal to extract the teeth and provide a comprehensive performance assessment. None of the analyzed methods provided satisfactory results and the authors conclude that an adequate method for the segmentation of dental X-Ray images, which can serve as a basis for automatic analysis, is still to be found.

In this paper, a novel method for automatic teeth segmentation in dental panoramic radiographs is presented. A 2-D coupled shape model based on [5] is used to segment and label 28 individual teeth. The 2-D coupled model is composed of a statistical shape model (SSM) for each tooth which is coupled with all other individual models using their spatial relation. This enables a more robust segmentation process using gradient image features (bottom-up) in combination with a priori statistical knowledge about the teeth in order to guide the segmentation process (top-down) [7]. A drawback of statistical models is that they rely on a good initial placement if local search algorithms like active shape models are used [4]. We propose to handle this by using a binary mask of the teeth area that is generated using a deep neural network [8]. The mask is then used for the initialization of the coupled shape model in terms of position and scale.

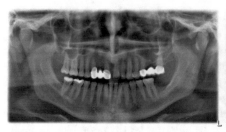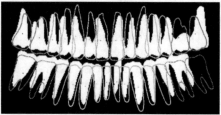

Fig. 1. A more difficult case with bridges and missing teeth (left) and the initial placement of the mean coupled model on the corresponding (cropped) binary mask (right).

2 Methods

2-D Coupled Shape Model. The presented method is based on a 3-D coupled shape model consisting of rigid model items and deformable model items [5]. It has already been successfully applied to CT images in order to segment different structures in the head & neck area [11,12]. To be able to apply the model to dental X-Ray images, the coupled shape model has been extended to support single 2-D images. Deformable 2-D model items and the corresponding 2-D transformations have been added that represent the contour of objects and their relative transformation to the center of the coupled model. These 2-D model items are represented as statistical shape models and are generated using a point distribution model (PDM) [2] and principal component analysis (PCA).

The contour of an individual item is represented by 100 landmark points and denoted as vector $c = (x_1, y_1, \ldots, x_{100}, y_{100})$. Procrustes alignment is used to transform all s training instances of a single item into a common coordinates system. The statistical information of these training instances is then extracted using PCA by computing eigenvectors e_m and their respective eigenvalues λ_m (with $\lambda_i > \lambda_{i+1}$) of the covariance matrix $S = \frac{1}{s-1} \sum_{i=1}^{s} (c_i - \bar{c})(c_i - \bar{c})^T$, where $\bar{c}$ is the mean shape. For each model item, only the first n eigenvectors required for capturing 95% of the shape variance are kept and the remaining ones are discarded. Every valid shape $\tilde{c}$ can then be approximated by a linear combination of these n principal modes: $\tilde{c} = \bar{c} + \sum_{i=1}^{n} v_i e_i$.

The coupled shape model is created by combining the relative pose of each model item in relation to the center of mass of the complete model and its shape information. The parameter vector p_j for an individual model item j consists of $4 + n$ entries, the 4 transformation parameters (2 for translation and 1 for rotation and isotropic scaling, respectively) and the n principal modes. By concatenating the parameter vectors p_j of all model items for a training instance k, the configuration vector f_k is generated. Again, PCA is used here to describe the space of all possible configurations over all training instances, which is later used during the adaptation process. Any possible configuration can then be described by a vector b as $\tilde{f} = \bar{f} + A \cdot b + r$, where $\bar{f}$ is the mean configuration and A is the matrix containing all eigenvectors of the covariance matrix of all possible configurations. For more details see [12].

The coupled shape model consists of 28 individual teeth and is trained based on 10 manually annotated panoramic X-Ray images. Wisdom teeth are not included in the model at the moment due to the limited amount of training data available. In order to adapt the model and segment the teeth in the panoramic image, a robust initialization of the coupled model onto the image is required.

Binary Mask Generation. The binary mask of the teeth area, which is used for the initialization process, is generated by a modified neural network (u-net model) proposed by Ronneberger et al. [8]. Simpler, threshold-based methods proved ineffective in producing reliable results for the initialization of the coupled model. The network was originally used to segment neuronal structures in microscopy images, but has also been successfully applied to bitewing radiographs [13]. The advantage of this kind of neural network is that it can be trained with a limited number of training data and still produce accurate segmentation results. This is achieved by relying on data augmentation to extend the training set and a specially tuned network architecture. For more details see [8]. The modified U-Net model used in this work has the same internal architecture as the original one, but was modified to work on input images with a resolution of 608×320 pixels and only uses half the amount of channels on each layer (i.e. 32 on the first layer instead of 64). With this design, the generated binary masks were robust and detailed enough to be used for the initialization process. Figure 1 shows a panoramic image and the corresponding (cropped) binary mask.

The network was trained on the same 10 training instances that were used for the coupled shape model. Image augmentation was applied to increase the number of training images to about 4000.

Model Initialization. The coupled shape model needs to be initialized on the input image in terms of position and scale. Both values are computed on the binary mask of the teeth area. For the position, instead of using a simple center of mass, which is easily affected by missing or broken teeth, the presence or absence of wisdom teeth and unusual teeth configurations, the x- and y-coordinates are computed separately. First, the bounding box of the binary mask is computed. The y-coordinate is then determined using a horizontal projection to identify the location of the 'valley' between upper and lower jaw. The x-coordinate is calculated by taking the average of the x-centroid of the bounding box area and its inverse. The scale value is initially approximated by the ratio between the sizes of the bounding box of the binary mask and the bounding box of the mean model. This value is then refined by placing the model according to previously computed position and maximizing the overlap between mask and model. Having both the values for position and scale, the coupled model can be initialized onto the input image. An example of an initialization is shown in Fig. 1.

Model Adaptation. After the initialization process, the model is adapted to the input image. The adaptation is done by minimizing an energy functional E. It depends on two parameters: (a) the transformation t describing the global position of the model in terms of translation and rotation and (b) the configuration

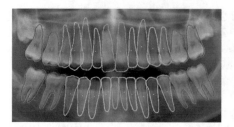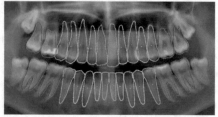

Fig. 2. Two examples of segmentation results.

vector f describing the configuration of the coupled model. The functional is given by $E(f,t) = E_{ext}(f,t) + \lambda E_{int}(f)$. The external term E_{ext} is responsible for ensuring that the contour of model items moves in the direction of strong image features (gradient features) whereas the internal energy term E_{int} restricts the model to stay within or close to the learned configuration space. The optimization process is done using a gradient descent optimizer. The transformation parameters t are optimized first, and then the configuration and transformation parameters f,t are optimized jointly.

The process of adapting the model to the image is separated into multiple steps. Initially, the model is adapted to the binary mask to ensure a good placement of all teeth before using the intensity image. Starting with only the 4 incisors, the set of model items (teeth) which are adapted to the image is gradually extended. Model items that are not adapted during an adaptation step are only changed passively through the learned (spatial) configuration. The gradual extension of the set of adapted items is done because the mean model is initialized according to its center of mass. Therefore, the teeth close to the center (the incisors) show good overlap with the input image while the teeth farther away from the center (e.g. molars) might not match as good, depending on the structure of the teeth in the input image. By adapting the outer teeth at a later time, they have already been (passively) moved closer to their correct position and more reliable image features will be found once they are adapted. The final adaption is then performed on the intensity image and the segmentation result of each individual tooth is stored as a binary image.

3   Experiments and Results

The presented fully automatic segmentation method has been evaluated on a separate test set of 14 manually annotated panoramic radiographic images (referred to as gold-standard segmentations), which were not part of the training set. The images each have a resolution of 2440×1280 pixels. The test set includes images of a variety of cases with several difficulties like completely- and partially missing teeth, artificial teeth, fillings and bridges. It also covers patients that have all, none or only some wisdom teeth.

First, the results of the automatic initialization have been assessed visually to determine if the model was positioned and scaled correctly. The placement was

Table 1. The average, minimum and maximum values for different metrics used for comparing the segmentation results to gold-standard segmentations.

	Precision	Recall	Accuracy	Specificity	F-Score	DICE
Avg.	0.790	0.827	0.818	0.799	0.803	0.744
Min.	0.404	0.440	0.582	0.647	0.417	0.381
Max.	0.883	0.914	0.887	0.862	0.886	0.824

considered as correct, if the incisor teeth of the mean model were overlapping with the corresponding structure in the binary mask. The position of the model after initialization was correct for 13 out of the 14 test cases. The incorrect placement was caused by an asymmetry in the binary mask.

Therefore, the centroid computed on the binary mask was shifted too far to one side causing a wrong overlap. The model was unable to recover from this incorrect initialization during the adaptation process, resulting in a DICE overlap of only 0.38 (cf. Table 1). Scale estimation was accurate enough for all cases to enable a working adaptation. However, in some cases the initial size of the model was too large, so that molar teeth were in between two teeth in the input image, causing an incorrect segmentation of these teeth as a result. Central teeth like incisors or canine were still segmented correctly.

Exemplary segmentation results are depicted in Fig. 2. The final segmentations are compared to gold-standard segmentations and evaluated in terms of precision, recall, accuracy, specificity, f-score and dice overlap. In order to receive meaningful results for specificity and accuracy, the evaluation is done on the minimum bounding box that covers both automatic- and gold-standard segmentation. For a single test instance, first the values for each tooth present in the test instance are computed. Then, the average over all these teeth is computed to get the result for that test instance. Finally, the average is computed over all 14 test instances. Table 1 shows the average values as well as minimum and maximum values for each category.

4   Discussion

The proposed approach combines a coupled shape model with a neural network to robustly segment teeth in panoramic radiographic images. Most state of the art methods rely only on information extracted from the image itself, which is directly influenced by image quality. The coupled shape model, however, employs a priori knowledge about the shape and spatial configuration of the individual teeth to guide the search for suitable image features which helps to handle the poor image quality of dental X-Ray images. The neural network provides a robust binary mask for calculating the necessary information for the initialization of the coupled model. Additionally, the mask is useful for an initial adaptation to ensure a good placement of individual teeth. This way, the parameters of the final adaptation on the intensity image can be chosen specifically to detect the correct tooth contour.

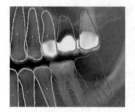 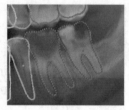 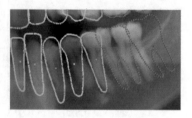

Fig. 3. Difficult cases: bridge and missing teeth (left), broken tooth (middle) and failed segmentation in case of a missing premolar tooth and no gap in this place (right)

Wisdom teeth have not been incorporated into the model at the moment. Their position and shape can vary highly from patient to patient and not all patients have them. There was simply not enough training data available to train a reliable shape model and get a meaningful estimate of the space of possible positions. Wisdom teeth will be added at a later point when sufficient training data is available. The approach is able to handle missing teeth, if the space originally occupied by the missing tooth is still visible so that the mean shape model of that tooth can be placed into the gap and subsequent teeth can be positioned correctly. In case the gap is too small or no longer present, subsequent teeth are labeled incorrectly. Partially missing or broken teeth are labeled correctly. However, due to their unnatural shape, segmentation accuracy is lower since the shape adaptation is limited to valid shapes given by the shape model. Post-processing steps would be required to tackle this problem. Fillings can influence the segmentation accuracy since the denser material appears brighter in X-Ray images and results in stronger gradient features. The contour might be placed incorrectly in cases were fillings do not match the true contour of the teeth. Figure 3 depicts some examples for the aforementioned cases.

Overall, the presented approach performs significantly better than any of the state of the art methods reviewed in [10]. None of the reviewed methods managed to achieve good results in both precision and recall. Watershed-based methods provided a high recall value of 0.816, but only a low precision of 0.478. The opposite is the case for splitting/merging methods with a precision of 0.816 and recall of only 0.081. The best methods according to the f-score value were local-threshold methods with a precision of 0.513 and recall of 0.826. The approach presented in this paper achieves an average precision of 0.790 together with a recall of 0.827.

5   Conclusion

In this paper an automatic approach for teeth segmentation in panoramic radiographic images was presented. It performs better than current state of the art methods and is able to handle difficulties like missing or broken teeth, filling and bridges. On a set of 14 test images the approach achieves an average DICE overlap of 0.744 and precision and recall values of 0.790 and 0.827, respectively.

Future work includes increasing the segmentation accuracy and robustness, extending the coupled shape model by using a larger set of training images and potentially including wisdom teeth into the model. Since the framework itself is generic, it can also be applied to other types of dental X-Ray images.

Acknowledgements. We thank Dr. Werner Betz, Goethe University Frankfurt for providing the panoramic radiographic images used in this work.

References

1. Amer, Y.Y., Aqel, M.J.: An efficient segmentation algorithm for panoramic dental images. Procedia Comput. Sci. **65**, 718–725 (2015)
2. Cootes, T.F., Taylor, C.J., Cooper, D.H., Graham, J.: Training models of shape from sets of examples. In: Hogg, D., Boyle, R. (eds.) BMVC92, pp. 9–18. Springer, London (1992). https://doi.org/10.1007/978-1-4471-3201-1_2
3. Hasan, M.M., Ismail, W., Hassan, R., Yoshitaka, A.: Automatic segmentation of jaw from panoramic dental x-ray images using GVF snakes. In: 2016 World Automation Congress (WAC), pp. 1–6, July 2016
4. Heimann, T., Meinzer, H.P.: Statistical shape models for 3D medical image segmentation: a review. Med. Image Anal. **13**(4), 543–563 (2009)
5. Jung, F., Steger, S., Knapp, O., Noll, M., Wesarg, S.: COSMO - coupled shape model for radiation therapy planning of head and neck cancer. In: Linguraru, M. (ed.) CLIP 2014. LNCS, vol. 8680, pp. 25–32. Springer, Cham (2014). https://doi.org/10.1007/978-3-319-13909-8_4
6. Lira, P.H., Giraldi, G.A., Neves, L.A.: Panoramic dental x-ray image segmentation and feature extraction. In: Proceedings of V Workshop of Computing Vision, Sao Paulo, Brazil (2009)
7. McInerney, T., Terzopoulos, D.: Deformable models in medical image analysis: a survey. Med. Image Anal. **1**(2), 91–108 (1996)
8. Ronneberger, O., Fischer, P., Brox, T.: U-Net: convolutional networks for biomedical image segmentation. In: Navab, N., Hornegger, J., Wells, W.M., Frangi, A.F. (eds.) MICCAI 2015. LNCS, vol. 9351, pp. 234–241. Springer, Cham (2015). https://doi.org/10.1007/978-3-319-24574-4_28
9. Said, E.H., Nassar, D.E.M., Fahmy, G., Ammar, H.H.: Teeth segmentation in digitized dental x-ray films using mathematical morphology. IEEE Trans. Inf. Forensics Secur. **1**(2), 178–189 (2006)
10. Silva, G., Oliveira, L., Pithon, M.: Automatic segmenting teeth in x-ray images: trends, a novel data set, benchmarking and future perspectives. Expert. Syst. Appl. **107**, 15–31 (2018)
11. Steger, S., Jung, F., Wesarg, S.: Personalized articulated atlas with a dynamic adaptation strategy for bone segmentation in CT or CT/MR head and neck images. In: Medical Imaging 2014: Image Processing, vol. 9034, p. 90341I. International Society for Optics and Photonics (2014)
12. Steger, S., Kirschner, M., Wesarg, S.: Articulated atlas for segmentation of the skeleton from head & neck CT datasets. In: 2012 9th IEEE International Symposium on Biomedical Imaging (ISBI), pp. 1256–1259. IEEE (2012)
13. Wang, C.W., et al.: A benchmark for comparison of dental radiography analysis algorithms. Med. Image Anal. **31**, 63–76 (2016)

Craniomaxillofacial Bony Structures Segmentation from MRI with Deep-Supervision Adversarial Learning

Miaoyun Zhao[1], Li Wang[1], Jiawei Chen[1], Dong Nie[1], Yulai Cong[2],
Sahar Ahmad[1], Angela Ho[3], Peng Yuan[3], Steve H. Fung[3],
Hannah H. Deng[3], James Xia[3(✉)], and Dinggang Shen[1(✉)]

[1] Department of Radiology and BRIC,
University of North Carolina at Chapel Hill, Chapel Hill, USA
dgshen@med.unc.edu
[2] Department of Electrical and Computer Engineering,
Duke University, Durham, USA
[3] Houston Methodist Hospital, Houston, TX, USA
jxia@houstonmethodist.org

Abstract. Automatic segmentation of medical images finds abundant applications in clinical studies. Computed Tomography (CT) imaging plays a critical role in diagnostic and surgical planning of craniomaxillofacial (CMF) surgeries as it shows clear bony structures. However, CT imaging poses radiation risks for the subjects being scanned. Alternatively, Magnetic Resonance Imaging (MRI) is considered to be safe and provides good visualization of the soft tissues, but the bony structures appear invisible from MRI. Therefore, the segmentation of bony structures from MRI is quite challenging. In this paper, we propose a cascaded generative adversarial network with deep-supervision discriminator (Deep-supGAN) for automatic bony structures segmentation. The first block in this architecture is used to generate a high-quality CT image from an MRI, and the second block is used to segment bony structures from MRI and the generated CT image. Different from traditional discriminators, the deep-supervision discriminator distinguishes the generated CT from the ground-truth at different levels of feature maps. For segmentation, the loss is *not only* concentrated on the voxel level *but also* on the higher abstract perceptual levels. Experimental results show that the proposed method generates CT images with clearer structural details and also segments the bony structures more accurately compared with the state-of-the-art methods.

1 Introduction

Generating a precise three-dimensional (3D) skeletal model is an essential step during craniomaxillofacial (CMF) surgical planning. Traditionally, computed tomography (CT) images are used in CMF surgery. However, a patient has to be exposed under radiation [1]. Magnetic Resonance Imaging (MRI), on the other hand, provides a safer scanning without radiation and non-invasive way to render CMF anatomy. However, it is extremely difficult to accurately segment CMF bony structures from MRI due to the

© Springer Nature Switzerland AG 2018
A. F. Frangi et al. (Eds.): MICCAI 2018, LNCS 11073, pp. 720–727, 2018.
https://doi.org/10.1007/978-3-030-00937-3_82

confusing boundaries between bones and air (both appearing to be black in MRI), low signal-to-noise ratio, and partial volume effect.

Recently, deep learning has demonstrated outstanding performance in a wide range of computer vision and image analysis applications. With a properly designed loss function, deep learning methods can automatically learn complex hierarchical features for a specific task. In particular, fully convolutional neural network (FCN) [2] was proposed to perform image segmentation by down-sampling and up-sampling streams. U-Net based methods further proposed skip connections to concatenate the lower fine feature maps to the higher coarse feature maps [3]. Nie *et al.* proposed a 3D deep-learning based cascade framework, in which a 3D U-Net is used to train a coarse segmentation and then a CNN is cascaded for fine-grained segmentation [4]. However, most of the previous works typically perform segmentation on the original MRI with low contrast for bony structures. Inspired by great success of Generative Adversarial Network (GAN) [5] in generating realistic images, we hypothesize that the segmentation problem can also be treated as an estimation problem, i.e., generating realistic CT images from MRIs and performing segmentation from the generated CT images. In this paper, we propose a framework of deep-supervision adversarial learning for CMF structure segmentation on the MR images. Our proposed framework consists of two major steps: (1) a simulation GAN to estimate a CT image from an MR image, and (2) a segmentation GAN to segment CMF bony structures based on both the original MR image and the generated CT image. Specifically, a CT image is first generated from a given MR image by a deep-supervision discriminative GAN, where a perceptive loss strategy is developed to obtain the knowledge from the real CT image *in terms of* both local detailed information and global structures. Furthermore, in segmentation task, with the proposed perceptive loss strategy, the discriminative GAN evaluates the segmentation results with the feature maps at different layers and the feedback structure information from both the original MR image and the generated CT image.

2   Method

In this section, we propose a cascaded generative adversarial network with deep-supervision discriminators (Deep-supGAN) to perform CMF bony structures segmentation from the MR image and generated CT image. The proposed framework is shown in Fig. 1. It includes two parts: (1) a simulation GAN that estimates a CT image from an MR image and (2) a segmentation GAN that segments the CMF bony structures based on both the original MR image and the generated CT image. The simulation GAN consists of the deep-supervision discriminators designed at each convolution layer to evaluate the quality of the generated image. In segmentation GAN, the deep-supervision perception loss is employed to evaluate the segmentation at multiple levels. Note that, for the discriminators of both parts, we utilize the first four convolution layers of a VGG-16 network [6] pre-trained on the ImgeNet dataset to extract the feature maps.

2.1 Simulation GAN

The simulation GAN for generating CT from MRI is shown in the upper portion of Fig. 1. Considering z as a ground-truth MRI patch, x as a ground-truth CT patch, and x' as a generated CT patch, we design a generator $G_c(z)$ to map a given MR image patch into a CT image patch. To make the generated CT image patch similar to the ground-truth CT image *in terms of* both local details and global structures, we design multiple deep-supervision discriminator $D_c^l(x)$, $(l = 1, 2, 3, \cdots)$. Here, $D_c^l(x)$ is a discriminator at the l-th layer of a pre-trained VGG-16 network, where each layer can extract features with different scales, from local details to global structures. Thus, each discriminator compares the generated CT with the ground-truth CT in different scales, resulting in an accurate simulation. To match the generated CT with the ground-truth CT, an adversarial game is played between $G_c(z)$ and $D_c^l(x)$. The loss function for the game is described as:

$$
\min_{G_c} \max_{D_c^l} \mathbb{E}_{x \sim p(x)} \left[\sum_l \sum_{i,j} \log \left(\left[D_c^l(x) \right]_{i,j} \right) \right]
$$
$$
+ \mathbb{E}_{z \sim q(z)} \left[\sum_l \sum_{i,j} \log \left(1 - \left[D_c^l(G_c(z)) \right]_{i,j} \right) \right] \tag{1}
$$

where $p(x)$ is the distribution of the original CT data, $q(z)$ is the distribution of the original MRI data, $\left[D_c^l(x) \right]_{i,j}$ is the (i, j)-th element in matrix $D_c^l(x)$, and L is the number of layers connected with discriminator.

2.2 Segmentation GAN

Similarly, with the generated CT x' from $G_c(z)$, we can construct a segmentation GAN $G_s(z, x')$, which learns to predict a bony structures segmentation y'. Then, the ground-truth y and the predicted segmentation y' are forwarded to the discriminator $D_s(y)$ to get an evaluation. Note that, different from the discriminator D_c^l in the simulation GAN, the discriminator $D_s(y)$ is only designed for the feature map at the last layer of the pre-trained VGG-16 net. The adversarial game for segmentation is as follows:

$$
\min_{G_s} \max_{D_s} \mathbb{E}_{y \sim p(y)} [\log D_s(y)] + \mathbb{E}_{z,x' \sim q(z,x')} [\log(1 - D_s(G_s(z, x')))] \tag{2}
$$

where $p(y)$ is the distribution of ground-truth segmentation images, and $q(z, x')$ is the joint distribution of the original MRI and the generated CT data. For the segmentation results, a voxel-wise loss is intuitively considered as follows:

$$
\mathcal{L}_{vox} = \mathbb{E}_{z,x' \sim q(z,x')} \| G_s(z, x') - y \|^2 \tag{3}
$$

Moreover, we also consider a perceptual loss L_{percp}^l to encourage the consistence of features maps from generated segmentation and ground-truth segmentation. To this end, the pre-trained part of the discriminator is utilized to extract multi-layer feature maps from the generated segmentation and ground-truth segmentation. Taking $\varphi_l(y)$ as the feature map of input y at the l-th layer of the feature extraction network, and N_l as the number of voxels in feature map $\varphi_l(y)$, we can obtain the perceptual loss for the l-th layer as follows:

$$\mathcal{L}_{percp}^l = \mathbb{E}_{z, x' \sim q(z, x')} \left[\frac{1}{N_l} \| \varphi_l(G_s(z, x')) - \varphi_l(y) \|^2 \right] \tag{4}$$

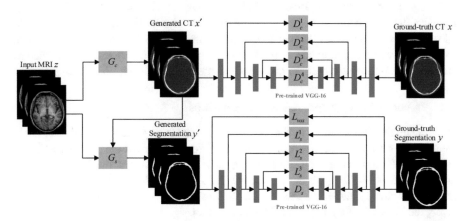

Fig. 1. The overview of the proposed Deep-supGAN. **Top:** CT generation net, where the generator G_c takes MRI patch z as input and generates the corresponding CT patch x', while the discriminator D_c^l takes generated CT patch x' and ground-truth CT patch x as input and produces classification (ground-truth = 1, generated = 0). **Bottom:** segmentation net, where G_s takes MRI patch z and generated CT patch x' as input and then generates the segmentation y', while D_s takes the generated segmentation y' and the ground-truth segmentation y as input and produces classification (ground-truth = 1, generated = 0).

In summary, the total loss function *with respect to* the generator is:

$$\min_{G_s} \mathbb{E}_{z, x' \sim q(z, x')}[-\log D_s(G_s(z, x'))] + \lambda_1 \mathcal{L}_{vox} + \lambda_2 \sum_{l=1}^{L} \mathcal{L}_{percp}^l \tag{5}$$

where parameters λ_1 and λ_2 are utilized to balance the importance of the three loss functions.

3   Experimental Results

3.1   Dataset

The experiments were conducted on the Alzheimer's Disease Neuroimaging Initiative (ADNI) database [7]. It consists of 16 subjects with paired MRI and CT scans. The MRI scans were obtained by a Siemens Triotim scanner, with a voxel size of 1.2×1.2 1 mm^3, TE 2.95 ms, TR 2300 ms, and flip angle 9. The CT scans were obtained from a Siemens Somatom scanner, with a voxel size of $0.59 \times 0.59 \times 3$ mm^3.

The preprocessing was conducted as follows. Both MRI and CT scans were resampled to size $152 \times 184 \times 149$ with a voxel size of $1 \times 1 \times 1$ mm^3. Each CT was aligned with its corresponding MRI. All intensities of MRI and CT were rescaled into $[-1, 1]$. To be compatible with VGG-16 net, both MRI and CT data were cropped into patches of size $152 \times 184 \times 3$ for training. The experiments were conducted on the 16 subjects in a leave-one-out cross validation. To measure the quality of the generated CT, we used the mean absolute error (MAE) and peak-signal-to-noise-ratio (PSNR). To measure the segmentation accuracy, we used Dice similarity coefficient (DSC). We adopted TensorFlow to implement the proposed framework. The network was trained using Adam with a learning rate of 1e-4 and a momentum of 0.9. In the experiments, we empirically set the parameters in the proposed method as: $L = 4$, $\lambda_1 = 1$ and $\lambda_2 = 1$.

3.2   Impact of Deep-Supervision Feature Maps

To evaluate the effectiveness of the deep-supervision strategy on the simulation GAN, we train the network with the discriminator in different layers of the pre-trained VGG-16 network. The results are shown in Fig. 2. It is obvious that the lower layer the discriminator is applied, the clearer the results will be. A quantitative comparison is shown in Table 1, indicating that, when the lower layer is connected with discriminator, the PSNR is bigger and the MAE is smaller.

To evaluate the effectiveness of the deep-supervision strategy on the segmentation GAN, we train the network with the perception reconstruction loss in different layers of the pre-trained VGG-16 network. As shown in Fig. 3, the results with higher layer connected with perceptual loss, $\mathcal{L}^2_{percp}$ and $\mathcal{L}^3_{percp}$, are more smooth and accurate in thin structures, as shown in the yellow rectangles. The DSC of different layer connected with perceptual loss is provided in Table 2, which again indicates that the deep-supervision perceptual loss enhances the performance greatly.

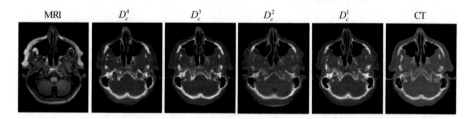

Fig. 2. CT generated by proposed Deep-supGAN with different layers connected with the discriminator. **Left to right:** original MRI, four CT images generated with the fourth, third, second, and first layer respectively connected with the discriminator, and ground-truth CT.

Table 1. PSNR and MAE with different layer connected with the discriminator.

Layer ID	1	2	3	4
PSNR	23.03	23.95	24.40	25.11
MAE (%)	1.99	1.61	1.45	1.23

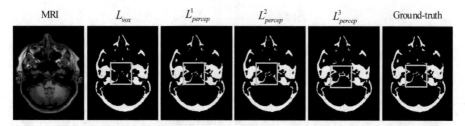

Fig. 3. Segmentation of proposed Deep-supGAN with different layers connected with the perceptual loss.

Table 2. DSC (%) of proposed Deep-supGAN with different layers connected with the perceptual loss.

Layer ID	$\mathcal{L}_{vox}$	$\mathcal{L}_{percp}^1$	$\mathcal{L}_{percp}^2$	$\mathcal{L}_{percp}^3$
DSC (%)	90.52	92.16	94.24	94.46

3.3   Impact of Generated CT

To evaluate the contribution of generated CT to the segmentation results, the segmentation results *only with MRI as input* (denoted as with MRI) is shown in Fig. 4. The segmentation result *with both original MRI and generated CT as input* (denoted as with MRI + CT) is more smooth and complete for thin structures, especially in the regions indicated by the yellow rectangles. The quantitative comparison in terms of DSC is shown in Table 3. It can be seen that the performance is significantly improved with the generated CT.

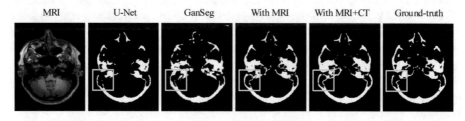

Fig. 4. Segmentation results by comparison methods. **Left to right**: Original MRI, U-Net, GanSeg, our method with MRI, our method with MRI+CT, and ground-truth.

Table 3. DSC (%) of compared methods on 16 subjects using leave-one-out cross validation.

Methods	U-Net [3]	GanSeg [8]	With MRI	With MRI + CT
DSC (%)	85.47	83.30	89.94	94.46

MRI   Scratch   VGG-16   CT

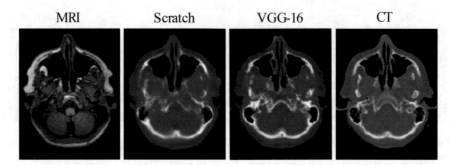

Fig. 5. The impact of pre-trained VGG-16 for generating CT. **Left to right:** original MRI, two CT images generated respectively by our method with discriminator (1) trained from scratch and (2) utilizing a pre-trained VGG-16, and ground-truth CT.

3.4   Impact of Pre-trained VGG-16 Network

Here we compare the generated CT with two different training settings: (1) learning the discriminator from scratch (denoted as Scratch) and (2) utilizing a pre-trained VGG-16 network (denoted as VGG-16) for the discriminator. As shown in Fig. 5, the CT generated with pre-trained VGG-16 is much clearer and more realistic than that trained from scratch.

3.5   Comparison with State-of-the-Art Segmentation Methods

To illustrate the advantage of our method on bony structures segmentation, we also compared it with two widely-used deep learning methods, i.e., U-Net [3] based segmentation method and Generative Adversarial Network based semantic segmentation method [8] (denoted as GanSeg, a traditional GAN with the generator designed as segmentation network). Comparison results on a typical subject are shown in Fig. 4. It can be seen that both U-Net and GanSeg failed to accurately segment bony structures, as indicated by yellow rectangles. Compared with these two methods, our proposed method can achieve more accurate segmentation. The quantitative comparison in terms of DSC is shown in Table 3. It clearly demonstrates the advantage of our proposed method in terms of segmentation accuracy.

4   Conclusion

In this paper, we proposed a cascade GAN network, Deep-supGAN, to segment CMF bony structures from the combination of an original MRI and a generated CT image. A GAN with deep-supervision discriminator is designed to generate a CT image from an MRI. With the generated CT image, a GAN with deep-supervision perceptual loss is designed to perform bony structures segmentation using both original MRI and the generated CT image. The combination of MRI and CT image can provide complementary information about bony structures for the segmentation task. Comparisons with the state-of-the-art methods demonstrate the advantage of our proposed method in terms of segmentation accuracy.

References

1. Brenner, D.J., Hall, E.J.: Computed tomography-an increasing source of radiation exposure. N. Engl. J. Med. **357**(22), 2277–2284 (2007)
2. Long, J., Shelhamer, E., Darrell, T.: Fully convolutional networks for semantic segmentation. In: Proceedings of the IEEE Conference on CVPR, pp. 3431–3440 (2015)
3. Çiçek, Ö., Abdulkadir, A., Lienkamp, S.S., Brox, T., Ronneberger, O.: 3D U-Net: learning dense volumetric segmentation from sparse annotation. In: Ourselin, S., Joskowicz, L., Sabuncu, Mert R., Unal, G., Wells, W. (eds.) MICCAI 2016. LNCS, vol. 9901, pp. 424–432. Springer, Cham (2016). https://doi.org/10.1007/978-3-319-46723-8_49
4. Nie, D., et al.: Segmentation of craniomaxillofacial bony structures from MRI with a 3D deep-learning based cascade framework. In: Wang, Q., Shi, Y., Suk, H.-I., Suzuki, K. (eds.) MLMI 2017. LNCS, vol. 10541, pp. 266–273. Springer, Cham (2017). https://doi.org/10.1007/978-3-319-67389-9_31
5. Goodfellow, I., Pouget-Abadie, J., Mirza, M.: Generative adversarial nets. In: Advances in Neural Information Processing Systems, pp. 2672–2680 (2014)
6. Simonyan, K., Zisserman, A.: Very deep convolutional networks for large-scale image recognition. arXiv preprint arXiv:1409.1556 (2014)
7. Trzepacz, P.T., Yu, P., Sun, J., et al.: Comparison of neuroimaging modalities for the prediction of conversion from mild cognitive impairment to Alzheimer's dementia. Neurobiol. Aging **35**(1), 143–151 (2014)
8. Luc, P., Couprie, C., Chintala, S.: Semantic segmentation using adversarial networks. arXiv preprint arXiv:1611.08408 (2016)

Automatic Skin Lesion Segmentation on Dermoscopic Images by the Means of Superpixel Merging

Diego Patiño$^{(\boxtimes)}$ ⓘ, Jonathan Avendaño$^{(\boxtimes)}$ ⓘ, and John W. Branch$^{(\boxtimes)}$ ⓘ

Universidad Nacional de Colombia, Faculty of Mines,
Calle 80 #65 - 223, Medellín, Colombia
{dapatinoco,jdavendanoo,jwbranch}@unal.edu.co

Abstract. We present a superpixel-based strategy for segmenting skin lesion on dermoscopic images. The segmentation is carried out by over-segmenting the original image using the SLIC algorithm, and then merge the resulting superpixels into two regions: healthy skin and lesion. The mean RGB color of each superpixel was used as merging criterion. The presented method is capable of dealing with segmentation problems commonly found in dermoscopic images such as hair removal, oil bubbles, changes in illumination, and reflections images without any additional steps. The method was evaluated on the PH2 and ISIC 2017 dataset with results comparable to the state-of-art.

1 Introduction

Melanoma is a type of skin cancer that can occur in any type of skin, and it is the leading cause of death among all skin cancer. A well-known criterion for early-stage melanoma detection is the "ABCDE" rule, which was designed for human-based visual analysis of a skin lesion. The "ABCDE" rule uses different visual cues to classify the lesion type: (A) Asymmetry, (B) irregularity of the Borders, (C) presence of specific Colors, (D) lesion shape and size, and (E) evaluation of the lesion evolution over time.

Early detection of malignant melanoma in dermoscopy images is crucial and critical since its detection in the early stages can be helpful to cure it. Computer Aided Diagnosis systems are becoming very helpful in facilitating the early detection of cancers for dermatologists. However, some challenges are present in this type of images that make difficult for computers to identify the lesion from healthy skin: presence of hair, changes in illumination, different types of skin, reflections, and oil bubble are some of the most common artifacts found in this type of images.

This paper focuses on constructing an accurate fully-automatic method to identify skin lesions in dermoscopy images to facilitate accurate, fast and more reliable identification and analysis. We used well-stated computer vision algorithms to segment skin lesion by first over-segmenting the original image and then merging the resulting regions into two types: skin lesion and healthy skin.

ⓒ Springer Nature Switzerland AG 2018
A. F. Frangi et al. (Eds.): MICCAI 2018, LNCS 11073, pp. 728–736, 2018.
https://doi.org/10.1007/978-3-030-00937-3_83

One fundamental difference of our approach compared to previous work is the fact that our segmentation method does not require a pre-processing step for correcting image artifacts like hair removal or illumination correction in contrast with most approaches in the literature. The stated work outputs a final binary mask containing the image's area where the lesion is located without the need for any user-defined parameter.

The segmentation strategy was tested on the PH^2 [1] and the ISIC 2017 challenge (part 1) [2] datasets. PH^2 consists of 200 images divided into three groups: common lesions, atypical nevi, and melanomas. ISIC, instead, has 2000 dermoscopic images with corresponding ground-truth segmentation. The experiments using our approach show comparable results with respect to previous works, achieving sensitivities and accuracy of around 92% in almost all tests, and demonstrate that our algorithm can be a suitable tool for the development of CAD support systems for the early detection of skin lesions.

The rest of this document is organized as follows: Sect. 2 reviews previous works on skin lesion segmentation. Section 3 presents a method for skin lesion segmentation based on superpixel approach. Section 4 experimental results are presented. Finally, Sect. 5 concludes the paper and states potential future work.

2 Related Work

Many segmentation algorithms have been proposed in the literature to deal with the problem of accurately segmenting skin lesion on dermatoscopic images while classifying several types of lesions [3–6]. Such approaches share a common structure that consists of first removing artifacts like hair and oil bubbles in the images, and then segment the skin lesion using different combinations of thresholding, clustering, and morphological operations.

One of the more representatives works on the subject is [7], where the authors defined a complete framework for skin lesion segmentation and classification based on Delaunay Triangulation. The polygons in such triangulation adapt to the lesion border according to a color criterion. In an early work, Sabbaghi et al. [8] also presented an interesting approach for this type of classification. They used QuadTree algorithm to subsequently group pixels with similar color properties and then analyze which color are present in each type of lesion. The authors did not perform any segmentation and do the classification using the whole set of pixels in the images.

Although Deep Learning is considered the state-of-the-art for a vast number of computer vision tasks, only in recent years deep learning methods have started being applied to skin-disease segmentation and classification using different architectures and schemes [9–12].

In this paper, we proposed a novel superpixel-based method for segmenting skin lesion on dermoscopic images without the need of pre-processing operations for artifacts removals such as reflections and hair. The main idea of our method is to over-segment the image into several superpixels, and then merge those which belong to the skin lesion to create a binary mask containing the area where the lesion is located.

3   Skin Lesion Segmentation

In this section, we describe our method for skin lesion segmentation on dermoscopic images. First, we use SLIC algorithm to obtain an over-segmentation of the original dermoscopic image (I). Later, a binary search is performed to find the best threshold to greedily merges all the superpixels into two regions: lesion and healthy skin. Finally, a post-processing stage is run to remove small superpixels and smooth the final segmentation.

3.1   Data Set

In order to test the proposed approach, we used the PH^2 [1] data set released by the Universidade do Porto, in collaboration with the Hospital Pedro Hispano in Matosinhos, Portugal. This data set contains 200 RGB dermoscopic images of melanocytic lesions, including 80 common nevi, 80 atypical nevi, and 40 melanomas. All images have manually generated ground-truth segmentation of the skin lesion of each image.

The method was also tested on the ISIC 2007 challenge dataset [2] which consist of 2000 dermoscopic images with corresponding manually generated ground-truth.

3.2   Superpixel Segmentation

Superpixels methods over segment an image by grouping pixels into units called superpixels. One of the most well-known algorithms for superpixel segmentations is Simple Linear Iterative Clustering (SLIC) developed by Achanta et al. in 2012 [13]. In SLIC the pixel grouping is done by clustering pixels with k-means algorithm using as features their color intensities plus their (i, j) coordinates of each pixel, weighted by a factor α. The parameter α helps to regularize the trade-off between spatial clustering and color clustering. Additionally, SLIC modifies the basic k-means algorithm applying some constraints to prevent that unconnected pixels could belong to the same superpixel.

For segmenting the skin lesion from the whole image, our method performs a SLIC superpixel segmentation on the RGB dermoscopic images. Ideally, in the over-segmented image, some superpixel's boundary should match partially the boundary of the object that is intended to segment.

SLIC requires a parameter k indicating the desired number of superpixels in the resulting image. A low value of k, although faster, leads to few and bigger superpixels where the superpixel's boundary does not entirely match the boundary of the object. With higher values of k, too much over-segmentation is done resulting in longer execution times with no significant improvement in the resulting segmentation. Figure 1 shows the resulting superpixel segmentation for two images and four different values of k. In our experiments we empirically set $k = 400$.

All original images have a dark shadow around the four corners of the images. This is an effect of the illumination setup in the dermatoscope device that was

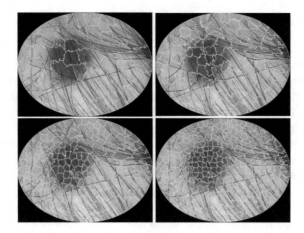

Fig. 1. SLIC segmentation for several k values. Left to right and top to bottom: $k = 100, 200, 400, 600$.

used to capture the images. To remove such effect, a binary mask is applied to the resulting SLIC segmentation. The mask is defined as the maximum ellipse inscribed in the image area.

3.3 Superpixel Merging

SLIC segmentation produces an over-segmented image with approximately k pieces. Hence, a merging operation must be done to separate the skin lesion (foreground superpixels) from the region containing pixels with no lesion (background superpixels). SLIC's output can be seen as a label image (L) where each integer label corresponds to one superpixel. From this representation, a Region Adjacency Graph (RAG) is constructed. Each node is equipped with a list of properties derived from its RGB intensity values: Mean color, total color, and pixel count.

Superpixel merging is then done by greedily combining pairs of nodes using the euclidean distance of the mean color of each node as criterion. If this difference is less than a threshold t, then the two nodes will merge, and a new node is created. The new node's properties are then calculated based on the merging nodes.

A binary search determines the optimal threshold by running the merging procedure with several values of t. Assuming RGB images with 3 channels, and intensity levels of each pixel in the range: $p \in [0, 255]$, the distance between the mean color of two different superpixels will in the interval $(0, 500)$. Therefore, the binary search will be constrained to such interval. The search converges when for a given t only two superpixels remain, or in the case that the maximum number of iterations is reached, or if $\Delta t < \epsilon$. To avoid trivial results with just one region, If the procedure result has only one superpixel, then it returns the last known threshold with at least two regions.

3.4 Post-processing

After merging with the optimal threshold, a post-processing step is performed to determine the final segmentation and smooth the results. First, All remaining regions with an area lower than 2% from the total area of the image are removed. Small superpixels remaining after merging are considered as noise because the two expected regions should be relatively significant areas corresponding to the lesion or healthy skin.

The merging produces a label image (L) where each superpixel is associated to an integer value. At this point, it is not possible to determine whether a label corresponds to background or skin lesion. Therefore, image O is created by applying adaptive equalization to a gray-scale version of the original image and subsequently segmenting it using an Otsu threshold. Each label in L is compared with O by calculating the Jaccard similarity index between the two areas. The label with the maximum Jaccard index is selected as the final segmented image after applying binary fill holes, and a morphological dilation with a disk-shaped structural element of radius 8.

4   Experimental Results

To compare our segmentation with other methods, we performed the same set of test presented in [7]. Hence, we used PH^2 ground-truth lesion segmentation to evaluate the outcome of our algorithm using four metrics: sensitivity, specificity, accuracy, and F-measure. Additionally, the data set was split into four subsets: all images, common lesions, atypical nevi, and melanomas. Tables 1a to d show the segmentation results as presented in [7], but extended with our results.

In each of the four tests, the presented strategy achieved significantly better sensitivity than previous works. This means that pixels belonging to a skin lesion are segmented correctly in a higher proportion compared with other methods (fewer false positives). A similar situation occurs with the F-measure metric. Also, better accuracy was also obtained in all test cases except with melanoma lesions.

However, specificity did not perform as well as the other three metrics. In all cases, specificity was slightly less than the highest value. This means our method tends to classify healthy pixels as lesion over-estimating the lesion area.

In previous works, hair removal is in many cases addressed with an extra preprocessing step before segmenting the lesion. This step involves the applications of different filters such as directional Gaussian filters [17] to the original image. In contrast, our strategy does not require any additional step since SLIC's superpixels fit the borders of the lesion avoiding hair areas. Figure 2 shows the segmentation results for three different images. Rows one and three correspond to Atypical nevi lesion, and row two is a melanocytic nevus.

Table 1. Segmentation results on the PH2 dataset.

(a) Using all 200 images (melanocytic nevi, dysplasic nevi, malignant lesions).

(b) Only 80 melanocytic nevi images (common healthy lesions).

Method	Sens.	Spec.	Acc.	F-measure	Method	Sens.	Spec.	Acc.	F-measure
JSEG[14]	0.7108	0.9714	0.8947 ± 0.0176	0.7554	JSEG[14]	0.6977	**0.9783**	0.9370 ± 0.0027	0.7265
SRM[15]	0.1035	0.8757	0.6766 ± 0.0346	0.1218	SRM[15]	0.0751	0.9332	0.7250 ± 0.0277	0.0611
KPP	0.4147	0.9581	0.7815 ± 0.0356	0.5457	KPP	0.3360	0.9566	0.7912 ± 0.0241	0.3960
K-means	0.7291	0.8430	0.8249 ± 0.0107	0.6677	K-means	0.7008	0.8767	0.8466 ± 0.8467	0.6004
Otsu	0.5221	0.7064	0.6518 ± 0.0203	0.4293	Otsu	0.4777	0.7832	0.6911 ± 0.0193	0.3658
Level Set[16]	0.7188	0.8003	0.7842 ± 0.0295	0.6456	Level Set[16]	0.7069	0.8262	0.7996 ± 0.0264	0.5856
ASLM[7]	0.8024	**0.9722**	0.8966 ± 0.0276	0.8257	ASLM[7]	0.8717	0.9760	0.9477 ± 0.0032	0.8690
Our method	**0.9104**	0.8973	**0.9039 ± 0.1419**	**0.8918**	Our method	**0.9212**	0.9642	**0.9524 ± 0.0637**	**0.9292**

(c) Only 80 dysplasic nevi images (atypical moles).

(d) Only 40 melanoma images (malignant lesions).

Method	Sens.	Spec.	Acc.	F-measure	Method	Sens.	Spec.	Acc.	F-measure
JSEG[14]	0.7435	0.9708	0.9236 ± 0.0065	0.7768	JSEG[14]	0.6746	0.9593	**0.7591 ± 0.0456**	0.7710
SRM[15]	0.1042	0.8954	0.6812 ± 0.0358	0.0919	SRM[15]	0.2234	0.7512	0.4148 ± 0.0366	0.2852
KPP	0.2895	0.9446	0.7512 ± 0.0261	0.3568	KPP	0.2648	0.7623	0.4324 ± 0.0336	0.3589
K-means	0.7650	0.8804	0.8501 ± 0.0065	0.6914	K-means	0.5971	0.4870	0.5524 ± 0.0211	0.6064
Otsu	0.5515	0.7579	0.6779 ± 0.0193	0.4372	Otsu	0.7073	0.7015	0.7249 ± 0.0214	0.7503
Level Set[16]	0.7364	0.8237	0.7985 ± 0.0346	0.6532	Level Set[16]	0.7141	0.7010	0.7313 ± 0.0230	0.7550
ASLM[7]	0.8640	**0.9733**	0.9271 ± 0.0099	0.8689	ASLM[7]	0.5404	**0.9597**	0.6615 ± 0.0506	0.6524
Our method	**0.9225**	0.9354	**0.9314 ± 0.0841**	**0.9112**	Our method	**0.8645**	0.6870	0.7519 ± 0.2216	**0.7779**

Table 2. Segmentation results compared with the state-of-the deep learning [12].

Method	Jaccard	Accuracy
Optimized single	0.836	0.949
Default augmentation	0.828	0.947
No noise or dropout	0.812	0.941
Ensemble of 10 U-Nets	0.841	0.951
State-of-art	**0.843**	**0.953**
Human expert average agreement	0.786	0.909
Our method	0.606	0.869

Moreover, experimental results also show that the performance of our method, although slightly lower, is comparable with those achieved by deep learning methods (as shown in Table 2), but without the use of artifacts like fine-tuning or data augmentation.

Although the algorithm does an acceptable job segmenting the images, a particular case occurs when the lesion consists of several unconnected regions.

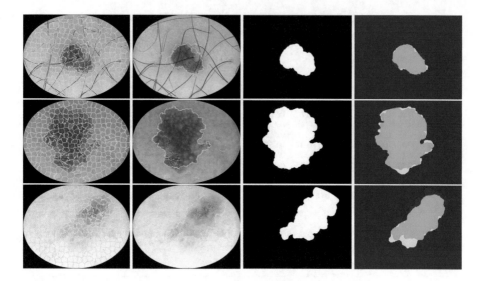

Fig. 2. Segmentation results for three different images. From left to right: Original image with SLIC segmentation ($k = 400$), Merged superpixels, final segmentation binary mask, and ground-truth comparison. TP=light blue, TN=dark blue, FN: yellow and FP: red.

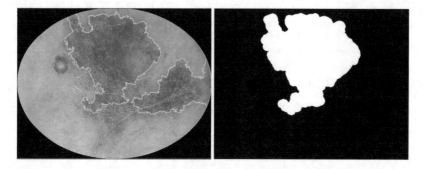

Fig. 3. Skin lesion with two unconnected regions. The segmentation algorithm only identified one of two parts.

In this case, the algorithm only chooses one region as the final segmentation as stated in Sect. 3.4, resulting in an incorrect binary mask (See Fig. 3).

The source code implementation of the presented method is publicly available at https://github.com/dipaco/mole-classification, and is entirely written in python 2.7. The implementation uses scipy and scikit libraries for its functionality. All tests ran on a desktop machine with an Intel Core i7 processor of 2.5 GHz.

5   Conclusions and Future Work

In this paper, we proposed a new fully-automatic strategy to segment skin lesion on dermoscopic images. Our method uses the SLIC algorithm to over-segment the image, and then merge the resulting superpixels to produce two regions: healthy skin and skin lesion. The merging criterion is based on the mean color intensity of each superpixel. Our method does not require any form of pre-processing of the original image before segmentation and can produce slightly better results than other approaches. In contrast with other works, our approach is able to deal with the presence of hair in the original image without any additional steps.

From Table 1a to d is possible to conclude that, for most methods, segmentation performance was low in cases where the images contained malignant lesions compared with the case of common and atypical nevi. Despite this, our approach achieved better sensitivity and F-measure, and the second-best accuracy on melanocytic images.

Future work will focus on adjusting the merging criterion to deal with cases where the lesion has more that one unconnected region.

References

1. Mendonc, T., Ferreira, P.M., Marques, J.S.: PH 2 - a dermoscopic image database for research and benchmarking. In: Annual International Conference of the IEEE Engineering in Medicine and Biology Society, PP. 5437–5440 (2013)
2. Codella, N.C.F., et al.: Skin lesion analysis toward melanoma detection: a challenge at the 2017 international symposium on biomedical imaging (ISBI), hosted by the international skin imaging collaboration (ISIC), pp. 1–5 (2017)
3. Celebi, M.E., Wen, Q., Iyatomi, H., Shimizu, K., Zhou, H., Schaefer, G.: A State-of-the-Art Survey on Lesion Border Detection in Dermoscopy Images. CRC Press, Boca Raton (2015)
4. Celebi, M.E., Stoecker, W.V., Schaefer, G.: Lesion border detection in dermoscopy images. National Institute of Health Public Access (2010)
5. Abuzaghleh, O., Barkana, B.D., Faezipour, M.: Automated skin lesion analysis based on color and shape geometry feature set for melanoma early detection and prevention. In: IEEE Long Island Systems, Applications and Technology (LISAT) Conference 2014, IEEE, pp. 1–6, May 2014
6. Barata, C., Celebi, M., Marques, J.: Melanoma detection algorithm based on feature fusion. In: Proceedings of the Annual International Conference of the IEEE Engineering in Medicine and Biology Society, EMBS November 2015, pp. 2653–2656 (2015)
7. Pennisi, A., Bloisi, D.D., Nardi, D., Giampetruzzi, A.R., Mondino, C., Facchiano, A.: Skin lesion image segmentation using Delaunay triangulation for melanoma detection. Comput. Med. Imaging Graph. **52**, 89–103 (2016)
8. Sabbaghi, S., Aldeen, M., Garnavi, R., Varigos, G., Doliantis, C., Nicolopoulos, J.: Automated colour identification in melanocytic lesions. In: 2015 37th Annual International Conference of the IEEE Engineering in Medicine and Biology Society (EMBC), pp. 3021–3024. IEEE, August 2015

9. Codella, N., Cai, J., Abedini, M., Garnavi, R., Halpern, A., Smith, J.R.: Deep Learning, sparse coding, and SVM for melanoma recognition in dermoscopy images. In: Zhou, L., Wang, L., Wang, Q., Shi, Y. (eds.) MLMI 2015. LNCS, vol. 9352, pp. 118–126. Springer, Cham (2015). https://doi.org/10.1007/978-3-319-24888-2_15
10. Li, Y., Shen, L.: Skin Lesion Analysis Towards Melanoma Detection Using Deep Learning Network. arXiv preprint (61672357) (2017)
11. Gao, M., Xu, Z., Lu, L., Harrison, A.P., Summers, R.M., Mollura, D.J.: Holistic interstitial lung disease detection using deep convolutional neural networks: multi-label learning and unordered pooling. eprint arXiv:1701.05616 (2017)
12. Codella, N.C.F., et al.: Deep learning ensembles for melanoma recognition in dermoscopy images. IBM J. Res. Dev. **61**(4), 5:1–5:15 (2017)
13. Achanta, R., Shaji, A., Smith, K., Lucchi, A., Fua, P., Süsstrunk, S.: SLIC superpixels compared to state-of-the-art superpixel methods. In: IEEE Transaction on Pattern Analysis and Machine Intelligence (2012)
14. Zhao, Q.: JSEG method implementation (2001). http://cs.joensuu.fi/zhao/Software/JSEG.zip
15. Boltz, S.: SRM method implementation (2010) http://www.mathworks.com/matlabcentral/fileexchange/authors/73145
16. Crandall, R.: Level set implementation (2000). https://github.com/rcrandall/ChanVese
17. Abuzaghleh, O., Barkana, B.D., Faezipour, M.: Noninvasive real-time automated skin lesion analysis system for melanoma early detection and prevention. IEEE J. Transl. Eng. Health Med. **3**(Oct 2014), 1–12 (2015)

Star Shape Prior in Fully Convolutional Networks for Skin Lesion Segmentation

Zahra Mirikharaji[✉] and Ghassan Hamarneh

School of Computing Science, Simon Fraser University, Burnaby, Canada
{zmirikha,hamarneh}@sfu.ca

Abstract. Semantic segmentation is an important preliminary step towards automatic medical image interpretation. Recently deep convolutional neural networks have become the first choice for the task of pixel-wise class prediction. While incorporating prior knowledge about the structure of target objects has proven effective in traditional energy-based segmentation approaches, there has not been a clear way for encoding prior knowledge into deep learning frameworks. In this work, we propose a new loss term that encodes the star shape prior into the loss function of an end-to-end trainable fully convolutional network (FCN) framework. We penalize non-star shape segments in FCN prediction maps to guarantee a global structure in segmentation results. Our experiments demonstrate the advantage of regularizing FCN parameters by the star shape prior and our results on the ISBI 2017 skin segmentation challenge data set achieve the first rank in the segmentation task among 21 participating teams.

1 Introduction

Skin cancer is the most common type of cancer in the world. Early detection of skin cancer can increase the five year survival rate of patients from 18% to 98% [1]. While skin cancer can be detected by visual examination, distinguishing malignant from non-malignant lesions is a challenging task. In recent years, computer aided diagnosis has been widely leveraged in automated assessment of dermoscopy and clinical images to assist dermatologists evaluation. Semantic segmentation, the task of labeling each image pixel with the class label of its surrounding object, is generally the first step toward the automatic understanding of images. Remarkable variations in the appearance of healthy and unhealthy skin, including color, texture, lesion shape and size originating from image acquisition and inter- and intra-class variation, complicates the skin lesion segmentation problem.

For decades, since the seminal work of Kass et al. [13], energy functional minimization techniques were the most popular approaches to solve image segmentation problems [15]. Imaging artifacts and variability in the appearance of image regions make the data fidelity term insufficient to achieve robust segmentation results. Therein, the segmentation that minimizes a weighted sum of

© Springer Nature Switzerland AG 2018
A. F. Frangi et al. (Eds.): MICCAI 2018, LNCS 11073, pp. 737–745, 2018.
https://doi.org/10.1007/978-3-030-00937-3_84

unary (data) and regularization energy functional terms is sought. Incorporating prior knowledge about the structure of target object in the objective function to regularize plausible solutions with anatomically meaningful constraints have been widely leveraged to obtain more reliable delineations [10, 17]. Active shape models (ASM) was one of the pioneering works to incorporate shape priors into deformable models [9]. To effectuate the shape prior, ASM and many other shape-encoding segmentation methods required an estimate of the object pose (i.e., the orientation, scale, and location of the target object in the image) [11, 22]. Some examples of priors which have been utilized in energy optimization based segmentation methods are shape models, topology preservation, moment constraints and geometrical and distance interaction between image regions.

Recently deep fully convolutional networks have achieved significant success in the task of semantic segmentation. Hierarchical extraction of features followed by skip connections and up-sampling operations was first introduced by Long et al. in an end-to-end trainable framework [14]. Despite the success of FCNs, they have indicated clear limitations in the dense per-pixel prediction task. Consecutive spatial pooling and striding convolutions in FCNs reduce the initial image resolution and lead to loss of the image fine structures. Some techniques have been proposed to address these limitations of FCNs. Learning multiple deconvolutional layers and concatenating low-level fine features with high-level coarse features through skip connections are commonly used to retrieve low-level visual features [20]. Dilated convolutional has also been introduced to aggregate multi-scale contextual information without losing image resolutions [24]. Although pixel-wise prediction benefits from these resolution enlarging techniques, they are only capable to partially recover detailed spatial information.

In the context of fully convolutional networks, leveraging prior information about the target object structure in the segmentation model has not been widely studied. By optimizing individual pixel level class predictions in the FCNs loss function, independent class labels are assigned to image pixels without considering high-level label dependencies. There have been some efforts towards structured prediction and leveraging meaningful priors into deep learning frameworks. Deeplab-CRF and CRF-RNN employ probabilistic graphical modeling either as a post processing step or by implementing recurrent layers in FCNs to enforce assigning similar labels to pixels with similar color and position and further improve the object boundaries [6]. Recently BenTaieb et al. proposed a new loss function to encode the geometrical and topological priors of containment and detachment in an end-to-end FCN framework [2, 27]. To leverage the shape prior in segmentation models, Chen et al. learn a shape constraint by a deep Boltzmann machine and then employ the learned prior in a variational segmentation method [5]. In addition, training convolutional auto-encoder networks to learn anatomical shape variations has demonstrated improvements in the robustness of FCN segmentation models [18, 19].

To the best of our knowledge, none of the existing works incorporates a star shape prior as a regularization term in the loss function of FCNs trained in an end-to-end fashion. The star shape prior was first introduced in the context of image segmentation by Veksler, where it was encoded as a regularization term into the cost function formulation of a graph-based (discrete) image segmentation approach [21]. Later, Chittajallu et al. incorporated three types of shape constraints including star shape prior into a Markov random field based segmentation model and applied their method to non-contrast cardiac computed tomography scans [7]. Yuan et al. extended the star shape prior to 3D objects and applied it to prostate magnetic resonance images [25]. Nosrati et al. derived a star shape prior in a continuous variational formulation and applied it to segmenting overlapping cervical cells [16]. Although the star shape prior clearly improved results for a variety of target objects, one limiting requirement of Veksler's approach and its variants, however, is the assumption that the center of foreground objects is known (e.g. provided by user interaction).

We aim to harness the powerful proven capabilities of deep learning in automatically extracting learnt (i.e., not hand-crafted) pixel-driven image features (i.e., likelihood) and augment it with demonstrably useful shape priors without requiring the knowledge of the target object pose. We propose to encode the star shape prior into the training of fully convolutional networks to improve segmentation of skin lesions from their surrounding healthy skin. Our idea is to formulate the star shape prior in the loss function of FCN frameworks to penalize non-star shape segments in prediction maps and preserve global structures in the output space. Integration of the star shape prior in the loss function makes it possible to train the whole FCN framework in an end-to-end manner. In contrast to Veksler's work and its variants, our approach to star shape prior in a deep learning setting not only eliminates the need for manually setting object centers, but also alleviates, at inference time, the computationally intensive optimization associated with the energy minimizing approaches. Our experimental results illustrate how imposing the shape prior constraint in deep networks refines skin lesion segmentation in comparison to using a single pixel level loss in FCNs.

2 Methodology

Our goal is to leverage the star shape prior into the learning process of an FCN to generate plausible segmentation maps (e.g. skin lesions) from their surrounding background without requiring additional training, user interaction, pre- or post-processing.

FCN's Pixel-Wise Loss. In FCNs, given a set of N training images and their corresponding ground truth segmentations, $\{(X(i), Y(i)); i = 1, 2, \ldots, N\}$, the deep network learns to take unseen image samples and generate a segmentation probability map, the same size as the input images that assigns a semantic label to each pixel. Learning the deep network parameters θ, is performed by maximizing the a posteriori probability of giving the true label to each image pixel given the input image. Maximizing the a posteriori probability is usually replaced by minimizing its negative log-likelihood function as a cost function L:

$$\theta^* = \arg\min_{\theta} L(X, Y; \theta). \tag{1}$$

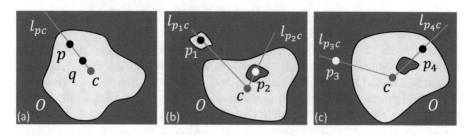

Fig. 1. (a) Star shape object O w.r.t. the supplied object center c (*red dot*). (b) Examples of the star shape constraint violation. (c) Examples of cases where conditions (i) and (ii) in (4) are required.

For binary dense class prediction, a binary cross entropy loss L_{ce} is generally deployed:

$$L_{ce}(X, Y; \theta) = -\sum_{i=1}^{N} \sum_{p \in \Omega} [y_{ip} \log P(y_{ip} = 1 | X(i); \theta)$$
$$+ (1 - y_{ip}) \log(1 - P(y_{ip} = 1 | X(i); \theta))] \tag{2}$$

where Ω is the pixel space, y_{ip} is the ground truth label of pixel p in image i and $P(y_{ip} = 1 | X(i); \theta)$ is the FCN sigmoid function output indicating the predicted probability of the pth pixel of the ith image being a skin lesion. The pixel-wise binary logistic loss L_{ce} penalizes the deviation of the predicted label for each pixel from its true label.

Star Shape Regularized Loss. Assuming c is the center of object O, object O is a star shape object if, for any point p interior to the object, all the pixels q lying on the straight line segment connecting p to the object center c are inside the object (Fig. 1(a)). This definition of star shape prior holds for a large group of object shapes including convex ones. To incorporate the star shape prior as a new regularization term, we augment the loss function in (2) with a new loss term to penalize line segments that violate the prior (e.g. Fig. 1(b)) in the prediction maps:

$$L(X, Y; \theta) = \alpha L_{ce} + \beta L_{sh} \tag{3}$$

where α and β are hyper-parameters setting the contribution of each term in the optimization function, L_{ce} is the binary cross entropy loss and L_{sh} is our star shape prior:

$$L_{sh}(X, Y; \theta) = \sum_{i=1}^{N} \sum_{p \in \Omega} \sum_{q \in l_{pc}} B_{pq}^{i} \times |y_{ip} - P(y_{ip} = 1 | X(i); \theta)|$$
$$\times |P(y_{ip} = 1 | X(i); \theta) - P(y_{iq} = 1 | X(i); \theta)|; \tag{4}$$

$$B_{pq}^{i} = \begin{cases} 1, & \text{if } y_{ip} = y_{iq} \\ 0, & \text{otherwise} \end{cases} \tag{5}$$

where l_{pc} is the line segment connecting pixel p to the object center c and q is any pixel incident on line l_{pc}. L_{sh} is trained to assign to all such q pixels a label identical to the label of pixel p as long as (i) p and q have the same ground truth labels ($B_{pq}^i = 1$) and (ii) the difference between the ground truth label and the predicted labels for p is non-zero ($|y_{ip} - P(y_{ip}|X(i); \theta)| > 0$). The 3rd term of (4) determines how labels of pixels internal to the lesion are penalized to ensure star shapes, whereas the first two terms of (4) are designed to allow discontinuities of pixel labels across the ground truth boundary of the lesion and ignore the star shape term when the given label is true. In Fig. 1(c), $p = p_3$ and $p = p_4$ are examples where the value of $\sum_{q \in l_{pc}} |P(y_{ip}|X(i); \theta) - P(y_{iq}|X(i); \theta)|$ is positive while their assigned labels should not be penalized. Condition (i) chooses a set of pixels q on $l_{p_3 c}$ and allows discontinuities between the background (p_3) and foreground assigned labels and, condition (ii) enforces the loss function not to penalize the label assigned to p_4.

In our implementation of (4), instead of penalizing the difference between the predicted probabilities and ground truth labels for all the points on the straight line l_{pc}, we only examine the m closest pixels to p on l_{pc} and compute the loss value per pixel p based on those m predicted probabilities. We also quantize, to a set of d directions, the possible angles of all lines passing through p. In the training of our deep network, we automatically find the star object center from binary ground truth maps. At inference time, we do not need to supply the center of star objects as prediction maps are achieved by a forward pass through the network whose parameters are already trained to generate segmentations.

3   Experiments

Data Description. We validated our proposed segmentation approach on dermoscopy data provided by the International Skin Imaging Collaboration (ISIC) at ISBI 2017 *Skin Lesion Analysis Towards Melanoma Detection Challenge* [8]. The data set contains 2000 training, 150 validation, and 600 test images. We first re-scaled all images to 192×192 pixels and normalized each RGB channel by the mean and standard deviation of the training data. To confirm the suitability of adopting the star-shape prior for this task, we calculated the percentage of segmentation mask pixels that violate the star shape definition to be only 0.14% over the whole dataset (0.05% of training, 0.3% of validation, and 0.38% of test image pixels). Figure 2 shows examples of rare pixels where the star shape constraint is violated.

Network Architecture. We exploited two state-of-the-art fully convolutional network architectures to evaluate our proposed new loss: (1) U-Net [20] (2) ResNet-DUC. ResNet-DUC deploys the FCN version of ResNet-152, pretrained on ImageNet as an encoder [12]. Instead of using multiple deconvolutional layers to decode low resolution feature maps into the original image size prediction maps, single Dense Upsampling Convolution (DUC) layer is used to reconstruct

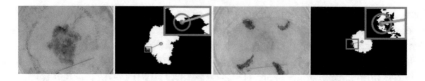

Fig. 2. Examples of skin lesion pixels violating the star shape constraint.

fine-detailed information from coarse feature maps [23]. Furthermore, dilated convolutions are used in the encoder to benefit from multi-scale contextual information from previous layers activations [24].

Implementation. We trained deep networks implemented with the PyTorch library, over mini-batches of size 12. We tuned all hyper-parameters on the validation set. Loss functions are optimized using the stochastic gradient descent algorithm with an initial learning rate of 10^{-4}. The learning rate was divided by 10 when the performance of model on validation data set stopped improving. Momentum and weight decay were set to 0.99 and 5×10^{-5}, respectively. For the implementation of the star shape regularized loss function, $\alpha = 1$, $\beta = 5$, $m = 6$ and $d = 8$. We first trained the deep network with binary cross entropy function for 5 epochs and then fine-tuned the network parameters with the proposed loss function. Training takes 2 days and test takes 1 s/image on our 12 GB GPU.

Results. We evaluated the performance of U-Net and ResNet-DUC trained with and without the star shape prior. As shown in Table 1, using our shape regularized loss function in the training of U-Net and ResNet-DUC, the Jaccard index is improved by more than 3% (row A vs. B and row C vs. D). We measured the statistical significance of our results by exploring the Jaccard index over the test data. We used the non-parametric Wilcoxon signed rank sum test and found that the results of U-Net and ResNet-DUC with and without incorporation of star shape prior are statistically significantly different at $p < 0.05$.

We compared our proposed method with 21 competing methods participating in the challenge. The ResNet-DUC architecture trained with our star shape regularized loss achieved the first rank based on the challenge ranking metric, Jaccard index. Table 1, rows E, F and G, show results of the first three ranked teams. Although all top three teams used FCNs to perform image segmentation, in contrast to our work, they employed various additional steps like averaging over multiple model results, multi-scale image input as well as pre- and post-processing approaches like inclusion of different color spaces in the input and multi-thresholding. Qualitative results of our proposed approach are presented in Fig. 3. Encoding star shape prior into the loss function results in smoother prediction maps with a single connected component as lesion for most cases.

Table 1. Segmentation quantitative performance. Bold numbers indicate the best performance. All values are in percentages.

	Method	Jaccard	Dice	Accuracy	Specificity	Sensitivity
A	U-Net [20]	70.5	79.7	91.8	97.8	77.0
B	U-Net + Star Shape	73.3	82.4	92.4	95.3	85.4
C	ResNet-DUC [23]	74.0	83.3	93.00	98.2	80.0
D	ResNet-DUC + Star Shape	**77.3**	**85.7**	**93.8**	97.3	**85.5**
E	Yuan et al. [26]	76.5	84.9	93.4	97.5	82.5
F	Berseth et al. [3]	76.2	84.7	93.2	97.8	82.0
G	Bi et al. [4]	76.0	84.4	93.4	**98.5**	80.2

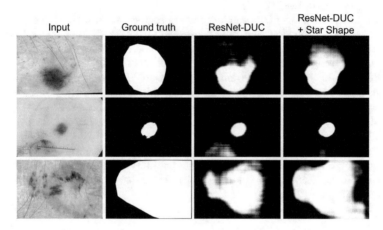

Fig. 3. Qualitative comparison of ResNet-DUC architecture results with and without star shape prior.

4   Conclusion

We encoded the star shape prior in the loss function of an end-to-end trainable fully convolutional network to generate more accurate and plausible skin lesion segmentations. In contrast to energy minimization approaches, our proposed framework does not require computationally expensive optimization at inference time nor a user-defined object centre. Our experiments indicated that leveraging the prior knowledge in fully convolutional networks yield convergence to an improved output space. In future works, we will extend to other prior information including but not limited to anatomically meaningful priors in fully convolutional networks trained for other 2D and 3D medical imaging applications.

Acknowledgments. We gratefully thank NVIDIA Corporation for the donation of the Titan X GPU used for this research.

References

1. Cancer facts and figures 2017 (2017). http://www.cancer.org/acs/groups/content/@editorial/documents/document/acspc-048738.pdf
2. BenTaieb, A., Hamarneh, G.: Topology aware fully convolutional networks for histology gland segmentation. In: Ourselin, S., Joskowicz, L., Sabuncu, M.R., Unal, G., Wells, W. (eds.) MICCAI 2016. LNCS, vol. 9901, pp. 460–468. Springer, Cham (2016). https://doi.org/10.1007/978-3-319-46723-8_53
3. Berseth, M.: ISIC 2017-skin lesion analysis towards melanoma detection. arXiv:1703.00523 (2017)
4. Bi, L., et al.: Automatic skin lesion analysis using large-scale dermoscopy images and deep residual networks. arXiv:1703.04197 (2017)
5. Chen, F., et al.: Deep learning shape priors for object segmentation. In: IEEE CVPR, pp. 1870–1877 (2013)
6. Chen, L.C., et al.: DeepLab: semantic image segmentation with deep convolutional nets, atrous convolution, and fully connected CRFs. arXiv:1606.00915 (2016)
7. Chittajallu, D.R., et al.: A shape-driven MRF model for the segmentation of organs in medical images. In: IEEE CVPR, pp. 3233–3240 (2010)
8. Codella, N.C.F., et al.: Skin lesion analysis toward melanoma detection: a challenge at the 2017 international symposium on biomedical imaging (ISBI), hosted by the international skin imaging collaboration (ISIC). arXiv:1710.05006 (2017)
9. Cootes, T.F., et al.: Active appearance models. IEEE TPAMI **23**(6), 681–685 (2001)
10. Cremers, D., et al.: A review of statistical approaches to level set segmentation: integrating color, texture, motion and shape. IJCV **72**(2), 195–215 (2007)
11. Freedman, D., Zhang, T.: Interactive graph cut based segmentation with shape priors. IEEE CVPR **1**, 755–762 (2005)
12. He, K., et al.: Deep residual learning for image recognition. In: IEEE CVPR, pp. 770–778 (2016)
13. Kass, M., et al.: Snakes: active contour models. IJCV **1**(4), 321–331 (1988)
14. Long, J., et al.: Fully convolutional networks for semantic segmentation. In: IEEE CVPR, pp. 3431–3440 (2015)
15. McInerney, T., Terzopoulos, D.: Deformable models in medical image analysis: a survey. MIA **1**(2), 91–108 (1996)
16. Nosrati, M.S., Hamarneh, G.: Segmentation of overlapping cervical cells: a variational method with star-shape prior. In: IEEE ISBI, pp. 186–189 (2015)
17. Nosrati, M.S., Hamarneh, G.: Incorporating prior knowledge in medical image segmentation: a survey. arXiv:1607.01092 (2016)
18. Oktay, O., et al.: Anatomically constrained neural networks (ACNNs): application to cardiac image enhancement and segmentation. IEEE TMI **37**(2), 384–395 (2018)
19. Ravishankar, H., Venkataramani, R., Thiruvenkadam, S., Sudhakar, P., Vaidya, V.: Learning and incorporating shape models for semantic segmentation. In: Descoteaux, M., Maier-Hein, L., Franz, A., Jannin, P., Collins, D.L., Duchesne, S. (eds.) MICCAI 2017. LNCS, vol. 10433, pp. 203–211. Springer, Cham (2017). https://doi.org/10.1007/978-3-319-66182-7_24
20. Ronneberger, O., Fischer, P., Brox, T.: U-Net: convolutional networks for biomedical image segmentation. In: Navab, N., Hornegger, J., Wells, W.M., Frangi, A.F. (eds.) MICCAI 2015. LNCS, vol. 9351, pp. 234–241. Springer, Cham (2015). https://doi.org/10.1007/978-3-319-24574-4_28

21. Veksler, O.: Star shape prior for graph-cut image segmentation. In: Forsyth, D., Torr, P., Zisserman, A. (eds.) ECCV 2008. LNCS, vol. 5304, pp. 454–467. Springer, Heidelberg (2008). https://doi.org/10.1007/978-3-540-88690-7_34
22. Vu, N., Manjunath, B.: Shape prior segmentation of multiple objects with graph cuts. In: IEEE CVPR, pp. 1–8 (2008)
23. Wang, P., et al.: Understanding convolution for semantic segmentation. arXiv:1702.08502 (2017)
24. Yu, F., Koltun, V.: Multi-scale context aggregation by dilated convolutions. arXiv:1511.07122 (2015)
25. Yuan, J., et al.: An efficient convex optimization approach to 3D prostate MRI segmentation with generic star shape prior. In: PROMISE Challenge, MICCAI (2012)
26. Yuan, Y., et al.: Automatic skin lesion segmentation with fully convolutional-deconvolutional networks. arXiv:1703.05165 (2017)
27. Zheng, S., et al.: Conditional random fields as recurrent neural networks. In: ICCV, pp. 1529–1537 (2015)

Fast Vessel Segmentation and Tracking in Ultra High-Frequency Ultrasound Images

Tejas Sudharshan Mathai[1]($\boxtimes$), Lingbo Jin[2], Vijay Gorantla[3],
and John Galeotti[1]

[1] The Robotics Institute, Carnegie Mellon University, Pittsburgh, PA 15213, USA
tmathai@andrew.cmu.edu
[2] Department of ECE, Carnegie Mellon University, Pittsburgh, PA 15213, USA
[3] Department of Surgery, Wake Forest Institute for Regenerative Medicine,
Winston-Salem, NC 27101, USA

Abstract. Ultra High Frequency Ultrasound (UHFUS) enables the visualization of highly deformable small and medium vessels in the hand. Intricate vessel-based measurements, such as intimal wall thickness and vessel wall compliance, require sub-millimeter vessel tracking between B-scans. Our fast GPU-based approach combines the advantages of local phase analysis, a distance-regularized level set, and an Extended Kalman Filter (EKF), to rapidly segment and track the deforming vessel contour. We validated on 35 UHFUS sequences of vessels in the hand, and we show the transferability of the approach to 5 more diverse datasets acquired by a traditional High Frequency Ultrasound (HFUS) machine. To the best of our knowledge, this is the first algorithm capable of rapidly segmenting and tracking deformable vessel contours in 2D UHFUS images. It is also the fastest and most accurate system for 2D HFUS images.

Keywords: Ultrasound · Vasculature · Segmentation · Tracking

1 Introduction

Ultra High Frequency Ultrasound (UHFUS) is a new advancement in non-invasive imaging, capable of operating above 50 MHz and resolving structures less than 0.03 mm. Potential clinical applications include vascular measurements for surgical procedures and disease diagnosis, with such measures including intimal wall thickness and variations in atherosclerotic plaque buildup [1]. It can be used to monitor hand transplant recipients [1], for whom the gold standard diagnosis using invasive histopathology is not practical due to suppressed immune systems [1]. However, UHFUS can only image through ~1 cm of tissue. Vessels can be visualized at this depth (see Fig. 1(a)), in contrast to skeletal structures, which are too deep to be imaged. When compared against traditional high frequency ultrasound (HFUS) (see Fig. 1(b)), substantially increased speckle noise is encountered with UHFUS at such shallow depths. The vessel measurements have naturally occurring sub-millimeter(mm) variations along their length, and

© Springer Nature Switzerland AG 2018
A. F. Frangi et al. (Eds.): MICCAI 2018, LNCS 11073, pp. 746–754, 2018.
https://doi.org/10.1007/978-3-030-00937-3_85

sub-mm displacements of the probe confound comparisons across time. Our motivation is that vessel tracking across B-scans with sub-mm precision should enable consistent comparisons. *In this work, the primary medical image computing (MIC) goal is the fast sub-mm 2D vessel contour localization.*

Traditional ultrasound based real-time vessel tracking has been researched before [2–5]. However, when tested on UHFUS images, these gradient-based edge detection approaches failed to detect and track the vessel boundaries in the presence of higher speckle noise. Furthermore, precise delineation of the deforming vessel is required for vessel-based measurements, whereas prior approaches [2–5] modeled the vessel as an ellipse without accounting for the deforming vessel contour. A recent approach in [5] was designed for a specific imaging setting of 55% maximum gain, but when applied to UHFUS sequences, it completely failed to track vessels regardless of gain settings (see Fig. 1(c)). A recent level-set based approach [6] designed for HFUS images ran slowly at 0.5 s per image.

In this paper, a fast GPU-based approach is presented to segment and track the deforming vessel contour in UHFUS images. It combines the robust edge detection capability of local phase analysis, with a distance regularized level set to accurately capture the vessel contour, and an efficient Extended Kalman Filter (EKF) to track the vessel. Validation on 35 UHFUS sequences showed that it successfully segmented and tracked vessels undergoing dynamic compression. Our algorithm achieved a maximum Hausdorff distance error of 0.135 mm, which was 6× smaller than the smallest vessel diameter of 0.81 mm. It also generalized to datasets acquired with different imaging settings and from a HFUS imaging system, with errors ~2× smaller than the state-of-the-art for HFUS [6].

Contribution. (1) We present the first system capable of rapidly segmenting and tracking a vessel contour in UHFUS images, and we demonstrate its high speed performance ($\geq$52 FPS). (2) We demonstrate the generality of our approach by applying it to datasets acquired from a traditional HFUS machine, and show that it is faster than the state-of-the-art approach for HFUS.

2   Methods

2.1   Data Acquisition

The Visualsonics Vevo 2100 UHFUS machine (Fujifilm, Canada) and a 50 MHz transducer (bandwidth extendable to 70 MHz) was used to acquire freehand ultrasound volumes. This UHFUS system has a physical resolution of 30 μm, and the pixel pitch is 11.6 μm between pixel centers. 35 deidentified UHFUS sequences were acquired over a wide range of gain values (40–70 dB), with the maximum gain value setting being 70 dB. The sequences contained a wide range of motions with the probe, such as longitudinal scanning, out-of-plane tissue deformation, beating vessel visualization, etc. Figure 1(a) shows an example ultrasound image of the proper palmar digital artery acquired with the UHFUS system. Each sequence consisted of 100 2D B-scans with dimensions of 832 × 512 pixels. To show the generality of our approach, 5 additional sequences were acquired from a traditional HFUS machine (Diasus, Dynamic Imaging, UK) using a 10–22 MHz transducer. The pixel resolution for the HFUS machine was 92.5 μm, and each sequence consisted of 250 2D B-scans of dimensions 280×534 pixels.

2.2   Noise Reduction and Clustering

Noise Reduction. In contrast to traditional HFUS, speckle noise is greater in UHFUS as seen in Figs. 1(a) and (b). To mitigate the effects of speckle during segmentation and speed up computation, the UHFUS B-scans were first down-sampled by a factor of 4 in each dimension (see Fig. 1(d)). Next, a bilateral filter [7] of size 5×5 pixels was applied to the downsampled image to smooth the small amplitude noise (see Fig. 1(e)), while preserving vessel boundaries that are crucial to our segmentation. The bilateral filtered image is represented by I_B.

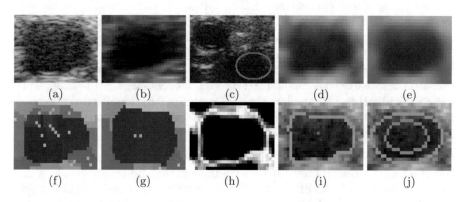

Fig. 1. Vessel imaged using (a) UHFUS, (b) HFUS; (c) Failed vessel detection result (red ellipse) of algorithm in [5] on an UHFUS image; (d) Downsampled image; (e) Bilateral filtered image (I_B); (f) With a kernel size 3×3, pixels in I_B are clustered into homogeneous patches in I_C, each with its own root (orange points); (g) I_C generated with 7×7 kernel; (h) Feature Asymmetry map (I_FA); (i) Initial boundary locations (green points) estimated from I_FA using the tracked point $\mathbf{s}^t$ (magenta); (j) Ellipse (green) fitted to green points in (i), and then shrunk (brown ellipse) to initialize the level set evolution.

Clustering. The approach published in [8], which has also shown applicability to MRI images, was used to produce an image I_C, where the pixels in I_B were clustered into homogeneous patches (see Figs. 1(f) and (g)). Each pixel in I_C can be represented by two elements: the mean intensity of the patch that it belongs to, and a cluster/patch center (root). For each pixel in I_B, the mean intensity and variance is found in a circular neighborhood, whose size varies depending on the size of the vessel. For small vessels in UHFUS images (≤ 70 pixel diameter or 0.81 mm), the neighborhood size was 3×3 pixels, while it was 7×7 pixels for larger vessels (>70 pixels). Each patch root in I_C has the lowest local variance amongst all the members of the same patch [8]. Roots in I_C were used solely as seeds to track vessels over sequential B-scans. As seen in Figs. 1(f) and (g), increasing the neighborhood size reduces the number of roots that can be tracked, which can cause tracking failure when large motion occurs.

2.3   Local Phase Analysis

Vessel boundaries in I_B were highlighted using a Cauchy filter, which has been shown to be better than a Log-Gabor filter at detecting edges in ultrasound [9]. We denote the spatial intensity value at a location $\mathbf{x} = [x\ y]^T$ in the image I_B by $I_B(\mathbf{x})$. After applying a 2D Fourier transform, the corresponding 2D frequency domain value is $F(\mathbf{w})$, where $\mathbf{w} = [w_1\ w_2]^T$. The Cauchy filter $C(\mathbf{w})$ applied to $F(\mathbf{w})$ is represented as:

$$C(\mathbf{w}) = \|\mathbf{w}\|_2^u \exp\left(-w_o\|\mathbf{w}\|_2\right), \qquad u \geq 1 \tag{1}$$

where u is a scaling parameter, and w_o is the center frequency. We chose the same optimal parameter values suggested in [9]: $w_o = 10$, and $u = 1$. Filtering $F(\mathbf{w})$ with $C(\mathbf{w})$ yielded the monogenic signal, from which the feature asymmetry map (I_{FA}) [9] was obtained (see Fig. 1(h)). Pixel values in I_{FA} range between $[0, 1]$.

2.4   Vessel Segmentation and Tracking

Initialization. As in [3,4], we manually initialize our system by clicking a point inside the vessel lumen in the first B-scan of a sequence. This pixel location is stored as a seed, denoted by $\mathbf{s}^0$ at time $t = 0$, to segment the vessel boundary in the first B-scan, and initialize the vessel lumen tracking in subsequent B-scans.

Initial Boundary Segmentation. $N = 360$ radial lines of maximum search length $M = 100$, which corresponds to the largest observed vessel diameter, stem out from $\mathbf{s}^0$ to find the vessel boundaries in I_{FA}. The first local maximum on each radial line is included in a set $\mathcal{I}$ as an initial boundary point (see Fig. 1(i)).

Segmentation Refinement. A rough estimate of the semi-major and semi-minor vessel axes was determined by fitting an ellipse [10] to the initial boundary locations in $\mathcal{I}$. Next, the estimated values were shrunk by 75%, and used to initialize an elliptical binary level set function (LSF) ϕ_o (see Fig. 1(j)) in a narrowband distance regularized level set evolution (DRLSE) [11] framework. As the LSF initialization is close to the true boundaries, the DRLSE formulation allows quick propagation of LSF to the desired vessel locations $\mathcal{D}$ (see Fig. 2(a)) with a large timestep $\Delta\tau$ [11]. The DRLSE framework minimizes an energy functional $\mathcal{E}(\phi)$ [11] using the gradient defined in Eq. (2). μ, λ, ϵ, and α are constants, g is the same edge indicator function used in [11], and δ_ϵ and d_p are first order derivatives of the Heaviside function and the double-well potential respectively. The parameters used in all datasets were: $\Delta\tau = 10, \mu = 0.2, \lambda = 1, \alpha = -1, \epsilon = 1$ for a total of 15 iterations.

$$\frac{\partial\phi}{\partial\tau} = \mu\mathrm{div}(d_p(|\nabla\phi|)\nabla\phi) + \lambda\delta_\epsilon(\phi)\mathrm{div}\left(g\frac{\nabla\phi}{|\nabla\phi|}\right) + \alpha g\delta_\epsilon(\phi) \tag{2}$$

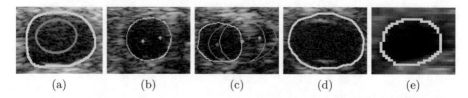

(a)   (b)   (c)   (d)   (e)

Fig. 2. (a) Refined segmentation (yellow contour) evolved from initial LSF (brown ellipse); Tracking under large motion - (b) In frame 87, s_{ekf}^{87} (blue) chosen over s_C^{87} (orange) to segment vessel (yellow contour), which is then fitted with an ellipse (green); (c) In frame 88, the EKF prediction s_{ekf}^{88} (red) is ignored as Eq. (7) is not satisfied. Instead, s_C^{88} (magenta) is chosen as it falls under the elliptical neighborhood (brown) of s_C^{87} (orange); (d) Successful contour segmentation (Adventitia) of UHFUS image in Fig. 1(c); (e) Successful segmentation of vessel in HFUS image shown in Fig. 1(b).

Vessel Tracking. To update the vessel lumen position s^t at time t to s^{t+1} at time $t+1$, two new potential seeds are found, from which one is chosen. The first seed is found using an EKF [5,12]. The second seed is found using I_C, and it is needed in case the EKF fails to track the vessel lumen due to abrupt motion. The EKF tracks a state vector defined by: $\mathbf{x}^t = [c_x^t, c_y^t, a^t, b^t]$, where $\mathbf{s}_{ekf}^t = [c_x^t, c_y^t]$ is the EKF-tracked vessel lumen location and $[a^t, b^t]$ are the tracked semi-major and semi-minor vessel axes respectively. Instead of tracking all locations in $\mathcal{D}$, it is computationally efficient to track $\mathbf{x}^t$, whose elements are estimated by fitting an ellipse once again to the locations in $\mathcal{D}$ (see Fig. 2(b)). The EKF projects the current state $\mathbf{x}^t$ at time t to the next state $\mathbf{x}^{t+1}$ at time $t+1$ using the motion model in [5], which uses two state transition matrices A_1, A_2, the covariance error matrix P, and the process-noise covariance matrix Q. These matrices are initialized in Eqs. (3)–(6).

$$A_1 = diag([1.5, 1.5, 1.5, 1.5]) \tag{3}$$

$$A_2 = diag([-0.5, -0.5, -0.5, -0.5]) \tag{4}$$

$$P = diag([1000, 1000, 1000, 1000]) \tag{5}$$

$$Q = diag([0.001, 0.001, 0.001, 0.001]) \tag{6}$$

The second seed was found using the clustering result. At s_C^t in the clustered image I_C^{t+1} at time $t + 1$, the EKF tracked axes $[a^{t+1}, b^{t+1}]$ were used to find the neighboring roots of s_C^t in an elliptical region of size $[1.5a^{t+1}, b^{t+1}]$ pixels. Amongst these roots, the root s_C^{t+1}, which has the lowest mean pixel intensity representing a patch in the vessel lumen, is chosen. By using the elliptical neighborhood derived from the EKF state, s_C^t is tracked in subsequent frames (see Fig. 2(c)). The elliptical region is robust to vessel compression, which enlarges the vessel horizontally.

The EKF prediction is sufficient for tracking during slow longitudinal scanning or still imaging as s_{ekf}^{t+1} and s_C^{t+1} lie close to each other. However, when large motion was encountered, the EKF incorrectly predicted the vessel location (see Fig. 2(c)) as it corrected motion, thereby leading to tracking failure. To mitigate tracking failure during large vessel motion, s_{ekf}^{t+1} was ignored, and s_C^{t+1} was updated as the new tracking seed according to the rule in Eq. (7):

$$
s^{t+1} = \begin{cases} s_C^{t+1} & if \quad \|s_{ekf}^{t+1} - s_C^{t+1}\|_2 > a^{t+1} \\ s_{ekf}^{t+1} & otherwise \end{cases} \tag{7}
$$

3 Results and Discussion

Metrics. Segmentation accuracy of the proposed approach was evaluated by comparing the contour segmentations against the annotations of two graders. All images in all datasets were annotated by two graders. Tracking was deemed successful if the vessel was segmented in all B-scans of a sequence. Considering the set of ground truth contour points as G and the segmented contour points as S, the following metrics were calculated as defined in Eqs. (8)–(11): (1) *Dice Similarity Coefficient* (DSC), (2) *Hausdorff Distance* (H) in millimeters, (3) *Definite False Positive and Negative Distances* (DFPD, DFND). The latter represent weighted distances of false positives and negatives to the true annotation. Let I_G and I_S be binary images containing 1 on and inside the area covered by G and S respectively, and 0 elsewhere. The Euclidean Distance Transform (EDT) is computed for I_G and its inverse I_G^{Inv} [13]. DFPD and DFND are estimated from the element-wise product of I_S with $EDT(I_G)$ and $EDT(I_G^{Inv})$ respectively (10)–(11). $d(i, G, S)$ is the distance from contour point i in G to the closest point in S. Inter-grader annotation variability was also measured.

$$
DSC = \frac{2|G \cap S|}{|G| + |S|} \tag{8}
$$

$$
H = \max \left(\max_{i \in [1,|G|]} d(i, G, S), \max_{j \in [1,|S|]} d(j, S, G) \right) \tag{9}
$$

$$
DFPD = \log \left(\|EDT(I_G) \circ I_S\|_1 \right) \tag{10}
$$

$$
DFND = \log \left(\|EDT(I_G^{Inv}) \circ I_S\|_1 \right) \tag{11}
$$

UHFUS Results. We ran our algorithm on 35 UHFUS sequences (100 images each), and the corresponding results are shown in Figs. 3(a)–(d). The two graders varied in their estimation of the vessel boundary locations in UHFUS images due to the speckle noise obscuring the precise location of the vessel edges, as shown in the inter-grader Dice score in Fig. 3(a), inter-grader Hausdorff distance in Fig. 3(b), and inter-grader variation between Figs. 3(c) and (d). Grader 2 tended to under-segment the vessel (G1vG2, low DFPD and high DFND scores), while grader 1 tended to over-segment (G2vG1, high DFPD and low DFND scores). As desired, our segmentation tended to be within the region of uncertainty between the two graders (see Figs. 3(c) and (d)). Accordingly, the mean Dice score and mean Hausdorff distance of our algorithm against grader 1

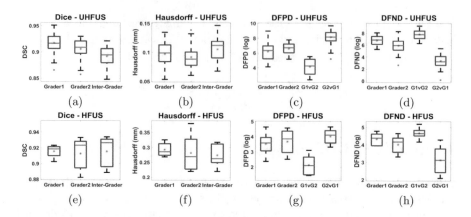

Fig. 3. Quantitative segmentation and tracking accuracy metrics for 35 UHFUS (top row) and 5 HFUS (bottom row) sequences respectively. The black * in each box plot represents the mean value of the metric. The terms 'G1vG2' and 'G2vG1' in figure represent the inter-grader annotation variability when grader 2 annotation was considered the ground truth, and vice versa.

$(0.917 \pm 0.019, 0.097 \pm 0.019\,\text{mm})$ and grader 2 $(0.905 \pm 0.018, 0.091 \pm 0.019\,\text{mm})$ were better than the inter-grader scores of $(0.892 \pm 0.019, 0.105 \pm 0.02\,\text{mm})$. *The largest observed Hausdorff distance error of* $0.135\,\text{mm}$ *is 6 times smaller than the smallest observed vessel diameter of* $0.81\,\text{mm}$. *Similarly, the mean Hausdorff distance error of* $0.094 \pm 0.019\,\text{mm}$ *is* ~7 *times smaller than smallest observed vessel diameter. This satisfies our goal of sub-mm vessel contour localization.* Tracking was successful as the vessel contours in all sequences were segmented.

HFUS Results. To show the generality of our approach to HFUS, we ran our algorithm on 5 HFUS sequences (250 images each), and the corresponding results are shown in Figs. 2(e) and 3(e)–(h). As opposed to UHFUS, lower DFPD and DFND scores were seen with HFUS, meaning a greater consensus in grader annotations (see Figs. 3(g) and (h)). Notably, our algorithm still demonstrated the desirable property of final segmentations that lay in the uncertain region of annotation between the two graders. This is supported by comparing the mean Dice score and mean Hausdorff distance of our algorithm against grader 1 $(0.915 \pm 0.008, 0.292 \pm 0.023\,\text{mm})$ and grader 2 $(0.912 \pm 0.021, 0.281 \pm 0.065\,\text{mm})$, with the inter-grader scores $(0.915 \pm 0.02, 0.273 \pm 0.04\,\text{mm})$. To compare against the 0.1 mm Mean Absolute Deviation (MAD) error in [6], we also computed the MAD error for HFUS sequences (not shown in Fig. 3). The MAD error of our algorithm against grader 1 was $0.059 \pm 0.021\,\text{mm}$, $0.057 \pm 0.024\,\text{mm}$ against grader 2, and $0.011 \pm 0.003\,\text{mm}$ between the graders. *Despite the lower pixel resolution (92.5 μm) of the HFUS machine used in this work, our MAD errors were* $\sim2\times$ *lower than the state-of-the-art* $0.1\,\text{mm}$ *MAD error in* [6]. Furthermore, only minor changes in the parameters of the algorithm were required to transfer the methodology to HFUS sequences; namely, the bilateral filter size was 3×3 pixels, $w_o = 5$, and $\Delta\tau = 8$. No other changes were made to the level set parameters.

Performance. The average run-time on an entry-level NVIDIA GeForce GTX 760 GPU was 19.15 ms per B-scan and 1.915 s per sequence, thus achieving a potential real-time frame rate of 52 frames per second. The proposed approach is significantly faster than the regular CPU- [6], and real-time CPU- [2–4] and GPU-based approaches in [5] respectively. Efficient use of CUDA unified memory and CUDA programming contributed to the performance speed-up.

4   Conclusion and Future Work

In this paper, a robust system combining the advantages of local phase analysis [9], a distance-regularized level set [11], and an Extended Kalman Filter (EKF) [12] was presented to segment and track vessel contours in UHFUS sequences. The approach, which has also shown applicability to traditional HFUS sequences, was validated by two graders, and it produced similar results as the expert annotations. To the best of our knowledge, this is the first system capable of rapid deformable vessel segmentation and tracking in UHFUS images. Future work is directed towards multi-vessel tracking capabilities.

Acknowledgements. NIH 1R01EY021641, DOD awards W81XWH-14-1-0371 and W81XWH-14-1-0370, NVIDIA Corporation, and Haewon Jeong.

References

1. Gorantla, V., et al.: Acute and chronic rejection in upper extremity transplantation: what have we learned? Hand Clin. **27**(4), 481–493 (2011)
2. Abolmaesumi, P., et al.: Real-time extraction of carotid artery contours from ultrasound images. In: IEEE Symposium on Compter Medical Systems, pp. 181–186 (2000)
3. Guerrero, J., et al.: Real-time vessel segmentation and tracking for ultrasound imaging applications. IEEE Trans. Med. Imag. **26**(8), 1079–1090 (2007)
4. Wang, D., et al.: Fully automated common carotid artery and internal jugular vein identification and tracking using B-mode ultrasound. IEEE Biomed. Eng. **56**(6), 1691–1699 (2009)
5. Smistad, E., et al.: Real-time automatic artery segmentation, reconstruction and registration for ultrasound-guided regional anaesthesia of the femoral nerve. IEEE Trans. Med. Imag. **35**(3), 752–761 (2016)
6. Chaniot, J., et al.: Vessel segmentation in high-frequency 2D/3D ultrasound images. In: IEEE International Ultrasonics Symposium, pp. 1–4 (2016)
7. Tomasi, C.: Bilateral filtering for gray and color images. In: ICCV (1998)
8. Stetten, G., et al.: Descending variance graphs for segmenting neurological structures. In: Pattern Recognition in Neuroimaging (PRNI), pp. 174–177 (2013)
9. Boukerroui, D., et al.: Phase-based level set segmentation of ultrasound images. IEEE Trans. Inf. Technol. Biomed. **15**(1), 138–147 (2011)
10. Fitzgibbon, A.: A Buyer's guide to conic fitting. BMVC **2**, 513–522 (1995)

11. Li, C., et al.: Distance regularized level set evolution and its application to image segmentation. IEEE Trans. Image Process. **19**(12), 3243 (2010)
12. Kalman, R.E.: A new approach to linear filtering and prediction problems. J. Fluids Eng. **82**(1), 35–45 (1960)
13. Maurer, C.: A linear time algorithm for computing exact Euclidean distance transforms of binary images in arbitrary dimensions. IEEE PAMI **25**(2), 265–270 (2003)

Deep Reinforcement Learning for Vessel Centerline Tracing in Multi-modality 3D Volumes

Pengyue Zhang[1,2]([✉]), Fusheng Wang[1], and Yefeng Zheng[2]

[1] Department of Computer Science, Stony Brook University, Stony Brook, USA
pengyue.zhang@stonybrook.edu
[2] Medical Imaging Technologies, Siemens Healthineers, Princeton, USA

Abstract. Accurate vessel centerline tracing greatly benefits vessel centerline geometry assessment and facilitates precise measurements of vessel diameters and lengths. However, cursive and longitudinal geometries of vessels make centerline tracing a challenging task in volumetric images. Treating the problem with traditional feature handcrafting is often ad-hoc and time-consuming, resulting in suboptimal solutions. In this work, we propose a unified end-to-end deep reinforcement learning approach for robust vessel centerline tracing in multi-modality 3D medical volumes. Instead of time-consuming exhaustive search in 3D space, we propose to learn an artificial agent to interact with surrounding environment and collect rewards from the interaction. A deep neural network is integrated to the system to predict stepwise action value for every possible actions. With this mechanism, the agent is able to probe through an optimal navigation path to trace the vessel centerline. Our proposed approach is evaluated on a dataset of over 2,000 3D volumes with diverse imaging modalities, including contrasted CT, non-contrasted CT, C-arm CT and MR images. The experimental results show that the proposed approach can handle large variations from vessel shape to imaging characteristics, with a tracing error as low as 3.28 mm and detection time as fast as 1.71 s per volume.

1 Introduction

Detection of blood vessels in medical images can facilitate the diagnosis, treatment and monitoring of vascular diseases. An important step in vessel detection is to extract their centerline representation that can streamline vessel specific visualization and quantitative assessment. Precise vascular segmentation and centerline detection can serve as a reliable pre-processing step that enables precise determination of the vascular anatomy or pathology, which can guide

Electronic supplementary material The online version of this chapter (https://doi.org/10.1007/978-3-030-00937-3_86) contains supplementary material, which is available to authorized users.

A. F. Frangi et al. (Eds.): MICCAI 2018, LNCS 11073, pp. 755–763, 2018.
https://doi.org/10.1007/978-3-030-00937-3_86

pre-surgery planning in vascular disease treatment. However, automatic vessel centerline tracing still faces several major challenges: (1) vascular structures constitute only a small portion of the medical volume; (2) vascular boundaries tend to be obscure, with presence of nearby touching anatomical structures; (3) vessel usually has an inconsistent tubular shape with changing cross-section area, which poses difficulty in segmentation; (4) it is often hard to trace a vessel due to its cursive lengthy structure.

Majority of existing centerline tracing techniques compute centerline paths by searching for a shortest path with various handcrafted vesselness or medialness cost metrics such as Hessian based vesselness [1], flux based medialness [2] or other tubularity measures along the paths. However, these methods are sensitive to the underlying cost metric. They can easily make shortcuts through nearby structures if the cost is high along the true path, which is likely to happen due to vascular lesions or imaging artifacts. Deep learning based approaches are proved to be able to provide better understanding from data and demonstrate superior performance compared to traditional pattern recognition methods with hand-crafted features. However, directly applying fully-supervised CNN with an exhaustive searching strategy is suboptimal and can result in inaccurate detection and huge computation time, since many local patches are not informative and can bring additional noise.

In this paper, we address the vessel centerline tracing problem with an end-to-end trainable deep reinforcement learning (DRL) network. An artificial agent is learned to interact with surrounding environment and collect rewards from the interaction. We can not only generate the vesselness map by training a classifier, but also learn to trace the centerline by training the artificial agent. The training samples are collected in such an intelligent way that the agent learns from its own mistakes when it explores the environment. Since the whole system is trained end-to-end, shortest path computation, which is used in all previous centerline tracing methods, is not required at all. Our artificial agent also learns when to stop. If the target end point of the centerline (e.g., iliac bifurcation for aorta tracing starting from the aortic valve) is inside the volume, our agent will stop there. If the target end point is outside of the volume, our agent follows the vessel centerline and stops at the position where the vessel goes out of the volume. Quantitative results demonstrate the superiority of our model on tracing the aorta on multimodal (including contrasted/non-contrasted CT, C-arm CT, and MRI) 3D volumes. The method is general and can be naturally applied to trace other vessels.

2   Background

Emerging from behavior psychology, reinforcement learning (RL) approaches aim to mimic humans and other animals to make timely decisions based on previous experience. In reinforcement learning setting, an artificial agent is learned to take actions in an environment to maximize a cumulative reward. Reinforcement learning problems consist of two sub-problems: the policy evaluation problem which computes state-value or action-value function based on a given policy; and the control problem which searches for the optimal policy. These two sub-problems rely on the behavior of agent and environment, and can be solved alternatively.

Previously, reinforcement learning based approaches have achieved success in a variety of problems [3,4], but its applicability is limited to domains with fully observed and low dimensional spaces and its efficacy is bottlenecked by challenges in hand-crafted feature design in shallow models. Deep neural network can be integrated into reinforcement learning paradigm as a nonlinear approximator of value function or policy function. For example, a stabilized Q-network training framework was designed for AI game playing and demonstrated superior performance compared to previous shallow reinforcement learning approaches [5]. Following this work, several deep reinforcement learning based methods were proposed and made further improvements on game score and computing speed in game playing scenario [6,7]. Recently in [8,9], deep reinforcement learning framework was creatively leveraged to tackle important medical imaging tasks, such as 3D anatomical landmark detection and 3D medical image registration. In these methods, the medical imaging problems are reformulated as strategy learning process in a completely different way, in which artificial agents are trained to make sequential decisions and yield landmark detection or image alignment intelligently.

3   Method

In this section we propose a deep reinforcement learning based method for vessel centerline tracing in 3D volumes. Given a 3D volumetric image $\mathbf{I}$ and the list of ground truth vessel centerline points $\mathbf{G} = [\boldsymbol{g}_0, \boldsymbol{g}_1, \ldots, \boldsymbol{g}_n]$, we aim to learn a navigation model for an agent to trace the centerline through an optimal trajectory $\mathbf{P} = [\boldsymbol{p}_0, \boldsymbol{p}_1, \ldots, \boldsymbol{p}_m]$. We propose to solve the problem as a sequential decision making problem and model it as a reward-based Markov Decision Process (MDP). An agent is designed to interact with an environment over time. At each time step t, the agent receives state s from state space $\mathcal{S}$ and selects action a from action space $\mathcal{A}$ according to policy π. For vessel centerline tracing, we allow an agent to move to its adjacent voxels, resulting in an action space $\mathcal{A}$ with six actions {left, right, top, bottom, front, back}. A scalar reward $r_t = r_{s,a}^{s'}$ is used to measure the effect of the transition from state s to state s' through action a. To define the reward for centerline tracing, we first calculate minimum distance from the current point p_t to a point on the centerline and denote the corresponding point as g_d. Then, we define a point-to-curve distance-like measure:

$$D(\boldsymbol{p}_t, \mathbf{G}) = ||\lambda(\boldsymbol{p}_t - \boldsymbol{g}_{d+k}) + (1 - \lambda)(\boldsymbol{g}_{d+k+1} - \boldsymbol{g}_{d+k-1})||. \qquad (1)$$

This measure is composed of two components balanced by a scalar parameter λ, where the first component is pulling the agent position towards the ground truth centerline and the second one is a momentum enforcing the agent towards the direction of the curve. k represents the forward index offset along the uniformly sampled curve (by default, $k = 1$). We also consider the reward calculation under two cases: when the current agent position is far from the curve, we want the agent to approach the curve as quickly as possible; when it is near the curve we also want it to move along the curve. Thus the step-wise reward is defined as

$$r_t = \begin{cases} D(\boldsymbol{p}_t, \mathbf{G}) - D(\boldsymbol{p}_{t+1}, \mathbf{G}), & \text{if } ||\boldsymbol{p}_t - \boldsymbol{g}_d|| <= l \\ ||\boldsymbol{p}_t - \boldsymbol{g}_d|| - ||\boldsymbol{p}_{t+1} - \boldsymbol{g}_d||, & \text{otherwise} \end{cases} \qquad (2)$$

where l is an empirically chosen threshold for the point-to-curve distance. Note that when $l \to \infty$ and $\lambda = 1$ we have simplified forward distance based reward as $r_t = ||\boldsymbol{p}_t - \boldsymbol{g}_{d+k}|| - ||\boldsymbol{p}_{t+1} - \boldsymbol{g}_{d+k}||$.

We use the long-term expected return $R_t = \sum_{\tau=t}^{\infty} \gamma^{\tau-t} r_\tau$ as discounted accumulated reward with discount factor $\gamma < 1$. The action-value function $Q^\pi(s, a) = \mathbb{E}[R_t | s, a, \pi]$ represents the expected future discounted reward selecting a in state s and then following policy π. An optimal action-value function is defined as $Q^\star(s, a) = \max_\pi Q^\pi(s, a)$, which represents the reward collected by the agent which starts from state-action pair (s, a) and acts optimally thereafter. The corresponding optimal policy is $\pi^\star(s) = \arg\max_{a \in \mathcal{A}} Q^\star(s, a)$. By the Bellman equation [10], the optimal action-value function satisfies a recursive formulation:

$$Q^\star(s, a) = \mathbb{E}_{s'}[r + \gamma \max_{a'} Q^\star(s', a')]. \qquad (3)$$

We parameterize and approximate the optimal action-value function by a deep neural network $Q(s, a; \theta) = Q^\star(s, a)$, where θ represents trainable parameters in the neural network. The optimal action-value target can be approximated as $y = r + \gamma \max_{a'} Q(s', a', \theta_{i'})$, where $\theta_{i'}$ is the network weights from some previous iteration $i' < i$. To avoid the correlation between sequence of observations which may cause instability in training, the target is updated every few iterations. Following the experience replay mechanism, we can cache a replay set D of length M and draw samples from D for network training. Then we can define the loss function as

$$\begin{aligned} \mathcal{L}_i(\theta_i) &= \mathbb{E}_{s,a,r} \left[\mathbb{E}_{s'}[y|s, a] - Q(s, a; \theta_i) \right] \\ &= \mathbb{E}_{s,a,r,s'} \left[y - Q(s, a; \theta_i) \right]^2 + \mathbb{E}_{s,a,r} \left[\mathbb{V}_{s'}[y] \right]. \end{aligned} \qquad (4)$$

With fixed parameters $\theta_{i'}$ from previous iteration, we can calculate the gradient with respect to θ_i and apply stochastic gradient descent afterward:

$$\nabla_{\theta_i} \mathcal{L}(\theta_i) = \mathbb{E}_{s,a,r,s'} \left[\left(r + \gamma \max_{a'} Q(s', a', \theta_{i'}) - Q(s, a; \theta_i) \right) \nabla_{\theta_i} Q(s, a; \theta_i) \right]. \qquad (5)$$

Training Details. For training reinforcement learning models in medical imaging problems, it is important to find a good probing strategy to avoid early overfitting and make the model robust. We train the model in an episodic manner, in which we start from one sample volume and accumulate samples in experience replay set. Then, we calculate a maximum returning action value based on the current neural network among all six possible actions. We apply a ϵ-greedy policy that takes the greedy action with probability ϵ and a random action with probability $1 - \epsilon$. To encourage exploration in early training epochs, we set ϵ as 1 at first and let it decrease to 0 at constant rate over training iterations. We also select starting point in a similar probabilistic way: given the ground truth path $\mathbf{G} = [\boldsymbol{g}_0, \boldsymbol{g}_1, \ldots, \boldsymbol{g}_n]$, we set the initial point $\boldsymbol{p}'_0$ as $\boldsymbol{g}_0$ with probability η and some random point along $\mathbf{G}$ with probability $1 - \eta$. Furthermore, we randomly select the starting point $\boldsymbol{p}_0$ in a local patch centered at $\boldsymbol{p}'_0$ with size $10 \times 10 \times 10$ voxels. The agent reaches a termination state in an episode when it reaches the last point in ground truth path $\mathbf{G}$ or the step number reaches the maximum episode length. Then, we starts a new episode in another volume.

Vascular Centerline Tracing. With an unseen test sample, we provide a starting point $\boldsymbol{p}_0 = \boldsymbol{g}_0$ at the vascular root to the system. We set the state as local volume observation $s_0 = \mathbf{I}_{\boldsymbol{p}_0}$ which is a 3D patch centered at $\boldsymbol{p}_0$, and feed it into the detection model. From the neural network we generate an action a_0 which moves the current point to $\boldsymbol{p}_1$. Then, the current state is updated as $s_1 = \mathbf{I}_{\boldsymbol{p}_1}$ and fed into the neural network to generate action again. We repeat this process until the path converges on oscillatory-like cycles. To further stabilize the tracing process, we also apply momentum on action-values from network output: $r_t \leftarrow \alpha r_{t-1} + (1 - \alpha) r_t$, where α is the momentum factor. The centerline tracing process stops if the agent moves out of the volume or if a cycle is formed, i.e., moving to a position already visited previously. We remove the cycle from the traced centerline path during detection.

We define a curve-to-curve distance metric to measure the tracing error. In our problem setting, the ground truth $\mathbf{G}$ consists of a list of 3D points $\boldsymbol{g}_i$ and the centerline is approximately represented as the set of concatenating segments $\mathbf{C} = \{c_{i,i+1}\}$ of adjacent points $\boldsymbol{g}_i$ and $\boldsymbol{g}_{i+1}$. We first compute the distance from a detected point $\boldsymbol{p}_j \in \mathbf{P}$ to the ground truth $\mathbf{G}$ by finding the minimum distance from $\boldsymbol{p}_j$ to any segments $c_{i,i+1} \in \mathbf{C}$ or points $\boldsymbol{g}_i \in \mathbf{G}$. Then, the distance from $\mathbf{P}$ to $\mathbf{G}$ is computed as the average distance from any point $\boldsymbol{p}_j \in \mathbf{P}$ to $\mathbf{G}$. The distance from $\mathbf{G}$ to $\mathbf{P}$ can be computed similarly and the curve-to-curve distance error is defined as the average of these two distances.

4 Experiment

4.1 Dataset

We evaluate the proposed approach on the problem of tracing centerline of tho-racic/abdominal aorta. We collected a dataset of 531 contrasted CT, 887 non-contrasted CT, 737 C-arm CT and 232 MR volumes from multiple sites over the world. These data represent different imaging modalities, scopes and qualities. All of the volumes are normalized to 2 mm isotropic resolution before experi-ments. We also map the intensity distribution of MR volumes to CT to make

760   P. Zhang et al.

sure they are equally bright. From the original 12-bit images, we clip and normalize the voxel intensities within [500, 2000]. We mix all volumes from different modalities and partition the dataset into training set and test set with 3:1 ratio on each modality. Ground truth annotations are provided by experts and reviewed by different people to ensure correctness.

4.2 Network Architecture and Implementation

We use a multi-layer neural network as a non-linear approximator for the action value function. The network consists of several convolutional, batch normalization, and fully connected layers. The first hidden layer is a convolutional layer with 32 filters of size $4 \times 4 \times 4$ and stride 2 followed by a batch normalization layer and a ReLU nonlinearity layer. The second hidden layer is a convolutional layer with 46 filters of size $3 \times 3 \times 3$ and stride 2. The following layers are two fully connected layers with 256 and 128 units, respectively. The last layer is also a fully connected layer with a probabilistic output for six possible actions.

The experiments was conducted on a server with one Nvidia Titan X GPU. We trained the model for 3000 epochs which takes about 64 h with an average running time of 77.13 s per epoch. The target network parameters were frozen and updated every 10,000 iterations. We used a set of 100,000 samples to store the history samples. The batch size was 8 and the learning rate was 0.0005 throughout the training process. The forward offset k was set as 1 and the detection momentum was set as $\alpha = 0.8$ based on our experiment. Other

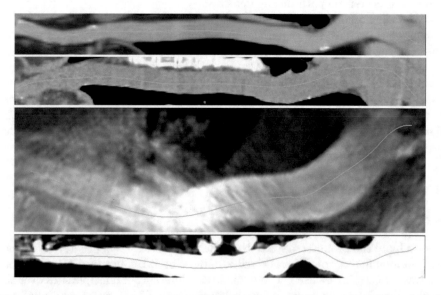

Fig. 1. Examples of traced aorta centerlines in the curved planar reformatting (CPR) view. From top to bottom: contrasted CT, non-contrasted CT, C-arm CT and MR. We recommend the readers to refer to the videos in supplementary material for better visualization effects.

parameters were set empirically as $\lambda = 0.5, \gamma = 0.9, \eta = 0.5$. Noticing that the exploration trend was gradually suppressed as the number of training iteration increased, we also gradually decreased the maximum length of each episode. The detected curve was represented as integer coordinates and then smoothed by B-spline interpolation. Over our experiment, we used volume patches with $50 \times 50 \times 50$ voxels as processing units.

4.3   Evaluation and Discussion

We evaluate the proposed deep reinforcement learning based 3D vessel centerline tracing approach on 3D medical volumes. The vessel centerline tracing results of our method is illustrated in Fig. 1. We observe that our deep reinforcement learning based model can trace the vessel centerline precisely. More importantly,

Table 1. Quantitative evaluation of different methods measured by the curve-to-curve distance in mm. A volume is considered as a failed case if the curve-to-curve distance is larger than 10.0 mm.

Modality	Method	Mean	Median	Std	80 percentile	Max	% failed
Contrasted CT	SL-CNN	8.62	4.67	10.94	5.35	49.38	11.11%
	DRL-1	5.71	5.43	2.42	5.90	25.67	1.39%
	DRL-2	4.77	4.79	0.44	5.15	6.04	**0%**
	DRL-3	4.04	**2.89**	5.54	3.26	38.30	2.78%
	DRL-4	**2.94**	2.93	**0.36**	**3.22**	**4.10**	**0%**
Non-contrasted CT	SL-CNN	4.84	4.59	2.31	4.91	33.78	1.35%
	DRL-1	4.98	4.97	0.52	5.34	7.32	**0%**
	DRL-2	4.75	4.75	0.43	5.11	6.18	**0%**
	DRL-3	3.04	3.01	**0.33**	3.27	**5.13**	**0%**
	DRL-4	**3.00**	**2.93**	0.65	**3.19**	11.31	0.45%
C-arm CT	SL-CNN	7.35	4.77	9.06	6.17	55.82	9.77%
	DRL-1	5.93	5.30	4.42	6.22	47.26	2.73%
	DRL-2	5.13	4.78	**2.85**	5.64	35.26	**1.17%**
	DRL-3	4.23	3.11	4.73	4.39	38.29	3.13%
	DRL-4	**3.72**	**3.09**	2.90	**4.18**	**33.08**	1.56%
MR	SL-CNN	14.85	6.17	11.86	27.44	40.49	43.10%
	DRL-1	6.68	5.85	**2.67**	7.37	**20.40**	8.48%
	DRL-2	6.56	5.20	5.47	6.00	30.73	**3.39%**
	DRL-3	**5.09**	3.31	5.89	**3.81**	29.38	6.78%
	DRL-4	5.51	**3.30**	6.89	4.09	38.88	8.48%
Overall	SL-CNN	7.07	4.64	8.18	5.31	55.82	9.53%
	DRL-1	5.63	5.09	3.73	5.82	47.26	2.43%
	DRL-2	5.06	4.78	**2.53**	5.30	**35.26**	**0.94%**
	DRL-3	4.02	3.17	4.40	3.69	38.30	2.43%
	DRL-4	**3.23**	**2.81**	2.86	**3.35**	38.88	1.86%

our method has nice generalization property and performs consistently over different imaging modalities. We compare the proposed method with a supervised 3D convolutional neural network (SL-CNN) based approach which shares the same network architecture with the proposed DRL method in Table 1. However, SL-CNN is trained with uniformly sampled patches from the training volume to predict moving actions as output labels. We apply the same detection process and hyper parameters for fair comparison. So, the only difference between the SL-CNN approach and DRL approach is how the action network is trained. We consider four variants of the proposed DRL methods with slightly different settings: For DRL-1, DRL-2 and DRL-3 we use the reward function with momentum. In DRL-1 we remove the vessel radius limit by setting $l = \infty$, while in DRL-2 and DRL-3 we set $l = 4$ and $l = 2$, respectively. In DRL-4, we remove the momentum term and simply use the forward distance based reward. The curve-to-curve distance is used to evaluate tracing accuracy of an algorithm. We observe that all the DRL based method can outperform SL-CNN by a considerable margin and they perform consistently over different imaging modalities. We can also observe that the proposed DRL-4 method with forward distance based reward function can achieve best tracing error while DRL-2 with momentum reward has fewest failed cases. The results also demonstrate that setting vessel diameter threshold parameter l can potentially improve the tracing performance. By using smaller vessel diameter threshold l as in DRL-3, the agent can trace the curve in a finer way but it is also more prone to early stop. DRL-2 will be used in practice since reducing failure rate is more desired for our vessel centerline tracing task. With the proposed DRL based method, we can provide fast vessel centerline extraction, with an average detection time of 1.71 s per volume.

5   Conclusion

In this paper, we propose a deep reinforcement learning approach for vessel centerline tracing in 3D medical volumes. By reformulating the problem as a behavior learning problem, we establish an interactive reinforcement learning model to train an artificial agent. The agent communicates with the surrounding environment and receives feedback from the environment to guide action selection in next steps. Using a deep neural network as a non-linear approximator for the action-value function, we can train the model in an end-to-end manner without any requirements for feature engineering. The proposed method is evaluated on over 2,000 3D medical volumes with four different modalities and demonstrates satisfying performance on all of the modalities.

Acknowledgement. This research is supported in part by grants from National Science Foundation ACI 1443054 and IIS 1350885.

References

1. Frangi, A.F., Niessen, W.J., Vincken, K.L., Viergever, M.A.: Multiscale vessel enhancement filtering. In: Wells, W.M., Colchester, A., Delp, S. (eds.) MICCAI 1998. LNCS, vol. 1496, pp. 130–137. Springer, Heidelberg (1998). https://doi.org/10.1007/BFb0056195
2. Siddiqi, K., Bouix, S., Tannenbaum, A., Zucker, S.: Hamilton-Jacobi skeletons. Int. J. Comput. Vis. **48**(3), 215–231 (2002)
3. Riedmiller, M., Gabel, T., Hafner, R., Lange, S.: Reinforcement learning for robot soccer. Auton. Robots **27**(1), 55–73 (2009)
4. Diuk, C., Cohen, A., Littman, M.L.: An object-oriented representation for efficient reinforcement learning. In: Proceedings of the 25th International Conference on Machine Learning, pp. 240–247, ACM (2008)
5. Mnih, V., et al.: Human-level control through deep reinforcement learning. Nature **518**(7540), 529 (2015)
6. Mnih, V., et al.: Asynchronous methods for deep reinforcement learning. In: International Conference on Machine Learning, pp. 1928–1937 (2016)
7. Silver, D., et al.: Mastering the game of Go with deep neural networks and tree search. Nature **529**(7587), 484–489 (2016)
8. Ghesu, F.C., Georgescu, B., Mansi, T., Neumann, D., Hornegger, J., Comaniciu, D.: An artificial agent for anatomical landmark detection in medical images. In: Ourselin, S., Joskowicz, L., Sabuncu, M.R., Unal, G., Wells, W. (eds.) MICCAI 2016. LNCS, vol. 9902, pp. 229–237. Springer, Cham (2016). https://doi.org/10.1007/978-3-319-46726-9_27
9. Liao, R., et al.: An artificial agent for robust image registration. In: AAAI, pp. 4168–4175 (2017)
10. Bellman, R.: Dynamic Programming. Courier Corporation, North Chelmsford (2013)

Author Index